A Handbook on Stuttering

A Handbook on Stuttering

Sixth Edition

OLIVER BLOODSTEIN
Ph.D., CCC-SLP, Honors of the ASHA
Brooklyn College of the City University
of New York

NAN BERNSTEIN RATNER
Ed.D.,CCC-SLP, ASHA-F
The University of Maryland,
College Park

THOMSON
DELMAR LEARNING™ Australia Canada Mexico Singapore Spain United Kingdom United States

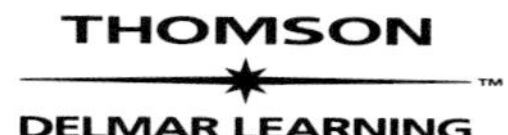

A Handbook on Stuttering, 6th Edition

by

Oliver Bloodstein
Ph.D., CCC-SLP, Honors of the ASHA

Nan Bernstein Ratner
Ed.D., CCC-SLP, ASHA-F

Vice President, Health Care Business Unit:
William Brottmiller

Director of Learning Solutions:
Matthew Kane

Managing Editor:
Marah Bellegarde

Senior Acquisitions Editor:
Sherry Dickinson

Senior Product Manager:
Juliet Steiner

Marketing Director:
Jennifer McAvey

Marketing Manager:
Christopher Manion

Marketing Coordinator:
Vanessa Carlson

Production Director:
Carolyn Miller

Senior Art Director:
Jack Pendleton

Content Project Manager:
Katie Wachtl

Printed in Canada
1 2 3 4 5 6 7 XXX 11 10 09 08 07

For more information, contact Delmar, 5 Maxwell Drive, Clifton Park, NY 12065-2919 Or you can visit our Internet site at http://www.delmarlearning.com

Library of Congress Cataloging-in-Publication Data
Bloodstein, Oliver.
A handbook on stuttering/
Oliver Bloodstein, Nan Bernstein Ratner.—6th ed.
p. cm.
Includes bibliographical references and index.
ISBN-13: 978-1-4180-4203-5
ISBN-10: 1-4180-4203-X
1. Stuttering. I. Ratner, Nan Bernstein.
II. Title.
[DNLM: 1. Stuttering. WM 475 B655ha 2008]
RC424.B54 2008
616.85'54—dc22

2007035428

Notice to the Reader

Contents

Foreword

A Handbook on Stuttering had its origin in 1959 as an 88-page booklet entitled *A Handbook on Stuttering for Professional Workers*. The National Society for Crippled Children and Adults (Easter Seal Society) had called on the American Speech and Hearing Association to prepare a publication on stuttering for distribution to physicians. The editor of the Association, Robert West, gave the task to me, a young colleague who had a special interest in stuttering. By that date a considerable amount of research on stuttering had gradually been done, small as it now seems. As I saw it, my task was to provide a brief summary of what we had learned from this research. In 1959 a review of research findings on stuttering was an innovation. Until then, most scholarly works on the subject had been merely compilations of the theories of various authorities. When Dr. West read my manuscript he sent me a cherished note that read, "Elegant! Much better than I could do." Unexpectedly, the booklet soon began to be adopted as a text in university courses on stuttering and was even translated into Japanese. In the research-oriented discipline that Robert West and Lee Edward Travis had pioneered, a publication surveying the research on stuttering clearly filled a need. As a result, the Easter Seal Society agreed to publish an expanded version in 1969 that would be more suitable as a textbook. That was the first edition of *A Handbook on Stuttering*. As the research findings grew, I continued to produce a new edition, each one thicker than the last, every six years. When I completed the fifth edition of the *Handbook* in 1995, I finally had no intention to revise it further. But by then it had been taken up by a new publisher, and Kalen Conerly, an acquisitions editor for Delmar, proposed that the *Handbook* be brought up to date once again by a coauthor. Nan Bernstein Ratner, my first choice, agreed to undertake the revision. Concerning her accomplishment I can say with all sincerity: Elegant! Much better than I could do.

Oliver Bloodstein
Brooklyn, New York, April 2007

Preface

In the decade that has passed since the last revision of *A Handbook on Stuttering*, at least 700 new studies of stuttering have been reported. It was certainly a large task to tackle this growth in knowledge, and so we are now two authors who bring you the most recent incarnation of the *Handbook*. As a team, we have endeavored to preserve the goal of all prior editions, to maintain a chronicle of the most important research in stuttering, while thoroughly updating the *Handbook* with the most recent advances in the field.

Advances in technology lie at many of the recent themes. In this edition of the *Handbook*, we discuss new work in genetics, which emphasizes the clear genetic contribution to some cases of stuttering. Brain imaging, in its very infancy in the last edition, now assumes a major role in modeling the nature of stuttering as well, but has also shown that biology is not destiny: many of the atypical activations seen when scanning the brains of people who stutter are altered dramatically by therapy that teaches a more fluent manner of speaking. Some conventional debates that have sought to describe stuttering as a monolithic disorder have been moderated: recent work suggests that the motor systems of individuals who stutter are particularly vulnerable to linguistic stressors, a finding that bridges research across a number of approaches to the problem of stuttering.

More integration is to be found in the many therapies that increasingly combine components to more effectively treat stuttering: it is now more common, rather than less, to see therapies that teach new ways of speaking partnered with therapies that directly address cognitive and emotional sequelae of stuttering. Older indirect methods of treating the very young child who stutters are being partnered, in many cases, with very direct intervention methods. The result is a rapidly growing body of clinical research that can quantify the short- and increasingly long-term outcomes of a variety of therapy approaches. The move toward Evidence-Based Practice in speech-language pathology, as in medicine, has increased the emphasis placed on documenting outcomes. Partnered with consistent expansion of the self-help and consumer advocacy movements among people who stutter and their families, and the explosive growth in Internet-based resources that can enable people to track and evaluate therapy, we will doubtless continue to see changes and improvements in the way therapy is conceptualized, administered, and evaluated. If there is a theme that unites these developments in theory, basic research, therapy, and consumer values, it may be one of more consensus on some issues, rather than less. We do not say that we have yet arrived at a single best model of the disorder or its best treatment, but many old arguments appear to be somewhat defused by growing evidence that a number of viewpoints have value in understanding and treating this disorder.

Over 35 years have elapsed since the National Easter Seal Society agreed to expand a booklet by the first author into a textbook for students and a resource for speech-language pathologists. The National Society ably saw *A Handbook on Stuttering* through four editions, despite the fact that book publishing was not part of its mission. Although the *Handbook* is now at home with Delmar, it has not changed its theme and purpose. As in previous editions, the book's endeavor is to guide the reader to the edge of our knowledge about stuttering and, where the edge is not well defined, to point out where the footing is insecure and where we stand on solid ground.

—Oliver Bloodstein and Nan Bernstein Ratner

About the Authors

Oliver Bloodstein is Emeritus Professor of Speech and former director of the program in speech-language pathology and audiology at Brooklyn College of the City University of New York. His career has been spent in research, teaching, and clinical work on stuttering and he has written extensively on the subject. He is a Fellow of the American Speech-Language-Hearing Association and the recipient of its highest award, the Honors of the Association.

Nan Bernstein Ratner, Ed.D., C.C.C. is Professor and Chairman, Department of Hearing and Speech Sciences, University of Maryland at College Park. With degrees in Child Studies, Speech-Language Pathology, and Applied Psycholinguistics, she is the editor of numerous volumes, and author of numerous chapters and articles addressing stuttering as well as child language acquisition/disorders. Dr. Bernstein Ratner is a Fellow of the American Speech-Language-Hearing Association. In 2006, she was presented with the Distinguished Researcher Award by the International Fluency Association. She is pleased to be joining with Oliver Bloodstein in this edition of the *Handbook*, since his work was the primary inspiration for her first research study and professional publication. She hopes someday to inspire others to the degree that he has inspired her.

As always, we dedicate this edition to the memory of those who have contributed so much to our understanding and treatment of stuttering, and who have inspired us to continue this venture:

WENDELL JOHNSON

ROBERT WEST

BRYNG BRYNGELSON

JOSEPH G. SHEEHAN

LEE EDWARD TRAVIS

DEAN E. WILLIAMS

CHARLES VAN RIPER

HUGO GREGORY

MARCEL WINGATE

Chapter 1

Symptomatology

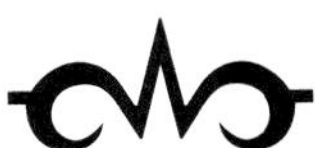

DEFINING STUTTERING

We start this book by attempting to define what we intend to describe and explain in the chapters that follow. Most of us believe we know what stuttering is, yet a great deal of disagreement generally results when we try to define it. Some of the disagreement stems from conflicting inferences about the underlying nature of the disorder that reveal themselves in our definitions. When we try to avoid this problem by adhering strictly to the description of behavior, other difficulties present themselves. Traditionally, stuttering has been viewed as a disorder in which the "rhythm" or fluency of speech is impaired by interruptions, or blockages. For many ordinary purposes, such a definition is adequate, and in this chapter we will discuss at some length those moments of interruption or blockage that are a dominant feature of the disorder. Yet it cannot be denied that what we identify as stuttering is sometimes evident not only in the intermittent impairment of fluency, but also in the rate, pitch, loudness, inflectional patterns, articulation, facial expression, and postural adjustments of the speaker and that there are stutterers[1] for whom its features are not always confined in an easily identifiable manner to discrete "moments."

[1] We recognize that "person-first" terminology (e.g., *person who stutters* rather than *stutterer*) has been adopted as an editorial policy by many professional groups (including APA, whose editorial style we follow in all other ways) since the publication of the last edition. However, we note that the two labels are not perceived differently by people who stutter, clinicians, or the public (see St. Louis, 1999), and that person-first language, by introducing a clause within a noun phrase, makes sentence processing more difficult for you, the reader. We concur with the notion that the term "stutterer" does not reduce a person to symptoms; as one of our colleagues says, he does not think it better to call him "a person who skis" rather than a "skier" or a "person who writes" rather than a "writer" or "author." For this reason, we will begin this edition of the text by noting that we intend to use a variety of labels to describe people who experience difficulty in speaking fluently, including the term "stutterer."

Furthermore, when, with our definition in hand we stride to the task of specifying just where or when a "block" has taken place, we find that it is not so simple. Research has shown that the most highly expert observers may have considerable difficulty in agreeing on whether an instance of stuttering has occurred on a given occasion, as we will see.

It is particularly important to point out in addition that conventional definitions of stuttering, even when considerably elaborated, do not adequately serve to differentiate it objectively from various other forms of disfluency that are regarded as distinct from the familiar clinical entity under discussion here. They are of notably little help in clarifying the relationship between stuttering and "normal" disfluency and so ride roughshod over some of the most critical questions that arise in developing a theory of stuttering. Johnson et al. (1959, chap. 8; Johnson 1961a) demonstrated that there is little the stutterer does, of a sort that can be conveyed by available descriptions of nonfluent speech behavior, that a typically fluent speaker does not also do to some extent and in some instances in equivalent measure. We will discuss this problem at some length in a number of places in this book.

THE MEASUREMENT OF STUTTERING BEHAVIOR

From a scientific standpoint, the problem of defining a phenomenon is intimately bound up with the question of the operations we use to measure it. Consequently, it will be useful to explore the measurable dimensions of stuttering. How does one express quantitatively such a concept as the degree, amount, or severity of stuttering behavior? In investigations of this problem so far, essentially five ways have been found for doing this.

Frequency of Stuttering Measurements

The frequency of stuttering, expressed as a number or percentage of moments of stuttering or of stuttered words or syllables, is one of the most familiar of such measures and has been extensively used in research on the variability of the disorder beginning with studies by Wendell Johnson and his associates at the University of Iowa in the 1930s. We may impart a rough notion of the frequency with which stutterers block by saying that, on the average, about 10 percent of words are stuttered in oral reading, but the variability of this measure, both from person to person and under different conditions, is quite high. To cite some representative data, thirty adult stutterers, reading "average factual prose" to two listeners, stuttered on a mean of 10.8 percent of the words and ranged from 0.0 percent to a frequency of 47.0 percent of words stuttered (Bloodstein, 1944). In clinical experience, it is not unusual to find both stutterers who have difficulty on a large majority of words in ordinary speaking situations and those who so rarely appear to block at all, most of their trouble consisting of the anticipation of difficulty, that Freund (1934a) referred to their problem as "inneres Stottern" (interiorized stuttering).[2] Variations in the frequency of stuttering from situation to situation are equally striking and will be discussed in Chapters 11 and 12.

The distribution of people who stutter with respect to frequency of stuttering is skewed, as Soderberg (1962b) and Johnson, Darley, and Spriestersbach (1963, p. 252) pointed out. That is, there are more "mild" than "severe" stutterers if the mean frequency of stuttering is arbitrarily taken as the line of demarcation for making such a judgment. To put it more succinctly, the median stutterer blocks less frequently than the average stutterer.

Special techniques that have been discussed for measuring the frequency of stuttering include electronic counters (Norcross & Andrews, 1973; Fowler & Ingham, 1986), time-expanded speech (Manning, Lee, & Lass, 1978; O'Keefe & Kroll, 1980; Kroll & O'Keefe, 1985), and automatic speech recognition (ASR) programs, such as those reported by Howell,

[2] See also Douglass and Quarrington (1952) on the subject of interiorized stuttering. However, even with the passage of so many years, this topic has not yet attracted a significant body of published research. "Covert" stuttering appears to be a well-recognized clinical phenomenon with sparse research documentation.

Sackin, and Glenn (1997). Some conceptual concerns in the development and application of such devices are summarized by Bakker (1999).

Agreement among different observers on the frequency of stuttering is not high, as an increasing body of research indicates.[3] Kully and Boberg (1988) found poor agreement among clinicians at nine treatment centers on counts of stutterings in the same recorded speech samples. Ingham and Cordes (1992) noted substantial differences between trained judges at both the same and different speech clinics. Thus, it appears that clinician training in precise definitions of the behaviors to be counted may make a difference: Yaruss, Max, Newman, and Campbell (1998) found relatively good correlation between "on-line" (live) and transcript-based counts for two clinicians in the same setting. Inversely, asking raters to judge "stuttering" or a more precise list of behaviors does not appear to improve reliability (Hubbard, 1998a). Ingham, Cordes, and coworkers have reported improved agreement in counts of time intervals containing stuttering, rather than the events themselves.[4]

Finally, the basic unit over which stutter frequency should be averaged (e.g., words vs. syllables) has been argued. Yaruss (2000) provides one of the most recent discussions regarding the utility and comparability of counts that are based on proportion of stuttered words, as opposed to stuttered syllables. While simple ratios of 1.4 to 1.5 syllables per word have been proposed for converting between these options in speech samples taken from English-speaking adults, Yaruss (2000) suggests a much lower value of 1.15 when comparing preschoolers' samples. Alternatively, Brundage and Bernstein Ratner (1989) found poor correlation between these measures in their speech samples from children who stutter and caution against using simple ratios to convert from one unit of measurement to the other. This would be particularly true in converting from words to syllables in languages with differing patterns of word formation (e.g., languages that typically have longer or shorter words in either adult or child speech).

[3] We return to this issue in Chapter 12.

[4] Cordes, Ingham, Frank and Costello Ingham (1992), Ingham, Cordes, and Gow (1993), Ingham, Cordes, and Finn (1993), Cordes and Ingham (1996), Cordes and Ingham (1999).

Mean Duration of Stuttered Events

The average duration of a stuttering block as judged by laboratory observers is about one second. Blocks tend to vary in duration only within a few seconds, although some appear to be extremely fleeting and those of severe stuttering events may occasionally be observed to continue for longer than a minute. Johnson and Colley (1945) found that the combined mean of the 10 longest blocks of each of 20 subjects in oral reading was 4.32 seconds. The combined mean based on the 10 shortest blocks in their sample was 0.41 seconds.

If measures of the duration of individual moments of stuttering vary so little, then, as might be expected, the *mean duration of stutters*, employed as a measure of amount of difficulty on a given reading or speaking task, varies still less. In a study referred to earlier (Bloodstein, 1944), thirty subjects ranged in mean duration of their stutterings from less than 0.05 seconds to 3.7 seconds in oral reading, the median subject having a mean duration of 0.9 seconds. Only 25 percent of the subjects had a mean duration of more than 1.4 seconds.

As Table 1-1 shows, mean duration of stuttered events does not appear to be related in any notable degree to other measures of severity of stuttering. The chief reason for this is its restricted range of variability. In general, one stutterer does not differ very much from another in the mean duration of blockages. This characteristic somewhat limits its usefulness as a measure of severity of stuttering.

Frequency of Specified Disfluency Types

Most conversational speech contains a considerable variety of interruptions or hesitations. This is true whether the speaker is regarded as a stutterer or a normal speaker, as Johnson and his students abundantly demonstrated, or is a "clutterer," or one who repeats syllables in a manner characteristic of certain types of neurological impairment.

TABLE 1-1 Coefficients of Correlation between Measures of Severity of Stuttering

	Reading	Speaking
Judges' Rating vs. Frequency of Stuttering		
Sherman, Young, and Gough (1958)	0.87	
Aron (1967)	0.57	
Riley, Riley, and Maguire (2004)	0.75	
Judges' Rating vs. Rate or Time*		
Sherman, Young, and Gough (1958)	0.76	
Minifie and Cooker (1964)	−0.69	
Aron (1967)	−0.89	
Young (1961)**		0.68
Young (1961)**		0.67
Prosek, Walden, et al (1979)	−0.80	
De Andrade, Cervone, and Sassi (2003)	NR	
Frequency of Stuttering vs. Rate or Time*		
Bloodstein (1944)	−0.88	
Dixon (1955)	0.89	
Sherman, Young, and Gough (1958)	0.76	
Aron (1967)	−0.72	
Andrews and Cutler (1974)		0.81
Prins, Mandelkorn, and Cerf (1980)		−0.69
Judges' Rating vs. Frequency of Specified Disfluencies		
Young (1961)**		0.87
Young (1961)**		0.85
Judges' Rating vs. Duration of Specified Disfluencies		
Riley, Riley, and Maguire (2004)		0.69
Frequency of Specified Disfluencies vs. Rate or Time		
Sander (1961)***	0.86	0.81
Young (1961)**		0.59
Mean Duration of Stutterings vs. Frequency of Stuttering		
Bloodstein (1944)	0.17	
Johnson and Colley (1945)	0.54	
Mean Duration of Stutterings vs. Rate or Time*		
Bloodstein (1944)	−0.46	

NR = not reported; correlation coefficients were not reported but correlation was reported as significant at $p < 0.0001$.
*Correlation coefficients are positive or negative depending on whether time or rate in words or syllables per minute was used.
**Disfluencies included part-word repetition, sound prolongation, broken utterance, and unusual stress.
***Disfluencies included Johnson's eight categories.

Convenient broad generic terms for the phenomenon of interruption in the smooth flow of speech are "disfluency" or "dysfluency."[5] It is clear, and of basic importance, that not every instance of disfluency is to be regarded as an example of the specific type of disorder to which we refer as stuttering.

Unfortunately, we have no satisfactory *objective* means of differentiating moments of stuttering from other instances of disfluency. Most typically, the identification of moments of stuttering involves the judgment of a listener, although self-judgment of stuttering has been found to be fairly reliable (O'Brian, Packman, & Onslow, 2004), and may in fact be a utilitarian component of therapy (see Chapter 14). However, speakers and listeners may agree more highly when rating words as fluent rather than when identifying stutter events (Tetnowski & Schagen, 2001). Thus, any measure of severity of stuttering that requires listener identification of stuttered moments is based upon an evaluative process subject to such troublesome uncontrolled variables as the standards, definitions, or criteria of the person who is doing the identifying. It should be clear that the measures already discussed—frequency of stuttering and mean duration of stuttered moments—belong in this category.

This raises the question whether there is any type of serviceable index that is free of the process of identification of stuttering. The problem is essentially one of finding an objectively measurable feature of speech that is highly related to subjective judgments of amount or severity of stuttering. One obvious possibility is that there are certain particular *aspects or kinds of disfluency* that might fulfill these requirements. We therefore turn briefly to some investigations that have been carried out on the subject of disfluency types and their relationship to judgments of stuttering.

Johnson et al. (1959, chap. 8; Johnson 1961a), with the help of his students and coworkers, gathered normative data on the disfluencies of stuttering and nonstuttering adults and young children through analysis of tape-recorded speech samples. For this purpose, he devised a system of classification of disfluent types of speech behavior consisting of eight categories: (1) *interjections* ("uh," "er," "well"), (2) *part-word repetitions* (repetitions of sounds or syllables of words), (3) *word repetitions*, (4) *phrase repetitions* ("I was I was going"), (5) *revisions* ("I was—I am going"), (6) *incomplete phrases* ("She was—and after she got there he came"), (7) *broken words* ("I was g—(pause)—oing home"), (8) *prolonged sounds*.

This scheme is usable in obtaining such measures of a speaker's disfluency as the total number of instances per hundred words read or spoken.[6] Similar normative data have been gathered on school-age children by F. H. Silverman (1974). More recently, Yairi and Ambrose (2005) summarize research done to construct a similar series of normative data for preschool-aged children. These data sort and weigh less typical disfluency types (called "stutter-like disfluencies," or SLDs) to create an expected disfluency rate for children aged 2–6 years of age. In conjunction with the normative data, these measures afford a basis for judging how usual or unusual the speaker's disfluencies may be. We discuss this type of weighting scale for early disfluency profiles in Chapter 12. In varying degrees, of course, the counting of "broken words" or of "prolonged sounds" also depends upon the perceptions and judgments of a listener.[7] But these are relatively descriptive terms compared with "stuttering," which is a highly inferential construct usually embodying the evaluational notion of failure or abnormality.

[5] Whether these two terms are mere spelling variants or should be used distinctively to refer to more typical and less typical fluency failures is a small but periodically interesting question that has been debated most recently, we believe, by Quesal (1988) and the second author (Bernstein Ratner, 1988). This book will use the term "disfluency" to refer to all moments of fluency breakdown.

[6] For a more complete description of procedures for obtaining such measures, see Darley and Spriestersbach (1978, chap. 9). Pauses were omitted for lack of a precise way of distinguishing hesitant pauses from meaningful ones.

[7] In fact, judges did not agree well in applying Johnson's categories to the disfluencies of young children in a study by Onslow, Gardner, Bryant, Stuckings, and Knight (1992).

The question is, can any useful *relationship* be found between the counting of types of disfluencies and the identification of stutterings? As might be expected, Johnson's classification of disfluencies appears to contain certain types that would probably not fit most listeners' definitions of stuttering and, conversely, there are aspects of stuttering not described by any of the features of disfluency in his list. Yet, on the whole, Johnson's stutterers proved to have much more disfluency than his normal-speaking subjects. While with respect to certain categories (e.g., revisions, incomplete phrases, and interjections such as "uh") the differences were small or nonexistent and the distributions markedly overlapping, with respect to others (notably, part-word repetitions and prolonged sounds) there were large differences between the two groups with little overlapping of distributions.

Johnson's findings suggest, in other words, that within his classification, there are certain descriptions that are distinctly typical of disfluencies likely to be considered stuttering. This view is strengthened by other research findings showing that listeners are likely to classify sound or syllable repetitions and prolonged sounds as stuttering, and revisions and interjections as normal disfluency (Boehmler, 1958; Williams & Kent, 1958; Schiavetti, 1975). One measure that attempts to separate "stutter-type" disfluencies from others is the index of disfluency used by Sander (1961), which has found some application in research. It is a count of disfluent words for which a disfluency is defined as one of the following: a sound, syllable, or word repetition, a sound prolongation, a broken word, or an interjection within a word.

The basic question of the relationship between stuttering and disfluency was attacked directly by Young (1961), who set out to determine whether judges' ratings of severity of stuttering in recorded speech samples could be adequately predicted from selected measures of disfluency and speaking time. Young found a relatively high degree of association (see Table 1-1) between ratings of stuttering severity and the frequency of occurrence of a category of disfluencies made up of syllable or sound repetitions, sound prolongations, broken words, and words involving "apparent undue stress or tension."

Despite this relationship for his speech samples as a whole, Young found that his measures did not permit the prediction of individual ratings of severity with a satisfactory degree of precision. When he examined the 10 speech samples that had resulted in the largest discrepancies between predicted and obtained ratings, Young made some interesting observations. In all 10 cases, the predictions had underestimated the actual ratings made by the judges. Each of the 10 samples appeared to be "characterized by some unusual and distinctive pattern" that had not been adequately represented in the frequency count of disfluencies. In particular, these patterns tended to include drawn-out repetitions of syllables, or "audible manifestations of excessive tension." Among other features evident in isolated cases were severe harshness and a rapidly rising pitch level during syllable repetitions.

Young's findings implied that much more work remains to be done on our descriptions of disfluency. At the same time, they offered the hope that as these descriptions become more refined, they will lend themselves to the development of increasingly useful measures of stuttering. The problem is apparently not that stuttering is indistinguishable from any other kind of disfluency, but that some of the differences are easily obscured by our rough-and-ready verbal classifications.

Most recently, Ingham and colleagues (see Einarsdóttir & Ingham, 2005) have suggested a return to a proposal voiced by Martin and Haroldson (1981) that listeners be allowed to self-define the percept of "stuttering." Rather than continuous attempts to create taxonomies of stuttered events, Einarsdóttir and Ingham propose that researchers work backwards from samples of speech behaviors that listeners agree are instances of stuttering to better specify what they have in common. However, it is not clear that all listeners reach agreement on this concept. Brundage, Bothe, Lengeling, and Evans (2006) found that highly experienced judges identified many more intervals of speech as "stuttered" than did less-specialized clinicians or student clinicians, who tended to be similar in their judgments.

As we develop more sophisticated methods for monitoring speech production, it may well be that objective means for isolating stutter events can be found, if the object is to verify specific moments for closer research scrutiny. For example, the findings of Kalotkin, Manschreck, and O'Brien (1979) suggested that electromyographic measures of masseter muscle tension during speech may be a useful indicator of severity of stuttering. Suter, Hutchinson, and Mallard (1979) identified visible concomitants of stuttering that appear to influence judgments of severity. Studies by Manning, Emal, and Jamison (1975) and Curran and Hood (1977b) began the investigation of the number of repeated units per speech repetition as related to judgments of severity of stuttering in adults.

We have been discussing the features of disfluencies that must be taken into account when we attempt to measure the frequency of "stuttering" as opposed to other kinds of disfluency. Note that our main concern here is with the measurement of stuttering in its developed form. The differentiation of stuttering from normal disfluency in early childhood is a question with special implications and difficulties, which we will take up in Chapter 12. Finally, as an increasingly large number of stutterers speak a first language different from that of their therapist or others in their community, it is of value that a small number of studies have begun to ask whether non-native speakers can reliably detect stuttering in a language they do not know or do not know well. The symptoms of stuttering appear to transcend the listener's knowledge of the sound system or words of an unfamiliar language—in other words, the ability to understand or predict what is being said. Van Borsel and Pereira (2005) found that both Dutch and Brazilian Portuguese speakers could identify stuttering in the other speaker group's language with good reliability; however, they were more accurate and agreed more highly when listening to native language speakers. Both Van Borsel and Pereira (2005) and Einarsdóttir and Ingham (2005), who report a similar pattern, suggest that availability of agreed-upon "exemplar databases" in a variety of languages that could then be used to train clinicians might improve agreement for frequency counts in stuttering, as well as refine our definitions of what constitutes a moment of stuttering.

Speech Rate

Our discussion of disfluency counts in the preceding paragraphs was prompted by the question of whether there are any measures of severity of stuttering that are independent of a listener's judgment of the occurrence of stuttering. Another type of objective measure is rate of speech production—for example, oral reading rate in words or syllables per minute, or of the time it takes a speaker to utter a given number of words. Stuttering, of course, tends to retard the speaker's speed of verbal output. In a study of oral reading rates of adult stutterers (Bloodstein, 1944), a mean rate of 123 words per minute was found in the reading of factual prose of average word length, with a range among thirty subjects of 42 to 191 words per minute. By contrast, the same material was read by normally fluent speakers in a previous study (Darley, 1940) at a mean rate of 167 words per minute, with a range of 129 to 222 words per minute. Extensive normative data presented by Johnson (1961a) for both reading and speaking show comparable differences as well as overlap in values between stutterers and nonstutterers.

From a practical standpoint, measures of rate have the advantage of being convenient to use. They take into account both frequency and duration of stutters and tend to be fairly highly correlated (see Table 1-1) with frequency. They are also influenced, however, by various factors that presumably do not enter into listeners' criteria for the occurrence of stuttering and are insensitive to any aspects of symptomatology that do not waste time, and so have usually been found to be only moderately related to judges' ratings of severity of stuttering. Young, in the study cited, found that speaking time did not contribute as much to the prediction of ratings of severity as did his count of specified disfluencies, except in the case of the more severe stutterers. On the other hand, Prosek et al. (1979) found reading rate, as well as frequency of pauses within sentences, to be more closely related to judged severity of stuttering than were other measures including frequency of stuttering.

From these observations and the data in Table 1-1 we may infer that speech rate is not so well correlated with any other measure of severity as to be considered merely its equivalent and yet is sufficiently related to other measures as to suggest that it may reflect an aspect of severity that they do not adequately take into account. For this reason, there has been a tendency to use speech rate in conjunction with other measures in which the amount or severity of stuttering has also been a variable. For the same reason, it lends itself to use in composite indices such as that proposed by Minifie and Cooker (1964).

Ratings of Severity

Listeners' ratings of stuttering severity constitute a frankly subjective measure reflecting the judgmental nature of the criteria that we use to define stuttering. There is perhaps no better evidence of that judgmental nature than the common practice of validating other measures of severity by comparing them with the results obtained on the same stutterers by means of listeners' ratings of severity. Of all measures, in short, this one has the highest "face" validity.

It is also by far the oldest and most familiar type of measurement in general use, in the sense that we employ it on every occasion in which we characterize stuttering as "mild," "moderate," or "severe." In the 1950s, this method underwent its first major development with the introduction of tape-recorded speech samples, multiple judges, and refined psychological scaling techniques developed by Sherman and others, and a considerable amount of work was then done in an effort to find the most advantageous ways of obtaining severity ratings for clinical and research purposes. Since that time, digital audio and video recording has accelerated our ability to conduct research in this area.

These investigations resulted in reliable methods for scaling the severity of stuttering in continuous speech, in short samples, or of individual moments.[8] Studies have shown that, by and large, the reliability of the measures is not critically affected by such factors as the type of scale used, the number of scale points, the definition of scale points, the addition of visual or "live" cues, the number of judges, their sophistication, or the kinds of instructions they receive.[9] In addition, work has been done on the measurement and improvement of observer agreement and on the control of observer bias in judging severity of stuttering.[10]

The scale of stuttering severity constructed by Lewis and Sherman (1951) using the method of equal-appearing intervals consists of a series of tape-recorded speech samples representing the whole range of severity from very mild to very severe. These samples form touchstones, as it were, with which the speech of a given stutterer may be compared. The scale affords a precise method of rating severity, though a study by Berry and Silverman (1972) suggests that the scale has ordinal rather than interval properties—that is, the intervals are not subjectively equal.

Having said this, interval-scaled severity rating schemes have experienced a recent return to popularity, especially in clinical research that has involved parents' monitoring of early stuttering and their child's response to treatment (see Yairi & Ambrose, 2005 and discussion of the Lidcombe Programme of Early Stuttering (Onslow, Packman, & Harrison, 2003) in Chapter 14). Recent work by O'Brian, Packman, Onslow, and O'Brian (2004) suggests that a nine-point stuttering severity scale correlates quite well with stuttering counts, except when a speaker has few, but very significant, stuttered events in his speech. For this type of speaker, estimated to be approximately 13 percent of the participants in the O'Brian et al. study, both types of measures might be most appropriate, especially in judging speakers' pre- and post-intervention profiles.

An alternative rating method is known as direct magnitude estimation. In place of a scale, raters use a single stimulus as a standard for comparison. Assigning any number (e.g., 10) to that standard, they then estimate the numerical magnitude of

[8] Lewis and Sherman (1951), Sherman (1952), Sherman (1955), Sherman and Trotter (1956), Sherman and McDermott (1958).

[9] Young and Prather (1962), Cullinan, Prather, and Williams (1963), Williams, Wark, and Minifie (1963), Martin (1965), Cullinan and Prather (1968).

[10] Young and Downs (1968), Young (1969a, 1969b, 1970).

other stimuli as proportions of the magnitude of the standard. Martin (1965) showed that the severity of stuttering could be rated reliably in this way. Results of a study by Schiavetti, Sacco, Metz, and Sitler (1983) suggested that direct magnitude estimation is a more valid method of rating the severity of stuttering than interval scaling. More recently, use of this technique produced interesting results (Lickley, Hartsuiker, Corley, Russell, & Nelson, 2005). Even the supposedly fluent speech of people who stutter was judged to be more disfluent than "matched" samples from typically fluent speakers, suggesting subtle differences between the fluent speech of stutterers and nonstutterers. Moreover, stutterers judged more speech samples as disfluent than did typically fluent speakers. We will return to this study to address implications of these findings for subclinical differences in speech production in people who stutter (Chapter 5) and models of stuttering (Chapter 2).

Summary Remarks

The preceding discussion has served to raise several fundamental questions. How is stuttering to be defined? What are its measurable dimensions? How is it to be differentiated from other kinds of disfluent behavior, including that of normal speech? We have seen that, except for the evaluation of a listener that stuttering has occurred, we as yet have no operational definition serving to characterize the stuttering response in a wholly satisfactory way. On the other hand, we can identify certain features of speech, notably sound or syllable repetitions, broken words, prolonged sounds, and signs of unusual effort or tension that are more closely related than others to what most listeners judge to be stuttering. There are thus hints that with further description we may eventually be able to define stuttering more adequately in terms of its observable features. Whether or not observable moments of stuttering will suffice to provide data to elucidate explanatory models of stuttering will be addressed in Chapter 2, where some, notably Anne Smith (Smith & Kelly, 1997; Smith, 1999), have argued that the external manifestations of stuttering provide little guidance in developing accounts of its nature and cause.

We can summarize the essential meaning of all we have said so far in this chapter by suggesting that, for investigators who are anxious to define carefully what they mean by stuttering, the best definition we appear to be able to offer at present is: whatever is perceived as stuttering by a reliable observer who has relatively good agreement with others. This, in turn, reminds us of other elusive definitions, such as what characterizes "art" or the essence of "true love."[11] Without trivializing the issue, if we want to be guided by a more "objective" definition, we must not ask questions about "stuttering," but about repetitions, prolongations, broken words, speech rate, and the like, and must be content with answers that are not about stuttering, but about repetitions, prolongations, and so forth. In this sense, stuttering is an abstract construct, whose nature is informed indirectly by these types of behavior counts, but is not limited to them.

In any consideration of the problem of defining stuttering it is, of course, also vitally necessary to keep distinct a number of different meanings with which the term may be used. For example, the question of whether a person "is a stutterer" (i.e., stutters habitually) is one on which it is generally fairly easy to obtain agreement, except with respect to young children (see Chapter 12), on the basis of observed speech behavior on a series of occasions, as well as the speech history, the conditions under which the behavior varies, the person's self-concepts, speech attitudes, methods of coping with the problem, and the like. Agreement that the person "is a stutterer," however, does not help much to answer the question of whether he or she has spoken in a stuttering manner in a given speech situation. That question, in turn, is not as difficult to answer as the question of whether the speaker has stuttered on a given word. The use of the term "stuttering" in each of these cases must not be allowed to become a source of confusion. If we are unable to define the moment of stuttering so as to differentiate it easily from other instances of speech interruption, this is a

[11] We thank Bob Quesal for this analogy.

curious and by no means trivial fact. But it does not rule out an operationally meaningful definition of stuttering as a disorder.

It is, of course, within the realm of possibility that not only incidents of stuttered speech, but even individuals who stutter, may prove impossible to characterize in every case with absolute unambiguity. If so, the prospect need not alarm us unduly. There is, as we shall see, more than one conceptual scheme available to stuttering theory that is compatible with the assumption that the population of "stutterers" is not separable from the normally fluent population in a sharply dichotomous way. As in other developmental disorders, such as childhood language impairment (Dollaghan, 2004), stuttering may lie on a continuum of behaviors, rather than defined by sharply delineated boundaries.

In this section, we have not explored specific assessment protocols or scales that may be used to measure stuttering frequency and severity for assessment and treatment purposes. In clinical practice, there are a great many such published devices, and their use is critical in establishing pre- and post-treatment fluency profiles. These measures will be addressed both here and in Chapter 14.

PHYSIOLOGICAL AND ACOUSTIC DESCRIPTIONS OF THE MOMENT OF STUTTERING

This section will address what we have learned about what happens in the moment of stuttering. The instruments and methods of the speech laboratory have been put to great use in the study of stuttering symptomatology. After a period of many decades during which such research was largely confined to the investigation of the stutterer's breathing patterns by relatively limited means, we now have considerable electromyographic, spectrographic, fiber-optic, radiographic, aerodynamic, and other kinds of data about the stuttering block. However, there has always been concern that we may learn as much, if not more, from studying the otherwise perceptually "normal" speech of people who stutter. This line of inquiry is pursued in great detail in Chapter 5.

Respiration

Disordered breathing is associated with stuttering so often and so conspicuously that it was one of the earliest factors to be investigated as a possible cause of stuttering. Pneumographic research was consequently conducted over a long period of time. Breathing curves during stuttering show a series of abnormalities, some of which are obviously parallel to audible or visible aspects of symptomatology. These include antagonisms between abdominal and thoracic breathing, irregularity of consecutive respiratory cycles, prolonged expirations or inspirations, complete cessation of breathing, interruption of expiration by inspiration, and attempts to speak on intake of air.[12] Perhaps for these reasons, the carbon dioxide concentration of air exhaled during moments of stuttering is markedly lower than during exhalation for fluent speech (Raczek & Adamczyk, 2004).

Phonation

Breath-holding, glottal fry, and stutterers' reports that their "throat closes tightly" are common clinical observations that point to the larynx as a site of abnormal activity during stuttering. As with the respiratory mechanism, various attempts have been made since the 19th century to identify the larynx as the primary source of difficulty for those who stutter.

In 1963, Chevrie-Muller reported a study of the vocal folds during stuttering by the technique of glottography. The method employed by Chevrie-Muller provided a continuous record of the size of the glottal opening by measuring the amount of light permitted to pass through it. She found many abnormalities including "breaks in the rhythm of

[12] Halle (1900), Ten Cate (1902), Gutzmann (1908), Fletcher (1914), Lambeck (1925), Hansen (1927), Travis (1927a), Fossler (1930), Steer (1935), Henrikson (1936), V. Travis (1936), Steer (1937), Morley (1937), Starbuck and Steer (1954), Umeda (1962b), Brankel (1961, 1963).

vocal fold vibration and a clonic fluttering of the folds in some but not all of her stutterers" (as cited by Van Riper, 1971, p. 150).

Janssen, Wieneke, and Vaane (1983) used glottographic recording to test the assumption that stuttering blocks are associated with slowness in initiating phonation, relative to the start of articulatory activity. Among five stutterers, this proved to be true of only two. Weiner (1984a) produced a series of glottograms corresponding to various types of stuttering by using a technique that measured the impedance of the glottis to an electrical current passing over it. Using the same technique, Borden, Baer, and Kenney (1985) found that after a stuttering block on initial /t/ in the word "two," almost all stutterers tended to build up voicing gradually instead of abruptly as in fluent productions of the word. They speculated that the speakers used this as a means of releasing themselves from the block. Borden, Baer, and Kenney also noted evidence of rigidity of the vocal folds during stuttering, as well as tremors that coincided with visible tremors of the lip.

Electromyography, the recording of electrical potentials from the muscles, was first used to observe a stutterer's laryngeal activity by Bar, Singer, and Feldman (1969). They reported an increase in the action potentials just before and during stuttering. Freeman and Ushijima (1975, 1978) took electromyographic (EMG) recordings simultaneously from six separate intrinsic laryngeal muscles of four stutterers. Their results showed high levels of muscular activity during stuttering, as well as simultaneous contractions of adductor and abductor muscles (see Figure 1-1). These observations—excessive muscular activity and poor coordination of antagonistic laryngeal muscles—were confirmed by Shapiro (1980) with four additional individuals who stuttered. Laryngeal hyperactivity was also reported by Thürmer, Thumfart, and Kittel (1983) in an electromyographic study of 42 stutterers. Metz, Conture, and Colton (1976) found a delay in laryngeal activity prior to disfluencies as measured electromyographically in two stutterers.

Conture, McCall, and Brewer (1977) used a fiber-optic technique to make direct visual observations of the glottis during stuttering in 10 adults stutterers. In 60 percent of the part-word repetitions, the vocal folds were in a state of abduction throughout the block, regardless of whether the repeated speech segment was voiced or unvoiced. In the remaining cases, the vocal folds were either adducted or alternately adducted and abducted. During prolongations of sounds, the position of the folds was always appropriate to the voicing characteristics of the sound. In a later fiber-optic study, Conture, Schwartz, and Brewer (1985) found that during voiced prolongations, the vocal folds were usually appropriately adducted, but that during sound or syllable repetitions and voiceless prolongations the folds were adducted, abducted, or in an intermediate position. Their observations appeared to show that stutterers do not "simply 'squeeze' their vocal folds together during all instances of stuttering"; the vocal folds either may be inappropriately adducted or abducted. Wolk (1981), using a similar technique with one subject, found a "shuddering" of the larynx, asymmetry of the arytenoid cartilages and vocal folds, and partial adduction of the folds, seeming to represent a conflict between adductory and abductory behavior, during all types of stuttering. In a more recent investigation of laryngeal activity during moments of stuttering using EMG, Anne Smith and her colleagues (Smith, Denny, Shaffer, Kelly, & Hirano, 1996) did not find higher levels of thyroarytenoid or cricothyroid muscle activity during disfluent speech than fluent speech in persons who stutter, nor did stutterers show unusually high levels of intrinsic laryngeal muscle tension when contrasted with that seen in people who do not stutter.

Thus, it is clear that the larynx is involved, along with other parts of the vocal apparatus, in the abnormality that we perceive as stuttering. However, whether the deviant activity of the larynx is "primary" in any sense is not a question that can be answered by descriptive studies of stuttering symptomatology. Such studies, and those described in the sections that follow, fail to distinguish among causes, features, and effects of stuttering. We will return to this question when we consider other types of investigations of laryngeal functioning in Chapter 5.

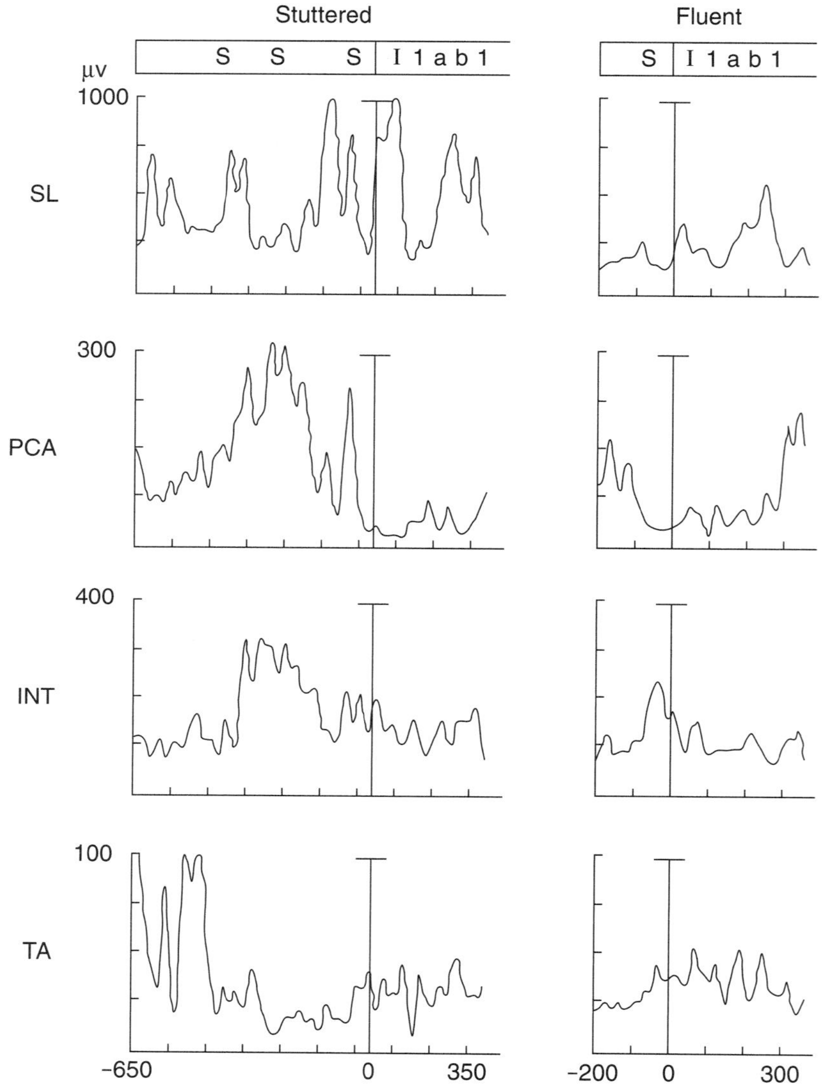

FIGURE 1-1 Comparison of muscle activity—superior longitudinal (SL), posterior cricoary-tenoid (PCA), interarytenoid (INT), and thyroarytenoid (TA)—for one subject's stuttered and fluent utterances of the world *syllable*. Note the simultaneous contraction of the PCA (abductor) and INT (adductor) muscles during stuttering, as well as the increased muscular activity. Reprinted with permission from "Laryngeal muscle activity during stuttering," by Freeman and Ushijim, *J. Speech Hearing Res., 21,* 538–62. Copyright 1978 by the American Speech-Language-Hearing Association. All rights reserved.

Articulation

Research has been done to examine the activity of the peripheral organs of articulation during stuttering, as well as to examine certain aspects of the stutterer's speech sound production. The earliest of these studies were kymographic investigations by Robbins (1935) and Cords (1936) concerned with durational aspects of speech sounds during stuttering blocks or in stuttered speech. Shaffer (1940) measured jaw movement during stuttered and nonstuttered productions of stop-plosive consonants in initial position in words. He found that stuttering was characterized, among other abnormalities, by longer time intervals between onset of jaw movement and onset of phonation, by more directional changes in jaw movement, and by longer intervals between initiation and first directional change of jaw movement.

Electromyographic Studies The development of electromyography permitted observations to be made of individual muscles of articulation during stuttering. Electromyographic studies of the masseter muscles by Travis (1934), Morley (1937), Steer (1937), and Williams (1955) showed that in stuttering there is frequent evidence of defective synchronization, as well as other abnormalities of the action potentials of the paired musculatures. In a different type of investigation, Sheehan and Voas (1954) used unilateral masseter action potentials to show that muscular tension appears to build up during stuttering, reaching its peak near the termination of the block.

Further studies were done on the orbicularis muscle by Tatham (1973) and Belyakova (1973) and on the masseter and geniohyoid muscles by Brankel (1963). In each case, the occurrence of stuttering was found to be recognizable in some manner in the electromyographic recordings. In a study by Shapiro (1980), four stutterers fitted with electrodes at the lip and tongue showed excessive muscular activity on stuttered words, poor coordination of muscles, and inappropriate bursts of activity during silence (see Figure 1-2). Craig and Cleary (1982) observed high levels of activity in the orbicularis oris in their three participants during stuttering, while Thürmer, Thumfart, and Kittel (1983) found excessive activity in the orbicularis oris and tongue in 42 adults who stutter.

A frequent observation, in studies of both the articulatory and laryngeal muscles, is that the same electromyographic phenomena that characterize overt stuttering may sometimes appear in the absence of any noticeable blocks (see especially Shapiro,

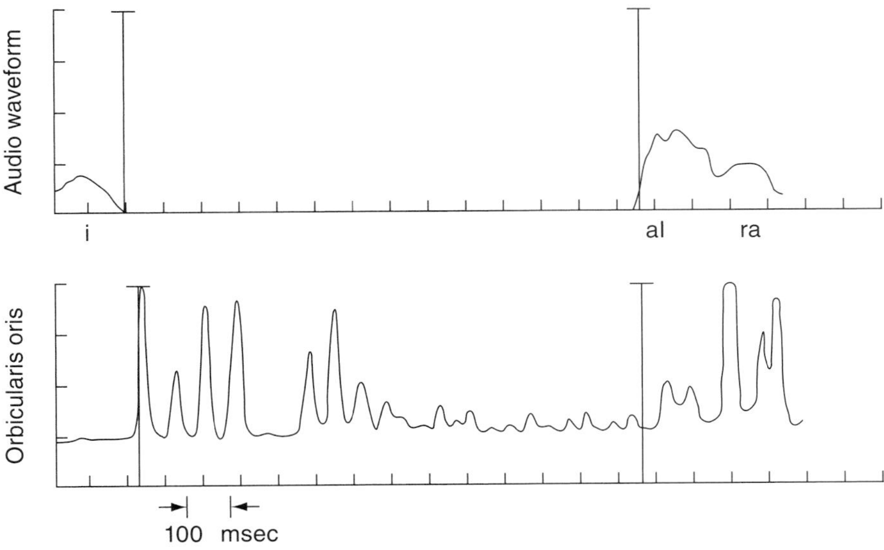

FIGURE 1-2 Abnormal supraglottal muscular activity during stuttering on "Ira." Reproduced by permission of the publisher from "An electromyographic analysis of the fluent and dysfluent utterances of several types of stutterers," by Arnold Shapiro, *Journal of Fluency Disorders, 5,* 203–31. Copyright 1980 by Elsevier Science Publishing Co., Inc.

1980; Freeman, 1984). The reverse—stuttering without evidence of increased muscular tension—as reported by McClean, Goldsmith, and Cerf (1984). In an electromyographic and strain-gauge study of the depressor labii inferior and mentalis muscles (antagonists in the elevation and depression of the lower lip) during stuttering on bilabial consonants by five speakers, the investigators failed to find simultaneous contraction of antagonistic muscles or increased levels of electromyographic activity.

Anne Smith (1989) correlated the activity of neck, jaw, and lip muscles during stuttering. She found little indication that the coordination of these muscles differed from that of normally fluent comparison speakers, but unlike any of the nonstutterers, 6 of 10 stutterers exhibited large rhythmic oscillations in muscle activity during stuttering. These occurred at the same frequency in all of the muscle groups, suggesting that they had a common source. In the same muscles, Smith, Denny, and Wood (1991) observed tremor-like oscillations and increased activity, which were not timed precisely with perceived stutters but occurred in their "neighborhood." Denny and Smith (1992) reported that neither the oscillations nor the high electromyographic amplitudes always occurred with stuttering, but appeared in varying degrees in different subjects; these findings were further detailed in an additional report (Smith et al., 1993).

Two lip muscles were the subject of a study of three stutterers and three comparison speakers by Guitar, Guitar, Neilson, O'Dwyer, and Andrews (1988). In articulating the initial /p/ of the words *peek, puck*, and *pack*, the normally fluent speakers typically activated the depressor anguli oris before the depressor labii inferior. The stutterers reversed this sequence most of the time when stuttering and half the time when not. The authors hypothesized that the stutterers were deliberately stiffening their lips in the expectation of stuttering. If so, this demonstrated what Van Riper (1937d; p. 66) described as one of the stutterer's "preparatory sets," namely the tendency to establish a focus of tension in the articulators in advance of the attempt on a difficult word.

Van Riper (1982, pp. 123–126) remarked on the occurrence of tremors in the speech muscles during stuttering and the role of strenuous postures of the articulators in precipitating them. Through the use of electromyographic recordings, Platt and Basili (1973) discovered that such tremors appear to be similar to those that are commonly produced by isometric contractions of muscles (i.e., co-contractions of antagonists). They found three stutterers who exhibited jaw tremors during stuttering and instructed the stutterers to produce contractions of the jaw muscles by opening and closing the jaw simultaneously without dental contact. The resulting tremors were compared with the stuttering tremors and found to be alike in frequency and amplitude. This lends support to Platt and Basili's parsimonious explanation that tremors in stuttering may result from isometric muscle status due to struggle.

Aerodynamic Studies Another approach to the description of stuttering has made use of devices for measuring intraoral air pressure and the rate of airflow from the oral cavity during speech. In a study of the stutters of eight adults, Hutchinson (1975) identified seven distinctive aerodynamic patterns. Repeated peaks in intraoral air pressure were associated with syllable repetitions. A gradual elevation of intraoral air pressure occurred with prolongation of a sound. Multiple elevations of intraoral pressure without airflow were associated with a silent block on a stop consonant. Prolonged airflow terminating in an excessive peak of airflow corresponded to a breathy articulation of a sound such as /w/, with an aspirated release. A sudden drop in air pressure and flow rate accompanied a brief silent interval. A prolonged peak of intraoral air pressure and absence of airflow signified the silent prolongation of an articulatory posture. Intraoral pressure elevations of low magnitude without airflow were observed on prolonged pauses between syllables.

These aerodynamic findings correspond in a predictable way to repetitions, prolongations, and other types of stuttering as they are conventionally described. But they also reflect a feature of stuttering that our unaided clinical observations are unable to penetrate—the underlying tension that appears to pervade the vocal mechanism during the block. Although we sometimes speak of tension among the features of stuttering as though we were employing a description, the tense state of muscles is something we must infer rather than anything we can observe directly. The electromyographic findings we have reviewed give us the most direct evidence of this state. Hutchinson's aerodynamic patterns do so less directly, but they graphically reveal the source of that tension to be the attempt that stutterers make to speak through an airway that they have constricted at some point.

Spectrographic Studies Acoustic investigation of stuttering done using spectrographic analysis has centered mainly around the transitions between speech sounds during part-word repetitions. Van Riper (1971, pp. 23–25) speculated that the stutterer's difficulty is not with sounds but with the transitions between them. He suggested that in stutterers' part-word repetitions, as distinguished from those of nonstutterers, the neutral vowel (schwa) is almost universally heard (e.g., *suh-suh-sandwich*) in place of the intended vowel that would be required by normal coarticulation. Neither perceptual judgments of trained observers nor spectrograms have wholly borne out this observation, however. In a perceptual and acoustic analysis, Montgomery and Cooke (1976) found that stutterers' part-word repetitions do not ordinarily contain the neutral vowel, but a vowel that often approximates that of the word being pronounced. Van Wyk (1978) reported an absence of formant transitions in the repetitions of eighteen stuttering children and adults, but perceptual and spectrographic analysis showed that the neutral vowel was not being used. Similar observations have been made by others.[13] Howell and his coworkers showed that what often strikes the ear as a neutralization of the vowel in stutterers' repetitions actually is occasioned by a decrease in the duration and amplitude of the vowel.[14]

Nevertheless, Stromsta and Fibiger (1981) produced evidence suggesting reduction of normal coarticulation during stutterers' sound repetitions. Spectrograms and electromyographic recordings were made from the upper lip of stutterers while they read a passage weighted with syllables that normally elicit anticipatory coarticulation of lip rounding (e.g., as in *Europe, screw*, where the rounded vowel typically affects articulatory posture for the consonant in advance). The spectrograms showed less coarticulatory labial activity during repetitions than on stutterers' fluent utterances or normally fluent speakers' productions of the same words.

Other Studies Wave form analyses have also been conducted on the characteristics of repetitions in young stuttering children and more typically fluent peers. In a series of studies, Ehud Yairi and colleagues (Throneburg & Yairi, 1994; Yairi & Hall, 1993) found that the inter-iteration interval (time between repeated segments) was noticeably shorter in repetitions produced by children who stutter than children who were considered typically fluent. Zebrowski (1994) found that there was a negative correlation between the rate of iterations and the number of repetitions seen in childhood stuttering—the longer the iteration duration, the fewer the number of repetitions per moment of stuttering. This work has been extended to examine its potential in predicting spontaneous recovery or chronicity in stuttering, as we discuss in Chapter 12.

Another technique applied in the study of articulatory dynamics has been the strain-gauge transducer, a device for converting mechanical movement into electrical signals. Hutchinson and Watkin (1976) used it to study the jaw movements of four stutterers at the terminations of blocks. In confirmation of clinical observations, they found that articulatory movement was abnormally rapid at the moment of release from the stuttering block. In addition, in a number of instances, the movement of the jaw was not coordinated with the onset of

[13] Hutchinson and Watkin (1974), Freeman, Borden, and Dorman (cited by Freeman, 1979; Harrington, 1987).

[14] Howell and Vause (1986), Howell, Williams, and Vause (1987), Howell and Williams (1988), Howell, Williams, and Young (1991), and Howell and Williams (1992).

vocalization, sometimes preceding and sometimes lagging behind it.

Zimmermann (1980a) used X-ray motion picture photography to observe movements of the lower lip and jaw during stuttering in two speakers and of the tongue as well in two others. His main finding was that there is a repositioning of the articulators preceding the release of a stuttering block. This usually takes the form of a lowering of the jaw and lower lip and a reshaping of the tongue toward its resting position.

In summary, instrumented laboratory studies to date have served mainly to confirm a number of significant clinical impressions. During stuttering there is abnormal function of essentially the whole speech system, including but not limited to the larynx. A notable aspect of that abnormal function is excessive muscular tension. Judging from the way in which stuttering is associated with elevations of intraoral breath pressure, at least part of that tension must result from efforts to force the outgoing breath stream past heightened resistance.

However, as Chapter 5 will show, most of the research focus over the past 20 years has been on the perceptually fluent speech of stutterers. As Anne Smith (1999) notes, trying to understand stuttering from measuring attributes of its breakdown can only bring us so far in understanding the disorder: she likens it to trying to develop a theory about the cause of volcanic eruptions from examining their lava flows. While the two are related, one needs to "dig deeper" to understand the major underlying phenomenon that sets eruptions off, in this case plate tectonics.

ASSOCIATED SYMPTOMS

There is much more to stuttering than repetitions, prolongations, or pauses. We must include in our description any number of associated features, often referred to as "secondary" symptoms. The concomitant features of stuttering are many and extremely varied. Their precise specification is difficult since it depends to a large extent on what is meant by the essential or integral features of stuttering. The term *associated* may be applied to aspects, attributes, or correlates of speech blockages or to clearly independent behaviors. We will use the term broadly and somewhat loosely here to stand for (1) visible or audible reactions accompanying or interspersed among stutterers' speech interruptions, (2) visceral or physiological correlates of stuttering, and (3) changes in stutterers' perceptions of their environment and in their subjective states when experiencing difficulty with speech.

Overt Concomitants

The observable concomitants of stuttering consist of a number of different kinds of reactions, chief among them being movements and interjections. We detail these in this section.

Associated Movements Stutterers often display visible tension in the face or such movements as a jerk of the head while speaking. These reactions may be simple and brief or complicated and bizarre. Most often, the mannerisms accompanying stuttering involve parts of the speech mechanism or related structures. Among the most frequent are eyeblink, wrinkling of the forehead, and sudden exhalation of breath. Also common are frowning, distortions of the mouth, quivering of the nostrils, and movements of the eyes, head, tongue, and muscles of respiration. It is difficult to catalog all of the acts or tension sites that may become associated with stuttering; any part of the voluntary musculature of the body may participate, including that of the hands, arms, legs, feet, and torso. Although these concomitants are usually closely associated with a stuttering block, they may appear independently of any readily observable interruption in speech. Such involuntary movements are noticeably more frequent in stuttered than fluent speech, and in people who stutter than those who do not, even when speaking fluently (Mulligan et al., 2001). While they could suggest underlying motor dysfunction in people who stutter, it appears to most researchers that these behaviors mark responses to the challenge of trying to produce fluent speech, rather than symptoms of disordered motor control.

A systematic classification of these visible concomitants of stuttering was made by Prins and Lohr

(1972) on the basis of a motion picture study. Riley (1972) devised a test of severity of stuttering in which ratings of such overt concomitants contribute to the total measure, along with frequency of stuttering and duration of the longest blocks. This measure has been revised over the years; its most recent version is the frequently employed *Stuttering Severity Instrument—3* (*SSI-3*, Riley & Riley, 1994).

Kraaimaat and Janssen (1985) and Janssen and Kraaimaat (1986) studied the temporal relationship of associated facial movements to the primary symptoms of stuttering. Jaw and mouth movements almost always occurred during moments of stuttering, while eyeblinking generally did not. Kraaimaat and Janssen speculated that jaw and mouth movements resulted from tension or struggle, whereas eyeblinks were avoidance reactions.

Interjected Speech Fragments Interjections (often called filled pauses in the speech production literature) take the form of sounds, syllables, words, or phrases, and, like the associated movements, they usually, but not necessarily, occur in immediate conjunction with observable stuttering events. Typical examples are "um," "er," "well," "like," "you know." They tend to be superfluous, as in "I'm g—er, well you see, I'm going home now," and they may be inappropriate as well (e.g., "I live at—in other words—19 Cadwallader Place"). Behaviors such as these may indicate the speaker's attempt to avoid a perceived likelihood of stuttering on the original target word (Manning, 2001). We note that filled pauses are common in the speech of fluent speakers and increase under conditions of higher task demand or other forms of attentional stress (Oomen & Postma, 2001). Thus, it is not surprising that, in a factor analysis of stuttering symptoms by Lewis (1991), interjections, word and phrase repetitions, and revisions separated themselves from other features, a division that Lewis interpreted as one between stuttering and its avoidance.

Vocal Abnormalities Stuttering is often accompanied by a variety of abnormal vocal and speech features. These may include rapid or slow rate, changes in vocal quality, odd inflections or sharp shifts in pitch level, and/or monotone. Quarrington and Douglass (1960) commented provocatively on the habitual tendency of some stutterers to suspend phonation, apparently in order to avoid audibility while stuttering.

Phonatory disturbances in the speech of stutterers, especially a frequent lack of normal pitch variation, were demonstrated by photo-phonographic techniques in early studies by Travis (1927b), Bryngelson (1932), and Adams (1955), and were studied spectrographically and oscillographically by Schilling and Göler (1961) and Luchsinger and Dubois (1963). Other intonational deviations were found by Stock (1966). Largely conflicting results were reported by Lechner (1979), however. She found that stutterers did not differ from nonstutterers in extent of pitch shifts and inflections or in rate of inflectional variations during speech. They differed from nonstutterers only in having more downward and therefore total inflections. Schäferskúpper (1982) also found more falling inflections in stutterers' conversational speech and fewer rising inflections. His subjects, 10- to 12-year-old children, accented the first word of a sentence more than twice as often as nonstutterers. Adams (1955), Schmitt and Cooper (1978), and Lechner (1979) did not observe any deviation in average pitch level or any unequivocal deviations in pitch range. A tendency toward higher pitch levels approaching statistical significance in 10- to 12-year-old stutterers' spontaneous speech was reported by Schäferskúpper and Simon (1983). It is not known how many of these reported abnormalities may be responses to certain therapeutic strategies of the "fluency-shaping" nature, which often instruct the stutterer to prolong speech segments and continuously link them (see Chapter 14).

Other Physical Reactions In severe stuttering, flushing, pallor, or perspiration may be visible as accompanying reactions. These are likely to reflect the stutterer's response to the challenge of speaking fluently.

The Meaning of the Overt Concomitants of Stuttering Some stutterers seem to show few of the associated symptoms that we have so far enumerated. Others exhibit a great many and may do so in highly individual combinations or patterns (Barr, 1940). They tend to be performed relatively automatically and unconsciously, particularly when they have persisted for some length of time. Most of them appear to be first adopted as devices for minimizing stuttering. In the effort to avoid or terminate blocks, the stutterer may discover by trial and error that blinking the eyes or taking a deep breath can be helpful expedients.

Since the effectiveness of such devices appears to lie in their ability to distract attention momentarily from the act of speaking, the eyeblink is no longer effective once it has lost its novelty, and the stutterer must then cast about for another contrivance. In this process, however, the outworn eyeblink often remains as a habitual part of the stuttering reaction. It appears to be in this manner that the complex symptom patterns of some stutterers develop. In a study of such patterns, Van Riper (1937a) found that in many cases, most of the overt abnormality of stuttering appears to consist of devices for concealing it.

Van Riper (1963) suggested a useful fivefold classification of such devices. The first category consists of symptoms of *avoidance*, by means of which feared words are avoided altogether. The most common examples are *word substitution* and *circumlocution*, which may become so awkward and extreme as to interfere with communication. A second category, symptoms of *postponement*, consists of maneuvers to delay the attempt on the feared word in the hope that the fear will subside sufficiently for the stutterer to say it normally. The speaker may pause strategically, repeat preceding words or phrases, or interject such expressions as "you know" or "well" in a pretense at thought. Third are symptoms of *starting*, tricks enabling the stutterer to say the feared word by making it easier to produce the difficult first sound. Adroitly timed grimaces or other associated movements may serve this purpose. A particularly common starter is an easy sound or syllable—for example "uh," prefixed to the feared word. Fourth are symptoms of *escape*. These embrace all of the stutterer's struggles to terminate the block. The person may attempt to "break" the block by means of a head jerk, gasp, or interjection; exhaust all breath and finish the word on residual air; or "back up and get a running start" on the word. The fifth category, symptoms of *anti-expectancy*, includes expedients the stutterer uses for preventing the anticipation of difficulty from arising. For example, the person may speak in a rapid monotone so that no particular word stands out to be feared or may attempt to distract attention from fear of stuttering by the use of almost any other unnatural speech pattern.

Van Riper's classification of concealment devices anticipates later discussions by virtue of the role it assigns to expectancy in stuttering behavior. It is cited here, however, because it exposes with particular clarity a valid sense in which many of the overt symptoms of stuttering may be regarded as "secondary" to or overlaid upon certain essential or "primary" symptoms.

Physiological Concomitants

Stuttering is accompanied by a variety of covert, internal bodily phenomena that must be observed indirectly by the use of suitable instruments for physiological investigation. A few are summarized here.

Eye Movements Unusual eye movements, associated mainly with the stuttering block, have been found during both the oral reading and spontaneous speech of stutterers (Jasper & Murray, 1932; Moser, 1938; Kopp, 1963). Some of the outstanding phenomena described are vertical "twitches" of the eyes, prolonged fixations, slow continuous or rapid "aimless" horizontal movements, and binocular incoordination exemplified by independent horizontal movements of the two eyes (temporary strabismus) or fixation of one eye and simultaneous vertical twitching of the other.

Cardiovascular Phenomena During speech, and just prior to speech under conditions likely to produce stuttering, there is often an acceleration of the heart and pulse rate.[15] In the most recent review of cardiac activity seen in stuttering, Alm (2004b) concluded, however, that stuttering is often associated with paradoxical slowing of heart rate, perhaps as a result of anticipatory anxiety over speaking and/or stuttering. Anticipatory anxiety can produce such symptoms.

Robbins (1920) also observed changes in blood distribution associated with stuttering in a plethysmographic study of a single stutterer, and this was confirmed by Kurshev (1968a) and Ickes and Pierce (1973) with groups of subjects. Such changes may become overt in severe instances as the pallor and flushing referred to earlier. In two stutterers, Wood et al. (1980) found lower blood flow during stuttering in Broca's area in the left cerebral hemisphere than in the corresponding area of the right hemisphere. We discuss a number of additional studies of cortical activity during speaking and stuttering in Chapter 4.

Uenishi et al (1973) reported changes in maximum blood pressure in stutterers during speaking and reading. Curiously enough, however, Dabul and Perkins (1973) found that when systolic blood pressure had been elevated by electric shock, stuttering served to decrease it.

Tremors Herren (1932) found that normal hand tremors of a rate of 8 to 12 per second were depressed during stuttering. A more rapid type of hand tremor (40 to 75 per second) tended to become more pronounced. Movement was recorded by means of a photographic procedure designed by Travis.

Cortical Activity Although the findings of electroencephalographic research on stuttering are difficult to interpret, there appears to be evidence from studies by Travis and Knott (1936), Travis and Malamud (1937), and Freestone (1942) that alpha-wave activity is intensified during the stuttering block. Fox (1966) found that stuttering produced more disruption in the regularity and interhemispheric synchronization of the waves than did nonstutterers' imitations of stuttering and thought it possible that this was due to a difference in emotional arousal. Sayles (1971), who searched for clinically abnormal wave patterns in stutterers, found a considerable number, but observed no tendency for the patterns to be related to moments of stuttering or speech activity in oral reading.

Of historical interest are some electroencephalographic findings of Boberg, Yeudall, Schopflocher, and Bo-Lassen (1983). During verbal tasks, normal speakers showed a suppression of alpha waves in the left cerebral hemisphere, a phenomenon evidently related to the greater role of the left hemisphere in speech processing in most individuals. Boberg and his coworkers failed to observe the expected interhemispheric difference in stuttering subjects during speech tasks in which stuttering presumably took place. However, the normal alpha relationship appeared after a three-week program of therapy in which the participants' stuttering was markedly reduced through the use of a slow speaking rate and easy vocal onsets. Additional studies that have examined brain activity preceding and following speech therapy are discussed in Chapter 4.

The development of functional brain imaging techniques (explored in greater detail in Chapter 4) has also enabled study of cortical activity during moments of stuttering. Roger Ingham and his colleagues (Ingham, Fox, Ingham, & Zamarripa, 2000) found that for four adult male stutterers, who were studied using positron emission tomography (PET), overt stuttering was marked by prominent activations in the medial supplementary motor area (SMA), right hemisphere Brodmann area 46, the anterior insula, and cerebellum (bilaterally) that were not seen during fluent speech production. Relative deactivations were also seen in the right secondary auditory area (Brodmann areas 21/22). Curiously enough, very similar activation and deactivation patterns were seen when the participants *imagined* stuttering, leading the authors to conclude that overt stuttering was not required to produce these aberrant patterns of cortical activity.

Biochemical Changes Moore (1959) reported that with increases in stuttering, there was a

[15] Fletcher (1914), Travis, Tuttle, and Cowan (1936), Moore (1959), and Brunner and Frank (1975). See Golub (1953), however, for contradictory evidence.

decrease in blood sugar and total protein. Edgren, Leanderson, and Levi (1970) found a greater increase in urinary excretion of adrenaline in stutterers than in nonstutterers after a period of public speaking. Following a speech situation, Chmelová, Kujalová, Sedláčková, and Zelený (1975) observed a rise in adrenaline, noradrenaline, dopamine, and 5-hydroxyindoleacetic acid.

Electrodermal Response Berlinsky (1955) failed to find a consistent relationship between stuttering symptoms and electrical conductance of the skin (Galvanic Skin Response: GSR). Kurshev (1969) studied GSR responses just prior to stutterers' attempts on words and found them to occur in advance of stuttering in many instances. Brutten (1963), using a photometric technique to measure palmar sweating, found that this reaction decreased concomitantly with decreases in the amount of stuttering, but contradictory results were obtained in subsequent research (Gray & Brutten, 1965; Adams & Moore, 1972).

Other Reflex Activity During the stuttering block there appears to be an inhibition of eyeblink (Amirov, 1962), an augmentation of the Achilles and patellar reflexes (Travis & Fagan, 1928), and a change in the impedance of the middle ear (Shearer, 1966). Gardner (1937) also reported a greater dilation of the pupils among stutterers than among normal speakers during speech and increases in dilated diameter during stuttering. On the other hand, pupillary contraction at the onset of speech was noted by Luchsinger (1943). Stuttering has been found to be accompanied by abnormal solar and oculocardiac reflexes (Sedláček, 1948) and by increased monosynaptic spinal cord reflex activity (Laštovka, 1970, 1979a, 1979b). Langová, Morávek, Široký, and Šváb (1975) reported an increase in the frequency and amplitude of the electronystagmographic response in stutterers during speech. In nystagmographic records of stutterers, Široký, Langová, Morávek, and Šváb (1978) observed many saddle-formed nystagmic jerks, which increased significantly during speech.

The Meaning of the Physiological Concomitants Although many of the changes just described were originally believed to be clues to an underlying physiological etiology of stuttering, they are now widely regarded simply as inward aspects of the symptomatology. In the first place, these manifestations are confined to the moment of stuttering and to a brief period just prior to it. Generally speaking, they are not present when the stutterer is silent or appears to be speaking normally. Furthermore, there is little evidence to suggest that any of these symptoms is a universal concomitant of all stuttered moments. Some systematic examination of this last point was done by Charles Strother as early as 1937.

Finally, many of these same physical changes have been observed to occur in normally fluent speakers under conditions of excitement or tension, while others may be produced in typically fluent speakers while responding in ways that simulate stuttering. For example, deep tendon reflexes increase with effort. Ainsworth (1939) found breathing abnormalities similar to those of stutterers in normally fluent speakers while they were listening to stuttering. Williams (1955) showed that the abnormal action potentials of the jaw muscles that occur during stuttering can be produced in nonstutterers by instructing them to imitate stuttering or merely to perform certain movements of the jaw.

In short, as a result of laboratory studies over many decades, the physiological symptoms of stuttering are now generally understood to be the visceral correlates of tension, exertion, or emotional arousal or to represent other indirect effects of stuttering or of some of its overt concomitants.[16] Some of these studies were focused in whole or in part on the period immediately preceding the stuttering block. We will therefore have occasion to refer to them again in somewhat more detail when we take up the question of fear and anticipation in relation to stuttering.

[16] Furthermore, the observations of Golub (1953) and McCroskey (1957) suggest that at least a few of these symptoms are to be found as accompaniments of speech in normal speakers and may therefore be "symptoms" of vocal expression rather than of stuttering.

Introspective Concomitants

The subjective evaluations that the stutterer makes while experiencing speech interruptions are, from our perspective, an exceedingly important part of the accompanying symptomatology of stuttering. These evaluations, as they are primarily conveyed through the introspections of older people who stutter, are chiefly of three types: (1) a sense of being frustrated in the attempt to speak, (2) feelings of muscular tension, and (3) emotional or affective reactions.

Feelings of Frustration in the Effort to Speak Stutterers in a block tend to experience the feeling of being physically halted in their attempt to speak. For a time, they are literally unable, by any ordinary definition of that word, to move or to control their speech mechanism for the purpose of articulating the intended word. Those having a more detailed awareness of the experience may report that their lips involuntarily "come together hard," that their tongue "sticks" to the roof of their mouth, that their "throat closes tightly," and the like. Even children may use the term "stuck" to convey their difficulty in speaking. It is noteworthy that stutterers generally appear to know precisely what word they want to say, but simply cannot say it.

This failure of the speech production system to do the speaker's bidding is often as baffling and disturbing to stutterers as an inexplicable spasm or paralysis might be. It is noteworthy that typically fluent speakers only experience anything similar to it in nightmares, when they attempt to call for help but find themselves unable to produce voice. They can, however, interrupt the stuttering reaction at short notice to perform some other activity, such as a protrusion of the abdomen, as Van Riper (1938) has shown. In fact, they often appear to be able to interrupt the "spasm" to produce a fluent utterance of an alternative word.

Feelings of Muscular Tension For most stutterers, the act of blocking is associated with some feeling of strain or tension. This is usually localized in the speech musculature (i.e., the muscles of articulation, phonation, or respiration), but in some cases may also be felt elsewhere in the body—for example, the arms, legs, or shoulders. In a group of adult stutterers, Snidecor (1955) found that tension was reported primarily in the jaws, the front of the mouth, the front of the throat, the chest, and the abdomen, with subsidiary foci often perceived in the inside or back of the throat and the front of the tongue.

Affective Reactions These vary widely in intensity and are of several types, depending upon whether they occur before, during, or after the stuttering block. The majority of stutterers do respond affectively to their disfluency.

Prior to the block, there is often an apprehension of impending difficulty, varying in severity from mild uneasiness to extreme panic, which is well known as anticipation or expectancy. It is typically one of the most unpleasant aspects of the disorder for stutterers and often the one that interferes most with communication. Anticipation may also occur independently of blocks, and it is not unusual for stutterers to experience the repeated threat of stuttering even in situations in which they have little or no overt speech difficulty. Conversely, some blocks seemingly occur with little or no overt speech difficulty. Further, some blocks seemingly occur with little if any prior awareness of their imminence on the speaker's part. By and large, however, older stutterers are able to predict the occurrence of their blocks with striking accuracy. An assumption long shared by a considerable number of speech pathologists is that the prediction itself frequently serves to precipitate the stuttering block. From this point of view anticipation is among the phenomena lying at the heart of the stuttering problem. We will discuss this question in some detail in Chapter 10.

During the stuttering block, the affective reactions, especially in severe stuttering, tend to be reported predominantly as confusion or mental "blankness." In extreme cases, stutterers may feel what they describe as a kind of momentary loss of "contact." Subjective reports such as these are illuminated by certain objective research findings. Herren (1931) found that voluntary movements of the hands (alternately flexing and extending the fingers about a rubber ball) tended to cease or become reduced in extent during stuttering blocks. Dewar, Dewar, and Anthony (1976) happened on the same phenomenon when they instructed stutterers to turn on a masking noise at the moment that they began to stutter; the stuttering caused delays in the operation of the hand-actuated device. Similarly, stutterers' finger-tapping rates appeared to be slowed down by stuttering in a study by Greiner, Fitzgerald, and Cooke (1986b). In a related observation, Ringel and Minifie (1966) demonstrated that stuttering tends to impair the ability to estimate the passage of time. Froeschels and Rieber (1963) reported that during the block stutterers gave evidence of a considerable inability to perceive auditory and visual stimuli—for example, the banging of a fist on a desk or the waving of a hand as signals to stop speaking. This was not confirmed in studies by Perkins (1969) or Hugo (1972), however; it may be that auditory and visual imperceptivity is one of the more extreme symptoms of stuttering. Kamhi and McOsker (1982) found evidence that stuttering during oral reading of a passage may interfere with stutterers' comprehension of the material read.

Following the block, affective reactions frequently verbalized by stutterers include frustration, exasperation, embarrassment, and feelings of anxiety about further stuttering. That there may also be some measure of relief or tension reduction immediately after a block was suggested by the results of a study by Wischner (1952a), in which stutterers used projective drawings to depict their behavior before, during, and after the moment of stuttering. Using a similar method, Sheehan, Cortese, and Hadley (1962) found evidence of shame and guilt following stuttering. Bar and Jakab (1969) found both types of reactions, with relief more characteristic of the drawings done by adults than of those done by children. Drawings of both adults and children who stutter thus show clear evidence of the affective and cognitive reactions to living with a stutter (Lev-Wiesel, Shabat, & Tsur, 2005; Stewart & Brosh, 1997) that are exemplified in Figure 1-3. For example, many such self-drawings are characterized by features that illustrate blocking of speech, such as tight collars, or other representations of impeded ability to act or speak.

"Real," Forced, and Faked Blocks Frankly, introspective studies of the stuttering block have rarely been done because of their obvious limitations, but a sidelight was thrown on this aspect of

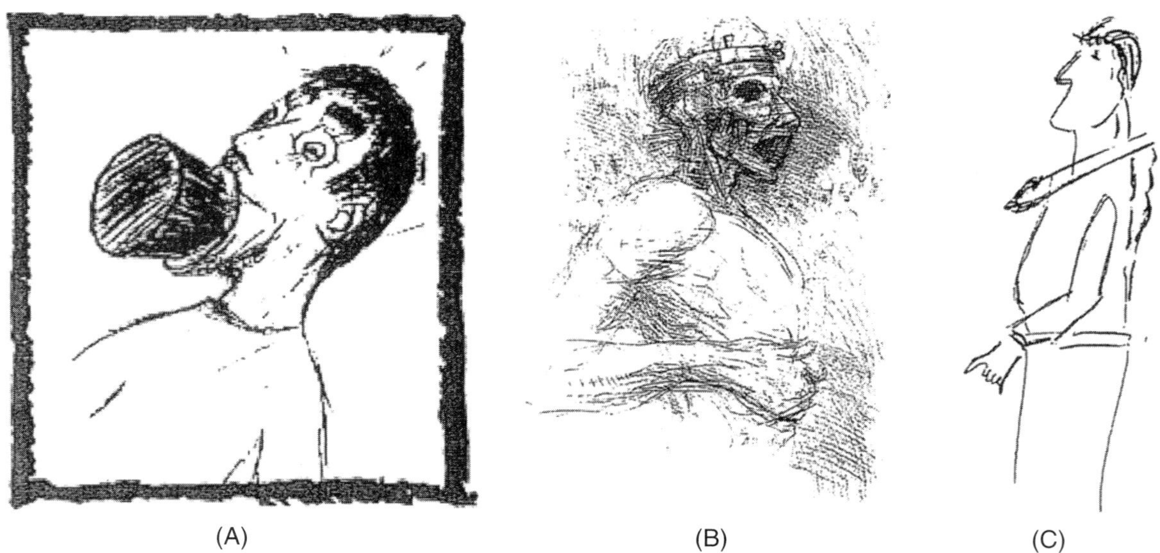

(A) (B) (C)

FIGURE 1-3 Self drawings of adults and children who stutter. From (A) Adrianna DiGrande (see Kuster, Lundberg, DiGrande & Andrews, 2000); (B) Stewart and Brosh (1997); and (C) Lev-Wiesel, Shabat, and Tsur (2005).

the problem in a study of stutterers' ability to throw themselves into blocks. Curious about Van Riper's observation that tense articulatory postures often seem to trigger involuntary tremors of the stutterer's jaw, tongue, or lips, Bloodstein and Shogan (1972) instructed adults who stutter to try to force themselves into blocks by exerting articulatory pressure on the initial sounds of isolated words. After each attempt, the speakers were asked whether the block they produced was real or fake and how they knew. Of twenty stutterers, all but three were able in at least a few instances to force themselves into what they regarded as real blocks. In general, however, articulatory pressure was not enough. In most cases, they were able to do this only on a word that began with a difficult or feared sound or by "thinking" of the word as difficult. None had notable difficulty distinguishing real stuttering from faked or imitated blocks. The two essential features of real stuttering referred to repeatedly were its tension and its involuntary quality. The following are a few of the comments that the participants offered to explain how they knew when blocks were real: "It's like a rock inside." "I could have stopped the others at any time, but not this one." "There's tension and heaviness." "When it's real it's like being drunk or like having your foot on the gas with no control—you can't control the speech. If I control the word it has weight. If not, it's like a balloon."

However, Kelly and Conture (1988) could find nothing in the spectrographic record to differentiate stutterers' imitated from their actual stuttering. In a study by Moore and Perkins (1990), listeners were also unable to distinguish a stutterer's real from her simulated stuttering with an accuracy much greater than chance. The stutterer herself was not much better at it when listening to the tape recording only an hour afterward. Such findings are particularly interesting when viewed in light of studies reported in Chapter 4 that show similar brain activation patterns for imagined and actual stuttered events (e.g., Ingham, Fox, Ingham, & Zamarripa, 2000).

ATTITUDES AND ADAPTATIONS

In addition to what is ordinarily considered stuttering behavior, there is a pattern of attitudes, assumptions, and habitual methods of attempting to cope with stuttering that tends to characterize the disorder in its fully developed forms. These aspects must be considered in connection with symptomatology, since they often constitute a major part of the problem of stuttering.

At the most basic level, we observe the attitudes that stuttering is shameful, that speech is unpleasant and threatening, and that people who stutter are for some unaccountable reason innately unable to speak in any other way. From these primary beliefs, there is likely to develop in time a systematic and detailed ideology or cognitive state regarding both speaking and stuttering. Specific words, sounds, and speaking situations may become "difficult" and eventually feared. Listeners may be perceived as critical, impatient, embarrassed, pitying, or amused to a degree that often seems to distort reality. The conviction of basic inability to speak normally may become elaborated in subtle ways until it amounts to what Williams (1957) referred to as stutterers' magical belief in a "something" inside that strives to prevent them from speaking. An increasingly rigid self-concept as a stutterer—first, last, and always—may be reinforced by an equally unrealistic concept of nonstutterers as people who are almost totally without speech hesitancy or anxiety.

Motivated by attitudes such as these, stutterers tend to acquire a variety of exaggerated and inefficient approaches to their problem. They are likely to form the habit of avoiding difficult words by using synonyms or circumlocutions, and some become extremely adept at this. They may anticipate difficult speech situations long in advance, may frequently avoid feared situations, and, in general, may severely restrict their verbal output and the range of their social relationships. Some stutterers attempt to avoid stuttering through behavior contrived to inhibit expectancy, as Van Riper (1963) pointed out—for example, by artificiality of manner, bravado, or clowning. Still other adaptations stem from a desire to alleviate what stutterers see as the social penalty for stuttering. For example, they may habitually avoid eye contact with the listener, avoid mentioning their stuttering or discussing it with others, or attempt to compensate for speech inadequacy by maladjustive efforts to gain approval in other ways.

Research on the Reactive Aspects of Stuttering

Although much of our knowledge of the reactive aspects of the problem is derived from clinical experience, an increasing amount of research has been devoted to the subject. In early studies, Johnson (1932, 1934a, 1934b) and Kimmell (1938) found evidence that college stutterers' attitudes toward stuttering tended to influence their personal, social, sexual, home, and school behavior and adjustment and even their choice of a vocation. Knott (1935) investigated stutterers' ratings of the unpleasantness of their stuttering experiences. A study by Frasier (1955) was concerned in part with some of the assumptions held by stutterers about the nature of their stuttering and the factors that cause their difficulty to come and go. Bloodstein and Bloodstein (1955) and Wingate and Hamre (1967) reported data on stutterers' conflicting interpretations of listeners' facial reactions. Nutall and Scheidel (1965) showed that stutterers frequently fail to appreciate the extent to which the nonstutterer, as well as the stutterer, may experience anxiety in speaking situations.

Over the years, investigators have continued to find evidence of stutterers' reactions to stuttering in unusual and varied ways. Yovetich, Booth, and Tyler (1977) gave stutterers the task of repeating speech heard in one ear while hearing a competing message in the other ear. When the competing message contained stuttering, the participants made more errors than nonstutterers, though they were more accurate than their typically fluent peers when the competing message was fluent. Brutten and Janssen (1979) studied the eye movements of stutterers during the silent reading of a passage they were about to read aloud. The stutterers exhibited more regressions and long forward jumps than nonstutterers, evidently related to the habit of looking ahead in search of danger.

Leith and Mims (1975) found that Caucasian stutterers generally tended to have overt speech repetitions and prolongations, while African American stutterers were more likely to have few of these features and more devices for avoiding, terminating, or concealing them. Leith and Mims related this finding to a difference between the groups in the social stigma they attached to stuttering. However, Olsen, Steelman, & Montague (1999) found no observable differences between racial groups when examining either behaviors or attitudes of school-aged African American and Caucasian children who stutter.

In a survey of the experiences of male and female stutterers by Silverman and Zimmer (1982), most participants reported that they took little part in classroom activities, tended to avoid speaking privately with instructors, took jobs for which they were overqualified, and expected limited vocational success. In a questionnaire study, Hohmeier (1987) gathered information about the vocational problems that stuttering created. Black (1937) was concerned with perceptions of the barriers that stuttering created to the enjoyment of leisure activities. In a more recent large survey of over 200 adults who stutter, it was found that 70 percent felt that stuttering limited career options, almost a third thought it impaired their actual job performance, and 20 percent reported turning down potential jobs or promotions because of their stuttering (Klein & Hood, 2004).

There is some evidence of a tendency for stuttering to be a more serious problem for males. Manning, Dailey, and Wallace (1984) investigated the attitudes of older stutterers, chiefly members of self-help groups, between 52 and 82 years of age. Most perceived their speech difficulty to be less severe and handicapping than it had been in early childhood, although their performance on attitude tests did not differ from that of younger participants. Leith and Timmons (1983) reported a study concerned specifically with stutterers' attitudes toward use of the telephone. The earliest age at which negative reactions to the telephone was recalled was approximately ten years. Craig (1990) also showed that stutterers' self-reported anxiety during a phone call to a stranger was greater than that of people who did not stutter.

Martens and Engel (1986) obtained objective evidence that many stutterers avoid words beginning with certain sounds. Resnick and Tureen (1990) found that stutterers rated their own stuttering as more severe than did a group of unsophisticated listeners. The degree to which children and adults who stutter (and their relatives) experience guilt and shame about their fluency has been explored by Bill Murphy, who draws on the scholarly literature that has investigated this problem in a number of other clinical populations (Murphy, 1999). Crichton-Smith (2002) used interviews from four adults who stutter to suggest that perception of others' negative reactions to their stuttering began in childhood, and resulted in significant feelings of isolation and limitation.

Nonverbal Behavior in Dyadic Communication Krause (1978, 1982) conducted a unique study of the nonverbal behavior of stutterers filmed in conversation with normally fluent partners, using a group of normally fluent dyads as a comparison condition. He reported several thought-provoking findings. Whereas the normally fluent dyads shared the floor equally, the stutterers used more floor time than their partners; this was also true of a subgroup of some ten stutterers who were judged by observers not to have stuttered on the film. The stutterers displayed relatively little of the "back-channel" behavior (smiling, nodding, and the like) so typically seen in nonstutterers while being spoken to. In general, the stutterers tended to keep their faces immobile. Compared with the nonstutterer dyads, the stutterers and their partners exhibited fewer of the simultaneous utterances ("simultalk") that frequently occur in ordinary conversation. There were also fewer of the turn-taking speaker switches that tend to accompany simultaneous interruptive speech. While these observations may be open to various interpretations, they clearly point to a disruption of the spontaneous interactive behavior that characterizes typical conversational relationships. Jensen, Markel, and Beverung (1986) also found some evidence of aberrant turn-taking behavior on the part of stutterers involving eye contact, body movement, and latency of response.

Reactions of Children Some special attention has been paid to the reactive aspects of stuttering in children, chiefly those of school age. In an early study of grade school stutterers' oral recitation problems, Knudsen (1939) found that about half of their group had attempted to avoid stuttering by giving the wrong answer or saying "I don't know" in response to questions in the classroom; some had even played truant in order to avoid recitation. Furthermore, large numbers believed they had concealed their stuttering from some of their teachers by remaining in the background. Pukacová (1974) found similar evidence of social speech fears in children. Silverman (1976a) found that by the time stutterers reached fourth to sixth grade, they tended to speak fewer words than nonstutterers when asked to tell a story. Silverman and Williams (1973) observed that stuttering children stopped to correct only half the number of oral reading errors that normally fluent children did, although the number of errors was about the same for the two groups. Similar findings were reported by Janssen, Kraaimaat, and van der Meulen (1983). Although unclear, the reason may reflect anxiety about stuttering or the diffident behavior of a reader who has no pretensions about doing well and is bent on completing the task as inconspicuously as possible. In a study of the eye movements of schoolchildren during silent reading, Brutten, Bakker, Janssen, and van der Meulen (1984) noted that stutterers exhibited more fixations and regressions. They related the observation to "searching and sorting" arising from concern about words and sounds. In a comparison of stutterers and nonstutterers aged 7 to 14 years, De Nil and Brutten (1991a) found more negative attitudes toward speech among the stutterers at all ages. The difference in attitudes appears to grow larger over the school years (Vanryckeghem & Brutten, 1997). In follow-up work that adapted their assessment device (*The Communicative Attitude Test [CAT]*) (Vanryckeghem, 1995; Vanryckeghem & Brutten, 1996; Vanryckeghem, Hylebos, Brutten, & Peleman, 2001) to use with preschool aged children (the *KiddyCAT*), Martine Vanryckeghem and colleagues (Vanryckeghem, Brutten, & Hernandez, 2005) found evidence of negative attitudes much earlier, in children as young as 3 years of age. Moreover, there is some evidence that negative communication attitude is correlated with severity of fluency breakdown, although the directionality of this relationship is unclear (Vanryckeghem & Brutten, 1996, 2007).

However, some children, and some adults as well, do not seem to be highly concerned about their stuttering. Silverman (1972a) asked a group of stuttering children to make three wishes. Of 62 children in second to fifth grade, only 4 made wishes that had anything to do with speech, and of these, 1 wished that he could go on with speech class as long as he lived. These observations were corroborated by Culatta, Bader, McCaslin, and Thomason (1985). Woods (1974) discovered that, while grade school stutterers tended to rate themselves as relatively poor speakers, this had little effect on their own estimation of their social position among their classmates. Bloodstein (1960a) and McLelland and Cooper (1978) found that, as might be expected, there appears to be an increase with age in reactive features of stuttering such as word substitutions, avoidance of speaking, self-perception as a stutterer, and communication fear. However, a Japanese study of school-aged children who stutter (Ota & Nagasawa, 2004a) found no differences between stuttering and nonstuttering children on measures of self-esteem, and noted that both fluent and stuttering children showed decreases in self-esteem over the period between third and sixth grade. The same team found that positive self-image in adulthood was related to perceptions of self-esteem in adolescence for those who stutter (Ota & Nagasawa, 2004b). Similarly, some school-aged children who stutter are less likely to withdraw from potential social interaction because of their stuttering than are adults (Green, 1998).

Reactions of Listeners Since the attitudes and adaptations of stutterers must be due in large measure to the reactions that they receive from others, it is relevant that a large amount of research over the years has been done on the behavior of people listening to stuttered speech, on prevalent attitudes toward stutterers, and on the effect of stuttering on listeners' perception of a message.[17] Despite a large amount of work that has suggested a physical underpinning for the disorder (see Chapters 4, 5, and 6), many adults unfamiliar with stuttering view people who stutter as inherently and excessively anxious and shy (Craig, Tran, & Craig, 2003). Recent work suggests that these listener attitudes are evident even when considering the communicative environment of young children who stutter. Children apparently begin to notice stuttered speech and evaluate it negatively between the ages of 3 and 5, as shown in a study that asked them to evaluate speech samples produced by puppets (Ezrati-Vinacour, Platzky, & Yairi, 2001), and this awareness begins to negatively affect preschoolers' attitudes toward children who stutter. For example, young stutterers are more likely than nonstutterers to be rejected or bullied by their peers (Hugh-Jones & Smith, 1999; Davis, Howell, & Cooke, 2002). By fourth and fifth grade, there are significant measurable negative reactions by children to stuttering speakers (Franck, Jackson, Pimentel, & Greenwood, 2003).

Among adults, for the most part, negative stereotypes of stutterers as nervous, fearful, and insecure have been found to be common. Krause (1978, 1982) noted that listeners tend to increase their head-nodding behavior in conversation with stutterers, engage in more "compulsive" smiling, and as a correlate of this behavior use fewer words expressing anger than when speaking with nonstutterers. In a study that examined the effects of personal experience on perceptions of stuttering, it was found that more positive perceptions were found in those who actually knew someone who stuttered (Klassen, 2002), implying that public education might reduce negative and inappropriate

[17] Rosenberg and Curtiss (1944), McDonald and Frick (1954), Yairi and Williams (1970), Woods and Williams (1971, 1976), Woods (1974), Duffy, Hunt, and Giolas (1975), Andrews and Smith (1976), Hulit (1976), Krause (1978), Phillips and Myers (1978), Turnbaugh, Guitar, and Hoffman (1979), Crowe and Walton (1981), Maxwell (1981), Turnbaugh, Guitar, and Hoffman (1981), Ragsdale and Ashby (1982), Silverman (1982), Hurst and Cooper (1983a) , Hurst and Cooper (1983b), Tatchell, van den Berg, and Lerman (1983), Cyprus, Hezel, Rossi, and Adams (1984), White and Collins (1984), McKinnon, Hess, and Landry (1986), Burley and Rinaldi (1986), Well and Terrell (1986), Yeakle and Cooper (1986), Horsely and Fitzgibbon (1987), Kalinowski, Lerman, and Watt (1987), Atkins (1988), Lass, Ruscello, Pannbacker, Schmitt, and Everly-Myers (1989), Collins and Blood (1990), Ham (1990a, c), Silverman (1990), Silverman and Paynter (1990), Patterson and Pring (1991), Bebout and Bradford (1992), Doody, Kalinowski, Armson, and Stuart (1993).

responses to stuttering. Despite this, it has also been found that even those who stutter view others who stutter less positively than they view fluent speakers (Lass, Ruscello, Pannbacker, & Schmitt, 1995).

Measuring the Reactive Aspects

Inasmuch as speech therapy for the stutterer has often been concerned in part with the removal of unfavorable attitudes and reactions, there has been some interest in the development of devices for their identification and measurement. We provide an overview of some of these instruments here.

Attitude Scales and Rating Sheets These measuring devices have consisted chiefly of self-administered scales for the rating of attitudes or reactions to stuttering and speaking situations. Initially, some use was made of the *Knower Speech Attitude Scale* and the *Knower Speech Experience Inventory*,[18] neither of which was designed specifically for administration to people with speech impairments. These tests were employed in research on stutterers by Brown and Hull (1942), who found them to be less "confident and enthusiastic in their use of speech" than nonstutterers and had made less use of speech in social situations. Naylor (1953) used the Knower tests for studying the relationship between stutterers' attitudes toward speech and various measures of severity of stuttering.

Of several early attempts to devise a specific measure of attitudes concerning stuttering the only one to come into significant use was the *Iowa Scale of Attitude toward Stuttering* devised by Ammons and Johnson (1944). This Likert-type scale consists of a series of statements (e.g., "A stutterer should not plan to be a lawyer") with which the respondent may indicate "moderate" or "strong" agreement or disagreement. A defect of many attitude inventories is that the approved or desirable choices are so obvious, but Robey (1976) found that scores on the *Iowa Scale of Attitude* were not correlated with measures of a response set toward acquiescent or socially desirable behavior.

[18]See Knower (1938).

Shumak (1955) reported normative data on a scale for measuring stutterers' reactions to speech situations, originally prepared for clinical use by Johnson in 1943.[19] The test consists of a list of 40 common speech situations, each of which the stutterer rates on a five-point scale with respect to (1) tendency to avoid the situation, (2) enjoyment or dislike of the situation, (3) the severity of stuttering in the situation, and (4) the frequency with which the situation is encountered. Further data for both stutterers and nonstutterers were obtained with this scale by Trotter and Bergmann (1957).

Lanyon (1967) described the construction of the *Stuttering Severity Scale*, a self-report inventory consisting of 64 true-false items for measuring the severity of stuttering, including behaviors such as avoidance, effort, and breathing difficulty as well as attitudes of worry, dissatisfaction, sensitivity, and the like. A factor analysis of stutterers' responses to the scale by Lanyon, Goldsworthy, and Lanyon (1978) showed that the behavioral and attitudinal items represented two distinct dimensions.

Woolf (1967) devised the *Perceptions of Stuttering Inventory*, consisting of 60 items representing struggle, avoidance, or expectancy. Stutterers judge whether the item is characteristic of their stuttering. Examples include: "Running out of breath while speaking," "Making your voice louder or softer when stuttering is expected," and "Avoiding asking for information." St. Louis and Atkins (1988) administered the inventory to normally fluent college students in order to gather comparison data for use with stutterers. This inventory has been used to assess treatment outcomes, as discussed in Chapter 14.

Erickson (1969) contributed an empirically derived *S-scale* for assessing the attitudes of stutterers toward verbal communication. Constructed with attention to factors of reliability and validity, the scale consists of 39 true-false items that were found to differentiate stutterers from nonstutterers—for example, "I usually feel that I am making a favorable impression when I talk," and "I dislike

[19]Shumak's speech situation rating sheet for stutterers is reproduced, with instructions for its use and interpretation, in Darley and Spreistersbach (1978, Chapter 10).

introducing one person to another." To facilitate comparison with nonstutterers' attitudes, the items make no mention of stuttering. Andrews and Cutler (1974) suggested a revision of the scale (the *S-24*) that they found to be more valid and reliable in repeated administrations to stutterers undergoing speech therapy. Quesal and Shank (1978) found that while persons with voice or articulation difficulties tended to have poorer communication attitudes as measured by the Erickson scale, stutterers' attitudes were poorer still. In a study by Cox, Seider, and Kidd (1984), stutterers scored lower than recovered stutterers, nonstuttering relatives, and typically fluent comparison speakers. E.-M. Silverman (1980) reported that a group of women who stuttered exhibited poorer attitudes on the Erickson scale than women who did not, but that they showed significantly more favorable attitudes than a group of male stutterers. An item analysis of the scale was reported by Jehle, Kühn, and Renner (1989), who administered it to a group of German stutterers and nonstutterers. Members of a national stutterers' self-help organization (the National Stuttering Project[20]) showed poorer speech attitudes than nonstutterers on the Erickson scale, but active members had more favorable scores than inactive ones (Miller & Watson, 1992). The scale was used more recently to investigate fluent high schoolers' attitudes toward their own speech and toward stuttering (Weisel & Spektor, 1998).

The *Stuttering Problem Profile* of Silverman (1980b) aims to identify behaviors to be modified and is based on the statements of 108 stutterers who were asked to tell how their problem had improved in therapy. The instructions ask stutterers to identify those statements that they would like to be able to make at the end of treatment. Sample items are: "I no longer have a great deal of difficulty speaking in school," "I am usually willing to use the phone," "I don't usually feel a great deal of tension and panic before speaking." Other items on the scale are deliberately designed not to reflect reasonably expected outcomes of speech therapy, such as "I am as cheerful as most people."

[20] Now the National Stuttering Association (NSA).

Brutten (1975) and Brutten and Janssen (1981) reported on the use of a *Speech Situation Checklist (SSC)* consisting of 51 situations that speakers rate on a five-point scale for the amount of anxiety experienced in them. A shortened version was developed by Hanson, Gronhovd, and Rice (1981). Brutten and colleagues have also utilized the *Behavior Checklist (BCL)* (Vanryckeghem, Brutten, Uddin, & Van Borsel, 2004) to examine ways in which adult stutterers deal with actual or anticipated moments of fluency disruption. In 2007, the SSC was combined with the *Communication Attitude Test* and the *BCL* to create the more inclusive *Behavior Assessment Battery* (Brutten & Vanryckeghem, 2007), which offers both adult and child versions of each section, with normative data for each component.

On a *Self-Efficacy Scale for Adult Stutterers (SESAS)*, devised by Ornstein and Manning (1985), stutterers rate each of 50 situations both for the confidence that they would enter the situation with a level of fluency and the confidence that they would maintain fluency in the situation. An adapted version of the *Scale* was used in a study that confirmed lower self-efficacy for speech in adolescents who stutter than in fluent teens (Bray, Lawless, & Theodore, 2003).

An *Inventory of Communications Attitudes* for adult stutterers was developed by Watson (1987, 1988) and Watson, Gregory, and Kistler (1987). Speakers rate 39 situations with respect to their enjoyment of the situation, their speech skills in the situation, how they believe others feel in the situation, their perception of other people's speech skills in the situation, and how frequently they meet the situation.

More recently, Yaruss and Quesal have developed a scale that combines many of the features of earlier scales. The new instrument, called the *Overall Assessment of the Speaker's Experience of Stuttering (OASES)* (Yaruss & Quesal, 2006) has published validity and reliability data, along with reference scores suggestive of severity levels for affective and cognitive components of stuttering in adults. An adaptation of the scale for child populations is in progress as of press time of this edition.

The *Wright-Ayre Stuttering Self-Rating Profile (WASSP)* (Wright, Ayre, & Grogan, 1998) is a hybrid rating scale that marks both frequency of stuttering behaviors as well as affective responses; it was originally developed as a baseline measure against which to measure therapy outcomes, as discussed further in Chapter 14.

Riley, Riley, and Maguire (2004) published a *Subjective Screening of Stuttering (SSS)*, disseminated currently in a research edition. The three areas screened by the *SSS* are perceived stuttering severity, the level of internal or external locus of control, and reported word or situation avoidance, each with a small number of items to be rated on a scale from one to nine. Pilot work with 16 adult stutterers revealed that for the sample, percent stuttered syllables correlated well with stuttering severity ($r = 0.75$) and less, but still significantly, with locus of control ($r = 0.43$) but did not correlate with avoidance. The *SSS* appears to be well correlated with older measures such as the *Perceptions of Stuttering Inventory (PSI)*.

Relatively less work has been done to explore attitudes in stuttering children, although this age group has attracted recent attention. Guitar and Grims (1979) reported preliminary work on a questionnaire on communication attitudes for children. Five stutterers, aged 5 to 10 years, did not differ from their normally fluent peers on this scale in a study by Devore, Nandur, and Manning (1984). Green (1999) found that, while adults' self-perceptions of stuttering severity predicted a lower level of social interaction in various situations, there was actually a positive association between perceived severity and participation in social interaction for children. Brutten's *Communication Attitude Test* for children did elicit unfavorable attitudes when administered to 6- to 14-year-old stutterers in both English and Dutch versions (De Nil & Brutten, 1986; Brutten & Dunham, 1989; Vanryckeghem & Brutten, 1992). This measure has been adapted for work with younger children between 3 and 6 years of age (the *KiddyCAT*; Vanryckeghem, Brutten, & Hernandez, 2005). Even at this young age range, scores for 45 children who stutter revealed significantly poorer speech-associated attitude than those of 63 comparison fluent peers. A finding from these studies relevant to assessment concerns addressed in Chapter 14 is that children's responses to these measures do not correlate well with parental report on the same attitudinal scale (Vanryckeghem, 1995); in general, parents often believe their stuttering children's communication-related attitudes to be poorer than they actually are, while parents of fluent children tend to believe their children's attitude to be more positive than they are by child report. As noted, this program of research on children's speech-related attitudes has resulted in an amalgamated assessment tool, the *Behavior Assessment Battery for Children Who Stutter* (Brutten & Vanryckeghem, 2006).

Speaking-Time Log The amount of time stutterers spend in speaking may frequently be taken as a basic measure of the extent to which the speech difficulty is handicapping. For clinical purposes, therefore, Johnson suggested the use of a personal log, kept by stutterers for varying periods of time to record each situation in which they spoke, together with an estimate of the time in which they spoke. Detailed suggestions for the use of such a log were given by Darley and Spriestersbach (1978, chap. 9). Trotter and Brown (1958) made use of this technique to demonstrate that there were often considerable increases in stutterers' verbal output after a period of therapy.

Measures of Anxiety There has been some interest in the objective measurement of speech-related anxiety under varying conditions. Brutten (1959) developed a photometric technique for measuring the palmar sweat response for this purpose and applied it in a number of research investigations on stuttering (Brutten, 1963; Gray & Brutten, 1965). Haywood (1963) showed that this method is apparently more sensitive to speech-related anxiety than are measures of heart rate or pulse pressure. However, physiological measures do not appear to correlate well with self-reported situational anxiety. Susan Dietrich (Dietrich & Roaman, 2001) asked adult stutterers to construct hierarchies reflecting their speaking-related anxiety. During reenactment of selected situations, skin conduction responses did not correlate well with their rankings. Using a very different kind of approach, Lerman and Shames

(1965) attempted to measure stutterers' level of anxiety in relation to a given speech situation by analyzing certain aspects of their language content as they talked about the situation.

A number of recent investigations have attempted to distinguish between state anxiety, which might logically be higher in speaking situations for those who stutter, and trait anxiety, a more stabile personality characteristic we will discuss further in Chapter 7. Most find evidence of elevated state anxiety in stutterers. In a study by Gabel and his colleagues (Gabel, Colcord, & Petrosino, 2002), stutterers self-reported speech-related anxiety during a series of speaking tasks that was higher than that reported by fluent comparison speakers, although no one speech condition differentiated the groups. Significant evidence of speech-related anxiety was obtained in a study that used the *Inventory of Interpersonal Situations (IIS)*, a social anxiety inventory (Kraaimaat, Vanryckeghem, & Van Dam-Baggen, 2002); in this study, half of the stutterers achieved scores that were well within the range of clinically socially anxious psychiatric patients. Ezrati-Vinacour and Levin (2004) used the *Trait Anxiety Inventory* and the *Speech Situation Checklist* with 94 adult male stutterers and found both state and trait anxiety to be elevated. Using the *Fear of Negative Evaluation (FNE) Scale* and the *Endler Multidimensional Anxiety Scales-Trait (EMAS-T)*, Messenger and colleagues (Messenger, Onslow, Packman, & Menzies, 2004) found adults who stutter to have substantially greater anxiety that was restricted to social situations. These results were consistent with those in an earlier study (Mahr & Torosian, 1999) that compared social phobics to stutterers; the primary differences between the groups were found only for speech-related social situations.

Measures of Depression Relatively little work has explored whether stuttering can lead to clinical depression. In a Chinese adult sample, a number of stutterers demonstrated signs of depression (Liu et al., 2001). However, in an adolescent American sample, self-efficacy, but not depression, differentiated between groups of stuttering and fluent teens (Bray, Lawless, & Theodore, 2003).

DEVELOPMENTAL CHANGES IN STUTTERING

In our discussion so far, we have been concerned chiefly with the features of stuttering as a fully developed disorder. Many of these features, however, appear to be acquired through a process of development that typically begins in early childhood, and stuttering in its earliest forms therefore tends to differ in certain respects from stuttering in older children and adults. Comprehensive studies of the development of all of the various features of stuttering are almost nonexistent. The information presented here is taken mainly from a report by Bloodstein (1960a) based on the first author's clinical examination of 418 stutterers aged 2 to 16 years, at the Brooklyn College Speech and Hearing Center from 1950 to 1956 (see Table 1-2).

Repetitions and Prolongations

As might be expected, repetitions and prolongations were observed at every age level. Before the age of 6 or 7 years, repetitions were a conspicuous feature of the child's stuttering and often involved whole words such as *he, I, but, and, in*, or *so*. Table 1-2 shows a steady decline in easy repetitions and prolongations as the sole symptoms of stuttering, but even at ages 2 and 3 years, they were the sole symptom in only 43 percent of the cases. Even at that early age, repetitions of words or sounds were by no means always slow and easy, and were often accompanied by additional features.

Hard Contacts

Tense and forceful attacks on words or syllables were very commonly observed during the interview at every age level. Table 1-2 shows only a slight tendency for these struggle reactions to increase with age. A striking fact was that they appeared in the Brooklyn group at the earliest ages. Of the nine

TABLE 1-2 Percentage of Subjects Exhibiting Each of Various Features of Stuttering Behavior at Age Levels from 2 to 16*

	Age Level						
	2–3 $N = 30$ %	4–5 $N = 74$ %	6–7 $N = 79$ %	8–9 $N = 60$ %	10–11 $N = 79$ %	12–13 $N = 47$ %	14–15–16 $N = 49$ %
Slow, easy repetitions	30	34	28	37	30	9	8
Easy repetition or prolongation as sole symptoms of stuttering	43	32	18	18	11	4	4
Hard contacts	40	32	44	45	53	51	53
Associated symptoms	33	39	57	58	57	64	65
Fluent periods	47	45	27	10	10	9	00
Difficult situations			27 (15)	67 (27)	71 (56)	75 (40)	72 (39)
Difficult words or sounds				82 (17)	62 (45)	72 (32)	73 (33)
Anticipation				38 (28)	45 (51)	62 (37)	71 (41)
Word substitution				48 (23)	65 (48)	66 (32)	83 (36)
Avoidance of speach	0	5	11	17	28	40	45

*Numbers in parentheses indicate the number of subjects on which the percentage was based where this differs from the total number (*N*) in the age group. From Bloodstein (1960a). Copyright 1960 by the American Speech-Language-Hearing Association. Reprinted by permission.

2-year-olds in the group, five exhibited signs of effort and strain and one had been observed to do so by the mother. To be sure, these may not have been typical cases; 2-year-olds are perhaps not likely to be taken to a speech clinic unless their stuttering is severe. They are, however, representative of what may be found in a clinical setting.

Although the child's stuttering was most often said to have begun with repetitions, in some instances the earliest symptoms were described as strenuous forcings. This was true in eight instances among 34 cases of children aged 2, 3, and 4 years in which parents gave "seemingly unequivocal descriptions . . . of the symptoms at onset." The records contained such reports as "Onset a few weeks ago. Forcing from the start. Mother is certain of that," or "Child taken for injection a month ago. Was very frightened. The next day he began to stutter with forcing, eyeblink, fist-clenching." Similar reports of severe stuttering at "onset" have been cited by Yairi and Ambrose (1992b).

Associated Symptoms

As shown in Table 1-2, the Brooklyn children who were observed to show the concomitant features of stuttering during the clinical interview rose steadily from 33 percent at ages 2 and 3 years to 65 percent at ages 14 to 16 years. The large percentage at the earliest age level is notable, even more so when we consider that stutterers may not exhibit secondary symptoms on all occasions. Among the symptoms noted in some cases at age 2 and 3 were eyeblinking, head jerking, violent gasping, clenching of the fists, exaggerated pausing, and "doubling up" of the body. The great majority of the secondary symptoms commonly seen in adults were to be observed in these children by age 5 (Bloodstein, 1960a). Tension in the respiratory muscles (gasping or rapid expulsions of breath) was observed in 13 percent of the 2- and 3-year-olds. Yairi, Ambrose, and Niermann (1993) noted frequent facial and head movements in the same age range. Schwartz, Zebrowski, and Conture (1990) observed associated symptoms (especially opening, closing, and movements of the eyes) in each of 10 children within 12 months of reported onset of stuttering. Conture and Kelly (1991) recorded facial, hand, arm, and head movements during the stuttering of thirty 3- to 7-year-olds.

Occurring as they do at all stages in the development of stuttering, associated symptoms may appear in conjunction with virtually any other feature of the problem. In the Brooklyn group, they sometimes accompanied the relatively simple repetitions of syllables or whole words of the youngest children. In many cases conspicuous secondary mannerisms were observed in the speech of children who were highly communicative and showed no outward sign of fear or shame because of their stuttering. A typical example was a boy of 11 whose symptoms included dilation of the eyes, frowning, repetition of "oh" before certain words, and speaking on residual air. In spite of his fairly severe stuttering, he spoke freely in all situations and resented the fact that his teacher did not call on him to recite in class (Bloodstein, 1960a). Another boy, aged 6 years, exhibited pausing, gasping, or rapid expulsions of breath before speech attempts, but evinced so little emotional reaction that both his mother and a speech clinician who had worked with the child thought that he was not aware of his speech difficulty.

Thus, secondary symptoms do not necessarily mean anxiety or embarrassment, or even a self-concept as a defective speaker. It is no doubt frustrating to children to be interrupted in their speech attempts, and so they can easily become conditioned to employ devices that temporarily help them to avoid or terminate blocks. We cannot know how much "awareness" this process requires; awareness has so many levels, and the word has so many meanings, that the question can have no simple answer.

Fluent Periods

As can be seen in Table 1-2, reports of intervals of normal speech decreased markedly past age 7 years and were nonexistent in the 14 to 16 age range. This emphasizes newer findings that suggest that permanent spontaneous recovery from stuttering is most likely to occur within a few years of its onset, rather than unpredictably through the individual's lifetime (Ramig, 1993; Yairi & Ambrose, 2005). However, "waves" of fluency can be seen in adults and children, often frustrating parents and the stutterer himself—why is it that sometimes speech is easy and other times it is so difficult for people who stutter? In preschool children, such temporary remissions can be very common and last for days, weeks, months, or even years. Following are two typical examples seen by the first author.

L. A. exhibited only phrase repetitions when he was interviewed at age 5–7. His first stuttering symptoms, consisting of rapid sound repetitions, were said to have appeared at age 3 for only about a week or two. At age 5 stuttering recurred in the form of sound repetition accompanied by severe eyeblinking. It became progressively more severe for several months but had become much milder again by the time the child was examined.

A. F. stuttered, blocking and repeating, at age 3 for two or three months, and then again at age 4.5 for a week. When seen again at age 6 he had been stuttering again, so badly that his teacher at school found it difficult to understand him, but there was no stuttering when he came for the interview.

In follow-up studies of preschool stutterers, Yairi and Ambrose (1992a) and Yairi, Ambrose, and Niermann (1993) found a distinct tendency for stuttering to disappear or decline markedly in severity several months after the initial diagnostic contact. Even children with severe stuttering accompanied by facial and head movements seemed to have recovered after six months. Thus, as we will explore further in Chapter 12, fluent periods mark much early stuttering as an ephemeral phenomenon, with a marked tendency toward spontaneous recovery as episodes come and go and often fail to develop into persistent cases. Risk factors for chronicity will be discussed in Chapter 12.

Difficult Situations

The data in Table 1-2 relating to difficult speaking situations are based upon the children's own reports. At age 7 years, the earliest age at which any children were questioned about this, about one-fourth spoke about specific situations, and the proportion remains at over two-thirds at all later ages. The outstanding situations are much the same at all age levels: recitation in the classroom, especially oral reading; going to the store; talking at home in the presence of company; and asking directions of strangers.

The remaining one-third of the group had nothing to say about specific occasions when they stuttered. At younger age levels, many of these children said that they stuttered whenever they "talked fast." Older children or teenagers in this category often spoke of stuttering when they were "nervous," "excited," or "talking fast."

Parents of children younger than 7 years were regularly asked about the conditions under which the children stuttered. They most often reported difficulty when the child was excited, enthusiastic, tense, upset, or "nervous," as when wanting something badly, being scolded, arguing with a sibling, or being "bothered" by other children. Another frequent report was about communicative urgency, as when the child had a lot to say, seemed to be trying to talk too fast, was telling a long story, or was fearful of being interrupted. Fatigue was also mentioned quite often.

Difficult Words or Sounds

As many as 82 percent of these children already regarded certain sounds or words as difficult to say by the earliest age at which they were questioned about this aspect (by 8 years of age), suggesting that it often develops earlier. In preschool children, parents sometimes reported noticing difficulty with particular words, in a few cases in children as young as 2.5 years. From age 8 years on, children commented that long words, words difficult to pronounce, their first or last names, or words with certain initial sounds or letters gave them particular trouble. However, at every age level at which the children were questioned, there were many who seemed to have no awareness of any words or sounds as especially difficult.

Anticipation

In response to the question, "Can you sometimes tell even before you say a word that you're going to stutter on it?" the answer "yes" rose steadily from 38 percent at ages 8 and 9 years to 71 percent in the 14 to 16 age group. One 13-year-old boy said, "I know when I'm going to stutter by my mouth becoming tense just before the word I'm going to block on."

A notable implication of the numbers in Table 1-2 is that at every age level there were numerous individuals who said they did not anticipate any of their stuttering moments, and this is in accord with a report of Silverman and Williams (1972b), who found that about one-fourth of school-age children were unable to predict the occurrence of any of their blocks by saying "yes" or "no" before their attempt on each word of a list. Because the relationship between the anticipation and occurrence of stuttering has certain theoretical implications (see Chapter 10), some clinicians have argued that children may in some sense anticipate their stuttering even when they are unable to signal their occurrence in advance. Bloodstein (1960a) found that each of 14 preschool children in the Brooklyn group exhibited the so-called consistency effect, blocking on the same words in repeated utterances of the same sentence, and thus inferred that even young children may anticipate their stutterings on a low level of awareness.

Word Substitution

The children who used synonyms to avoid difficult words increased from 48 percent to 83 percent between 8 and 16 years of age. It can be presumed that many children substitute words before the age of 8 years. One mother noticed her 6-year-old doing this, and two parents reported the use of circumlocutions by a 4-year-old and a 3-year-old. Even children as young as 2.5 years may appear to demonstrate word avoidances. The second author observed a case where within weeks of the emergence of stuttering, the toddler boy began to associate struggle with attempts to talk about his "blankie" and started to refer to it by its color ("green") instead. His mother astutely concluded that he had developed responses to his stuttering and sought clinical advice.

A distinction must be made between many of the substitutions of children and those of older stutterers. The majority of the school-aged children who were questioned said that they used substitutions only occasionally after the attempt on a word failed. For the most part, this was not the continual search for synonyms in response to anticipation of stuttering that characterizes so many fully developed cases. That development was not evident in the Brooklyn group before the age of 15 years. For most of the children, word substitution did not seem to be a reliable indicator of fear or shame; it appeared to be merely a reaction to speech frustration.

Avoidance of Speech and Other Signs of Emotional Reaction to Stuttering

Of all the items in Table 1-2, perhaps the only one that can be taken at face value as an indication of strong emotional reaction to stuttering is habitual avoidance of speaking. This was already manifest in a few children by age 5 years and increased steadily to 45 percent in the oldest age group. Occasional avoidance of speech occurred in a few children even younger than 5 years. Two 2-year-olds were said to have stopped talking for a few days after their first experience of stuttering. One child of 3 years sometimes gave up speech attempts, another sometimes asked his mother to speak for him, and a third at times refused to speak to adults when his stuttering was severe. But fairly consistent avoidance of speech was first reported at age 5 years, in most cases at school. At every age level, children avoided classroom recitation more often than any other situation, usually by not volunteering to speak, saying that they didn't know the answer or pretending to be unprepared. Other situations that were avoided increasingly with age were errands requiring speech, talking to adult strangers, and using the telephone. Only a few children showed any tendency to withdraw from social contacts with others of their own age, but many said that at times they let their friends do the talking.

As is evident from Table 1-2, large numbers of the children did not systematically avoid any speech situations. The assertion that this was so came from both the children themselves and their parents. An 8-year-old girl who stuttered severely was said to talk "constantly," to be "popular," and to have been elected president of her class. A 10-year-old boy with severe stuttering had a reputation as a "talker" and frequently volunteered to speak in class, as did a 15-year-old with conspicuous secondary symptoms. It was not that these children were content with the way they spoke. Given a choice, they would rather not have stuttered. But they stood in sharp contrast to those of their age mates who were panicked and tormented by their stuttering and sought every avenue of escape from speaking in class.

The emotional reaction to stuttering that avoidance of speaking expresses was often confirmed by vivid indications of other kinds. Many of the preschool children were said to have reacted to some of their severe stuttering blocks by hitting themselves on the mouth, crying, laughing, looking down and blushing, placing their hands in front of their face, hitting the wall with their hands, or saying "I can't talk," "Why can't I talk?" "Help me talk," "My goodness," "I'm doing it again," or "I'll tell you later." By about 3 years of age, about half the children had exhibited some such behavior.

These early reactions of very young children had two distinctive characteristics. First, they usually occurred sporadically; for the most part, the child talked freely and happily even while stuttering. And second, the behavior occurred in response to a specific stuttering event, usually of some severity. The children were not complaining about being afflicted with defective speech. Rather, they were simply upset by the frustration of being blocked in their efforts to communicate. In other words, there was as yet no evidence of a clear self-concept as a stutterer. Expressions of such a self-concept first began to appear in a few of these children at 4 years of age, when one child said, "Mommy, why can't I talk like other children?"; another asserted that he "talked funny"; and a third on leaving the speech clinic was heard to say, "Is my talking fixed now?" From 4 years of age on, increasing numbers of children asked "Why do I talk this way?" "When am I going to stop doing this?" and "Why was I born this way?" By the age of 7, a few children were beginning to ask to be taken to a doctor and one 7-year-old girl asked, "Will I stutter after I get married too?"

From 9 to 16 years of age, the verbal reactions were essentially similar to those that accompany fully developed stuttering. Children and teenagers more and more frequently admitted that they were frustrated, concerned, or embarrassed by their stuttering, that they mentally rehearsed speaking situations, that they were resentful of the unfavorable reactions of some of their listeners, and that they found it difficult to discuss their stuttering with others.

THE QUESTION OF DEVELOPMENTAL PHASES

In view of the observable changes that appear in so many aspects of stuttering over time, a question that naturally arises is whether it is possible to demonstrate that the problem, when persistent, follows a predictable course from its inception in childhood to its full-blown development in adolescents and adults. Are there identifiable stages of stuttering? No conceptual scheme of this sort has yet been generally accepted, and in fact only a few have been proposed. We review these here.

"Primary" and "Secondary" Stages

An early view that was given wide currency by Froeschels, Bluemel, and others and which undoubtedly reflects an important core of accurate observation is that much of the stuttering of young children consists of simple repetitions of sounds, syllables, or words unaccompanied by signs of effort or emotion. Froeschels (1921) depicted the development of stuttering as a process in which simple repetitions became more rapid, irregular, forced, and finally "inhibited" by progressive stages under the pressure of social penalty. Bluemel (1932) termed the incipient stage of the disorder "primary" stuttering. He noted that it often consisted of the repetition of the first word or syllable of the sentence and that it frequently had a tendency to disappear and return repeatedly over a period of months or years. He observed that a "secondary" stage of stuttering began after a "lapse of several years" or much sooner in cases in which the child is "made conscious of his stammering as a social defect." He described secondary stuttering as characterized by the child's consciousness of the impediment, physical effort, the use of starters, synonyms, and other attempts to control or conceal stuttering, anticipation, and above all fear—of letters, words, people, and speech situations.

Van Riper (1954, chap. 9) sought to refine Bluemel's concept of primary and secondary stuttering by adding a "transitional" stage. Later, he proposed an additional modification of the scheme in which simple, effortless repetitions and prolongations at normal tempo (primary stuttering) are followed by a stage of faster, longer, and less regular repetitions and prolongations with occasional reactions of surprise, then by struggle reactions accompanied by feelings of frustration, and finally by secondary stuttering characterized by fear and avoidance (Van Riper, 1963, p. 327ff.).

Four Phases in the Development of Stuttering

A developmental framework for stuttering proposed by the first author (Bloodstein, 1960b) emerged from a survey of the clinical case histories of a series of 418 stutterers, ranging in age from 2 to 16 years, whom he had examined at the Brooklyn College Speech and Hearing Center over a six-year period. When these 418 stuttering problems were viewed with attention to all of their elements—observable symptoms, reactions, adaptations, and conditions under which stuttering occurred—the great majority seemed to adhere to at least an approximate degree to one of four recurring patterns. Each of the four was a familiar type of clinical presentation. Each had a distinctly different typical age of occurrence, despite extreme overlapping of the age ranges represented, so that they were clearly in a sequential relationship to each other. It was thus possible to discern a broad trend conveniently described in terms of four major phases. These are summarized here.

It must be cautioned that the process of development as outlined here appears to be typical, *not* universal. It is, moreover, a continual and gradual process. The four descriptions that follow are best seen as descriptions of reference points along a continuum. Many stutterers correspond in an approximate way to one of these four "phases"; others are more accurately described as being in transition between one phase and the next.

Phase One The preschool period, roughly between the ages of 2 and 6 years, is one in which a large number of stutterers are seen. During this early period, there are six characteristics that may be said to typify most stuttering cases.

1. *The difficulty has a distinct tendency to be episodic.* One of the best indications that stuttering is still in its most rudimentary form is that it appears for periods of weeks or months between long interludes of normal speech. During this phase, there is a high percentage of spontaneous recoveries from stuttering that consist essentially of cases in which episodes of stuttering have failed to recur. How high this percentage is can be very difficult to determine, but appears to be roughly 80 percent of cases. It is not improbable that single episodes of stuttering so mild and brief that they are overlooked or soon forgotten are exceedingly common during these years. The program of research conducted by Ehud Yairi and his colleagues (Yairi & Ambrose, 2005) would seem to strongly support these impressions; specific patterns of remission will be discussed further in Chapter 12.
2. *The child stutters most when excited or upset, when seeming to have a great deal to say, or under other conditions of communicative pressure.*
3. *The dominant symptom is repetition.* This must be hastily qualified. Practically any of the integral or associated symptoms of stuttering may be seen in some of the youngest stutterers, and in some cases there seems to be little or no repetition. For the most part, however, the more severe symptoms appear briefly and intermittently in these children, and relatively simple repetition is far more common. In some cases repetition is practically the only symptom to be observed. While much of it consists of repetition of initial syllables, as it does in older stutterers, there is also usually a conspicuous tendency to repeat whole words, especially monosyllabic words.
4. *There is a marked tendency for moments of stuttering to occur at the beginning of the sentence, clause, or phrase.* In some of the youngest children stuttering seems to be limited almost entirely to the first word of the sentence. We will enlarge on this pattern in discussion of language factors that appear to affect early stuttering in Chapter 12.
5. *In contrast to more advanced stuttering, the interruptions occur not only on content words, but also on the function words of speech—the pronouns, conjunctions, articles, and prepositions*; in fact, they are much more likely to occur on such words, as we discuss in Chapter 12. Stuttering on such words often tends to consist of whole-word repetitions. In short, there is frequent repetition of such words as "like," "but," "and," "so," "he," "I," and "with."
6. *Most of the time, children in the first phase of stuttering show little evidence of concern about the interruptions in their speech.* This is not to say that they are completely unconscious of them. It is commonplace for children as young as 2 or 3 to show acute frustration when they stutter by refusing to speak, crying, beating the wall with their hands, or saying, "Why can't I talk?" Such reac-

tions are usually brief and sporadic, however, in contrast to the chronic fear and embarrassment of many older stutterers. Furthermore, the characteristic reaction of the Phase One stutterer may be epitomized by saying that when there is any reaction at all it is apparently in response to the immediate experience of being thwarted in efforts to communicate rather than to the ramified implications of the knowledge on the part of the child that he or she "is a stutterer."

Phase Two The second phase in the development of stuttering is marked by the following features.

1. *The disorder is essentially chronic.* There are few if any intervals of normal speech.
2. *The child has a self-concept as a person who stutters.*
3. *Stuttering occurs chiefly on the major parts of speech—nouns, verbs, adjectives, and adverbs.* There is much less tendency to stutter only on the initial words of sentences and phrases, and whole-word repetitions are no longer quite as common.
4. *Despite a self-concept as a stutterer, the child usually evinces little or no concern about the speech difficulty.* There is an absence of such features of more advanced stuttering as conscious anticipations of stuttering, substitution, circumlocution, avoidance of speaking, and word, sound, and situation fears.
5. *The stuttering is said to increase chiefly under conditions of excitement or when the child is speaking rapidly.*

This description of Phase Two is, of course, an abstraction that fits few people who stutter perfectly. Because the developmental process is continual, many children whom one would be inclined to classify in this or any other "phase" of stuttering exhibit some of the attributes of later or earlier forms of the disorder. Perhaps the single outstanding characteristic by which Phase Two may be recognized as a familiar clinical entity is the tendency of children, by their own reports and that of others, to stutter chiefly when they "talk fast and get excited," even though they may long since have passed the age limits of Phase One.

Phase Two stutterers are to be found for the most part among children of elementary school age. The age limits of this stage are very broad, however, and there are individuals who exhibit its principal characteristics as early as age 4 and as late as adulthood.

Phase Three The third phase of stuttering has the following typical features.

1. *The stuttering comes and goes largely in response to specific situations.* Among the situations the person often reports to be especially difficult are classroom recitation, speaking to strangers, making purchases in stores, and using the telephone.
2. *Certain words or sounds are regarded as more difficult than others.*
3. *In varying degrees, use is made of word substitutions and circumlocutions.* This tends to be done only occasionally and more often as a reaction to frustration, or its imminence, than in actual fear of stuttering.
4. *There is essentially no avoidance of speech situations and little or no evidence of fear or embarrassment.*

In addition, anticipation of stuttering as a highly conscious process sometimes begins to develop while the disorder is still in this form. The distinguishing feature of this phase of stuttering is the tendency to speak freely in virtually all situations despite the fact that the person may exhibit all of the other attributes of fully developed stuttering and may even stutter quite severely. When there is a reaction to the speech difficulty, it is likely to be a reaction of irritation rather than of shame or anxiety.

Phase Three stuttering is encountered at all ages from about 8 to adulthood. It appears to be most common in late childhood and early adolescence.

Phase Four At the apex of its development, stuttering is marked by the following features.

1. *Vivid, fearful anticipations of stuttering.*
2. *Feared words, sounds, and situations.*
3. *Very frequent word substitutions and circumlocution.*
4. *Avoidance of speech situations, and other evidence of fear and embarrassment.*

Phase Four stuttering is typically seen in later adolescence and adulthood, although it may be recognized in children as young as 10 years of age. Its distinctive aspect is the emotional reactions by virtue of which it tends to become a serious personal problem. Stutterers in this phase may become acutely conscious of the reactions of others to their speech, and they may be victimized by a tendency to exaggerate and misinterpret these reactions. They are likely to be unusually sensitive to the stigma involved in being regarded as a person who stutters, to shrink from discussing their speech difficulty with others, and to go to extreme lengths to maintain a pretense as a normal speaker. All of this, together with avoidance of speaking, tends to impair their capacity for spontaneous and constructive social relationships and in some cases may even serve to isolate them to some extent from others.

Van Riper's Four Tracks

Whatever regularities exist in the development of stuttering, as we have noted, there are also differences among stutterers in the manner in which the problem undergoes changes. Van Riper (1982, chap. 5) offered a descriptive scheme that placed particular stress on the developmental variability of stuttering. In his own cases, including forty-four that he was able to observe longitudinally, he discerned four alternate paths or "tracks" along which the disorder appeared to develop. While many clinicians have observed individuals who are described by such tracks, there has not been any demographic analysis of the relative frequency of any of these groupings.

Track I In by far the largest group of children, Van Riper found the symptoms to consist initially of effortless, unhurried repetitions of syllables and words, marked by extreme fluctuations and long remissions. Onset was gradual. As the disorder progressed the repetitions became more rapid and irregular, and there appeared, in sequence, prolongations, tension and forcing with intermittent evidence of concern on the part of the child, associated movements, word and situation fears, and avoidance.

Track II In a second large group, consisting chiefly of children who were late in beginning to talk, the stuttering was said to take the form of rapid, irregular syllable and word repetition from the beginning. Later, silent intervals, revisions, and interjections appeared, and the pattern took on many of the aspects of cluttering. Thereafter, the pattern changed relatively little. Word and sound fears were generally mild and tended to develop late.

Track III A third group was made up of a small number of children who were said to have begun to stutter with sudden inability to speak, or complete blockage. Very soon, this was followed by severe forcing and struggle, breathing abnormalities, signs of frustration, associated facial and other tensions, fear, and avoidance. In most cases, the severe struggle reactions abated after a while and were followed first by prolongation and then by syllable repetition.

Track IV Van Riper assigned a final track to a few children who were reported to have begun to stutter rather suddenly with repetition of phrases, words, and later syllables. They tended to stutter openly with few avoidances and showed little change in their stuttering over the years.

SUMMARY REMARKS

We have attempted to convey the complexity of stuttering in this first chapter of the text. Stuttering seems obvious to most people who stutter and those who listen to them, but elusive in its defining characteristics. It is very difficult to define exactly what behavioral features capture the distinction between stuttering and more typical disfluency. Adding to the complexity of the disorder is the fact that many of its features are somewhat hidden: physical, physiological, and psychological (affective and cognitive) concomitants very typical in stuttering are rarely perceptible to those interacting with the person who stutters. However, it is this characteristic complexity that guides the many topics we cover in the 13 chapters that follow.

Chapter 2

Theories of Stuttering

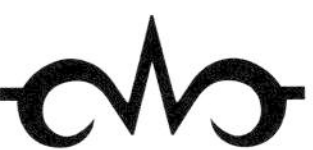

In this chapter, we will summarize and evaluate some of the many theories about the cause of stuttering. As we will show, such theories are plentiful. They can be grouped by emphasis, such as whether they primarily focus on the underlying cause of the disorder or the moment of speech breakdown, or whether they view stuttering as a physiological disorder or one best described by learning theory, for example. Over time, although numerous very specific models have been advanced, many tend to build on and refine theories first advanced many years before. We will attempt to group theories conceptually in the sections that follow, as well as track the historical roots of their development.

THEORIES OF ETIOLOGY VERSUS CONCEPTS OF THE MOMENT OF STUTTERING

For a proper understanding of the array of formulations that have been elaborated about stuttering, it is important to keep in mind that they are not all theories in the same sense of the word. Some, like Johnson's view that stuttering is caused by its own diagnosis, offer an account of the *etiology*, or so-called onset of stuttering. That is, they attempt to generalize about the conditions under which the disorder initially comes about. A second type of theory is concerned primarily with the nature of discrete instances of stuttering behavior. Like Coriat's theory that stuttering is a symbolic sucking activity, its emphasis is on a conceptual model of the individual *moment* of stuttering. Needless to say, some theorists have dealt with both the moment of stuttering and the etiology of stuttering in systematic detail. But this is not always so. And it is clarifying in any case to keep the two aspects of their theoretical formulations distinct. A theory that explains one may or may not be compatible with explaining the other.

There is still a third type of theory, in our view, whose basic contribution lies in a reformulation of a previous theory of either the etiology or the moment of stuttering, in terms of a new frame of reference. Theories that apply learning theory or cybernetics to stuttering would be in this category, as might psycholinguistic theories that have attempted to expand on models of hemispheric control of speech. It is only by keeping these three kinds of theories clearly separated that we will be able to appreciate the important connections existing among them and the contributions each of them has to make to our understanding of stuttering.

There are some challenges in developing viable theories. First, what causes stuttering to emerge may or may not play an important role in describing stuttering as it develops over the lifespan. It is almost certainly the case that the characteristics of adult stuttering bear little resemblance to those observed in children close to onset of symptoms: learning, experience, and adaptation to the disorder will shape the speaker continuously. How soon these factors begin to change the person who stutters is not clear, but we have seen toddlers show signs of avoidance (a cognitive feature of the disorder) as well as struggle within less than a week after adults noticed the stuttering behavior, as noted in Chapter 1. This "evolutionary" quality of chronic stuttering is important for both theories and therapies, and the studies that we report elsewhere in this book that attempt to evaluate them. When we study adults, we may not be able to generalize back to their childhood state to understand how they began to stutter. Moreover, what starts stuttering may or may not have relevance to its most effective treatment as symptoms of the disorder change over time.

Second, theories must account for the features of stuttering itself: the qualities that distinguish stuttered events from normal nonfluencies. This is nontrivial: many theories will predict that the speaker cannot maintain fluency, but few appear to explain the unique characteristics of the stuttering moment.

Third, the theory should be able to predict the distributional characteristics of stuttering: its patterns near its onset and as it develops, and conditions under which stuttering is exacerbated and ameliorated.

Fourth, theories must account for the fact that the onset of stuttering is typically reported to be in the years between 2 and 4. This makes it unique among all other developmental communication disorders, for which earlier symptoms and indicators are becoming increasingly evident.[1] In other words, there is relative continuity in the prelinguistic and early linguistic behaviors of children who have other speech and language disorders, while stuttering shows apparent marked discontinuity. One day the child appears to be normally fluent, and over a relatively short period of time, this normal profile converts into something that is categorically perceived to be atypical. In virtually all cases attested to, stuttering begins after the child has demonstrated fluent and capable speech and language performance. What could trigger breakdown of the child's early communicative system? Certainly, many of the theories we discuss in this chapter have seized on this particular feature of the disorder to investigate possible influences of the environment on the onset of stuttering. As we will note, another remarkable aspect of early stuttering is the child's typical awareness of communicative difficulty, a profile not apparent in children with language or articulation problems.

Fourth, theories of the nature of stuttering must account for the fact that approximately 80 percent of children who begin to stutter will stop spontaneously, while 20 percent of cases will persist. What

[1] For example, childhood articulation and language problems are now known to have precursor symptoms, even before the acquisition of early linguistic milestones, such as reduced quantity and quality of babble (Rescorla & Bernstein Ratner, 1996), as well as perceptual performance limitations (Newman et al., 2006).

differentiates these two groups of individuals? We take these challenges to be the minimal (rather than exhaustive) list of facts that theories of stuttering should be able to account for.

CONCEPTS OF THE MOMENT OF STUTTERING

We shall begin by putting aside the matter of the etiology of stuttering for a moment to consider the nature of the discrete stuttering response itself. When we ask what the moment of stuttering represents, we find several hypotheses from which to choose. Almost all contemporary points of view about stuttering behavior are represented by three major concepts. These we will term the *breakdown, repressed need*, and *anticipatory struggle* hypotheses.[2]

The Breakdown Hypothesis

Some theories appear to view the stuttering block as a momentary failure of the complicated coordination required among the systems involved in speech production. In the context of such theories, the words *breakdown, disorganization, disintegration*, and *disruption* are often used to describe what is believed to be happening when the person stutters.

One might object that this is less an explanation than a description, and a rather figurative one at that. That is, regardless of the reasons for its occurrence, it is no more than self-evident that the stuttering block entails a breakdown of speech function. The hypothesis, however, contains an additional element that elevates it above mere description. This is the specification of varied forms of "environmental" pressure as precipitating agents. Thus, the breakdown has been considered to be the effect of emotional or psychosocial stress (which can include speech anxiety) or language formulation demand on the rapid, smooth, complex neuromuscular adjustments required for normally fluent speech production. It would be more accurate, perhaps, to call it the *breakdown-under-stress hypothesis*. When translated into therapy goals, such a model calls for assisting stutterers in some way to cope with the external pressures that presumably precipitate their speech disruptions, and it is perhaps in terms of this type of clinical rationale that the hypothesis is best distinguished pragmatically from others.

Those who adhere to this point of view have had much to say about the possible reasons for which a child's speech originally becomes inclined to "fall apart," as it were, and we shall develop some of the implications of this hypothesis at greater length when we consider various theories of the etiology of stuttering in which the breakdown concept is embedded.

The simple notion of the moment of stuttering as a physical breakdown has often been elaborated in unique ways. Some well-known examples include the theories that the block is an expression of cerebral interhemispheric conflict (Travis, 1931), a miniscule convulsion (West, 1958), or a perseverative neurological response similar to the perseverative motor behavior of some brain-injured patients (Eisenson, 1958, 1975). Van Riper (1971, chap. 15), Adams (1974), and Perkins et al. (1976) each viewed stuttering as a failure of coordination of respiration, phonation, and articulation. More specifically, Zimmermann (1980c) suggested that brain stem reflexes affecting the speech production mechanism may become abnormally facilitated or inhibited when the movement of these structures exceeds certain ranges of velocity, displacement, or positioning. Moore and Haynes (1980) theorized that stuttering is a linguistic segmentation dysfunction due to right-hemisphere processing of language. A variety of other conceptions of the stuttering block as a breakdown in speech coordination emerged in the last decades of the twentieth century, due in part to a renewal of interest in organic factors in stuttering.[3] The role of speech motor control in stuttering

[2] All of these have their roots in a long history of thought about stuttering in the course of which counterparts of many modern views have reappeared many times. A valuable account of the extensive earlier developments in Europe and the United States was contributed by Freund (1966, pp. 1-47).

[3] See Zimmerman, Smith, and Hanley (1981), Andrews, Craig, Feyer, Hoddinott, Howie, and Neilson (1983), Kent (1984), MacKay and MacDonald (1984), Yeudall (1985), Stromsta (1986), Harrington (1988), Nudelman, Herbrich, Hoyt, and Rosenfield (1989), Perkins, Kent, and Curlee (1991).

has been the focus of a number of researchers who have undertaken a variety of programmatic analyses of speech motor timing and coordination in more recent years (see, for example, Kent, 2000; Smith & Kleinow, 2000; McClean & Runyan, 2000; Peters, Hulstijn, & van Lieshout, 2000; Ludlow & Loucks, 2003; Max, Caruso, & Gracco, 2003)[4] and has led to additional formal models of the disorder as one primarily based on difficulty in retrieving or executing speech motor commands (e.g., Venkatagiri, 2005).

The Repressed Need Hypothesis

Since the advent of psychoanalysis, various attempts have been made to characterize the stuttering act as a neurotic symptom of unconscious needs that are treated most appropriately by psychotherapy. Far from being seen as a type of failure, stuttering is viewed in this frame of reference as an integrated, purposeful activity that a person performs because of an unconscious wish to do so. Over a period of several decades in the last century, such writers as Brill (1923), Coriat (1928, 1943), Fenichel (1945, chap. 15), Glauber (1958), and others advanced psychoanalytic concepts of the moment of stuttering, albeit differing somewhat in their emphases. A fairly comprehensive notion of this viewpoint may be conveyed more clearly by enumerating the varied types of needs that stuttering has been said to satisfy.

First, it has been said to satisfy an infantile need for oral erotic gratification. In stuttering, the immature sexual pleasure of nursing, biting, and oral incorporation of objects that the person enjoyed as an infant is unconsciously perpetuated, according to this theory, together with the pleasure of complete dependence upon and identification with the mother.

Second, the act of stuttering has been regarded as an attempt to satisfy anal erotic needs. The function of the anal sphincter is symbolically "displaced upward," according to this view, and in stuttering, the person seeks to re-experience those anal gratifications said to characterize the infantile libido in a certain phase of its development.

Third, stuttering has been viewed as a covert expression of hostile or aggressive impulses that the person fears to express openly. Stuttering may be considered aggression in the sense that it is painful to the listener. It may also be regarded as aggression in the less obvious sense that stutterers, in "chewing up" their words, are symbolically attempting a cannibalistic destruction of their listeners, starting with their parents. Above all, stuttering is frequently seen as the persistence of a peculiarly anal kind of aggression characteristic of infantile levels of personality development. In this last sense, the stutterer's fluctuating "forcing out" and "holding back" of words may represent a hostile expulsion and retention of feces.

Fourth, stuttering may represent the unconscious desire to suppress speech. It is in this form that the need hypothesis has perhaps been most extensively developed (Fenichel, 1945, chap. 15). According to this reasoning, speech stoppages result from a conflict between all of the conscious pressures and needs that force stutterers to speak and their unconscious wish to be silent. For what reason do they need to be silent? A number of different answers are possible. To begin with, children may unconsciously fear that, in speaking, they will reveal certain forbidden wishes or feelings. For example, they may block in order to prevent themselves from saying unacceptable words. In the main, however, stutterers are thought to want to suppress speech because of what the act of speaking means to them. Speaking may represent oral gratification about which they may feel guilt. Speaking may also be seen as an aggressive act for which stutterers may fear retaliation. Such aggression may be predominantly oral or anal. In the Oedipal phase of psychosexual development, speech may be seen by boys as an exhibitionistic kind of behavior and as an act of competition with the father. To girls, speech may symbolize a usurpation of the male role. In all of these cases, the impulse to speak may be intermittently thwarted by guilt and anxiety.

[4] We address the findings of these investigations in Chapter 4.

This brief account does not do justice to the great subtlety with which psychoanalytic ideas about stuttering have been elaborated. The possible shades of meaning of stuttering to the psychoanalyst have not been exhausted here. Nor must it be assumed that the various unconscious needs that have been mentioned are mutually exclusive. Stuttering is frequently seen as satisfying a number of such needs simultaneously (Glauber, 1958). Writers differ chiefly in the amount of emphasis they give to different factors of unconscious motivation. Although the basic needs of classical Freudian theory, sex and aggression, predominate in most systematic psychoanalytic discussions of stuttering, there is also abundant reference to other unconscious uses of stuttering—for example, to gain attention, sympathy, or isolation, to provide an excuse for failures, or to avoid the necessity for coping with life's problems. Barbara (1954) contributed an extended analysis of the stutterer's personality employing the concepts of Karen Horney and Alfred Adler; Murphy and FitzSimons (1960) suggested some interpretations influenced by Harry Stack Sullivan. More recently, Gemelli (1982a, 1982b) reiterated and extended the psychoanalytic theory of stuttering as a childhood neurosis along classical Freudian lines. For a detailed history of psychoanalytic thinking about stuttering, see Bloom (1978).

Repressed need theories found support chiefly in the clinical observations and case findings of psychoanalysts, rather than speech scientists. Objective scientific corroboration of any of these theories of the moment of stuttering is largely lacking and is made extremely difficult by the very nature of the process by which psychoanalysis obtains its data. The studies that have been done on the stutterer's personality have *not* shown them more likely to be emotionally disturbed or markedly neurotic people, as we will see in Chapter 7. Neither have the end results of psychoanalytic treatment of stutterers afforded persuasive evidence for the repressed need hypothesis. Meta-analyses such as that by Andrews et al. (1983) indicate that neither psychoanalysis nor various other forms of psychotherapy have as yet proved very effective in modifying stuttering behavior. Psychoanalysts, however, tend to attribute this to an unusual amount of resistance to therapy on the part of the stutterer. Stuttering has sometimes been compared to obsessive-compulsive neurosis in this respect.

We think it is very important to note that, while this class of theories has lost appeal in mainstream American and Western European speech-language pathology, it is very much in evidence if one examines consumer and professional websites in other countries (Bernstein Ratner, 2005b). In addition, as we show in Chapter 7, mainstream medical classification and billing systems maintain the overall concept of stuttering as a form of psychopathology despite research that continually weakens the viability of this theory.

The Anticipatory Struggle Hypothesis

Although there remain a number of other ways of conceiving of the moment of stuttering, they all appear to be so similar that they may be placed under a single general heading. The underlying idea common to all of them is that *stutterers interfere in some manner with the way they are talking because of their belief that speaking is difficult*. This idea, termed here the *anticipatory struggle hypothesis*, has been, in one or another of its forms, one of the most widely employed explanations of the moment of stuttering and has exerted a strong influence on theory, treatment, and research.

As long as any serious professional concern about the problem of stuttering has existed, there appears to have been a perception that a very significant feature of the disorder was the tendency of stutterers to have difficulty whenever they expect to stutter and, inversely, to speak fluently when not "thinking" about their speech. In this respect, stuttering is similar to the mistakes that may occur in typing or playing a musical instrument in front of an audience, or to the stiffness that may hamper some graduates' walking while crossing the stage to receive their diploma. The central thesis, succinctly stated, is that it is the anticipation of stuttering that leads to stuttering. But why should this be?

An analogy will serve to amplify this hypothesis. Most people are likely to have little difficulty keeping their balance while walking the length of a narrow plank lying upon the ground. Place the same plank 20 feet in the air, however, and the task assumes an entirely different character. We may describe what happens to the manner in which people walk under such conditions by saying that they now anticipate falling off the plank, try hard to avoid this, and ultimately may come to be in real danger of falling off as a result of their struggle to stay on. The effects of anxiety on motor function have been documented by other disciplines, and thus are plausible as a mechanism by which otherwise well-coordinated behavior may be destabilized (see, for instance, Balaban & Thayer, 2001).

In the course of its long history, the anticipatory struggle hypothesis has been reiterated many times in a variety of ways. It will be helpful to examine various alternative statements of the hypothesis carefully.

Early Formulations The early literature on speech disorders contains numerous references to stuttering as stemming from "fear," "doubt," or anticipation of speech difficulty. This simple and somewhat empty kind of statement became more elaborate as researchers and clinicians began to grope for formulations that explained more fully how a belief in the inability to speak normally might lead to stuttering. Boome and Richardson (1931, p. 99) and Gifford (1940, p. 30) inferred that stuttering was due to faulty autosuggestion. Freund (1966) developed a conception of stuttering as an "expectancy neurosis," analogous to disturbances such as male sexual impotence that tend to be made more severe by the fear that they will occur.[5] Others referred to it as an anxiety neurosis, or speech "phobia."

Failure of Automaticity A distinctive form of the hypothesis stated that stuttering resulted from the attempt to exercise conscious control over the automatic processes of speech. The idea occurs widely in earlier writings on stuttering, where it is often accompanied by the analogy of the centipede who was crippled by the injunction to explain how it walked. The notion has come down through the years, and has been experimentally validated in tests of skilled motor performance in other fields (e.g., Masters, 1992). West (1931) offered the hypothesis in more refined form when he stated that stutterers tend to create difficulty for themselves by voluntarily producing individual speech movements rather than by initiating "automatic serial responses." Later, he contributed a more extended discussion of stuttering as articulatory "dysautomaticity," postulating its relationship to genetic factors, however, rather than to the learning of fear or anticipation.[6] Mysak (1960) made use of the concept of "deautomaticity" in a servo-theory context, as will be seen.[7]

This general version of the anticipatory struggle hypothesis is an important one, since it calls attention to the interesting fact that both stuttering and what appear to be other stutter-like phenomena are likely to occur in serially ordered activities (such as speech, walking, typing, or playing musical instruments) that appear to be implemented through integrated patterns or series of acts that, by some mechanism, appear to be evoked as wholes rather than as chains of individual responses. To put it in another way, interruptions produced by fear or anticipation seem to take place readily in the course of behavior demanding extensive motor planning (Frick, 1965). Perhaps the most pertinent example is the stutter-like difficulty reported to occur in some cases in the manual communication of the deaf (Silverman & Silverman, 1971; Montgomery & Fitch, 1988). Cases of stutter-like difficulty in the playing of musical instruments have been documented by Silverman and Bohlman (1988) and Meltzer (1992).

Anticipatory Avoidance The anticipatory struggle concept is perhaps best known in the special form in which Wendell Johnson developed it in a

[5] Freund (1966) has summarized much of his earlier thinking, as well as that of others, on the relationship between expectancy and stuttering.

[6] See West, Ansberry, and Carr (1957, p. 255), West and Ansberry (1968, chap. 5).

[7] The concept of automaticity also emerges when researchers consider the integrity of speech-motor control in stutterers, and the degree to which task demand may destabilize motor behavior, as we discuss in later sections of this chapter.

series of writings spanning three decades.[8] In accordance with this view, the very things that stutterers do in order not to stutter *are* their stuttering. Stuttering is, then, little more than the effort to avoid stuttering. Stated somewhat more elaborately, it is an "anticipatory, apprehensive, hypertonic avoidance reaction." That is, stuttering is what happens when a person anticipates stuttering, dreads it, and becomes tense in the attempt to avoid it. In a phrase, stuttering is "what the speaker does while trying not to stutter again." From this point of view, stuttering is not a symptom of a constitutional abnormality or an emotional disorder, but a consequence of certain inappropriate perceptual and evaluative reactions to speech that a speaker has learned from the social environment. Considerable research has been done on the moment of stuttering, using Johnson's anticipatory avoidance theory as the primary impetus, and we shall therefore refer to it again in Chapter 10.

Approach-Avoidance Conflict Stuttering may be represented as the resultant of a conflict between opposing wishes to speak and to keep silent. This view was developed extensively by Sheehan (1953, 1958a) in a learning theory context to be considered later in this text. At this point, it will be sufficient to indicate how the conflict idea is related to certain others that we have already mentioned.

From a practical standpoint, the conflict hypothesis may be reduced to the statement that stuttering results from the desire to avoid speaking. (The conflicting desire to speak may be regarded as implicit, since without it there would merely be silence.) In contrast to Johnson's view of stuttering as the avoidance of *stuttering*, then, the conflict theory depicts it as the avoidance of *speaking*. This is quite a different notion, and we may be inclined to raise the question whether it belongs logically among anticipatory struggle concepts at all. The answer seems to be *yes* and *no*, depending on what reason is given for the avoidance of speaking. If it is because of the wish to avoid expected stuttering or any other real or imagined difficulty or failure in speech, we are clearly dealing with a form of anticipatory struggle hypothesis. But if, like Fenichel, we believe that stutterers wish to avoid speech because they unconsciously regard it as a hostile act, or if, like Glauber, we see stuttering as a kind of mutism or articulatory spasm designed to block unconscious expressions of biting or sucking, the conflict motif is more reasonably regarded as belonging to the repressed need hypothesis.

Preparatory Set Van Riper (1937d; 1954, pp. 429–43) developed his concept of the role of the preparatory set in stuttering primarily as a therapeutic tool (see Chapter 14) and did not appear to place much emphasis on its theoretical implications. Yet, when seen in the proper light, it proves to be a highly descriptive statement of the anticipatory struggle hypothesis. Van Riper pointed out that, in advance of the attempt on a word perceived as difficult or feared, stutterers tend to place themselves in a characteristic muscular and psychological "set," which determines the form of the subsequent stuttering block. This set has essentially three identifiable features. First, stutterers establish an abnormal focus of tension in their articulators. Second, they prepare themselves to say the first sound of the difficult word as a fixed articulatory posture rather than as a normal movement blending with the rest of the word. That is, in their lack of conviction that they will be able to say the feared initial sound, they may prepare themselves to say "b" rather than "boy." This can only result, however, in failure to produce the word in a normal way. Third, they may adopt this unnatural posture of the articulators appreciably before they initiate voice or airflow, resulting in a silent "preformation" of the sound.[9] Having done all of these things because of their anticipation of difficulty on the word, it is apparent that they have effectively destroyed their chances of saying it normally. Conversely, it may be hypothesized that if

[8] See especially Johnson and Knott (1936). Johnson (1938), Johnson et al. (1956, pp. 216, 217), Johnson et al. (1967, p. 240).

[9] The relatively large body of data showing aberrant coordination of respiratory, laryngeal, and articulatory gestures in the speech of adults and older children who stutter (see Chapter 5) is relevant to the evaluation of this version of the hypothesis.

they did none of these things, they would not stutter on the word.

Tension and Fragmentation Finally, we may note that practically all of the integral features of stuttering behavior are reducible to the surface effects of two underlying forms of behavior—tension and fragmentation. Whenever we are faced with the threat of failure in the performance of a complex activity demanding accuracy or skill, we are likely to make use of abnormal muscular tension. We are also apt to produce a portion of the act separately and sometimes repeatedly before we complete it. In stuttering, the underlying tension produces prolongations and hard attacks. The repetitions of stuttering may be interpreted as a fragmentation of speech units somewhat analogous to the behavior of dart throwers rehearsing the initial part of their throw. Such an interpretation is useful in explaining why it is almost always the first sound of the word that the stutterer repeats, as well as certain other puzzling features of its distribution in the speech sequence. We will develop this model more fully later.

Compatibility of Alternative Statements of the Anticipatory Struggle Hypothesis We have examined a number of different ways in which essentially a single general conception of the moment of stuttering has been expressed. Some of them are undoubtedly to be preferred to others for various reasons. But it will in all probability have occurred to many readers that some of these statements differ from others only in their concern with different temporal phases of the hypothetical anticipatory struggle act. We might say that there occurs, in sequence, (1) a suggestion, in the form of some outside stimulus, of imminent difficulty in speech; (2) an anticipation of failure; (3) a feeling of need to avoid it; (4) abnormal motor planning for the voluntary articulation of the speech activity; (5) the mustering of certain preparatory sets for this purpose; and (6) the production of tension and fragmentation, which interfere with the normal process of speech.[10]

[10] It is interesting to note that, for virtually each step in this sequence, there is one corresponding and unique therapy that has been used with stutterers.

THEORIES OF THE ETIOLOGY OF STUTTERING

So far we have been concerned only with the moment of stuttering. In light of what has been surmised about it, we may now go on to examine various inferences about the conditions under which this behavior first arises. Various schemes have been proposed for classifying theories of the etiology of stuttering. None of them is completely satisfactory; the thinking that has been done on the subject of stuttering tends to defy the simple logic of mutually exclusive categories. It may not be difficult to see, however, that in our prior review of concepts of the moment of stuttering, we have been afforded a convenient means of making such a classification. Any satisfactory theory of the etiology of stuttering carries with it, either explicitly or by implication, an assumption about the nature of the individual stuttering events. Taking our three major hypotheses about the moment of stuttering as a basis, therefore, we may classify virtually all etiological theories as breakdown, repressed need, or anticipatory struggle theories.

Breakdown Theories: The Dysphemic Viewpoint

At present, most theories that regard stuttering behavior as a breakdown of speech function under some type of pressure are associated with the view that constitutional or organic factors are involved in its etiology. The reason for this is not difficult to see. There was a time in the history of modern thinking about stuttering when it was believed by many that a child's speech might begin to go to pieces for no reason other than environmental stress. That is, it was often suggested that stuttering resulted simply from the impact of shock, fright, illness, injury, or the like. Even today, expressions of this type are heard occasionally, with terms such as *emotional pressures* or *insecurity* used in place of terms such as *shock* or *fright*. To most serious workers on the problem of stuttering, however, it is now clear that the vast majority of children who have pneumonia or fall off bicycles even repeatedly do not stutter as a result.

It is equally apparent that most children with emotional difficulties do not stutter. This difficulty may be glossed over by saying that some people have a "weakness" in the "area of speech" that causes them to react to such stresses by stuttering, but this is, after all, only a figure of speech and serves chiefly to raise questions about the form in which such a weakness might manifest itself.

For this reason, more recent breakdown theories have gone to considerable pains to show why speech disintegrates under stress in some cases and not in others. For the most part, they have done so by asserting that children must be predisposed in some way to breakdown before their speech can give way under stress, and the more satisfactory of these theories attempt to explain both the nature of this predisposition and the reason why its effects appear to be confined to speech. While it is possible to assume, as did Bluemel (1957), that children are made prone to disorganized speech by the nature of their personality, on the whole, the predisposition is believed to take a genetic, or constitutional, form.

The hypothesis that stuttering is basically an organic disorder is at least as old as Aristotle, who speculated that there was something wrong with the stutterer's tongue. It is now well known that stuttering cannot be attributed to any gross structural abnormality of the articulators, but it is interesting that as recently as 1841, the Prussian surgeon Johann Dieffenbach was performing tongue operations for stuttering. Dieffenbach believed that by removing a wedge-shaped section of the base of the tongue, he could stop the muscular spasms of the glottis that he thought were the cause of stuttering. His operation at first appeared to be a sensational success, evidently because of the powerful suggestion it produced, but the improvement in his patients proved to be temporary.[11]

The point to be emphasized is that more modern constitutional theories of stuttering differ in certain fundamental respects from the naive speculations of Aristotle and Dieffenbach. The first and most important difference is that today's theories are *predisposition* theories. They adopt the assumption familiar to medical science that a disorder may be a joint product of a hereditary predisposition and environmental precipitating factors.

According to this point of view, which was first developed in detail by West and some of his students, certain persons have an inherited predisposition to breakdown in speech function. This predisposition takes the form of a pervasive constitutional abnormality, once termed "dysphemia," whose exact nature has not yet been established. Dysphemia was, then, considered to be an inner condition of which stuttering is an outward symptom. Given a sufficient amount of dysphemia, the symptom we perceive as stuttering may be precipitated by illness, emotional disturbance, or the stress of other accidental environmental circumstances during childhood. A child who is heavily predisposed to stutter, as indicated by an extensive family history of the disorder, might never become a stutterer in a favorable environment. On the other hand, a child who is subjected to many serious environmental pressures might stutter even though lightly predisposed by heredity to do so. Clearly, it is not difficult to explain on the basis of this type of reasoning why so many persons with a family background of stuttering have no speech difficulty and why those who stutter often have no known stuttering relatives or ancestors.

Research to date has produced no conclusive evidence regarding the precise description of dysphemia, if such a thing exists, or the manner in which it predisposes a person to stutter. In the past, it was common to look for organic causes in easily identifiable organs such as the tongue, the respiratory system, the larynx, or even the thymus gland. Interest in the larynx as a source of stuttering, in fact, enjoyed a revival in the 1970s. For the most part, however, the predisposing cause of the stutterer's difficulty is now sought—and this is a second important distinction of present-day constitutional theories—not in the peripheral organs of speech, but in subtle aspects of speech motor control or speech-language processing. It is at this point that the dysphemic point of view about stuttering becomes divided into many different theories. A number of these are noteworthy because they have

[11] See Rieber and Wollock (1977).

had a wide influence on current thinking or have provided an impetus for research.

Stuttering as an Outcome of Aberrant Cerebral Dominance Few theories of stuttering are as well known as the theory that children are predisposed to stutter by a conflict between the two halves of the cerebral cortex for control of the activity of the speech production system.[12] Sometimes known as the "handedness theory," it was advanced in an attempt to account for some assumptions about stutterers' lateral dominance that have since been largely rejected. In the late 1920s, it was widely believed that an unusual number of stutterers were left-handed or ambidextrous or had been shifted to right-handedness in childhood, and there had been some convincing clinical reports of onset of stuttering after enforced change of handedness.

The great virtue of the cerebral dominance theory was that it offered a single, clear explanation for all of these alleged facts. Its authors, Dr. Samuel T. Orton and Prof. Lee Edward Travis, took note of the fact that the right and left halves of the tongue, jaw, and other "midline" speech structures received their motor nerve impulses from separate sources in the two cerebral hemispheres. They reasoned that, for purposes of smooth, fluent speech, these two streams of impulses needed to be accurately synchronized. What mechanism was responsible for this synchronization? Orton and Travis hypothesized that one cerebral hemisphere was "dominant" over the other for the purpose of timing the nerve impulses. The non-dominant hemisphere, they argued, accepted the temporal rhythm of innervation established by the dominant one. If, however, one hemisphere were not sufficiently dominant over the other, they would tend to function independently, actions of the two halves of the speech musculature would be poorly synchronized, and a predisposition to speech breakdown would exist.

Cerebral dominance had long been a familiar concept in other areas of research in communication disorders. It had been established that, in cases of acquired aphasia, the precipitating injury was usually to be found in the left half of the brain in right-handed persons, while there was speculation[13] that in left-handed aphasics, the injury was in the right half of the brain. From this had grown the basically correct belief that one cerebral hemisphere tends to become specially developed for the formulation and comprehension of language and for the purpose of establishing lateral preference.

According to the Orton-Travis theory, it was this very same side of the cerebral cortex that was dominant for the purpose of "motor lead control." This was an essential element of the theory because it explained how handedness might be related to stuttering. In the first place, children who were innately ambidextrous could be seen to be lacking, presumably by heredity, in a safe margin of cerebral dominance. In the second place, training "naturally" left-handed children to use the right hand meant reducing their margin of cortical dominance by exercising their minor hemisphere at the expense of the major one. And in the third place, left-handed persons might become predisposed to stutter even when not deliberately shifted because they were subject to so many pressures exerted by a right-handed society to use the right hand.

The Orton-Travis theory met with one of the most favorable receptions ever accorded a theory of stuttering, and the literature in such fields as medicine, psychology, and education still makes scattered references to it as a current point of view about stuttering. The great vogue it enjoyed in the 1930s, however, has long since passed. A considerable amount of laterality research done since then has failed to show convincingly that stutterers are particularly distinguished either by left-handedness or ambidexterity, as was once thought. Also, evidence eventually accumulated that the vast majority of children whose handedness is changed by parents or teachers do not stutter. Finally, there were the disappointing results of therapy. The cerebral dominance theory had some obvious clinical implications. Strict unilaterality was to be enforced in all of the stutterer's activities. Furthermore, if right-handed stutterers seemed to be natively

[12] See Travis (1931).

[13] In the days before brain imaging techniques were available.

left-sided as determined from case history or by certain types of laterality tests, they would need to learn to exercise their natural dominance by changing to the use of the left hand. At the time that the popularity of the theory was at its height, a great many apparently right-handed stutterers were judged to be innately left-handed and rigorously trained in sinistrality. At first, the results seemed to be good and were sometimes reported in enthusiastic terms. The initial promise of this therapy was not fulfilled, however, and it fell into disuse.

We note, however, that subtle asymmetries in cortical structure and function continue to emerge in stuttering research (see Chapter 4), particularly with the advent of sophisticated brain imaging and recording techniques. Whether such phenomena are cause or effect in stuttering, and their potential role in the etiology or phenomenology of stutter events, has yet to be determined, although "normalization" of lateralization patterns has been seen following various forms of therapy that did not target handedness (e.g., De Nil, Kroll, Lafaille, & Houle, 2003; Neumann, Preibisch, Euler, von Gudenberg, Lanfermann, Gall et al., 2005).

What is essentially a modified version of the Orton-Travis model has been offered by Webster (1993, 1997) and Forster and Webster (2001). Using results from bimanual coordination and visual field tasks, Webster proposed that stutterers have a "labile system of hemispheric activation" that leads to inappropriate over-activation of the right hemisphere for tasks normally handled by the left hemisphere. This, in turn, interferes with efficient left hemisphere control of speech-motor function, which is relatively deficient in people who stutter, according to his research and others, discussed in much greater detail in Chapter 4.

Kent (1984), in turn, proposed that underdevelopment of the left hemisphere leads to difficulties in encoding rapidly changing temporally-sequenced events, such as those involved in speech articulation. He thus views stuttering as a disorder in central control of timing for aspects of speech production, which must integrate rapid segmental planning demands (presumed to be the primary responsibility of the left hemisphere) as well as the prosodic parameters (intonation, stress) of utterance generation (more heavily controlled by the right hemisphere).

Other Physiological Theories A second conception of the nature of dysphemia that had considerable influence was developed over a period of years by West. According to this theory, the source of stuttering lies in a basic difference between stutterers and nonstutterers in metabolic factors and their tissue chemistry. The speech interruptions are triggered by social and emotional pressures, but the stutterer's neurophysiological capacity for speech is rendered vulnerable to the disruptive effects of such pressures by a biochemical imbalance.

West regarded dysphemia as genetically intertwined with a predisposition to certain other conditions, notably allergy, left-handedness, delayed speech and language development, twinning, and respiratory disease. He eventually formulated a concept of stuttering as a convulsive disorder related to epilepsy and particularly akin to an epileptiform disorder of childhood known as pyknolepsy (West, 1958).[14] According to this concept, the stutterer is a basically seizure-prone person in whom outright convulsions are held in check by a relatively large amount of blood sugar. The convulsive tendency is, however, reflected in stuttering. As noted earlier, West's theory in one of its later forms viewed the moment of stuttering as a kind of miniature seizure that principally affects the speech-motor system and is precipitated by emotional stress. This theory was supported by a number of observations purporting to show elevated blood sugar levels in stutterers, a high incidence of stuttering among persons with epilepsy, and a rareness of stuttering among those with diabetes. There are conflicting research findings on all of these points, however, and none of them has thus far been generally accepted as fact.

---

[14] In this regard, it is interesting that some have sought to find relationships between stuttering and Tourette's Syndrome, a tic disorder (Pauls, Leckman, & Cohen, 1993; Abwender et al., 1998; Ludlow & Loucks, 2003; Van Borsel, Goethals, & Vanryckeghem, 2004; De Nil, Sasisekaran, Van Lieshout, & Sandor, 2005).

Perseverative Theory Another viewpoint that relates to the concept of dysphemia was suggested by Eisenson (1958, 1975). Eisenson believed that stuttering is based upon a constitutional predisposition to motor and sensory perseveration. His investigations reported in 1936 and 1938 showed that, on the average, stutterers were inclined to perseverate more than nonstutterers in performing certain psychomotor tasks. Subsequent research by other investigators, including two studies by King (1961) and Martin (1962), produced inconsistent results. However, researchers in the area of acquired neurogenic disorders have noticed similarities between behaviors in such cases and those seen in developmental stuttering (e.g., Christman, Boutsen, & Buckingham, 2004).

Hormonal Theory The concept of cerebral dominance made its appearance again in a theory proposed by Norman Geschwind to account for a number of developmental disorders.[15] On the strength of some evidence, Geschwind hypothesized that the male sex hormone testosterone tends to retard neuronal development in the fetal brain. Because the right hemisphere develops earlier than the left, the effect is more pronounced in the left hemisphere. The male fetus is exposed to higher levels of testosterone than the female, so excessive delays in the development of the left hemisphere will be more common in males. As a result, according to Geschwind's theory, males will be more prone to developmental disturbances of left-hemisphere functions, including those of speech and language. On this basis, Geschwind saw relationships among maleness, left-handedness, and such disorders as dyslexia, delayed speech and language development, and stuttering.

As a theory of stuttering, this concept is somewhat incomplete, since it says nothing about why some children stutter while others have dyslexia or delayed speech, but do not stutter. Moreover, there is an absence of convincing evidence that stutterers differ from others in handedness.[16] The theory accounts for the preponderance of males who stutter, however, as well as for the high incidence of delayed speech and language among stutterers (see Chapter 8). It also fits well with research reports suggesting that many stutterers show atypically high levels of activation in the right hemisphere during speech and language processing (see Chapter 4), as well as a small number of reports describing structural asymmetries that are also discussed in that chapter. However, we note that a number of the assumptions underlying the model have been questioned in the years since it was proposed (Bryden, McManus, & Bulman-Fleming, 1994).

Psycholinguistic Models: Stuttering as a Speech-Language Encoding Disorder We consider the models discussed in this section *psycholinguistic* (Bernstein Ratner, 1997), in the sense that fluency failure is presumed to result from weakness in encoding the syntactic, lexical, phonological, or suprasegmental targets in speech production. We differentiate them from the hypotheses discussed in the preceding section because the actual physiological substrates of speech production are less critical to the models than abstracting the stages and processes presumed to underlie encoding of linguistic plans. In this vein, a number of researchers have considered the possibility that stuttering has a relationship to deficits in the language abilities of some young children that precipitate fluency breakdown, which is then subject to principles of response and learning discussed in other sections of this chapter. We may contrast these two foci by juxtaposing a current "boxes and arrows" schematic, psycholinguistic model of language production (Levelt, 1989) with its potential cortical substrates (see Figure 2-1).

One psycholinguistic model (Bloodstein, 2002, 2006) focuses on children's acquisition of syntax. As Bluemel had done many years earlier in his concept of primary and secondary stuttering, Bloodstein

[15] See Geschwind and Galaburda (1985), later called the Geschwind, Behan, and Galaburda Model.

[16] See Chapter 4. Geschwind and Behan (1982) found dyslexia and stuttering more common among highly left-handed than among highly right-handed individuals.

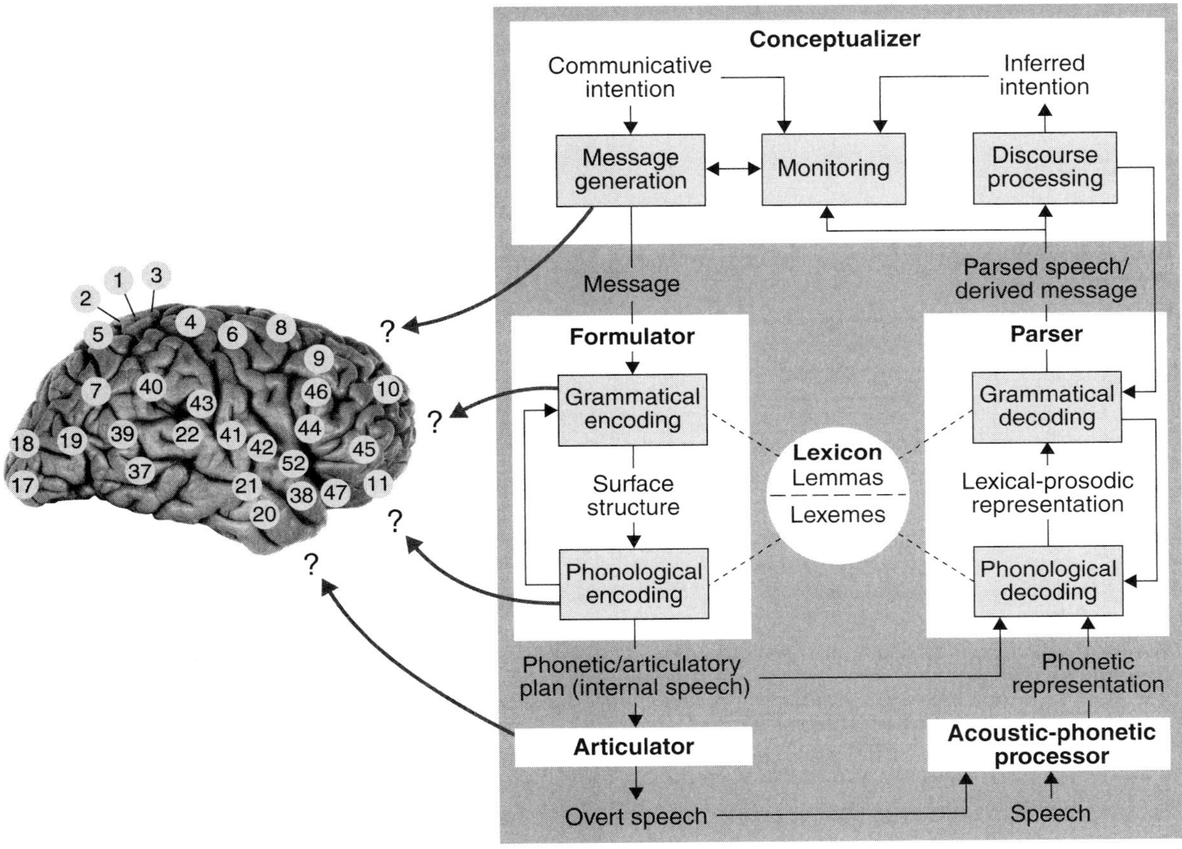

FIGURE 2-1 How stages of processing reflect actual brain mechanisms or areas of involvement (shown by numbered Brodmann areas) is as yet unclear. Levelt's psycholinguistic model of language production and comprehension (WEAVER++). Numbers represent hypothesized Brodmann areas underlying model components. Adapted from Levelt, 1989.

(2002) asserted that a transient incipient phase of stuttering was clearly distinct from its developed form. He suggested that, whereas developed stuttering is largely a difficulty in the initiation of words, incipient stuttering is a difficulty in ability to encode syntactic units. This theory is consistent with similar proposals offered by Bernstein (1981) and Bernstein Ratner (1997).

The hypothesis that stuttering originates in a child's uncertain mastery of syntax appears to provide a unifying explanation of an array of observations about incipient stuttering (see Chapters 8 and 12).

1. Incipient stuttering occurs regularly on the first word of an utterance or phrase, and virtually never at the end.[17]
2. The stuttering frequently takes the form of repetitions of whole words, which are themselves produced fluently.
3. Much of this repetition is of function words, which usually initiate syntactic structures.

[17] Indeed, in a recent reanalysis of a cohort of children near stuttering onset followed by Bernstein Ratner (2005a), fewer than 10 such events were observed over a body of several hundred stutters produced by 15 children. Even fewer were observed in single-word utterances.

4. In its form and distribution, incipient stuttering closely resembles the normal disfluencies of young children in the early years of language acquisition.
5. Incipient stuttering is almost never observed on one-word utterances.
6. Early stuttering does not appear to be influenced by word-related factors such as word length or grammatical function.
7. The frequency of incipient stuttering tends to increase with the length and grammatical complexity of utterances.
8. The onset of stuttering is rarely reported before 18 months, when children have generally begun to speak in multiword phrases.
9. The age range in which stuttering is usually said to begin, 2 to 5 years, is the interval in which most children are learning syntax.
10. By age 6, when the essentials of syntax have been acquired, a large number of children have spontaneously recovered from stuttering.
11. Studies have shown young children who stutter to be inferior to fluent speakers in various language skills, though there have been conflicting findings.
12. Incipient stuttering is more prevalent among boys than girls.

Many of these phenomena are discussed in further detail in Chapter 12. The broad implication of a syntax-based theory of the etiology of stuttering is that a small proportion of the human population is born not quite proficient in that innate proclivity for the effortless acquisition of syntax that most children demonstrate. If this is so, stuttering may be a reminder of how recently our genus acquired that aspect of language that most distinguishes us from animals' syntax. Stuttering may be a price we pay for the incalculable benefits of syntax.

Other Specific Psycholinguistic Accounts

While Bloodstein and Bernstein Ratner specifically target syntactic encoding as the "core" precipitating task that triggers stuttering onset, other models focus on alternative linguistic stages at which fluency failure might emerge during speech/language production. Most also reference the findings we discuss in Chapter 8 that have suggested some, albeit subtle, degree of atypical or depressed language ability in stutterers.

The first of the theories in this section target phonetic, phonological, or suprasegmental aspects of speech production. Harrington (1988) combined aspects of auditory feedback theory with syllable planning to suggest that stutterers have asynchronous perception of accented (stressed) vowel production; in this model, rules for realizing linguistic stress run afoul of speaker perception of their execution. His account attempts to place the development of stuttering within what was then known about children's perception and realization of linguistic rhythm.

Wingate (1988) offered his "fault-line" hypothesis, suggesting that stuttering emerged from a phonological encoding deficit that causes the speaker's difficulty in transitioning between syllable onsets and rimes. This failure "stalls" the speaker at the syllable onset.

The neuropsycholinguistic (NPL) model (Perkins, Kent, & Curlee, 1991) combined available models of speech production with known neurological substrates of segmental (linguistic) and paralinguistic (prosodic) processes to create the first fully fledged model of stuttering integrated with "box and arrow" psycholinguistic models of language encoding. Using "slot and filler" models of speech production,[18] they hypothesized that fluency breakdowns of any sort result when segmental and suprasegmental/paralinguistic information arrive dys-synchronously, as in the case where a syllable frame has been specified but its precise phonetic/phonological contents are not yet available, or its inverse, when adjustments to vocal prosody are still in progress when phonetic segments are forwarded for integration. However, the distinction between normal fluency failures and stuttering requires an additional component—the speaker's self-perception of time pressure and loss of

[18] Prosodic frames into which segmental information is inserted (Shattuck-Hufnagel, 1983; see additional discussion of such models in Bernstein Ratner, 1997).

control. The model considers this more likely when delays occur in forwarding the prosodic/paralinguistic envelope into which the segments of speech must be integrated. Rate of speech undoubtedly affects the coordination of these systems, which are also viewed as susceptible to deficiencies in temporal patterning or inefficient neural resources. The model also incorporates an expansion of Sheehan's approach-avoidance theory in positing that loss of control is also a function of conflict between the feelings of dominance and submissiveness in interaction, which is realized in adjustments to paralinguistic features of the utterance.

Karniol (1995) combined data from a single case study of a bilingual child stutterer with an extensive literature review to propose that stuttering emerges from a problem in Supra-segmental Sentence Plan Alignment (SPA), whereby the speaker experiences difficulty in aligning the segmental (lexical and syntactic) and suprasegmental (prosodic: stress, intonation) features of utterance constituents. She noted that this was most likely to emerge in the early stages of syntactic development when the child's preliminary suprasegmental plans generated in midstages of sentence production (as in most current models of speech production) require readjustment due to later stage syntactic or lexical revision of the sentence plan prior to articulation.

The Variability or V-Model (Packman, Onslow, Richard, & van Doorn, 1996) targets difficulty in the speaker's ability to encode suprasegmental variability (transitions between and among targets differing in stress value) as the locus of failure in stuttering. Specifically, the authors posit that, "the speech neuromotor systems of stutterers are destabilized by the variability of movement required to produce syllabic stress" (Packman & Lincoln, 1996, p. 47). The model proposes that early repetitive behavior in children who begin to stutter represents an attempt to regularize speech rhythm, in much the same way as speaking to a metronome or other syllable timing mechanisms do for adults. In some children, this timing difficulty (learning that some syllables must be de-stressed while others carry stress), resolves with language learning. In others, the problem persists, and the child's perception of the repetition as aberrant cause reactive struggle.

Still other models (the Execution and Planning Model, EXPLAN; Howell, 2004) combine hypotheses about the likely "epicenter" of planning difficulty (potentially phonetic or lexical complexity) with dys-synchrony in the planning and execution of utterance constituents.[19] Specifically, the model distinguishes between linguistic planning and motor execution of utterance components, which are presumed to overlap in spontaneous language production, allowing the planning of upcoming words or constituents during the motor output of preceding elements. The model is being tested to identify the most likely source of planning difficulty (leading to unavailability of the motor execution plan when the system is ready for it, as in the case of "a segment [that] takes a long time to plan, [while] the previous words in the section being executed take a short time to execute" (Howell & Dworzynski, 2005, p. 344). The preponderance of tests of the model to date has examined potential phonetic and phonological determinants of linguistic planning complexity and their effects on speech fluency.[20]

Perhaps the most influential psycholinguistic model in recent years has been the Covert Repair Hypothesis (Postma & Kolk, 1993; Kolk & Postma, 1997), which adopts Levelt's well-developed model of normal speech production (later called WEAVER++, a computer simulation; Levelt, Roelofs, & Meyer, 1999) and targets the "internal monitor" in that model as a likely culprit in producing symptoms that resemble those seen in stuttering. It is beyond the scope of this chapter to summarize the extensive experimental and naturalistic data that argue for a pre-articulation, internal monitor that checks for the well-formedness of intended speech output (see Berko Gleason & Bernstein Ratner, 1998, for such coverage). Postma and Kolk suggest that the likely consequences of an internal monitor that attempts to repair utterances that either have real or perceived errors before overt

[19] See also Howell and Au-Yeung (2002).

[20] See interchange between Bernstein Ratner (2005a) and Howell and Dworzynski (2005).

articulation would result in the blocks and repetitions that are the hallmarks of stuttered speech. They use results from prior work to suggest that the monitor detects legitimately poorly formed output (due to poor phonological encoding skills) and is not merely hyperfunctional, responding inappropriately to well-formed utterance plans.[21] The model is quite specific in predicting where in the speech production process various encoding errors might arise, and their resulting disfluency characteristics (see Tables 2-1 and 2-2).

Although the Levelt model is based on adult speech and language performance, there has been work to extend its prediction to children. Notably, Yaruss and Conture (1996) found that nonsystematic speech errors (slips of the tongue) did bear a relationship to stuttering children's disfluency, although systematic mispronunciations and phonological errors did not. There has also been a companion suggestion that at stuttering onset, stuttering results from over-attentive *post*-articulatory monitoring of normal disfluencies, exacerbated in young children who stutter because of their linguistic encoding difficulties (an "overt repair" hypothesis; Bernstein Ratner, 1998).

The "Vicious Circle" model (Vasić & Wijnen, 2005) combines elements of these models with the hypothesis that the internal monitor in adults who stutter is indeed hyperfunctional, and overly scrutinizes well-formed output in a psycholinguistic "twist" on anticipatory struggle hypotheses. Experimental data from their team suggest that simple dual-task assignments divert the resources allocated to the monitor, and thereby depress stuttering rates, a finding consistent with some known factors that moderate stuttering frequency (see Chapter 10).

Yet another model of stuttering invokes WEAVER++, although its emphasis is more consistent with our earlier group of models that target the phonological/phonetic systems as the core of the stuttering block. Venkatagiri (2005) implicates another feature of Levelt's model in modeling stuttering breakdown and its development in childhood. Motor encoding of utterances in this model is proposed to rely on a "mental syllabary," in which the most common syllables of a language are stored in memory as units to facilitate faster phonetic realization than would be possible with phoneme-by-phoneme encoding. In turn, the syllables are represented by "gestural scores" that specify the necessary involvement of each of five potential articulatory subsystems (glottis, velum, tongue body, tongue tip, and the lips). In stuttering, Venkatagiri hypothesizes that parts of the motor plan may be retrieved asynchronously from memory, leading to the array of behaviors that characterize the moment of stuttering.

Finally, although we discuss the Dynamic-Multifactorial model (Smith, 1999) in a following section, we note that this model includes a level of linguistic demand in its specification of conditions under which speech production instability is likely to arise and lead to stuttering (see Chapter 8 for experimental findings regarding interactions among cognitive, linguistic, and motor demands and stuttering). Likewise, Bosshardt's (2006) proposal that the neural systems subserving speech and language production are less modularized in stutterers than in typically fluent speakers, and thus more susceptible to task demand (see more on this model in the next section), specifies levels at which processing is vulnerable in people who stutter, including semantic and phonological encoding.

The Demands and Capacities Model (DCM) Starkweather (1987) has elaborated the point of view that stuttering results when demands for fluency from the child's social environment exceed the child's cognitive, linguistic, motor, or emotional capacities for fluent speech. According to this formulation, either low innate capacity or excessive speech and language pressures may cause fluency to disintegrate. Unlike most breakdown theories, it does not assume that organic deficits are a necessary condition for stuttering. The concept invokes environmental factors that have more often

[21] However, Lickley, Hartsuiker, Corley, Russell, and Nelson (2005) found stutterers to judge fluency of utterances more severely than nonstutterers; they hypothesize that stutterers' internal monitors become finely attuned to subtle deviations in intended speech output, whether or not they result in disfluencies or errors perceptible to listeners.

TABLE 2-1 Specification of Disfluency Types and Their Origins in the Covert Repair Hypothesis

Internal error source	Covert repair strategy	Resulting disfluency type
	Restart strategies	
Semantic or syntactic formulation	Restart the phrase	Phrase repetition
Lexical retrieval	Restart the previous word	Word repetition
Phonemic encoding error detected *before* word execution has begun	Restart syllable from beginning	Block
Phonemic encoding error detected after initial sound has been produced	Restart syllable from beginning	Prolongation *or* (sub) syllabic repetition
	Postponement strategies	
Semantic, syntactic, or lexical formulation	Hold execution and reformulate	Unfilled pause (>200 msec)
Phonemic encoding error detected *after* initial sound(s) produced	Prolong current sound until correct continuation sequence retrieved *OR* Hold execution of next sound	Prolong non-initial sounds in target syllable (typically vowel prolongation) *OR* Block in mid-syllable (broken word)

Source: Adapted from Postma & Kolk (1993).

TABLE 2-2 Covert Repairing in Intra-syllabic Interruptions*

Erroneous plan: SIT	Intended syllable: SIP
Executed part of the syllable upon error detection/interruption	Observed (intrasyllable) disfluency
– (no audible sound yet)	[3] ##..SIP (block)
S	[4] SSSIP (prolongation)
S	[5] S..S..SIP (repetition)
SI	[6] SI..SIP (repetition)
SI	[7] SIIIP (drawl)
SI	[8] SI#_P (broken word)
SIT	SIT..SIP (error + overt self-repair)

* The relation between how far a syllable is executed at the moment of interruption, and the type of resulting disfluency.
# Means a tense pause.
_ Means a clear silence.
Source: Adapted from Postma & Kolk (1993).

been considered in connection with anticipatory struggle theories, but the failure of the child's capacity for fluency to meet demands imposed upon it is assumed to lead directly to disorganization or breakdown of speech (see also Adams, 1990, and Starkweather & Gottwald, 1990). The model appears to capture the philosophy behind much of the basic research into cognitive, motor, and linguistic function in people who stutter: that at some level, stuttering reflects a weakness in the speech/language system that leaves it vulnerable to certain task demands. It is, of course, the specification of these demands that is so crucial to the refinement and thus the viability of the theory. Crucially, the Demands and Capacities Model (DCM) allows the potential for different mixes of speech, language, and motor limitations and environmental demands to create each individual case of stuttering. This tenet of the model has been criticized for rendering it untestable, since it does not require each person who stutters to demonstrate specific weaknesses or environmental pressures consistent with other stutterers.22

A model advanced by Hans-Georg Bosshardt and somewhat related conceptually to the underlying premise of the DCM places the basic limitations within the context of generalized task demand (see summary in Bosshardt, 2006). Using data from a series of monitoring and dual-task studies, Bosshardt suggests that a number of demands can affect the speed, fluency, and content of adult stutterers' speech output. However, Bosshardt's proposal is specific to cognitive processing load, which is presumed to impact speech production facility differentially in people who stutter than in those who are typically fluent. Results from a programmatic series of studies suggest that fluency in people who stutter is adversely impacted by increased cognitive loading and attentional processing demands. When faced with dual task conditions that impose an increased cognitive processing load, "either the disfluency rate increases or linguistic productivity decreases" (Bosshardt, 2006, p. 381). Additionally, his work suggests that the neural systems that support speech/language processing are more vulnerable to disruption under elevated demand in people who stutter because the cortical mechanisms underlying perception and production are less well-differentiated (or "modularized") than in normally fluent individuals.

Repressed Need Theories

We have considered the psychoanalytic assumption that the moment of stuttering represents an attempt to fulfill some type of unconscious neurotic need. On this assumption, the question of how stuttering originally develops becomes the question of how children acquire such needs and under what conditions they first try to satisfy them by stuttering. The answer we are given within the framework of classical Freudian theory is that these are essentially the same needs that underlie any other symptoms of psychosexual fixation and are brought about by the same conditions. Broadly speaking, the fixations are thought to stem from early conflicts over the satisfaction of the special psychic needs of infancy—chiefly oral and anal eroticism, dependence, aggressiveness, and self-assertion. Such conflicts are generally considered to grow out of disturbed parent-child relationships and to be related to abnormal feeding or nursing behavior of the mother, excessively harsh or early weaning or toilet training, parental domination, overprotection or overanxiety, or other traumatic features of the family environment that frequently go back to the parents' own neurotic conflicts.

Psychoanalytic writers for the most part have not been concerned with the special antecedent conditions leading to stuttering, as opposed to those leading to other forms of neurotic behavior, although a notable attempt to describe a specific family "constellation" for stuttering was made by Glauber (1958). From this point of view, there as yet appears to be little in the way of a unique psychoanalytic theory of the etiology of stuttering, to say nothing of competing theories of this kind. The important contributions of psychoanalysis have been the conceptual models of the moment of stuttering considered earlier in this chapter.

Anticipatory Struggle Theories

In our earlier discussion of the anticipatory struggle hypothesis, we reviewed a series of statements about the moment of stuttering that said, in effect, that stutterers interfere with the way they speak because of their belief in the difficulty of speech and their anticipation of speech failure. The question of the etiology of anticipatory struggle reactions is, then, the question of how children acquire such beliefs

---

[22] An entire issue of the *Journal of Fluency Disorders* (2000, volume 25, number 4) was devoted to scrutiny of the DCM.

and anticipations. The explanations that have been called on to account for this are essentially three in number and differ in the respect that they consider the causative factor of central importance to be (1) the child's excessive hesitations and repetitions (primary stuttering), (2) the parents' high standards of fluency (diagnosogenic theory), or (3) communicative failures or pressures, broadly viewed.

The Theory of Primary and Secondary Stuttering In Chapter 1, we had occasion to refer to an early view that stuttering arises as a reaction to unusual but relatively simple repetitions in a child's speech, termed *primary stuttering*. In accordance with this view, first advanced in somewhat different forms by Froeschels and Bluemel, stuttering first appears in the form of speech repetitions that occur without effort or awareness on the part of the child. This stage of the disorder was held to be essentially a normal phenomenon of early childhood and one that tends to disappear of its own accord if the child is prevented from learning that he or she is speaking differently. Sooner or later, however, it was argued, many primary stutterers are urged to "think" before they speak, to take a deep breath or to "stop and start over" so often that they become guilty and apprehensive about their mild speech interruptions.[23] The more serious form of the disorder was then believed to develop from the child's efforts to avoid primary stuttering. This advanced form, marked by strenuous blockages, fear, embarrassment, and various concomitant symptoms of effort and emotion, was characterized as *secondary stuttering*.

According to this theory of the development of stuttering, then, it is only some time after its onset, in a so-called secondary stage, that anticipatory struggle behavior emerges as children begin to react with anticipation, fear, and avoidance to their primary stuttering. In its incipient stage, it was considered to be something quite different. Primary stuttering was usually held to be a type of disintegration or breakdown, and both genetic and environmental factors were suggested as its chief cause. Van Riper, once its principal exponent, stated that in some instances the etiology was primarily constitutional, in others neurotic, and in still others stemmed from a home environment marked by frequent interruption, unresponsive listeners, demands to confess guilt orally, or other "fluency disruptors."

The theory that Weiss (1964) advanced regarding the relationship between stuttering and cluttering is also of interest here, in view of Weiss's identification of cluttering with primary stuttering. Cluttering, as it is usually described, is a disorder of fluency marked by monotonous, rapid, jerky, repetitive, indistinct utterances with frequent telescoping of words, unaccompanied by fear, anticipation, any sense of difficulty with specific words or sounds, or even a detailed awareness of speaking abnormally.[24] It has long been noted (e.g., Freund, 1934b) that stuttering and cluttering do not infrequently appear in the same person. In 1934, Weiss advanced the hypothesis that stuttering essentially always has its onset as a reaction of effort or struggle for the purpose of overcoming cluttering. Later, Weiss (1964, p. 71), perhaps employing a broader definition of cluttering than is usual, reflected that the difference between cluttering and Bluemel's primary stuttering was largely one of nomenclature.

As we noted in Chapter 1, knowledge of the early development of the symptoms of stuttering on the basis of scientific observation is still meager, but has been growing. While there is little doubt that relatively simple repetitions with little consistent emotional reaction are a feature of the speech of some young children who are regarded as stutterers, others appear to show a complex array of speech disfluencies that distinguishes their speech from that typically regarded as normal, and some also appear to show awareness and struggle. We will need much more research on the early presenting symptoms of stuttering, and perhaps even child and

[23] In 2003, the Stuttering Foundation of America reported the results of a study showing that this advisement is still the predominant response of adults when asked how they would respond to a child who stutters.

[24] Problematically, for the evaluation of this hypothesis, cluttering is itself poorly understood, and has been less well-researched over the years than stuttering (see a special issue of the *Journal of Fluency Disorders*, 1996, combined issues 3/4) that discusses this problem.

environmental characteristics that precede the onset of disfluency in order to evaluate the strength of such hypotheses.

Diagnosogenic Theory An alternative theory about the manner in which children learn to have anticipatory struggle reactions in their speech was offered by Johnson in 1942. This is the theory that the disorder is usually caused by a parent's inaccurate diagnosis of normal disfluencies in the child's speech as stuttering. As we have seen, Bluemel, Froeschels, and others had already identified developed stuttering, whether correctly or not, as a reaction to the relatively simple repetitions often noticeable in the speech of young stutterers. Froeschels, among others, had noted the similarity of these repetitions to those of many children considered normally fluent during their early stages of speech development. It remained for Johnson to make a final leap. Primary stuttering was not merely similar to normal childhood nonfluency, nor was it late-persisting or excessive normal nonfluency. The two were simply one and the same. According to Johnson's theory, it was not excessive hesitancy that usually caused a child to develop anticipatory reactions of struggle or avoidance, but abnormal parental reactions to this hesitancy. What others had termed primary stuttering was not a disorder to be treated. It was a normal attribute of speech. In order to prevent it from giving rise to stuttering, one needed to alter parents' evaluations of it.

Johnson was led to his conclusions while assisting in a study of young stuttering and nonstuttering children conducted under the direction of Lee E. Travis at the University of Iowa between 1934 and 1939. In the course of this investigation, he was struck by the fact that it was not always easy to distinguish the stutterers from the nonstutterers by listening to their speech. This led him to question the parents of the stutterers systematically about the nature of the speech interruptions that they had originally diagnosed as stuttering. Johnson found that the great majority of the descriptions that parents offered were confined to brief, "effortless" repetitions of syllables, words, and phrases of which the child was apparently "unaware," and he inferred that these descriptions were essentially similar to those that might have been made of the speech hesitations of most ordinary children.[25] Johnson's findings, as he summarized them some time later, may stand as a formal statement of his theory:

1. Practically every case of stuttering was originally diagnosed as such, not by a speech expert, but by a layman—usually one, or both, of the child's parents.
2. What these laymen had diagnosed as stuttering was, by and large, indistinguishable from the hesitations and repetitions known to be characteristic of the normal speech of young children ...
3. Stuttering ... as a definite disorder was found to occur, not before being diagnosed, but after being diagnosed. (Johnson, 1944)

Having been evaluated as a stutterer, in Johnson's view, the child was indeed likely to begin speaking differently in response to the parental anxieties, pressures, help, criticism, and correction that tended to go along with such a diagnosis. Thus, as Johnson put it, stuttering generally began "not in the child's mouth but in the parent's ear." This was not, however, because the parents were necessarily as aberrant in their perceptions of reality as this might seem to imply. Johnson believed that in most cases, they were essentially ordinary people whose concern about their child's speech hesitations, though exaggerated, was simply a reflection of rather unrealistic standards of speech and somewhat anxious, perfectionistic parental attitudes and child training policies broadly characteristic of our culture.

This is one of the best known of modern theories of stuttering, and various attempts have been made by researchers to evaluate it. So far, some evidence has accumulated that most young children are relatively disfluent and that some parents of stutterers can be characterized as dominating, overanxious, or perfectionistic. But Johnson's basic premise

[25]The findings of this study (Johnson et al., 1942) were presented in more detail in a subsequent publication (Johnson, 1955a) and also form the basis for Study I in his later and more extensive report of investigations of the onset of stuttering (Johnson & Associates, 1959).

that, "on the date of original diagnosis, stuttering children may speak in a manner that is not always to be clearly differentiated from that of other children of like age who have not been diagnosed as stutterers" has been exceedingly difficult to verify. Attempts to confirm it, based upon intensive interviewing of parents in cases of recent onset of the problem, or to find differences that systematically distinguish parents of young stutterers from those of normally fluent children have yielded results that must be regarded as highly equivocal at best.[26] We will return to this question in Chapters 9 and 12.

Theory of Communicative Pressure So far we have considered two ways in which anticipatory struggle reactions have been theorized to develop—chiefly through fear and avoidance of so-called primary stuttering and chiefly through fear and avoidance of "normal" disfluency. If stuttering is based upon the child's belief in the difficulty of speech, however, there would appear on the surface to be no clearly visible reason for supposing that there might not be other sources of such convictions from which stuttering might stem, and scattered references in the literature on stuttering have hinted strongly of such sources. An approach of this kind to the problem of the onset of stuttering was made by Bloodstein (1958, 1975) on the basis of a clinical study of 108 stuttering children. In essence, this viewpoint states that what is first identified as stuttering usually begins as a response of tension and fragmentation in speech, not sharply different from certain types of normal disfluency, and is brought about largely by the provocation of continued or severe communicative failure in the presence of communicative pressure.

This hypothesis finds its most significant elaboration with reference to the variety of factors that may contribute to a child's conviction that speech demands unusual effort or precautions. On the basis of clinical evidence, it appears possible that delayed language or articulation development, or practically any other kind of verbal weakness or impediment to communication may render children more or less chronically subject to the threat of speech failure to the degree that their attempts at speech may become more tense and fragmented than those of ordinary children who experience such difficulties in mild and intermittent form.

Such provocations might be assumed to be particularly likely to take effect if the children are subject, to a greater degree than average, to unrealistically high parental standards of speech or to other speech pressures such as competition with siblings more advanced in speech-language development, excessive praise for good speech, or identification with linguistically sophisticated adult language models. Finally, the likelihood cannot be ignored that there are certain personality and temperament traits (e.g., the tendency to be unusually sensitive, fearful, dependent, perfectionistic, easily frustrated, or too anxious for approval) that render a child more vulnerable to the provocations and pressures that may lead to anticipatory struggle behavior. In a similar vein, linguistic immaturity has been coupled with the child's temperament in Edward Conture's Communication-Emotional Model of Stuttering (Conture et al., 2006; Karrass et al., 2006; see Figure 2-2), as well as Barry Guitar's (2006) integrated model based on Grey's Behavioral Inhibition System model. In Guitar's view, separate constitutional predispositions may underlie primary and secondary stuttering. Motor and/or linguistic deficits may underlie the first, while temperament is the primary contributor to the second.

Such theories may perhaps be summarized most succinctly by the statement that stuttering is caused by the child's perception of communicative failure. From certain standpoints, it may be seen as a generalization of the two anticipatory struggle

[26]After Johnson's death, it was disclosed (Silverman, 1988) that there had been an attempt by one of his students (Mary Tudor, unpublished University of Iowa MA thesis, 1939) to experimentally test the diagnosogenic theory by providing misleading feedback to normally fluent children. Analysis of the primary data from the thesis leads to the conclusion that inappropriately labeling the study children as stutterers did not, in fact, create stuttering (see Ambrose & Yairi, 2002 and Goldfarb, 2006 for rather exhaustive discussion). Additional evidence relevant to the viability of the diagnosogenic theory is discussed in Chapter 10 (Stuttering as a Response) and Chapter 14 (Treatment). In particular, the success of recently popularized response-contingent therapies for preschool stuttering, such as Lidcombe (see Chapter 14), seriously weakens the plausibility of the diagnosogenic theory.

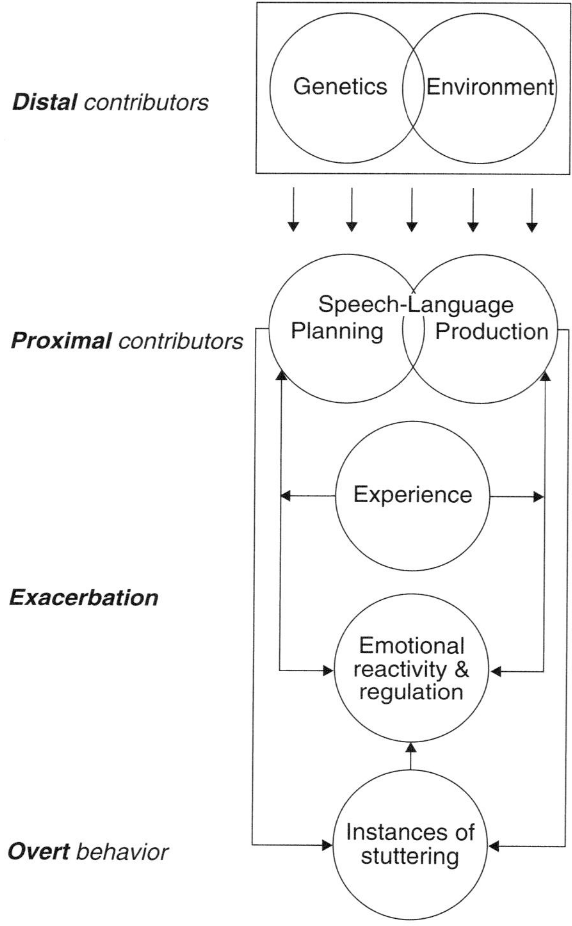

FIGURE 2-2 Conture et al.'s Communication-Emotional Model of stuttering (2006, p. 19). By permission of Lawrence Erlbaum Associates.

theories that we previously described. They differ from them, however, in requiring neither that a diagnosis of stuttering nor the occurrence of excessive repetitions in a child's speech is necessary in order for anticipatory struggle reactions to develop. Furthermore, they posit that incipient stuttering in its clinical form differs only in degree from anticipatory struggle reactions to be found in the speech of most children and so does not draw the sharp line between stuttering and normal disfluency that is required by the assumption that the one is the avoidance of the other. We will consider these issues further in Chapter 12.

THEORIES THAT SHIFT THE FRAME OF REFERENCE

A useful approach to the problem of stuttering is represented by the kind of theory that reformulates an existing concept about the disorder in terms of some new theoretical framework of scientific thinking. Such approaches to stuttering frequently present earlier theories in new relationships to other viewpoints and observations or reword them in new language with a desirable gain in verifiability.

Learning Theory Interpretations

Chief among such frames of reference that have held considerable appeal for theorists in the area of stuttering have been the stimulus response theories of learning that emerged through several decades of laboratory experimentation with animals in the latter half of the twentieth century. These learning theories have lent themselves to a number of systematic statements about stuttering. In general, the aim of such statements has been to make use of the relatively precise language of the behavioral sciences in order to try to define the process by which stuttering is learned and maintained by identifying the motivational factors, stimulus variables, and reinforcing conditions.

Stuttering as an Instrumental Avoidance Act

Much of the initial interest in the learning approach to stuttering was stimulated by the work of Wischner (1947, 1950, 1952b) within the framework of Clark L. Hull's theory of learning. Wischner based his formulations chiefly on two observations that had been the subject of considerable earlier research. One of these was the adaptation effect and the other was the phenomenon of expectancy or anticipation, which he equated with anxiety.[27]

[27]Adaptation and expectancy are discussed in Chapters 10 and 11.

Drawing an analogy between the tendency for stuttering to decrease with successive readings of the same passage (adaptation) and the experimental extinction of a learned response, he performed further adaptation studies that demonstrated what appeared to be analogues of such conditioning phenomena as spontaneous recovery, disinhibition, and conditioned inhibition.

One of the central problems in the application of learning principles to stuttering is to explain the nature of the reinforcement that causes it to persist in the face of repeated punishment. Wischner posited that this reinforcement consisted chiefly of a reduction in the stutterer's anxiety following the block. Prior to the moment of stuttering, there was a building up of expectancy, or fear. The immediate effect of stuttering was a reduction of this tension. Although the block obviously had punishing consequences, Wischner pointed out that these did not follow as immediately on the termination of the block as did the anxiety reduction. Consequently, the stuttering behavior was reinforced rather than extinguished.[28]

In general, Wischner likened stuttering to the so-called instrumental avoidance act, of which animal learning research has afforded many examples. A guinea pig may be placed in a cage constructed so that it will revolve when the animal runs and may be given an electric shock intermittently through the grillwork of the cage, preceded each time by the sound of a buzzer. If the apparatus is wired so that the electric current is shut off whenever the cage is in motion, the animal will quickly learn to escape the shock by running in response to the sound of the buzzer. This type of learned avoidance response has a peculiar feature distinguishing it from ordinary instrumental acts, such as learning to secure a pellet of food by depressing a bar. *It is unusually difficult to extinguish.* The bar-depressing act may be eradicated simply by withholding the food pellets. No such effect on the guinea pig's running response is produced by eliminating the shock, however, unless the animal accidentally fails to run and thereby "discovers" that the grill is no longer charged. Wischner stated that, from this point of view, there appeared to be a significant parallel between stuttering and the running behavior of the guinea pig. What is generally termed stuttering behavior, as Johnson had pointed out, may consist of little or nothing but stutterers' efforts to avoid stuttering. If stutterers could bring themselves to attempt their feared words without such efforts, they would be able to say them fluently. Like the guinea pig, however, they do not stop running long enough or often enough to acquire the conviction that the grill is not "hot."

Wischner's main analysis clearly consisted in part of a reformulation of Johnson's concept of the moment of stuttering as an anxiety-motivated avoidance reaction. In discussing the origin of the disorder, Wischner suggested that it was to be found in some kind of painful, anxiety-producing stimulation. He referred to Johnson's diagnosogenic theory as a tenable hypothesis from this standpoint, suggesting that the original instigators of anxiety in the stutterer might be parental disapproval of normal disfluency.

Stuttering as Approach-Avoidance Conflict Sheehan (1953, 1958a) viewed stuttering primarily as the result of a conflict between opposing drives to speak and to hold back from speaking and developed an interpretation of the moment of stuttering based on Neal E. Miller's research and theoretical formulations on approach-avoidance conflict in animals. Miller (1944) showed that, as a hungry rat approaches a food trough at the end of a runway, its motivation to reach the food steadily increases. It is possible to measure the strength of its approach drive, and to show by means of a sloping line precisely how it increases with nearness to the goal. If electric shock is substituted for the food, the rat flees. The farther it gets from the feared object, however, the weaker becomes its motivation to avoid it, and this declining avoidance drive may also be represented by a sloping line, or gradient. If electric shock and food are now combined, together with the appropriate cue-stimuli by which the rat may recognize their presence, the element of conflict

[28] See Wischner (1952a), Sheehan and Voas (1954), Luper (1956), Sheehan, Cortese, and Hadley (1962) for experimental findings related to the fear-reduction hypothesis regarding the reinforcement of stuttering.

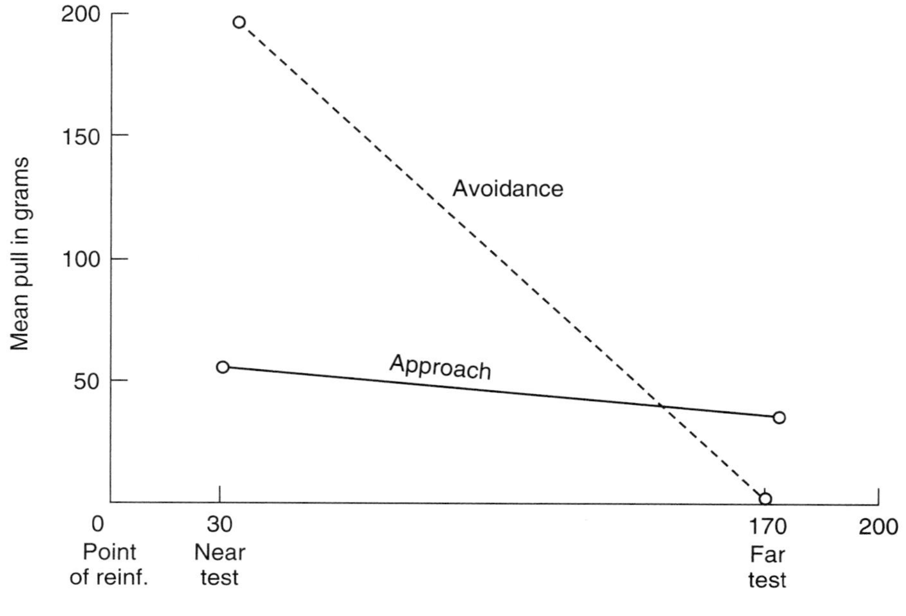

FIGURE 2-3 Gradients of approach and avoidance as determined by Miller. The approach gradient shows the force with which rats deprived of food for 48 hours pulled against a restraining harness at various distances from the point at which they had been fed. The avoidance gradient shows the force with which rats pulled away from the point at which they had previously been given a strong electric shock. Adapted from Miller, 1944.

is introduced. In such a situation, the approach and avoidance drives are present together, and it is possible to represent this by showing both gradients superimposed on the same field (Figure 2-3). Since the gradients slope in the same direction (both approach and avoidance increasing with nearness to the goal) they would appear as close parallel lines or the same line, except for one all-important fact. *The gradient of avoidance is steeper than the gradient of approach.*[29] As a result, if the opposing drives are of about the same average strength, at a certain distance from the goal the two gradients will intersect. This fact has some rather significant implications. Before the point of intersection is reached, the approach gradient is higher than the avoidance gradient, and the rat could be expected to run toward the goal. Once the animal had passed the intersection, however, it would find itself in a zone in which the strength of avoidance exceeded the strength of approach, and it could therefore be expected to turn and run the other way until approach exceeded avoidance again. This is precisely how Miller's rats behaved. They ran back and forth, vacillating within progressively narrower limits until they came to rest where the gradients apparently crossed, unable to go forward or back.

In Miller's description of the oscillatory behavior and fixations of these animals, Sheehan found a parallel to the speech hesitations of stutterers. He stated that stuttering was basically an approach-avoidance conflict. Whenever stutterers' urge to speak was distinctly stronger than their desire to

[29]This simply means that, within any given unit of distance from the goal or feared object, the amount of change in the strength of avoidance is greater than the amount of change in the strength of approach.

avoid speech, they spoke fluently. When avoidance of speaking was the clearly dominant drive, they were silent. But when their approach and avoidance drives were in relative equilibrium, so that the gradients crossed, they stuttered. Unlike the rat, however, the stutterer does not remain fixated for an indefinite time. How could the termination of the block be accounted for? Sheehan offered the hypothesis that once the blocking had begun to take place, the fear that had elicited it became reduced, the avoidance drive was consequently decreased, and so the conflict was temporarily resolved. Sheehan theorized further that the stutterer's conflicting feelings of approach and avoidance toward speech tended to be complicated by similar attitudes toward silence, and he pointed out that this, too, had its counterpart in the laboratory in the condition that Miller termed "double approach-avoidance conflict."

As we have already said, in a conflict analysis of stuttering behavior, the fundamental question of why the act of stuttering occurs finally reduces itself to the question of the reasons for which a person might wish to avoid speech. Sheehan postulated five distinct "levels" on which speech avoidance drives might operate. He stated that these drives might emanate from (1) reactions to specific words, resulting principally from past conditioning to phonetic factors, (2) reactions to threatening speech situations, (3) guilt and anxiety concerning the emotional content of speech, (4) feelings of anxiety in the stutterer's relationships with listeners, especially when these are seen as authority figures, and (5) the ego-defensive need to avoid competitive endeavors posing "threat of failure or threat of success."

This clearly suggests that stuttering may have its origin both in the learning of speech anxieties and in unconscious personality factors. Sheehan's formulations made little explicit reference to events surrounding the onset of stuttering. The essence of their contribution to stuttering theory is in the development of Miller's approach-avoidance conflict structure as a model of the moment of stuttering. The unique feature of this model, which Sheehan fully exploited, lies in its ability to adapt itself to both the repressed need and anticipatory struggle concepts of stuttering behavior, and so by implication to admit a very broad array of logically possible etiologies. Sheehan (1970, 1975) later extended his theory still further by viewing the stutterer's difficulty as an approach-avoidance conflict between alternate roles assumed as a stutterer and as a normal speaker.

Perkins (1953) pointed out that the logical implication of the conflict hypothesis was that the stuttering block itself was not learned behavior. Since it was the involuntary result of the learned avoidance and approach drives, he believed that the block itself was not dependent on reinforcement and should not be subject to extinction by nonreinforcement. Both Sheehan (1951) and Perkins (1953) attempted to determine the effect on stuttering of nonreinforcement, which they defined by a procedure in which a person repeated each stuttered word until they could say it normally, and obtained somewhat conflicting results.

Stuttering as Operant Behavior In 1958, Flanagan, Goldiamond, and Azrin announced that they had been able to reduce the stuttering of three laboratory volunteers very markedly by presenting a 105 dB blast of tone immediately after each occasion on which the stutterers blocked, and to increase the frequency of stuttering by briefly turning off a continuous tone each time they stuttered. Not long afterward, they reported that they had produced speech blockages at a high rate in a normally fluent speaker by similar use of continuous electric shock (Flanagan, Goldiamond, & Azrin, 1959). These reports suggesting that stuttering and normal disfluency could be brought under "operant control" did much to arouse interest in investigating these behaviors by applying the conditioning principles of B. F. Skinner.

In Skinner's system of behavioral analysis, a central role is played by the kind of response, termed an operant, that is capable of being increased or decreased through its consequences as they affect the organism. In terms of a reference experiment, such as that in which a rat learns to press a lever when the response produces a pellet of food, operant conditioning is identical with what other psychologists termed instrumental conditioning, or instrumental act learning, but Skinner developed a distinctive conceptual scheme for its laboratory investigation. An outstanding feature distinguishing this scheme from theories of learning such as that of Hull is its strict renunciation of terms referring to hypothetical states inside the organism, such as *drive* or *anxiety*. While Hull described a reinforcement as "positive" or "negative" based on typical perceptions of its nature, Skinner eschewed such value judgments, because they required knowing the subject's state of mind during reinforcement. Rather, he defined reinforcements as positive when they increased behaviors and negative when they decreased the frequency of behaviors—in other words, the valence of the reinforcement was determined by observing its effects. In either view, an important aspect of the laboratory description of operant conditioning is the precise schedule on which it is administered.

Shames and Sherrick (1965) attempted to view stuttering behavior in the light both of the diagnosogenic theory and of certain psychodynamic inferences about stuttering. Asserting that there is "no single, simple contingency for stuttering," they suggested that it is maintained by both positive and negative reinforcements on complex, multiple schedules. In large part, the paradigms they proposed as worthy of investigation were suggested by Johnson's theory of the etiology of stuttering.

They hypothesized that when a child's nonfluent responses are punished, the child may respond by changing the form of nonfluency to struggle or silence. This change is reinforced by the termination of the aversive stimuli of nonfluency (negative reinforcement), but may occasion new punishment. Further cycles of change in the response may then take place, reinforced in each case by the termination of aversive stimuli coming from the listener (negative listener reactions), and are also occasioned by the fact that stutterers tend to become their own listeners. In the process, the original simple repetition degenerates through negative reinforcement into the abnormal response forms that are characteristic of stuttering. At the same time, however, there are certain positive reinforcements for stuttering. The child may gain attention or may use stuttering as an excuse for failure or inadequacy. Shames and Sherrick speculated that the cycles of change cease when a "dynamic equilibrium" evolves in which the positive reinforcements for a particular pattern of stuttering are stronger than its aversive consequences or the negative reinforcements for further change.

Approaching the problem from a somewhat different point of view, Shames and Sherrick posited that normal disfluency is also operant behavior and that stuttering and normal disfluency are in certain respects similar and continuous rather than completely separate classes of responses. On this assumption, any contingencies observed to influence the frequency of disfluencies in children's speech may be similar to those that control stuttering as a clinical disorder. Shames and Sherrick called attention to several ways in which disfluency may come to be reinforced by its contingent consequences.

For example, in a group situation, speech repetitions were found to occur frequently when the normal-speaking child tries to gain attention by directing the activities of another child, obtaining an object possessed by someone else, criticizing another child, or the like (Davis, 1940). These examples belong for the most part to a type of verbal behavior that Skinner termed *manding*. They tend to occur on occasions of aversive stimulation or in states of deprivation, and as a consequence the listener frequently does something for or gives something to the child. In this way, not only the verbalization but the repetition as well is reinforced. This reinforcement is likely to be particularly strong because of the variable schedule on which it is usually given; responses that are intermittently reinforced are particularly resistant to extinction. Furthermore, if an unresponsive listener delays the reinforcement until the child has repeated the "manding" verbal behavior several times, the child is in effect being taught to repeat. Shames and Sherrick offered similar operant analyses of the increased repetition that might be observed in children when confessing guilt, speaking to interrupting listeners, competing with other speakers, or attempting to hold the listener's attention during pauses.

Various other researchers have made use of the operant model in connection with stuttering. For the most part, however, they have been less concerned with etiological theories than with experimental demonstrations of the operant nature of stuttering and disfluency. The result has been a considerable amount of research on punishment in relation to stuttering, which we will review in Chapter 11, and the development of operant treatments for stuttering, especially in its early stages (see Chapter 14).

Stuttering as Conditioned Disintegration Brutten and Shoemaker (1967), in contrast, theorized that stuttering in its integral aspects is a failure or disruption of fluency resulting from emotional arousal that has become associated with speech and speech-related stimuli through a process of classical conditioning. From this point of view, the stuttering block represents not operant, but respondent, behavior.

Most investigators of the learning process recognize at least a rough distinction between two kinds of learning, one based on operant or instrumental conditioning and the other on respondent or classical conditioning. Classical conditioning is represented by the well-known Pavlovian experiment in which a dog learns to salivate in response to a bell after several contiguous presentations of the bell with food. The fundamental point of contrast with operant learning is that the salivation is not instrumental in securing a reward. The dog gets the food whether performing the response or not, unlike the rat who is learning to operate a lever in a Skinner box. From the standpoint of the method used to bring learning about, in instrumental conditioning the basic contingency is between a response and a consequence. In classical conditioning, it is between two stimuli, one (e.g., food) having the power to elicit the response as an unlearned organismic reaction and the other a "neutral" stimulus having no such power until it is associated with the first.

How broad a role classical conditioning plays in shaping human behavior is a matter of theory. It appears to be widely agreed, however, that it plays an important part in the learning of anxiety reactions or other motivational states of autonomic arousal. Through classical conditioning, for example, a child who has once or twice responded autonomically to the doctor's needle may show a similar response to the doctor, or (by "higher-order" classical conditioning) to the doctor's driveway, and (by stimulus generalization) to white-coated persons anywhere.

This is the significance that classical conditioning has for stuttering from the point of view of Brutten and Shoemaker. They based their theory on the observation that, in normally fluent speakers, stress may produce autonomic reactions capable of disrupting speech fluency. If a child repeatedly encounters stress in a given situation, the negative emotional arousal may become a conditioned response to neutral stimuli in the situation. This marks the onset of the initial stage of stuttering. The child now regularly experiences emotional arousal with its attendant fluency failure each time the situational cues are present, instead of infrequently and sporadically as is usually the case. Furthermore, these cues, still chiefly situational in nature, increase in number through higher-order conditioning and stimulus generalization. Brutten and Shoemaker suggested that a further, or "advanced," stage of stuttering comes into being through penalties the child receives for abnormal speech behavior. As a result of such punishment, the act of speaking itself, or the words employed, come to elicit conditioned negative emotion, and in time the conditioned stimuli for fluency failure may for this reason consist increasingly of speech-associated cues (i.e., words, listeners, and the like).

In support of their basic premise that stress, occasioned by the threat of painful stimulation, tends to increase disfluency, Brutten and Shoemaker pointed to observations by Hill (1954), Stassi (1961), and others. Perhaps the most direct experimental support for their theory came from Hill's work. In a study of normally fluent speakers, Hill found that, when a red light that served as a signal for speech had been paired with electric shock on several occasions, the light by itself produced disorganized speech responses often "indistinguishable from what is generally termed stuttering."

It should be noted that Brutten and Shoemaker regarded the so-called secondary features of stuttering as instrumental escape or avoidance mechanisms for coping with fluency failures or the noxious states resulting from them. This, however, is the only role they assigned to operant conditioning. Their theory therefore presents us with a useful and relatively clear-cut question, whether the integral symptoms of stuttering represent classically or instrumentally conditioned behavior, assuming that they represent one or the other. Brutten and Shoemaker actually referred to their conception of stuttering as a "two-factor theory," since it holds that the integral and associated symptoms are learned through two different kinds of conditioning. There does seem to be some evidence that the distinction between the two types of symptoms is not one of outward appearance alone,[30] but there is as yet no satisfactory answer to the question whether they represent two different types of conditioning.

Finally, it is of interest that it is clearly a breakdown concept of the moment of stuttering that is expressed in this theory, and, unlike other learning-oriented viewpoints, it owes less to Johnson's thinking than to that of West. The development of stuttering is ascribed, not to speech anxiety, but to stress in essentially any form, and constitutional predisposition, in the form of innate susceptibility to conditioning and autonomic reactivity, is considered to play a part.

West observed that, in time, speech anxiety came to be a major source of the stress that precipitated moments of breakdown in speech. This, too, has its counterpart in Brutten and Shoemaker's observation that, as stuttering develops, the autonomic reactions disruptive of fluency become increasingly conditioned to speech-associated stimuli as a result of speech-related punishment. A major important difference lies in the role assigned to learning. The dysphemic viewpoint that was widely influential some years ago contained a notable gap. It never explained convincingly how the chronic tendency to speech breakdown that was postulated to underlie stuttering blocks could have been initiated by a single original episode of breakdown in early childhood, as though speech were a strut that, once broken, remained irreparably weak. In transferring the breakdown concept to a learning frame of reference, Brutten and Shoemaker bridged the gap effectively through the medium of stimulus substitution by classical conditioning.

Cybernetic Models of Stuttering

As we all learned as schoolchildren, the widespread replacement of hand tools with power-driven machines that began in the nineteenth century is commonly regarded as an industrial "revolution." What is less evident to most is that it was followed by a second development in the use of mechanical devices that was no less revolutionary than the first. This was the introduction of machines and computers that regulate themselves by automatic control systems or servomechanisms. Analogies between mechanical and computational servosystems and human perceptual and physiological function quickly followed. The term cybernetics refers to systems of control and communication in machines and in living organisms.

Automatic Control Systems The basic principle of a servomechanism is that of *feedback*. An ordinary machine consists of an effector unit producing output in the form of some type of work and a device for regulating or controlling it. In a servosystem, the essential added feature is a means for feeding back part of the output of the machine and allowing it to play on the control mechanism in such a way that what the machine does is regulated by its performance. A simple example of a servomechanism is the one that regulates the usual type of home heating system. The heating unit is controlled by a temperature-sensitive device, or thermostat, that automatically turns on or shuts off the unit when its output, the temperature of the room, differs by a certain amount from a desired output as represented by the setting on the thermostat. A system of this sort obviously depends upon its ability to perform a

---

[30] The integral and secondary features of stuttering have been reported to load differently in a factor analysis of stuttering phenomena (Prins & Lohr, 1972), to vary in frequency differently in the course of repeated readings of the same material (Sakata & Adams, 1972; Webster & Brutten, 1972), and to respond differently to contingent stimuli and instructions to avoid stuttering (see Chapters 10 and 11).

simple internal handling of information. The invention of computers made possible the development of a large variety of complex servomechanisms for such purposes as automatic control of industrial processes and automatic guidance of space vehicles.

The major components of an automatic control system may be described in general terms. The system contains a *sensor*, through which part of the output of the machine is converted to a form in which it can be fed back as information to the *controller* unit. The controller unit contains a *comparator*, which compares the actual output with some intended performance in the form of instructions that have been stored in the controller as a unit of input. The difference between these two sets of data emerges from the comparator as an error signal. This is mixed with the input signal to produce an effective driving signal, which modifies the action of the *effector* unit so that its output more nearly equals the intended output.

Cybernetic Theories of Speech An exceedingly interesting fact about the principle of feedback is that its significance extends substantially beyond the realm of mechanical devices. Wiener (1948) coined the term *cybernetics* to cover the broad application of automatic control principles and a related development known as information theory to engineering, biology, and the behavioral sciences. Some notable examples of biological systems that are illuminated by servo theory are the kinesthetic and proprioceptive mechanisms for automatic control of motor activity and the various internal homeostatic mechanisms for regulating body temperature, blood pressure, water balance, and the chemical contents of the blood and alveolar air.

The normal production of speech is an automatic process whose dependence on feedback had long been taken for granted. Although the extent of this dependence is no longer accepted without question, it should come as no surprise that a number of cybernetic models of speech have been proposed and elaborated over the years. A basic first-level schematic of the speech mechanism as a servosystem was drawn by Fairbanks (1954). In Fairbanks' model (Figure 2-4), the effector unit corresponds to the parts of the speech mechanism and their motor innervation. The major sensor is the ear, which senses the output of the effector unit through two channels, symbolizing air and bone conduction. The hypothetical controller unit is obviously some feature of the brain. Fairbanks deliberately refrained from speculating about its precise identity. He hypothesized that at a given moment during speech, its storage contains a unit of input that corresponds to as much as we can "hold in mind" of what we intend to say. This unit of input is continually compared with feedback about the output. The error signal that results from this comparison is a measure of the amount by which the speech unit displayed in the storage device has not yet been realized. The error signal is sent to the mixer, where it contributes to the effective driving signal. Simultaneously, it is also sent to the storage, where it signals the storage to continue to display the speech unit, or, when the error signal is about to equal zero, to display the next unit. Fairbanks pointed out that the source of input to the controller was a language system, not shown in his diagram, which originates messages. His model was concerned only with the speech production system.

Delayed Auditory Feedback (DAF) and "Stuttering" in Normal Speakers At about the same time that Fairbanks offered his feedback theory of speech, attention was being drawn to the possibility that a link existed between feedback and stuttering. This came about principally as the result of an observation that was first made by Lee (1950a, 1950b, 1951) and that has been confirmed by a large number of further investigations by others. It became possible, by means of a suitably designed magnetic-tape recorder, to return a subject's vocal output to the subject via earphones with a brief delay in transmission (such delays are now induced via digital signal processing). The basic observation with which we are concerned is that, when normal speakers' air-conducted auditory feedback is delayed by a time interval of the order of 0.2 seconds and amplified sufficiently to compete with their normal bone-conducted feedback, verbal output appears to suffer markedly (this phenomenon can be observed

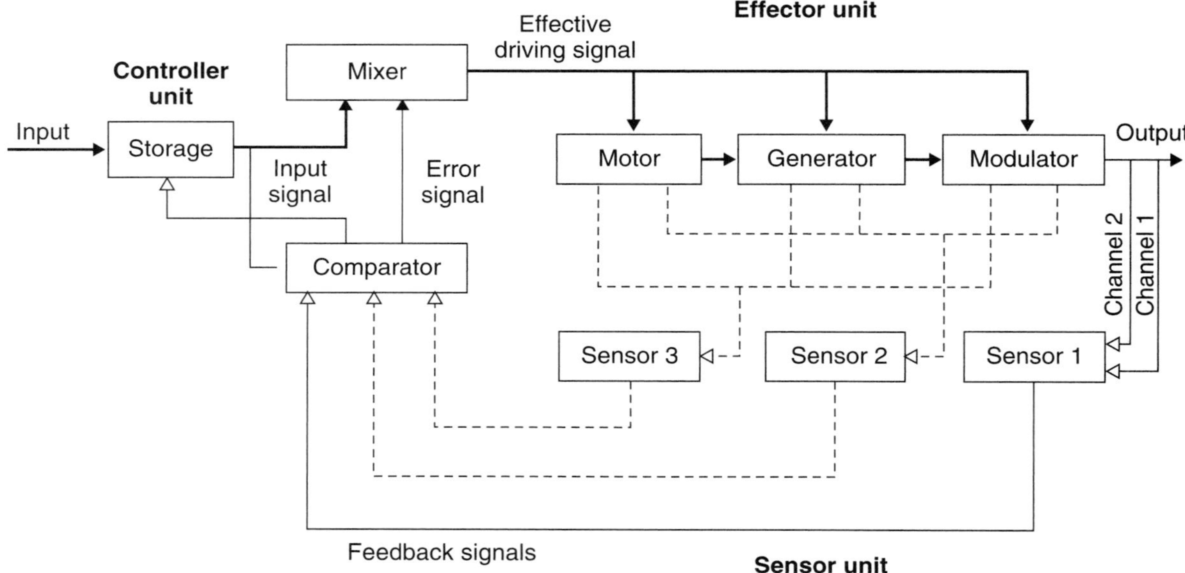

FIGURE 2-4 Fairbanks' model of an automatic control system for speaking. The respiratory, phonatory, and articulatory parts of speech mechanism are represented as motor, generator, and modulator respectively. Part of their audible output is conducted to the speaker's ear (sensor 1) by means of two channels (air and bone conduction). A hypothetical comparator unit compares the feedback signals from the sensor with an input (from a language system, not shown) representing an intended message unit. The difference, representing the amount by which the intended message unit has not yet been completed, is fed to the mixer where it is combined with the input signal and serves to modify the operation of the effector so that its output more closely approximates the intended message unit. The portions of the model represented by broken lines represent tactile and proprioceptive feedback mechanisms providing information about the operation of the effector, but not about its output. Reprinted with permission from Fairbanks, G. Systematic research in experimental phonetics: 1. A theory of the speech mechanism as a servosystem. Journal of Speech and Hearing Disorders, 19, 133–39.

when listeners "call in" to radio programs and fail to turn down their own radios while attempting to talk "on the air"). This disintegration may take the form of slowed speaking rate, articulatory inaccuracy, and disturbances of fluency, including, in some cases, blockings and repetition of syllables that may offer a realistic imitation of clinical stuttering. In addition, there is often an increase in loudness and pitch, which Fairbanks (1955) inferred was the result of the speakers' struggle to resist the interference with their response.

It is, of course, in the repetitions that we are most interested. Fairbanks and Guttman (1958) found that in a relatively small number of speakers, the characteristic response was frequent repetition and that the repetition consisted almost entirely of simple double articulations. Several explanations of these repetitions have been offered over the years. Lee (1950a) initially compared them with the behavior of an unstable electronic circuit oscillating with feedback that the first chance disturbance has set off. More generally, they are regarded as a direct effect of the misinformation that Delayed Auditory Feedback (DAF) gives speakers about their speech output. Lee (1950b) conjectured that the "unsatisfied monitor" of the speech circuit causes the loop to "continue for an extra turn or two" until the missing feedback returns. In short, if you say it and you don't hear it, you think you haven't said it, so you say it again. Fairbanks and Guttman

(1958) offered a somewhat different explanation. They inferred that, in a rapid sequence of serial speech responses, each response cannot be evoked individually. It must therefore be cued automatically by feedback from the preceding response. If so, delayed feedback from the first response dominates the feedback complex during a second response, and will trigger a repetition of the second response.[31]

Speech Behavior under DAF as an Analogue of Stuttering Lee referred to his effect as an "artificial stutter" and expressed the view that it might have significant implications for speech therapy. Soon afterward, Fairbanks (1955) and other investigators of the DAF phenomenon were similarly intrigued by its hypothetical relationship to stuttering. Chase (1958) discovered that most speakers could repeat a speech sound faster under DAF than with normal feedback and suggested that the factors responsible for this might also be at work in some types of stuttering. In the meantime, experiments had shown that many stutterers speak more fluently under conditions of loud white noise (see Chapter 11), and it was tempting to speculate that the noise served to mask out the stutterer's innately deviant auditory feedback.

Clearly, the interest that developed in the Lee effect as an analogue of stuttering rests on what may be nothing more than a chance resemblance between two unrelated kinds of behavior. Attempting to gauge the extent of this similarity, Neelley (1961) found that listeners were usually able to distinguish the speech of normally fluent speakers under DAF from the speech of stutterers. Additionally, stutterers reported that their habitual stuttering and their speech behavior under DAF were different kinds of experiences. Neelley also tried to determine whether normally fluent speakers' errors under DAF tended to occur consistently on the same words and to decrease in frequency with successive readings of the same material, as is characteristic of stuttering.[32] He found far less consistency and adaptation in the typically fluent speakers under DAF than in his stuttering participants in an ordinary reading situation. Neelley concluded that his findings as a whole tended to discredit the hypothesis that stuttering is related to delayed auditory feedback. This conclusion has been countered by Yates (1963), Beech and Fransella (1968, p. 169), and others with the argument that behavior that has been subject to change and development over many years is bound to differ in many respects from similar behavior when it is exhibited by laboratory subjects for the first time.

Brandt and Wilde (1977) found that, like stuttering, normally fluent speakers' disfluency under DAF was reduced when people read in unison with another voice and when they timed their speech to the beat of a metronome. Borden, Dorman, Freeman, and Raphael (1977) observed both similarities and differences between normally fluent speakers under DAF and stutterers in the electromyographic recordings from laryngeal and articulatory muscles. Venkatagiri (1980, 1982a) found that, like stutterings, the DAF disfluencies of normally fluent speakers showed a distinct adaptation effect over successive readings and occurred more often on content words than on function words and more often on long words than on short words. Unlike stuttering events, they did not occur preponderantly on the first syllables of words or the first words of sentences.[33] Although the consistency effect was present, it was considerably smaller than it is in the case of stuttering.

[31] Fairbanks and Guttman showed that, given certain assumptions, this explanation implies that a single repetition will temporarily restore the normal phase relationship between response and feedback. The explanation was therefore consistent with their observation that the repetitions of normally fluent speakers under DAF generally consist of simple double articulations except in rare instances that "give the impression of wild and uncontrolled oscillation of the vocal mechanism." It should be noted, incidentally, that the syllable repetitions of stutterers consist largely of double and triple articulations that appear with about equal frequency (see the normative data gathered by Johnson, 1961a).

[32] Consistency and adaptation effects in stuttering are discussed in Chapter 10.

[33] See Chapter 11. Venkatagiri comments, "These differences, however, are not unexpected. . . . In order to delay the feedback, the speech must be produced in the first place." How stuttering can occur on initial syllables poses a problem for the delayed auditory feedback theory.

Perturbed auditory feedback has been used as the basis for additional models of stuttering over the years and has received additional attention with the advent and broad advertisement of portable altered feedback devices for the treatment of stuttering (see Chapter 14). As noted in Chapter 4, there may be a relationship between responses to DAF and atypical anatomic asymmetry in cortical regions subserving speech and language (Foundas et al., 2004) for a subset of individuals who stutter.

Another proposal that utilizes speakers' responses to altered auditory feedback to model the underlying deficit in stuttering has been offered by Saltuklaroglu, Kalinowski, and Guntupalli (2004). These authors suggest that the reason why altered auditory feedback ameliorates symptoms of stuttering is that it engages the cortical "mirror neuron" system, which is activated in response to the motor activity human and nonhuman primates observe in their environment. In this case, an exogenous signal activates the mirror neuron system, which facilitates accurate speech gesture encoding. However, their model does not posit a causal role for the mirror neuron system in the proximal cause of stutters, which they view as potentially likely to emerge from problems in "sensory to motor integration of speech gestures." (p. 446) Thus, this particular interpretation of servosystems theory may intersect with the class of physiological models discussed earlier in the chapter.

Stuttering as "Verbalizing Deautomaticity"
Whether or not stuttering is related to delayed auditory feedback is not crucial to a theory of stuttering based on automatic control principles. Mysak (1960, 1966) brought a wide range of concepts about stuttering within the scope of servo theory by a cybernetic interpretation of the view that stuttering is basically a failure of the automaticity of speech. Mysak proposed the hypothesis that a disturbance in essentially any of the feedback circuits of the servosystem that maintains the automatic flow of verbal communication may result in stuttering. Extending Fairbanks' model to include language as well as speech, he discussed the various parts of the system in which the disturbances may occur.

1. They may occur in a hypothetical integrator unit in which thought and language connections are made. For example, unconscious guilt about verbal expressions of hostility may cause blocks or hesitations as the speaker "feels the need to guard against the automatic processing of his thoughts into words." Mysak refers to psychoanalytic concepts of stuttering and to Sheehan's conflict theory in this connection.
2. Disturbance may occur in that part of the speech controller (transmitter, in Mysak's terminology) in which word patterns are formulated internally as commands to the effector unit. As examples, Mysak cites the repetitive speech disruptions that have been observed to accompany such disorders as Parkinsonism and pseudobulbar palsy and the interference with speech that Penfield and Roberts noted on electrical stimulation of certain areas of the brain in their well-known studies. West's theory of stuttering as an epileptiform disorder of speech is also noted here.
3. Reformulating Johnson's views in terms of servo theory, Mysak suggests that the overmonitoring of fluency by "another communication system" may cause the development of a predicted fluency error signal in a child's speech comparator. As a result, the child's system may engage in an intentional scanning of its output for nonexistent error signals in a manner that interferes with speech automaticity.
4. Stuttering may originate in the sensor unit, as indicated by the effects on speech of disturbances in auditory feedback.
5. Finally, speech automaticity may be affected by disturbances in a feedback loop involving the listener. That is, if children repeatedly receive listener reactions indicating that their message has not been understood, they may come to anticipate such feedback and to "habitually reformulate or repeat" their utterances.

It is clear that in Mysak's theory, stuttering is defined very broadly. The possibility must be considered, however, that such a broad definition is inherent in the servo model. That is, if stuttering results from the breakdown of an interdependent circuitry that functions as a whole, then from the standpoint of the model there may be little justification for making sharp distinctions based on the cause or locus of the disturbance.

The Adaptive Model Theory A much more specific theory has been proposed by Peter and Megan Neilson (see Neilson & Neilson, 1987; Neilson, Neilson, O'Dwyer, and Summers, 1992; Neilson & Neilson, 2005) that specifies the consequences of impairment in various stages and functions involved in purposeful motor movements, such as sensory analysis, motor planning, and motor execution. They have developed a computational model and simulations of how human motor movement is implemented and self-corrected under various feedback conditions. In particular, they view fluent speech as too rapid a process to rely primarily on auditory feedback, and posit it to be more dependent on feedforward control. In a feedforward system, a central controller considers a number of factors that govern how the speech production system will execute target trajectories to produce desired acoustic output. These factors include inherent time delays that characterize communication among the systems required to produce and monitor speech output, the nonlinear dynamic interactions that characterize muscle control systems and biomechanical loads, and external factors that mediate how the vocal tract changes shape, and translates force and movement commands. This system also has the capability to construct what is called "an inverse internal model" of desired acoustic output. In other words, the system can reason backwards from the acoustic characteristics of speech (either one's own, or someone else's), to compute the speech motor commands that were used to generate them. That this system is in place early in life is clear, as infants learn to produce sounds, especially vowels, that are characterized by the appropriate patterns of formants required for their identification, even though the infant vocal tract is not like those of the adults providing the speech models. The infant and developing child learn to model the appropriate vocal tract configurations that yield the desired, corresponding acoustic patterns, and over time, the system develops the ability to generate a set of practiced trajectories that correspond to desired outputs. Gradually, the system becomes adept at comparing output commands to an efferent copy of the commands that generate hypothetical results from them; when the two don't match or are perturbed for some reason, adjustments can be made quickly by a typically fluent speaker.[34] The system is also a parallel transmission system:[35] while the feedforward controller is executing one response, the gesture trajectory generator is at work planning the next response. Feedback from the inverse modeling component of the system can confirm or contrast with the planned output of the feedforward system. The model proposes that stuttering represents an intermittent flaw in the neural processes that are involved in creating or realizing these complex motor activities (see Figure 2-5).

Earlier work by the team (Neilson, Quinn, & Neilson, 1976) had found that adults who stutter were relatively poorer at trying to use motor responses (a cursor) to generate a tone (fed to one ear) that would match an auditory model presented to the other ear. Thus, stuttering could be viewed as a consequence of a system that has difficulty making sensory to motor and motor to sensory transformations. Max, Guenther, Gracco, Ghosh, and Wallace (2004) posit a weakness in the feedforward system that makes the stutterer inappropriately dependent on auditory and somatosensory feedback, an inherently less successful system. Like the Neilsons, they have computationally simulated the consequences of such feedforward and feedback patterns in a neural network model called DIVA (Directions into Velocities of Articulators).

[34] An additional detailed discussion of the Neilson and Neilson model, with a schematic of its components, can be found in Guitar, 2006, pp. 108–11.

[35] In a parallel model, multiple stages of planning and execution can occur simultaneously or overlap in time; such models contrast with serial transmission models, in which one stage must be completed before the next may begin.

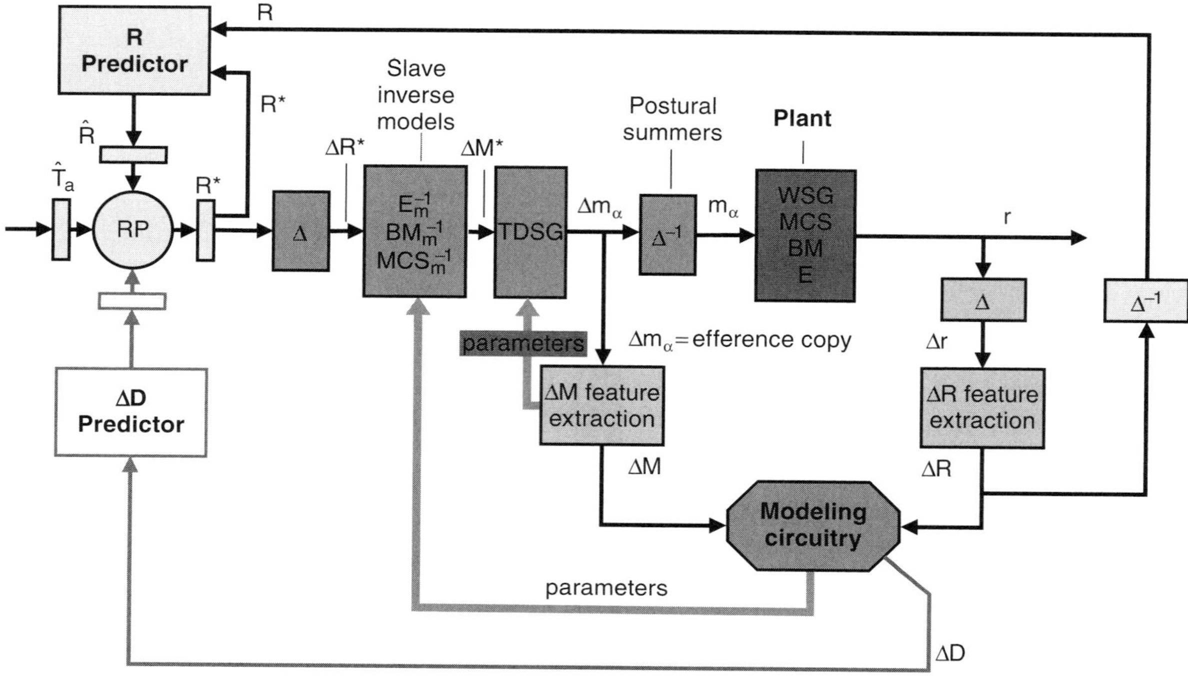

FIGURE 2-5 A computational model of adaptive sensory-motor processing. Adapted from Neilson and Neilson, 2005.

Stuttering as a Nonlinear Emergent Phenomenon Anne Smith and her colleagues (Smith & Kelly, 1997; Smith, 1999) believe that stuttering is best modeled within a multifactorial, nonlinear, and dynamic framework. Rather than the types of multifactorial models discussed elsewhere in this chapter, such as Demands and Capacities, theirs seeks experimental specification of the interactions among systems that support speech-language production and consequences across systems of changes in various parameters. The model is based on principles in nonlinear dynamics, in which even small changes in a single parameter can have large consequences on complex behavior. In this regard, Smith also centers on the notions of stability and instability in complex systems, and has provided experimental evidence of destabilization of speech motor gestures under conditions of increased linguistic formulation stress in stutterers (see Chapter 8). In view of the types of theories we have offered in the chapter, Smith is almost uniquely unconvinced of the value of centering on the moment of overt stuttering itself, since it may reflect only the end point of less easily observed problems in the stability of normally well-patterned and regular articulatory, vocal or respiratory movements. The model therefore concentrates on what might be called intrinsic factors in the beginning stages of stuttering: how weaker language representations in people who stutter interact to reduce automaticity and stability of speech patterning. Later-developing systems and behaviors may result from maladaptive responses to real or anticipated fluency failure that can be further shaped by experience. For example, tremor observed in some of Smith and her colleagues' studies (e.g., Smith, 1989; Kelly, Smith, & Goffman, 1995) appears only in older children and adults, rather than younger children who stutter, and may be conditioned by autonomic arousal that accompanies actual or perceived speech difficulty.

CONCLUDING OBSERVATIONS

Types of Theories Reviewed

We may conclude this chapter by calling attention once more to two distinctions we have made. First, there is the very fundamental one that exists between conceptual models of the stuttering moment and theories about the conditions under which the disorder develops. With regard to the moment of stuttering, there appear, broadly speaking, to be three major hypotheses, which view it respectively as a breakdown under stress, the fulfillment of a neurotic need, and an anticipatory reaction of struggle or avoidance. These three descriptions subsume a large variety of interpretations of the act of stuttering. In the effort to find the most accurate model, analogues of stuttering have been discerned in, to mention a few examples, the convulsive seizure; perseverative reactions of individuals with acquired brain injury; the compulsive act of emotionally disturbed individuals; sexual impotence; writer's cramp; the posture of runners on their mark; the behavior of golfers rehearsing the start of a swing; the physical tremors of rage or fear; the oscillatory breakdown of a mechanical device pushed beyond its capacity by internal damage or external stress; and the behavior of a rat as it runs from danger, is caught immobilized between two feared goals, or presses a bar to gain a pellet of food.

Theories of the etiology of stuttering are conveniently classified as breakdown, repressed need, or anticipatory struggle theories, depending upon the model of the moment of stuttering adopted (or incorporated, as in models that address more than one, such as the neuropsycholinguistic model). Breakdown theories of onset attribute the disorder to the effects of early environmental stress and usually assign an important role to constitutional predisposing factors. The principal issues that they raise concern the precise nature of these organic factors and the extent to which the incidence of stuttering is influenced by heredity. Repressed need theories about the etiology of stuttering tend to merge with theories of the etiology of neurotic behavior generally. They raise the question of whether stutterers typically possess a neurotic type of personality and why they choose stuttering as a symptom. Current theories of the etiology of stuttering as anticipatory struggle behavior ascribe it to perceived penalties for normal disfluency or to pressures extending to a broader range of possible speech failures. Among the issues they raise, perhaps the most fundamental is the specific nature of the relationship, if any, that exists between early stuttering and normal disfluency, and whether they lie on a continuum of normal fluency or represent distinctly different entities.

Having made a distinction between theories of the moment of stuttering and theories of etiology, we may say that any adequate theoretical formulation about stuttering provides both. Above all, a theory of the etiology of stuttering tends to make a marked impression of incompleteness unless it is accompanied at least implicitly by a consistent conceptual model of the stuttering act to bridge the gap between the conditions under which the disorder is said to develop and the precipitation, at any later point, of a discrete example of the behavior. Lacking this particular kind of elaboration, the mere statement that stuttering is "due to" insecurity or "caused by" an enlarged thymus gland, delayed myelinization of cortical areas, or the like, is somewhat like the representation of a body without a visible connection between head and torso. In this sense, we note that some would say that the etiology of stuttering is "genetic," but this says little about the conditions that cause its symptoms to emerge, persist or remit, or the underlying neurophysiological substrates of the behavior itself.

The converse of this, a theory that is incomplete because it is wholly concerned with the stuttering moment, perhaps does not strike us quite so unfavorably. It will be recalled, for example, that some of the systematic discussions of stuttering in terms of learning theory that we have reviewed have given scant attention to the etiology of the disorder. Perhaps the reason for the greater acceptability of such theories is that with a proper understanding of the moment of stuttering it would be possible, in principle, to devise effective therapeutic measures in the absence of essentially any notion of its etiology.

The second distinction we have made is between theories that are indigenous to their frame of reference and those representing old theories shifted to a new conceptual orientation. The new frameworks have been provided chiefly by theories of learning and to a lesser extent by cybernetic theory. Learning interpretations of stuttering have represented it as an instrumental avoidance response reinforced by anxiety reduction as an approach-avoidance conflict, as positively and negatively reinforced operant behavior, and as classically conditioned disintegrative emotional arousal. They have drawn chiefly upon Johnson's diagnosogenic theory, upon psychoanalytic concepts of stuttering, and upon dysphemic breakdown theories. The basic research issue that the conflicting formulations have served to raise concerns the nature of the reinforcement by which stuttering is maintained.

A frequent advantage in the use of new frames of reference is the gain in verifiability that a reformulation in more rigorous terms may bring about. A theory may be poor not because it is untrue, but because it is logically incapable of verification as stated. For example, the conceptions that stuttering is due to "habit," to "nervousness," or to children's attempts to talk faster than they can think—or to think faster than they can talk—are so ambiguous in their terminology that it is possible neither to prove them nor to dispose of them. In its proper frame of reference, however, the meaningless question of whether stuttering is a "habit" becomes the question of whether it is a conditioned operant, a formulation that suggests certain observations that might be employed to answer it. In the same vein, many of the newer formulations of stuttering, such as psycholinguistic or cybernetic models, make testable claims about the language and speech motor capabilities of stutterers that can be evaluated either experimentally or through computer simulations.

Multicausality

To some researchers, the complexity of the stuttering problem has appeared to justify the question whether stuttering has not one but many causes. When we consider the varied meanings with which the term multicausal may be used in connection with stuttering, however, it becomes evident that such a question needs considerable refinement before it can be answered. Perhaps some clarification may be gained by noting that the concept of multicausality appears in discussions of stuttering in three general forms that may be referred to for convenience as the *no-model, single-model*, and *multi-model* forms.

No-Model Multicausality The impressive accumulation of plausible theories about the etiology of stuttering sometimes evokes the reaction that there must be "some truth" in all of them. Those who find this an easy solution to the problem must be prepared to answer the objection that we as yet have essentially no conclusive evidence to show that *any* of the current theories of stuttering is wholly or partially valid, let alone to support the somewhat improbable conclusion that they all are. There is, however, an even more basic deficiency inherent in such casual appeals to the concept of multicausality. Let us take as a fabricated example the simple assertion that stuttering may be caused in some cases by an organic predisposition, in others by a parental misdiagnosis of stuttering, and in still others by neurotic insecurity fostered by disturbed family relationships. As it stands, such a proposal is essentially empty because it offers no model of the *moment* of stuttering to make the assumption of a multiplicity of causes necessary or plausible. Hence, it is open to the same criticism that may be made of any theory of the etiology of stuttering that fails to erect a bridge between the cause of the disorder and the precipitation of the individual instance of speech interruption. We are left to wonder how all these disparate things eventually result in the repetitions or prolongations of speech sounds so classically and uniquely identified as stuttering.

Single-Model Multicausality The term *multicausal* has sometimes been used to characterize theories of somewhat broad scope that offer a single model of the moment of stuttering. Examples are Sheehan's conflict theory, Mysak's deautomaticity theory, Eisenson's perseverative theory, and various others. Through their single concept of the stuttering moment, such theories often seek to unite several viewpoints or various observations on the etiology of stuttering by showing how they all add up to conflict, or to deautomaticity, or whatever. Despite this fact, we have grounds for questioning whether the term *multicausal* has unambiguous meaning as applied to such theories.

In the first place, it is obvious that multicausality may refer either to the interaction of multiple factors that contribute jointly to the etiology in a given case or to the notion of different etiologies in different cases. We pass over this ambiguity, however, to deal with a more serious one. In the case in which we assume a single model of stuttering behavior, *the extent to which stuttering is a multicausal phenomenon appears to be merely an artifact of the level of abstraction on which we happen to be discussing its causation.*

An analogy will suffice to make this clear. Does the motor disorder known as athetosis have one or more than one cause, and if several, how many? Ignoring certain areas of doubt or controversy, we could obviously set down a fairly long but not endless list of "textbook" causes, including birth injury, anoxia, maternal disease, and the like. But each of these causes has causes, and if we pursued these branching pathways for any distance we would soon have to admit that athetosis has a practically limitless number of "causes," or, to put it somewhat differently, it is highly improbable that any set of causal circumstances will ever exactly duplicate themselves from case to case.

Instead of being more specific, however, we can, if we choose, be more abstract and reduce our original list of causes to a smaller number of more general ones in almost any way we please. In fact, if we are willing to be abstract enough we can say that athetosis has just one possible cause—damage to certain parts of the extrapyramidal motor tract of the central nervous system. Clearly, any question about the number of "causes" of athetosis is meaningless unless we can somehow specify the level of generality or abstractness on which we are asking it.[36] Similarly, hoarseness has a great variety of causes; yet it also has just one cause: aperiodic vibration of the vocal folds.

This is not to say that it is not useful to describe differences in the factors or sets of circumstances that may lead to athetosis or hoarseness. In this book we shall, in fact, place considerable emphasis on different circumstances as they relate to the etiology of stuttering. The point we are making here is simply that when they are seen in their proper light essentially all theories that imply a single, unique model of the stuttering block must in some sense be both unicausal and multicausal. To say that stuttering has multiple causes with this type of concept in view is to add relatively little to our understanding. What we need to know in addition is the nature of the immediate *single* cause of stuttering and precisely how it is related to the numerous more remote causes.

Multi-Model Theories Finally, it is possible to suppose that stuttering in one person represents an act of oral gratification, in another the effort to keep from stuttering again, and in still a third a disruption due to internal delayed auditory feedback. In other words, we may say that stuttering has multiple causes because what appears to be a single type of speech difficulty actually represents several basically different forms of abnormal speech behavior having little or no relationship to each other beyond their superficial similarity. In one sense, whether or not this is true may depend on how broadly we define the term *stuttering*. To many clinicians and researchers, it seems unlikely that any and all types of speech interruption are symptoms of a single underlying disorder. Freund (1966, chap. 17) distinguished "common" stuttering systematically from certain hysterical symptoms resembling it, from the "stuttering" that appears to be associated with certain types of brain damage and from the disfluencies belonging to the symptomatology of cluttering.[37] Few would be inclined to quarrel with the mutual differentiation of these phenomena. Not all would use the term *stuttering* for all of them at the present time, but that is a

[36] Korzybski (1941, p. 433) expressed this succinctly by saying that "cause" is a multiordinal term (i.e., a term that has different meanings on different levels of abstraction).

[37] See also Johnson et al. (1967, p. 241) for a similar differentiation.

matter of definition. We will return to this subject shortly.

A more controversial issue arises when the multi-model hypothesis is invoked in connection with "common" stuttering in an attempt to account for some of its obscurities. The idea that what we ordinarily call stuttering represents two or more separate and unrelated disorders can hardly be dismissed as impossible and must always be kept in view. For example, De Nil (in press) has accumulated an impressive collection of fluency samples from individuals having a wide array of neurological impairments that all bear close resemblance to developmental stuttering. Should they be included in developing a model of developmental stuttering? To do so may seem less than parsimonious, and requires the assumption that a number of totally separate underlying causes produce symptoms that quite by chance strongly resemble each other. Before we advance such a theory we should be sure that it does not merely reflect a failure to generalize far enough about our "separate and unrelated" disorders to unite them with reference to one ultimate concept of the moment of stuttering.

In addition, it cannot be insisted too strongly that a theory stating that we have in stuttering not one but several distinct clinical entities is meaningless unless it provides hypotheses about the procedures or observations for their differential diagnosis on the basis of differences in the symptomatology, in the conditions under which the difficulty varies, in the pattern of distribution of stutterings in the speech sequence, or in some other observable features of the behavior. In short, if the hypothesis is that different etiologies give rise to different forms of stuttering, then one must attempt to theorize about the respects in which the forms are actually different. Without such operational definitions of the separate clinical entities that we are postulating, we do not have a multi-model theory, but only the surmise that it might be possible to advance one. This surmise has been made rather frequently, but theories of this type are as yet essentially lacking.

The Search for Subtypes of Stutterers In place of multi-model theories, all we have are a few widely scattered research efforts to identify etiological subtypes of stutterers. Berlin (1955) and Andrews and Harris (1964, chap. 6) tried to do it largely on the basis of features of individuals' case histories, while Prins and Lohr (1972) based their attempt on visible and audible features of their stuttering. Two of these studies employed factor analysis. In each instance little difficulty was found in isolating clusters of characteristics that seemed to belong together, but their etiological significance is an open question. Belyakova (1973) reported quantitative differences in the electromyographic recordings from the orbicularis oris muscle during stuttering in patients who exhibited signs of "diffuse organic lesions of the central nervous system" and patients whose stuttering represented "neurotic reactions." Riley and Riley (1980) factor analyzed the performance of stuttering children on tests of motor coordination, psycholinguistic abilities, and severity of stuttering. The analysis yielded factors that could be presumed to be related to the development of stuttering, notably oral motor ability, language skills, and auditory perceptual ability. Subgroups of stutterers were not identified, however (Riley & Riley, 1984).

Preus (1981) made a comprehensive search for subgroups among 100 stutterers using seventy variables related to symptomatology, reactive aspects, language development, frequency of stuttering under various conditions, intellect, signs of brain damage, general anxiety, and emotional adjustment. He could find no evidence that stuttering is an "aggregation of separate disorders." In a subsequent study, Preus (1983) reported some success in distinguishing a "neurogenic" and a "psychogenic" subgroup as defined by Halstead's *Impairment Index* (suggesting cerebral dysfunction) and the *Minnesota Multiphasic Personality Inventory*.

Schwartz and Conture (1988) subgrouped 43 young stutterers on the basis of disfluency types and the number and variety of associated behaviors. They found a number of clusters and partial support for differentiating between a predominantly "clonic" and a predominantly "tonic" type of stutterer.

Poulos and Webster (1991) used family history of stuttering as a basis for subgrouping 169 stutterers.

Like West, Nelson, and Berry (1939), they found that those without such a history were considerably more likely to have suffered birth injuries or other early conditions suggesting possible brain damage. Janssen, Kraaimaat, and Brutten (1990) noted some possible differences in type of stuttering between study participants with and without a family background of stuttering.

Finally, Yairi and Ambrose (2005) propose subgrouping stutterers not only on the basis of family history, but chronicity, having discovered some behavioral profiles more consistent with recovery in childhood than persistence into adulthood. Similarly, Alm and Risberg (2007) could also distinguish between groups of adult stutterers who had positive and negative histories of early brain injury and differing profiles for their study measures.

Cluttering The hasty, repetitive, hesitant pattern of speech known as cluttering is another type of disfluency believed to differ in etiology from the common variety of stuttering it often resembles. A number of efforts have been made to differentiate it objectively from stuttering. Langová and Morávek (1964) found differences between stutterers and clutterers in brain waves and in the effects of drugs on their speech. They also observed that delayed auditory feedback had a more deleterious effect on the speech of those regarded as clutterers, as did Hutchinson and Burk (1973). Rieber, Breskini, and Jaffe (1972) found higher mean pause times in stutterers than clutterers during oral reading, and Rieber (1975) reported lower reading rates in stutterers. Five clutterers studied by Dewar, Dewar, and Barnes (1976) were aided far less by masking noise than were a group of stutterers. Rieber, Smith, and Harris (1976) found that word length and word position in the sentence influenced stuttering and cluttering similarly, but that stuttering was more closely associated with the initial sound of the word. St. Louis, Hinzman, and Hull (1985) found less complex and complete utterances in the speech of "possible clutterers," whom they defined as children judged to be disfluent in articulation, but not stutterers.

Summary Remarks

We may sum up this discussion of the concept of multicausality in stuttering by saying that our chief concern has been to show, not that the concept is erroneous, but that it is all too easy to adopt it without proper regard for its implications. Multicausality has so many possible meanings that we simply are not conveying very much information about stuttering when we say, without extensive further qualification, that it has "multiple causes." Furthermore, when we do make the appropriate qualifications we find that, depending on the kind of multicausality we are talking about, the extent to which it applies to stuttering is partly a matter of the level of abstraction that we choose or of how broadly we define "stuttering." It is possible to define a type of multicausality in stuttering that is neither meaningless nor trivial, and which can be supported through empirical experimentation or neural network simulations.

Chapter 3

Prevalence and Incidence

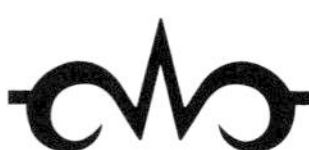

In the last chapter we reviewed theories of stuttering. The next chapters will be devoted to a survey of the research on stuttering in which we will be concerned with what we can infer about the validity of these theories.

There are a number of important questions about stuttering for which answers are to be sought chiefly by the operation of counting heads of persons who stutter. Such surveys have constituted a significant portion of the research on stuttering. Surveys of populations selected in various ways have resulted in information about the relationship between stuttering and such variables as age, sex, familial background of stuttering, and factors of social and cultural environment. Perhaps the major interest of this research derives from the fact that most of it has been focused on the broad question of the relative influences of heredity and environment in relation to stuttering. This focus, on the relative contributions of "nurture" and "nature," is not unique to stuttering (see Bronfenbrenner & Ceci, 1994), and has preoccupied many researchers working in the fields of speech and language acquisition and developmental disorders of communication (see Gilger, 1995; Gilger & Rice, 1996; Dale, Dionne, Eley, & Plomin, 2000; Fisher, Plomin, DeFries, Craig, & McGuffin, 2003).

We may establish a basic point of reference by first raising the question of how prevalent stuttering is in a population generally representative of our culture at a randomly selected moment in our time.[1] A precise answer to such a question presents

[1] *Prevalence* is defined as the frequency with which a condition may be observed in a population at a given period of time, while *incidence*, also important for our discussions, reflects the proportion of the population that has experienced periods of stuttering at any point in their lives. Given the high remission rate of developmental stuttering, the prevalence rate is only approximately 20 percent of the incidence rate.

considerable obstacles. Almost all attempts to achieve a reasonable approximation of it have dealt with the question of the number of stutterers to be found in populations of children attending school. Tables 3-1 and 3-2 present the findings of surveys of this kind done chiefly in the United States and Europe. Whatever variations are to be seen in these findings must be evaluated in the light of all of the factors by which such data may be influenced. In addition to any inherent differences in the nature of the populations sampled, the studies shown differed with respect to the size of the sample, the methods by which the sample was surveyed, and, inevitably, the criteria on the basis of which perceptual judgments of stuttering were made. The fact that these surveys were carried out in different eras during a span of many years introduces still a further possible source of variation about which little is known. All these things considered, the data are in general quite consistent. They point to a prevalence of stuttering of approximately 1 percent or somewhat more in the European populations studied and to somewhat less than 1 percent in the United States. It is not clear why these numbers vary, although they may be due to sampling error or to methodology. For example, in a Spanish study (Ardila et al., 1994) where college-aged students were asked to self-report if they demonstrated "syllabic iterations (kind of

TABLE 3-1 Prevalence and Sex Ratio of Stuttering among American Schoolchildren

	N	Population and grades sampled	Percentage of stutterers	Sex ratio
Hartwell (1893)	129,060	Boston, K-12	0.77	3.0:1
Conradi (1904)	87,440	Six American Cities,[a] 1-12	0.87	3.0:1
Blanton (1916)	4,862	Madison, Wis., 1-8	0.72	3.4:1
Wallin (1916)	89,057	St. Louis, Mo., K-12	0.77	2.6:1
Root (1926)	14,072	S. Dakota, 1-8	1.20	2.2:1
McDowell (1928)	7,138	New York City, 1-8	0.87	2.9:1
Louttit and Halls (1936)	199,839	Indiana, 1-12	0.77	3.1:1
Burdin (1940)	3,602	Indianapolis, 1-4	0.53	NA
Mills and Streit (1942)	4,685	Holyoke, Mass., 1-6	1.47	5.3:1
Schindler (1955)	22,976	Iowa,[b] 1-12	0.55	2.8:1
Hull (1969)	6,287	Rocky Mountain Region, 1-12	0.30	6:1
Gillespie and Cooper (1973)	5,054	Tuscaloosa, Ala., 7-12	2.12	2.7:1
Leavitt (1974)	10,445	New York City, 1-6[c]	0.84	6.3:1
Leavitt (1974)	10,449	San Juan, P.R., 1-6	1.50	2.9:1
Brady and Hall (1976)	187,420	Illinois, Pennsylania, K-12[d]	0.35	3.9:1
Hull et al. (1976)[e]	38,802	U.S., Nationwide, 1-12	0.80	3.0:1
Leske (1981)	7,119	U.S., 1-6[f]	2.00	2.6:1
Boyle et al. (1994)[g]	17,110	U.S Nationwide, 1-17	1.89	NA

[a] Mllwaukee, Cleveland, Louisville, Albany, Kansas City, and Springfield, Mass.
[b] Analysis of data from survey of urban and rural schools of five counties conducted from 1939 to 1942.
[c] Puerto Rican children.
[d] Included were 3,514 pupils with mental retardation.
[e] Cited by Leske (1981).
[f] Health examination survey, 1963–1970, National Center for Health Statistics.
[g] 1988 National health interview survey.

TABLE 3-2 Prevalence of Stuttering among Schoolchildren in Other Countries

	N	Population	Percentage of stutterers
Westergaard (1898)*	34,000	Denmark	0.61
Lindberg (1900)*	212,000	Denmark, Rural	0.90
Lindberg (1900)*	85,000	Denmark, Urban	0.74
Von Sarbo (1901)*	231,468	Hungary	1.02
Rouma (1906)	14,235	Belgium	1.40
Ballard (1912)	13,189	London	1.20
Watzl (1924)**	136,000	Vienna	0.60
Parker (1932)	32,123	Tasmania, Australia	1.27
McAllister (1937)	5,705	Glasgow	1.00
McAllister (1937)	38,736	Ayrshire	0.94
McAllister (1937)	21,452	Dunbartonshire	1.00
Wohl (1951)	20,101	Dunbartonshire	1.30
Morgenstern (1956)	29,499	Scotland	1.20
Seeman (1959)**	26,000	Prague	0.55
Petkov and Iosifov (1960)	45,068	Bulgaria	1.70
Aron (1962)	6,581	Johannesburg Bantu	1.26
Andrews and Harris (1964)	7,358	Newcastle Upon Tyne	1.20
Okasha, Bishry, et al. (1974)	8,494	Egypt	0.93
Glogowski (1976)	875,384	Poland	1.82, 1.72***
Ralston (1981)	1,999	British West Indies	4.70
Månsson (2000)[a]	1,021	Bornholm, Denmark	5.18
Okalidou and Kampanaros (2001)[b]	676* 437**	Patras, Greece	2.2 (girls = 1.3 and boys = 0.9)* 0.9 (girls = 0.7 and boys = 0.2)**
Craig et al. (2002)	2,553	New South Wales, Australia	0.9
Craig and Tran (2005)	1,881 (age 11–20)	New South Wales, Australia	0.5
Craig and Tran (2005)[c]	1,638 (age 2–10)	New South Wales, Australia	1.4
Van Borsel et al. (2006)	21,027	Belgium	0.58

*Cited by Conradi (1904).
**Cited by Van Riper (1971, p. 39).
***Two studies, the first in 1964 and the second in 1970–71.
[a]Total incidence over a nine-year period, following children born in 1990–91.
[b]Two studies, the first in *1998–99 and the second **2000–01. Results based on survey of kindergarten teachers using communication checklist for preschool teachers.
[c]Prevalance rates in the Craig and Tran (2005) study are based on results from Craig et al. (2002) and Craig et al. (2003).

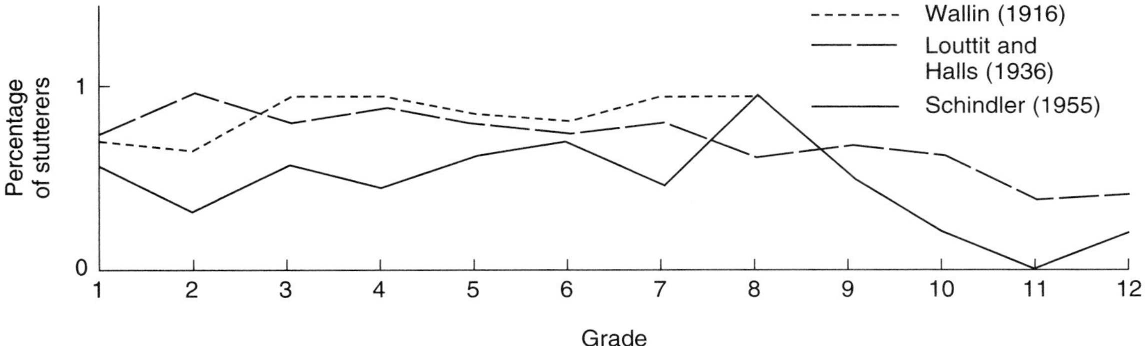

FIGURE 3-1 Prevalence of stuttering in schoolchildren by grade. The prevalence appears to remain relatively constant through the elementary grades.

stuttering)," almost 2 percent reported that they did so at least several times per week. Månsson (2000) reported an incidence rate for stuttering on the Danish island of Bornholm of about 5.2 percent, but more than 70 percent of the cases were reported to resolve within two years after onset, which would lower the prevalence rate in a school-aged sample to a level consistent with most previous studies. Other studies completed in Australia tend to center around the more typical value of ~1 percent (although the most recent, McKinnon, McLeod, and Reilly [2007] obtained a value of 0.33 percent of primary school-aged children, a value they themselves thought somewhat low). Craig and Tran (2005), in their summary of recent Australian prevalence studies, note that describing point prevalence relative to age can greatly inform the life-span characteristics of stuttering—many children who stutter appear to spontaneously recover, as we will discuss in further detail. Prevalence rates varied from a high of ~1.4 percent for the 2–10 year old sample to a range between 0.4 percent and 0.8 percent for older age groups. Whatever the true number, which may vary as a function of genetic susceptibility in a population, as we will discuss, stuttering is a relatively low-incidence communication disorder.[2]

[2]This, in turn, has ramifications for studying it, adequately testing treatments of it, and even teaching student clinicians how to treat it (Bernstein Ratner, & Tetnowski, 2006).

AGE VARIABLES

Prevalence with Grade Level

Having established a general estimate of the prevalence of stuttering as about 1 percent or less, we may now raise the question whether it changes in any significant fashion with age. For many years, the answers depended in large part upon surveys of school populations. The results of several surveys that have compared the percentages of stutterers to be found on various grade levels are shown graphically in Figure 3-1. It is clear that the prevalence of stuttering does not vary appreciably from grade to grade, with the possible exception of a gradual decline as the high school years are reached. A more recent survey by Brady and Hall (1976) produced a similar graph, including the same decline in the upper grades.

Stuttering, then, seems to differ markedly from infantile articulatory difficulties, which drop very sharply in prevalence during the first few grades of elementary school. At first glance this is puzzling. We have long had evidence that many children "outgrow" stuttering, just as they do articulatory difficulties, after episodes of brief duration. Why, then, is there no drop in the figures? A reasonable hypothesis is that additional instances of stuttering develop for a considerable period of time during childhood. In other words, the stability in the prevalence of stuttering depicted in Figure 3-1 might hide the fact that throughout the early years the disorder is passed about to an extent, new cases arising to take the place of those that disappear. Another possibility is that most of the recovery from stuttering occurs in the years prior to school enrollment, on which most of these numbers are based. In order to select between these options or others, there are evidently two processes we must explore further. One is the reported onset of stuttering as it relates to the age of the child. The other is the process of spontaneous recovery from stuttering.

Reported Age at Onset

Historically, most of our information about the ages at which children are said to begin to stutter comes from systematically gathered reports of parents, usually made many weeks or months afterward. Those who have gathered this information generally tend to emphasize that in the majority of cases the parent has perceived the onset of stuttering as gradual and is frequently vague and uncertain about the date of its occurrence. The data summarized in Table 3-3 must be examined with this in view. Above all we must keep in mind that any unqualified statement we make about the date of onset of stuttering begs some controversial questions about the identification of stuttering in young children and how it is to be differentiated from normal disfluency. Consequently, we need to face the fact that all we can be sure we are talking about here is the age at which the onset of stuttering was first perceived or reported by a parent.

It is apparent from Table 3-3 that the earliest age of onset of stuttering was quite consistently recalled in older studies as about 18 months, apparently with the beginning of speech in sentences. Of particular interest are the reports of the latest age of onset, which vary from age 7 to 13. Such information must be evaluated in the light of the age range of the subjects in each study since this obviously places a limit on the latest as well as the average age at which onset is observed. Nevertheless, there is clearly a decline in the frequency of new cases as we approach the upper age limit of the children investigated in these studies. It is also significant that the average age at onset as usually recalled is distinctly closer to the earliest than to the latest age. Year for year, onset is reported more frequently in the earlier than in the later years of childhood. A large proportion of cases begin with the beginning of speech, according to several investigators. Thereafter, the decline in frequency of reported onset with age takes place at a decreasing rate, following a negatively accelerated growth curve, as Andrews and Harris (1964, p. 113) pointed out, and new cases may therefore continue to appear for a considerable time.

Of exceptional interest are some findings reported by Andrews and Harris (1964, p. 31) since they were based not on parents' recollections, but on direct observation of 1,000 children in the city of Newcastle Upon Tyne, England, who were followed from birth to age 16 years in a longitudinal study of childhood disorders conducted by the University of Durham and the city Health Services.[3] By the conclusion of the study a total of 43 cases of stuttering had been identified (see Figure 3-2). Sixteen represented transient episodes (less than six months' duration), occurring between ages 2 and 4 years. Of the remaining 27 cases, 5 were first observed at age 3 years, half had begun by age 5 years, and the last appeared at age 11 years. There was a progressive decrease in frequency of onset with age.

A multifaceted research program coordinated by Ehud Yairi of the University of Illinois (with colleagues Nicoline Ambrose, Elaine Paden, Ruth Watkins, and Nancy Cox) has both confirmed and questioned some traditional views of the typical onset profiles of children who stutter, and their patterns of recovery or persistence. Their data, combined with other studies that have made aggressive attempts to locate children close to the onset of stuttering symptoms and to verify the child's

[3]This study should not be confused with one cited in Table 3-5 (Andrews & Harris, 1964, p. 113). The 1,000-family survey referred to here has also been reported by Morley (1957, pp. 13–56) and others. Ingham (1976) has pointed out that there was an attrition of subjects and a reduced frequency of contacts during the later years of this study. It remains, however virtually the only long-term longitudinal study of stuttering onset and recovery available prior to the Yairi project spanning the period of 1990–2000.

TABLE 3.3 Age at Reported Onset of Stuttering

	N	Age range of subjects in years	Mean or median[a] age of onset in years	Range and distribution of ages at onset
Meltzer (1935)	50	8–16		"Onset of Speech" to 13 years. Onset after 8 years in more than one-third of cases.
Millsen and Johnson (1936)	56	3–22	3	From 18 months to 8 years. Onset by age 3 years in 70 percent of cases.
Berry (1938c)	430	9–10	4.86	Latest age at onset was 9 years.
Johnson (1955a)	46	2–9	3	From 2 to 9 years. 75th percentile 3 years, 2 months.
Darley (1955)	50	2–14	3.87[b]	From 15 months to 9 years.
Johnson and Associates (1959)	150	2–8	3.53[b]	From 18 months to 7 years. 90th percentile 5.33 years.
Andrews and Harris (1964)	80	9–11	5	From 2 to 9 years. 75th percentile 6 years.
Dickson (1971)	369	[c]	3	From 18 months to 10 years. Onset by age 3 in almost half the cases.
Preus (1981)	98	16–21	4–5	More than a third began at age 2 or 3, another third by age 5, four after age 10.
Selder, Gladstien, and Kidd (1983)	437[d]	—	5.17	From 1:5 to 43, 50% by age 4:5, 90% by age 8.
Yairi and Ambrose (1992)	87 (59 male, 28 female)	2–6	2.73	25–41 months
Yaruss, LaSalle, and Conture (1998)	100 (85 males, 15 females)	2–6	2.76 (males); 2.5 (females)	Range 11.29 months (males); Range 10.05 months (females)
Bernstein, Ratner, and Silverman (2000)	15 (12 males, 3 females)	Approximately 2–4	2.67	24–44 months
Månsson (2000)	12	Approximately 5	2.75	24–42 months
Buck, Lees, and Cook (2002)	61 (42 males, 19 females)	2.9–6.6	3.03	NA
Yairi and Ambrose (2005)[f]	163	1.9–6.25	2.8	16–69 months

[a]Ages without decimal places are medians, except for Dickson's, which is the mode.
[b]As reported by the mothers. The mean age of onset reported by fathers was six months later in Darley's study, but comparable to that of the mothers in the study by Johnson and Associates.
[c]Kindergarten through 9th grade.
[e]Subjects were 305 stutterers and their recovered and persistent first-degree stuttering relatives.
[e]Children born in 1990 and 1991 in Bornhom, Denmark, were used in the study; these children were assessed for speech and language at age 3, and children who demonstrated signs of disfluency were followed for the next 9 years. Result represent the information provided at the evaluation when children were approximately 5 years old.
[f]Age of onset is based on parent interviews.

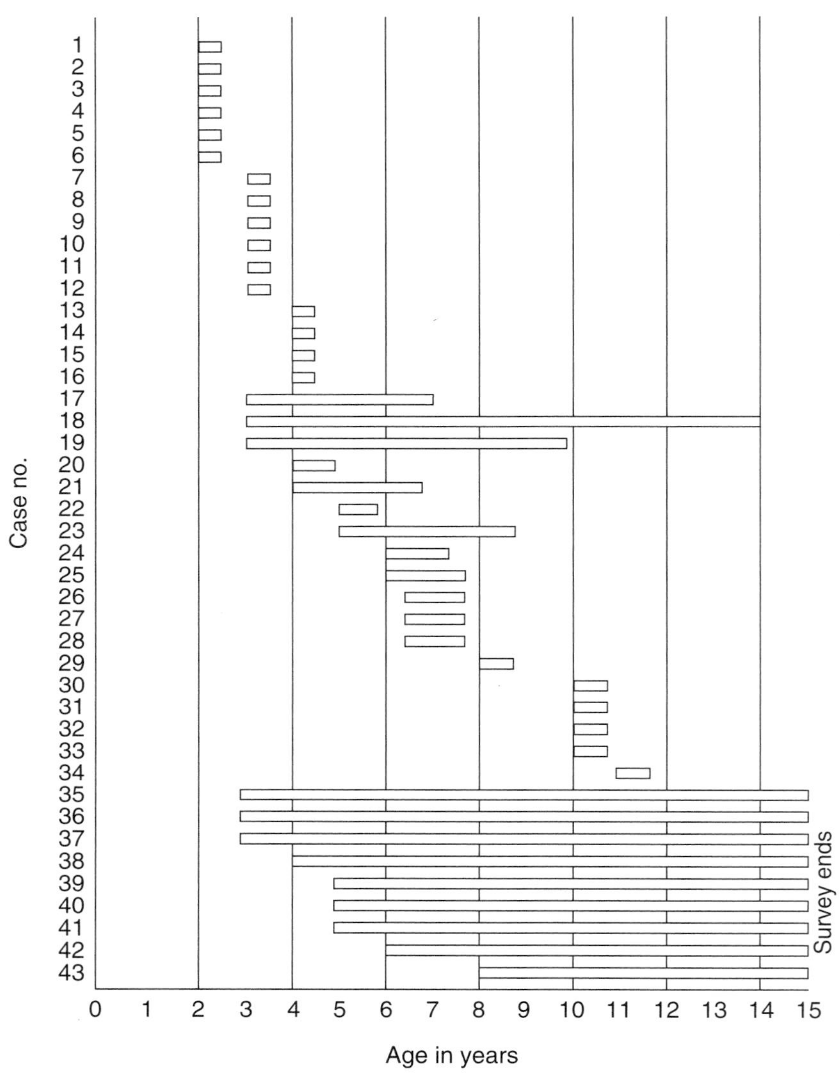

FIGURE 3-2 Onset and duration of stuttering of forty-three children identified as stutterers in a longitudinal survey of 1,000 children, all those born within the city limits of Newcastle Upon Tyne, England, during May and June of 1947, who were followed from birth to age sixteen years. Redrawn from Andrews, G., Epidemiology of stuttering. In Curlee, E. F., and Perkins, W. H. (eds)., *Nature and Treatment of Stuttering: New Directions.* Copyright 1984 by Allyn and Bacon. Reprinted by permission.

speech characteristics, suggest a narrower age range for typical stuttering onset. For example, Yairi and Ambrose (2005) report a mean age of onset of 33 months, with over 85 percent of onsets prior to 42 months of age and very few onsets prior to age 2. These findings are echoed by Månsson (2000), who reported an identical mean age of onset, and by Yaruss, LaSalle, and Conture (1998) who found the similar range of 30 months (for girls) to 36 months (for boys). Bernstein Ratner and Silverman (2000) found a similar onset pattern for their small sample of children specifically recruited in a study of stuttering close to onset. It appears that when studies directly target parents and pediatricians to report stuttering immediately after symptoms are noted that the typical age range for stuttering onset is actually much narrower than that reported in earlier studies.

Thus, while we may conclude that stuttering may develop at any age during childhood, the younger the child the more likely is the occurrence of an identifiable episode of stuttering, and some children apparently stutter with their first attempts to say sentences, which is now usually reported by parents to be at around age 2.5 years (~30 months), given advancements in parental report forms used to track children's language development (Bates, Dale, & Thal, 1995; Rescorla & Achenbach, 2002). It is unclear how much historical patterns and emerging demographics reflect growing awareness and willingness of parents to report their children's speech development and speaking difficulties. But it does appear that new cases may appear up to about 9 years of age, and some arise later. In a few instances, the onset of stuttering is even reported in adolescents or adults, although not all workers agree that this is basically the same kind of difficulty as is ordinarily referred to as stuttering.[4,5] Following the preschool years, there is little evidence of any pronounced vulnerability to stuttering at one age or another; the curve seems to be all downward. Andrews (1984a) estimated, "On the basis of data presently available, half the risk of ever stuttering is passed by age 4, three-quarters by age 6, and virtually all by age 12."

[4]For example, there are reports of observable disfluency patterns in children with language disorders (see Boscolo, Bernstein Ratner, & Rescorla, 2002) that are clearly atypical, but lack some of the behavioral and most of the affective components of what we have defined as stuttering in the first chapter.

[5]At least some cases of adult-onset stuttering appear to have an abrupt psychogenic origin different from those that develop during childhood. For example, Deal (1982) studied the case of a depressed 28-year-old who was addicted to heroin and who began to stutter after a suicide attempt. He stuttered in singing, unison reading, and even in miming speech movements. Another ambiguity about stuttering that appears to begin in adulthood is the uncertainty of determining whether it is not a recurrence of a forgotten early episode of stuttering.

Pattern at Onset

A number of recent studies have also examined whether stuttering onset was sudden or gradual, which can have ramifications for models of its presumed etiology. Yairi and Ambrose (2005) found that nearly 30 percent of their cases had onsets reported as sudden, as did 33 percent of cases reported by Månsson and 53 percent of cases reported by Buck, Lees, and Cook (2002).

Spontaneous Recovery

Concomitant with the incidence of new cases of stuttering during childhood, and offsetting it, there is a continuous tendency for stuttering to disappear of its own accord. Of those who at any time begin to stutter, a large proportion will stop by the time they reach adulthood. Estimates of the percentage who recover, varying from 36 to 79 percent, are shown in Table 3-4. Almost all are based on study participants' recollections of recovery. We have only a few large-scale, longitudinal studies to consult. In the first longitudinal investigation reported by Andrews and Harris, the percentage of stutterers who were recovered by 16 years of age was 79.1. This includes early episodes of brief duration. There is also a report by Fritzell (1976), who followed the progress of 90 stutterers, most of whom originally ranged in age from 7 to 9 years, and found that 10 years later, 46.7 percent no longer stuttered.

The estimated percentages of recovery shown in Table 3-4 are not really comparable with each other, chiefly because they are based on markedly different age groups. They suggest, however, that at almost any age level those who stutter are matched by at least an equal number who recall or are reported as having stuttered at one time. The older the group surveyed, the higher is the proportion of recovered stutterers likely to be found, as Dickson (1971) and Cooper (1972) showed, and by adulthood, the percentage of recovered stutterers may be as high as 80 percent. Some researchers are skeptical about a figure so high when based upon survey respondents' diagnoses of themselves as recovered stutterers. Young (1975c) suggested that

TABLE 3-4 Incidence of Stuttering (percentage of those who have stuttered at any time) and Rate of Recovery

	N	Population	Percentage of lifetime incidence	Percentage rate of recovery
Quinan (1921)	100	Male Adults, Over Age 44	5.0	
Millsen and Johnson (1936)	8,000	Council Bluffs, Iowa, Kindergarten through High School	2.5	42.3
Voelker (1942)	96	Nonstuttering University of Iowa Students	10.4	
Villarreal (1945)	271	Nonstuttering University of Texas Students	14.0	
Hertzman (1948)	4,213	Cincinnati Junior and Senior High School Students	5.8	
Glasner and Rosenthal (1957)	996	Anne Arundel County, Md., First Grade Entrants	15.4	54.2
Andrews and Harris (1964)	1,000	Newcastle Upon Tyne children followed from Birth to age 16	4.9[a]	79.1
Andrews and Harris (1964)	206	Newcastle Upon Tyne adults	4.8	
Sheehan and Martyn (1970)[b]	5,138	Berkeley and UCLA entering Freshmen and Graduate Students	2.9	78.9
Dickson (1971)	3,923	Buffalo, Kindergarten through Junior High School	9.4	54.4
Cooper (1972)	5,054	Tuscaloosa, Alabama, Junior and Senior High School Students	3.7	36.3
Porfert and Rosenfield (1978)	2,107	University of Massachusetts Students	5.5	61.7
Selder, Gladstien, and Kidd (1983)	1,857	First-Degree Relatives of Adult Stutterers	13.9	51.0
Culton (1986)[c]	30,586	University of Alabama Freshmen 1971–1983	0.7	58.8
Ramig (1993)[d]	19	Retrospective study of children who were diagnosed with stuttering years earlier and whose parents rejected the recommendation to receive treatment, original ages 3–8 years old		9.5
Janssen et al. (1996)[e]	106	Relatives of 106 stuttering children		Female: 6 Male: 14.3
Watkins and Yairi (1997)[f]	32	Children included in the Stuttering Research Project at the University of Illinois		Early recovery: 31.25 Late recovery: 31.25 Total: 62.25

Yairi and Ambrose (1999)	84	Children included in the Stuttering Research Project at the University of Illinois		73.8
Kloth et al. (1999)	23	Children with family histories of stuttering originally viewed as non-stutterers at the beginning of the longitudinal study		70
Rommel et al. (2000)	65	German-speaking children who stutter, examined at age 5 and tracked for six-month intervals over several years		77.4
Månsson (2000)	1,021	Bornholm, Denmark, children followed from birth to age 5	5.09	71.6
Felsenfeld et al. (2000)	1,567 pairs and 634 singles	Twin sample from the Australian twin registry aged 17–29 years old	8.8	NA
Ryan (2001)	22	2–5-year-old children with no intervention		68
Kalinowski et al. (2005)	2,036	School aged children who stutter, ages 5–11 years		Median recovery rate 13.9

[a] Based on an *N* of 875, the median number in the study as attrition took place (Andrews, 1984a).
[b] Includes date of previous surveys by Sheehan and Martyn (1966) and Martyn and Sheehan (1968).
[c] Includes date of Cooper, Paris, and Wells (1974).
[d] 21 families total did not pursue treatment. However, 19 parents responded to the survey; of those, 17 were formally assessed, confirming the parents' impressions.
[e] 77 mothers and 29 fathers of children who stutter reported female and male members of the family who stuttered.
[f] Early recovery was considered to be within 18 months of onset; late recovery was between 18–36 months.

some of these individuals may not be distinguishing adequately between stuttering and normal disfluency, and such doubts are given some substance by the finding of Lankford and Cooper (1974) that two-thirds of the parents of 68 self-diagnosed, recovered stutterers of junior and senior high school age said, when interviewed by telephone, that they did not believe their child had ever stuttered. Although these inconsistencies suggest the need for more research, it is quite possible that we are dealing here with the kind of question that can have no exact answer. If, as is possible, mild episodes of troublesome disfluency are commonplace during childhood, the question of precisely how many children recover from "stuttering" ultimately becomes a matter of what we are willing to define as stuttering. There are likewise ambiguities about the term "spontaneous recovery." Shall we apply it to a person who still stutters occasionally under stress? Does it exclude someone who has received speech therapy at some time?

At what age does spontaneous recovery take place? Studies of recovered adults by Wingate (1964), Shearer and Williams (1965), and Martyn and Sheehan (1968) showed that the age varied within a very broad range, although there was a considerable tendency to recall recovery between about ages 13 and 20 years. In one of these studies, the earliest age at which recovery was reported by these adults was 9 years. In another, it was 5. When parents are the informants, however, the age is pushed back considerably. In his study of schoolchildren, Dickson (1971) found the peak age of spontaneous recovery to be 3.5 years, with the great majority of former stutterers having recovered by age 6. In most cases the stuttering had lasted no more than two years, often no more than a few months. Moreover, Glasner and Rosenthal (1957) found that as many as 8.3 percent of 996 children about to enter first grade in Anne Arundel County, Maryland, were said to have already recovered from stuttering, and over a third of the stutterers identified during the Newcastle Upon Tyne 1,000-family survey had recovered from transient episodes by age 4 years (see Figure 3-2).[6] Evidently, a very large group of children who recover from stuttering in the early years will have no knowledge of it in later life. Inferences based on the recollections of older individuals about the ages at which recovery takes place must therefore be viewed with caution.

Better estimates of more typical recovery patterns have emerged with longitudinal research such as that reported by Yairi and Ambrose (2005) and demographic studies in which the same children may be tracked over time, such as in the Danish study by Månsson (2000), a study of high-risk Dutch children (Kloth, Kraaimaat, Janssen, & Brutten (1999), and a study of German children conducted by Rommel, Häge, Kalehne, and Johannsen (2000). In these cases, we may be more certain that the same criteria are being used to define and classify the children, and results tend to confirm the impression reported previously that most cases last no more than two to three years, with very frequent recovery in the first few months after symptoms emerge. In the Yairi corpus, 31 percent of children (whose mean age at onset was 3 years) had recovered within two years, 63 percent by three years post-onset, 74 percent by four years, and almost 80 percent by five years after stuttering onset. In the Månsson cohort, more than 71 percent of children had stopped stuttering within two years after their initial identification. The Dutch children in the Kloth et al. study were being tracked prospectively because at least one of the parents was an adult stutterer. Seventy percent of them were found to have recovered without intervention within four years after identification. Consistent with these trends, in a small sample of 22 2- to 3-year old children reported by Ryan (2001), almost 70 percent recovered without intervention by the two-year follow-up. In the Rommel et al. sample, children were identified relatively later than in these other studies, at around age 5. Three years later, 71 percent were found to have recovered. This pattern contrasts with that found by Ramig (1993), who found relatively little recovery for children first identified later, between almost 5 and 8 years of age.

[6]Furthermore, in a study of 8,000 elementary and high school children in Council Bluffs, Iowa, Milisen, and Johnson (1936) found that practically all of the former stutterers were reported to have recovered by age 8 years.

It appears from all available findings that some degree of recovery may occur at any age, however. Seider, Gladstien, and Kidd (1983) reported that among 132 stutterers' relatives who had recovered from stuttering, the ages of recovery ranged from 3 to 38 years. Shames and Beams (1956) gathered evidence indicating that stuttering may continue to become less prevalent even in older age groups. As we might expect, however, the younger the person, the better are the chances of recovery. The data of Seider, Gladstien, and Kidd show a decreasing probability of recovery with age. In an analysis of findings from several studies, Andrews, Craig, Feyer, Hoddinott, Howie, and Neilson (1983) estimated that at age 16 years, 75 percent of those stuttering at age 4 years, 50 percent of those stuttering at age 6 years, and 25 percent of those stuttering at age 10 years will have recovered. In the sections that follow, it may be worthwhile to consider potential differences between spontaneous recovery that occurs within the first two years of its onset, in young children, and that reported in older speakers, some of whom have been studied by researchers. Not as much information yet exists to track the youngsters seen by the University of Illinois, German, and Dutch teams into adolescence and beyond to ascertain later patterns of recovery.

Predictors of Recovery in Young Stutterers

Much of what is currently known about predictors of persistence and recovery in young children who have been diagnosed with stuttering at an early age (under the age of 6) is summarized in Yairi and Ambrose (2005). Their data reflect analysis of behaviors seen in 70 recovered and 19 persistent children identified shortly after stuttering onset. The first of these is gender. While 84 percent of the young girls recovered, only 77 percent of the boys recovered. Additionally, girls tended to recover almost six months earlier (post-onset age) than did boys. The second of these was age at onset of symptoms. Recovered children were an average of 32.6 months of age at onset, while persistent children were somewhat older, 36 months of age. However, these children had also been stuttering somewhat longer (an average of 7 months, as opposed to 4 months). Family history of persistence and recovery also related to eventual outcomes: children who had close relatives who were persistent stutterers were more likely to be persistent stutterers, while children whose family histories included relatives who had recovered from stuttering were more likely to follow this pattern. Although group averages for language abilities showed both persistent and recovered children to have average to above-average language abilities, children who recovered scored higher on both the expressive and receptive portions of the *Preschool Language Scale*. A surprising "non-contender" for predicting outcome was the pattern of stuttering when first referred to the study. Although the two groups obviously diverged over time in the frequency of stuttering behaviors, little distinguished their stuttering profiles at first evaluation. It is possible that subtle articulatory differences can differentiate persistent and recovered children close to onset; Subramanian, Yairi, and Amir (2003) found slight differences in second formant transitions in the speech of the two groups.

Recovery in Older Speakers

Although a very large proportion of stutterers recover at some time, it is noteworthy that among adults who regard themselves as recovered, at least half report a slight, occasional tendency to stutter, particularly when the recovery has been relatively late (Wingate, 1964; Shearer & Williams, 1965; Anderson & Felsenfeld, 2003). Dickson (1971) also found this to be true of some children. In addition, clinical observation suggests that recovered stutterers may bear a certain risk of developing stuttering again in later life.[7] A case study by Mouradian, Paslawski, and Shuaib (2000) documents the return of stuttering following a stroke.

Patrick Finn has extensively investigated the process of self-recovery in a cohort of 15 adults

---

[7]The German speech pathologist Erwin Richter (1982) relates that he stuttered as a young man, then spoke fluently for 28 years and all but forgot about his speech difficulty until the age of 57 years when he stuttered again for 9 or 10 months.

who self-identified as having recovered from stuttering without professional assistance (Finn, 1996, 1997; Finn & Felsenfeld, 2004; Finn, Howard, & Kubala, 2005). Finn (1997) found that, despite self-evaluation as recovered, listeners could distinguish their speech from that produced by speakers with no history of stuttering. Post-hoc analysis showed that when the speech of those who still reported a slight tendency to stutter (TS) under stressful conditions was removed, the remaining speakers' speech was indistinguishable from normal fluency. Both groups reported mean age of recovery to be in the late teen years, between an average of 18–19 years of age. Both groups described their speech and attitudes toward speaking as generally normal, although the TS speakers could articulate conditions under which they felt likely to stutter and had to monitor their speech. In extensive interviews, neither group articulated views consistent with the general handicaps typically associated with stuttering. The major evident theme in stories of self-recovery was self-guided change (Finn & Felsenfeld, 2004).

A few other attempts have been made to learn something about the conditions under which stuttering disappears in older speakers, chiefly by gaining the viewpoints of the individuals themselves and by examining their histories.[8] Among the factors to which recovery is frequently attributed by people are speaking more slowly, relaxing, acquiring new attitudes toward self or speech problem, speaking more, and speech therapy. Adults studied by Milisen and Johnson (1936) more frequently gave such reasons as enforced left-handedness, removal of tonsils, clipping of the lingual frenum, treatment by a chiropractor, and parental admonitions to repeat stuttered words or to "stop and start over." None are obvious agents of fluency change, except the last, but only when used systematically with very young children, as in the Lidcombe program (discussed in Chapter 14). Both then and more recently, many were unable to offer any explanation at all. Almost all in earlier studies tended to recall their recovery as having been gradual. In a sample of six recovered stutterers, Anderson and Felsenfeld (2003) could identify some overlapping themes, which included increased confidence and increased motivation for change. Some also articulated specific changes in speech that they made in their successful efforts to gain fluency, such as speaking more slowly, more loudly, or more carefully. It should be noted, however, that the majority of their recovered stutterers had received fluency intervention at some point in their lives, but recovered while not in therapy.

From the standpoint of sex ratio, familial incidence, reaction to their difficulty at the time they were experiencing it, and other basic features of the problem, they did not seem easily distinguishable as a group from those whose stuttering fails to disappear. The one factor that seemed to make a difference is severity of stuttering; the more severe cases tended to be more persistent (Sheehan & Martyn, 1970; Dickson, 1971). Presumably because recovered stutterers had less severe problems, Sheehan and Martyn found that they had less often received formal speech therapy. However, it must be said that severity has not been found to be a marker of persistent stuttering when applied to the cohort that recovers within the first two years after onset of stuttering (e.g., Yairi & Ambrose, 2005).

Cox and Kidd (1983) could find no evidence from familial data for supposing that persistent and recovered stuttering are transmitted differently as two genetic subtypes of differing severity. A few studies suggest that, although speech fluency is improved or normalized in speakers reporting self-recovery, some physiologic markers associated with symptomatic stuttering (see Chapter 4) may still be evident. For example, Ingham, Ingham, Finn, and Fox (2003) reported cortical activation during PET scanning that was intermediate between patterns seen in fluent speakers and currently stuttering adults. Forster and Webster (2001) found performance by recovered stutterers on motor control tasks to resemble that seen in nonstutterers; however, performance on divided visual field tasks were more comparable to that seen in adults with chronic stuttering, and appeared to reflect atypical hemispheric dominance.

[8] Milisen and Johnson (1936), Wingate (1964), Shearer and Williams (1965), Sheehan and Martyn (1966, 1970), Lankford and Cooper (1974), Fritzell (1976).

Lifetime Incidence

We have been examining the hypothesis that the essentially constant level that the prevalence of stuttering maintains through the school years represents an equilibrium resulting from two opposing processes in which stuttering develops in some children while it simultaneously ceases in others. We may make a final check on this. If it is true, then the lifetime incidence of stuttering (i.e., the percentage of the population who have stuttered at any time in their lives) should be appreciably higher than the prevalence of stuttering—the percentage who are stutterers at a given time. Estimates of the lifetime incidence of stuttering are summarized in Table 3-4. Although they vary widely, they are all well above the prevalence of stuttering, which is roughly 1 percent of the population. It should be noted that almost all the estimates are based on adults' recollections and that most of the data were obtained from college or university populations.

The disparity among some of the entries under "percentage of incidence" in Table 3-4 is quite large. The Voelker and Villarreal studies, which used exactly the same procedure, found a far higher incidence than did other comparable investigations. Most of the other comparable reports shown in Table 3-4 are in fair agreement, six of them clustering closely at about 5 percent. The 15 percent incidence given by Glasner and Rosenthal needs to be viewed separately. It represents the percentage of 5- and 6-year-old children whose parents said they were stuttering or had stuttered at some time, and apparently reflects the unusual tendency for brief outbreaks of stuttering to occur in preschool children. About half of this 15 percent had already recovered. As we have seen, this early, transient stuttering tends to be forgotten by those who did it. It is therefore a reasonable hypothesis that at least half the incidence found by Glasner and Rosenthal must be added to the incidence found in other studies to give a complete picture.

Thus, it would seem that a plausible figure for the lifetime incidence of all those who at some time either consider themselves or are considered by their parents to be stutterers is at least as high as 10 percent, which is approximately the figure that Dickson was given by parents. One difficulty with this guess is that it must be reconciled with the 4.9 percent finding of the Newcastle Upon Tyne 1,000-family survey in which subjects were studied by direct observation beginning at birth. This unique study made use of periodic checks by health visitors, following which all reports of speech difficulty were confirmed through examinations by speech therapists. A series of early, mild, and transient cases was identified (see Figure 3-2). It seems possible, however, that a considerable number of early episodes of stuttering are so slight and of such brief duration that they might not be confirmed by such a procedure. Glasner and Rosenthal simply questioned the parents. Which method is preferable may be solely a matter of whether there is any interest in stuttering that is mild and short-lived. From this standpoint, the question of the exact size of the longitudinal incidence of stuttering, like that of the exact percentage of spontaneous recovery, may have no absolute answer. As we shall see later, it may be a tenable hypothesis that very minor experiences of stuttering in young children are so widespread that they blend imperceptibly with what is generally regarded as normal disfluency.

Summary

We may now summarize the major facts we have established about the manner in which the prevalence of stuttering varies with age. Stuttering is found on all age levels beginning with the onset of speech. It is almost always reported to begin at some time before adolescence, most commonly in the early years. The older the child, the less likely the development of stuttering. There is a marked tendency for children to recover spontaneously after periods of stuttering of extremely variable duration, and this process continues at a steeply decreasing rate from the earliest childhood through adolescence and beyond. Much of what we know about stuttering in relation to age level may be summed up succinctly by saying that there appears to be some justification for the inference that has sometimes been drawn that stuttering is essentially a disorder of childhood.

THE SEX RATIO

Few facts about stuttering are as thoroughly documented as its unequal sex distribution. The data in Table 3-1 are representative and show a consistent ratio of boys to girls among American schoolchildren of approximately 3:1. A ratio of about 3:1 has also been reported for stuttering schoolchildren in Poland by Glogowski (1976) and in Egypt by Okasha, Bishry, Kamel, and Hassan (1974). These are all prevalence figures, relating to the ratio of boys to girls at a given time. To obtain an estimate of the sex ratio in the lifetime incidence of stuttering, Kidd, Kidd, and Records (1978) investigated the first-degree relatives (fathers, mothers, sisters, and brothers) of 511 stutterers and found a ratio of 2.93:1 among those who had ever stuttered. In a large-scale point prevalence study (see Craig & Tran, 2005, for details), the gender disparity was evident even in the youngest group (2–10 years), in which male prevalence was ~2 percent but female prevalence was only ~0.8 percent.

There is evidence that the sex ratio increases with age. Questionnaire data on schoolchildren gathered from 43 towns and cities in the White House Conference Survey of 1930 disclosed 10,268 stutterers in a sex ratio that rose steadily from 3.1:1 in first grade to 5.5:1 in eleventh and twelfth grade.[9] Glasner and Rosenthal (1957) found a ratio of only 1.4:1 among preschool stutterers. In principle, such a change in ratio might be caused either by an increasing preponderance of boys with age among new cases or by a tendency for girls to recover from stuttering with relatively greater frequency than boys. The latter is more strongly supported by the longitudinal work of the Illinois project (Yairi & Ambrose, 2005). Moreover, the ratio does not remain entirely stabile over the lifespan: Craig and Tran (2005) report ratios (male:female) of 3:1 for 2–10 year old cohorts, 4:1 for 11–20 year olds, 2:1 for stutterers between 21–49 years, and only 1.4:1 for those over age 50. It is not clear why the gender ratio narrows so much for the oldest age group.

The question of why there is a sex ratio in stuttering has been subject to almost as varied speculation as the cause of stuttering itself. At a relatively early date, some researchers regarded it as evidence of a sex-limited genetic predisposition to stuttering (West, 1958; Berry & Eisenson, 1956, chap. 11). It was frequently pointed out in this connection that there is more infant mortality, more birth injury, and greater susceptibility to most childhood diseases among males than females and that the sex ratio in stuttering may be viewed as directly or indirectly reflecting the broad congenital vulnerability of the male constitution.

Others, particularly Johnson and his students, stressed environmental explanations. Schuell (1946, 1947) found what appeared to be relevant differences in parental attitudes and reactions to boys and girls. She gathered evidence appearing to show that boys tend to compare unfavorably with girls in physical, social, and language development and that they are less sheltered than girls and encounter more unequal competition, insecurity, and frustration, especially in relation to language situations. She speculated that these factors tended to result in speech that was more hesitant and therefore more frequently lent itself to a diagnosis of stuttering by parents. Little sex difference appeared in the normal speech hesitancy of children in an extensive normative investigation by Johnson and Associates (1959, chap. 8).[10] Consequently, Johnson eventually surmised that it was not a difference in the fluency of boys and girls that accounted for the sex ratio in stuttering, but a difference in the manner in which parents perceived, evaluated, and reacted to the hesitancies of boys as opposed to those of girls (Johnson & Associates, 1959, p. 240).

There is little adequate evidence with regard to this hypothesis. Bloodstein and Smith (1954) found that, when listeners were presented with recorded speech samples previously judged to be ambiguous

[9]Louttit and Halls' (1936) breakdown by grade and sex of 1,519 stutterers in the public schools of Indiana does not show this systematic variation in sex ratio with age. An analysis by Schuell (1946) of over 1,000 stutterers' records in the files of the University of Iowa Speech Clinic does show it very clearly, but the nature of such data as Schuell's does not permit separation of factors that influence the incidence of stuttering from those influencing referrals to a clinic.

[10]Similarly, Brutten and Miller (1988) found no difference between normally fluent male and female first graders in frequency of disfluency.

with respect to the sex of the child, they did not classify significantly more of the children as stutterers when told they were listening to boys than when told they were listening to girls. Unfortunately, this procedure leaves much to be desired as an analogue of the diagnosis of stuttering in actual children by their parents.

Of possible relevance to Johnson's theory are some observations relating to differing social attitudes toward the stuttering of males as compared with females. E.-M. Silverman and Van Opens (1980) presented grade school teachers with anecdotes about children with various speech and language difficulties. When the anecdote concerned a child with disfluency, the teachers were more likely to recommend referral for remediation if the child had a boy's name than if the child had a girl's name. No such difference appeared in the case of lisping, hoarseness, or language disorders. E.-M. Silverman (1982) also found that university students had stronger negative stereotypes of male stutterers than female stutterers, and an interview study of adult stutterers by E.-M. Silverman and Zimmer (1982) revealed a tendency for stuttering to be a somewhat more serious problem for men than for women.

Outside the context of the diagnosogenic theory, attempts have been made to relate the sex ratio to slower early language development in males and to their greater proneness to articulatory errors, reading problems, and most other difficulties of speech and communication (West & Ansberry, 1968, p. 126; Bloodstein, 1958, p. 38). Clarice Tatman, in a personal communication to the first author, made the interesting suggestion that the sex ratio might be due in part to the difference between masculine and feminine roles with regard to speech. In general, girls are not expected to be as outspoken and self-assertive as are boys. Consequently, in many situations of anxiety, guilt, or tension, she believed that a girl may be permitted to take refuge in silence while a boy is more likely to feel compelled to speak under pressure.

Goldman (1967) sought to provide some evidence in support of the hypothesis that the sex ratio is related to greater environmental pressures on males. Reasoning that the lower socioeconomic segment of southern African American society possesses a matriarchal structure that often tends to impose less responsibility on the males than on females, he studied the sex ratio in a sample of 694 stutterers identified in a statewide survey of school-age children in Tennessee. There was a sex ratio of only 2.4:1 among the African American children, as opposed to 4.9:1 among the Caucasian children. Goldman then compared the sex ratio in stuttering among African American children from what he termed "matriarchal" and "patriarchal" home environments, which he differentiated on the basis of the presence or absence of a "stable and consistent male figure in the home." Among 77 stutterers from "patriarchal" home environments, he found a sex ratio of 3.5:1, while among 38 from a "matriarchal" environment it was 1.1:1.

Eisenson (1966) attempted to refute the environmental hypothesis by pointing out that the sex ratio appears to exist even among stuttering children to be found in Israeli kibbutzim, communal institutions where, at the date of Eisenson's observations, children generally saw their parents for only three hours a day and received "relatively objective upbringing" by nurses and teachers with "no conscious differences in the treatment of the children along sex lines." In the kibbutz visited by Eisenson, the stutterers consisted of 12 boys and 3 girls.

On the basis of a genetic study of 2,524 first-degree relatives of stutterers, Kidd, Kidd, and Records (1978) concluded that the sex ratio is best explained by some type of sex-modified inheritance. They proposed a model in which both genes and environment contribute to the liability to stutter and in which males have a lower threshold of susceptibility than females. The difference in threshold might be either biological or social. MacFarlane, Hanson, Walton, and Mellon (1991) studied a five-generation family with a high incidence of stuttering and found that the data met all criteria for sex-modified genetic transmission.

Some "odds" related to the transmission of stuttering by gender have emerged. Andrews et al. (1983), in combining data from earlier studies, estimated that stuttering men have a 22 percent risk of having a stuttering son and a 9 percent risk of having a stuttering daughter, while stuttering women have an elevated risk of having stuttering children, 36 percent for their sons and 17 percent for their daughters. Yairi and Ambrose (2005), using a much smaller sample, found a similar pattern of risk, while Janssen, Kloth, Kraaimaat, and Brutten (1996) could not discern elevated risk for the children of female stutterers in their sample of 106 adult stuttering probands.

It may be relevant to consider Geschwind's theory that the sex ratio in stuttering is due to higher levels of testosterone in the male fetus than in the female (see Geschwind & Galaburda, 1985). As noted in Chapter 2, Geschwind suggested that testosterone retards the development of the left cerebral hemisphere, thus increasing the risk of speech and language disturbances, including stuttering.

The meaning of the sex ratio has intrigued experts since the beginning of modern scientific curiosity about speech disorders. With the differences between boys and girls extending to so many factors of physiology, development, and social environment, however, all too many explanations of the sex ratio are possible, and it would unfortunately be difficult to think of a theory of stuttering that could not be reconciled with it.

THE INFLUENCE OF HEREDITY

There are several areas of research on the incidence of stuttering in which the focus of interest is on the question of whether heredity plays an important role in the disorder. They include the incidence of stuttering in the families of stutterers, in twins, and in families that adopt children who grow up to become stutterers.

Familial Incidence in Stuttering

The tendency for stuttering to appear in successive generations of the same family has served to provoke speculation about a genetic basis of stuttering for many years. In clinical practice, cases are occasionally encountered in which a large number of the person's relatives on the maternal or paternal side have been stutterers for several generations. The literature contains an abundance of reports of large proportions of stutterers giving a history of stuttering in the family background, these proportions generally ranging from about one-third to two-thirds of cases. For example, Buck, Lees, and Cook (2002) found 72 percent of a sample of 61 children to have positive family histories of stuttering, while Yairi and Ambrose (1992a, 1992b) found that about two-thirds of a sample of 87 children who stuttered reported a positive family history. The findings summarized in Table 3-5 represent the studies that have employed control data. They show that the proportion of nonstutterers who report a family history of stuttering tends to be much smaller than that of stutterers, ranging from 5 to 18 percent. On the basis of pooled data from several studies, Andrews et al. (1983) estimated that the incidence of stuttering among first-degree relatives of stutterers is more than three times that in the general population.

Genetic Interpretations

Many researchers have long accepted a genetic explanation of the familial incidence of stuttering as the simplest and most satisfactory. They have had difficulty, however, in establishing the manner of transmission. The question is complicated by the fact that we are concerned with the transmission, not of stuttering itself, but of a trait that might or might not be expressed or manifested in stuttering by the person who possessed it, depending upon environmental circumstances. A chapter by Ehud Yairi and Nicoline Ambrose (2005) provides a useful overview of some of the basic concepts necessary to an understanding of genetic studies in fluency and other communication disorders, and emphasizes the complex interaction between genes and behavior, an emerging discipline now called behavioral genetics (see Gilger, 1995; Gilger & Rice 1996; Dale, Dionne, Eley, & Plomin, 2000; Fisher, Plomin, DeFries, Craig, & McGuffin, 2003, for discussion relevant to communication disorders).

Pedigree Studies

Genetic investigations of stuttering have been conducted for well over half a century. Evidence obtained by Meyer (1945), Andrews and Harris (1964), and Kidd, Kidd, and Records (1978) from

TABLE 3-5 Percentage of Stutters and Nonstutterers Reporting Familial Histories of Stuttering

	N	Stutterers	Nonstutterers
Bryngelson and Rutherford (1937)	74, 74	46.0	18.0
Wepman (1939)	250, 250	68.8	15.6
Bryngelson (1939)	78, 78	54.0	6.0
West, Nelson, and Berry (1939)	204, 204	51.0	18.1
Johnson et al. (1942)	46, 46	32.6[a]	8.7[a]
Meyer (1945)	100, 246	61.0	6.5
Darley (1955)	50, 50	52.0	42.0
Johnson and Associates (1959)	150, 150	23.3	6.0[b]
Andrews and Harris (1964)	80, 80	37.5	1.3
Martyn and Sheehan (1968)	85, 277[c]	32.9	6.1
Mann (cited by Howle, 1976)	49, 49	31.9[d]	10.2[d]
Profert and Rosenfield (1978)	44, 1,965	29.5	5.0
Accordi et al. (1983)	2,802, 1,602	50.0	6.6
Goldberg and Culatta (1991)	693	46.5	NA
Poulos and Webster (1991)	169	66	NA
Janssen, Kloth, Kraaimaat, and Brutten (1996)[e]	2296	11.6	88.4
Drayna, Kilshaw, and Kelly (1999)[f]	482	46.5	53.5
Månsson (2000)	12	67	NA
Buck et al. (2002)[g]	61	72	NA
Viswanath, Lee, and Chakraborty (2004)	56	84	NA
Yairi and Ambrose (2005)[h]	123 families of children who stutter	69 (overall) 88 (families of persistent stuttering children) 63 (families of recovered stuttering children)	NA

[a]Represents the percentage who had stuttering relatives outside the immediate family.
[b]As reported by the mothers. The percentage as reported by the fathers was 5.3.
[c]The 85 subjects in the experimental group consisted of both recovered and active stutterers.
[d]Represents the percentage who had stuttering offspring.
[e]106 children at high risk of stuttering were identified and the parents of these children were studied: 77 stuttering fathers, 29 stuttering mothers. These parents reported on the presence of stuttering at any time in 2296 first-, second- and third-degree relatives.
[f]More than 100 small to medium-sized unrelated families with multiple cases of persistent stuttering were chosen to represent the adult population of familial stuttering.
[g]Retrospective analysis of records of children who attended Michael Palin Centre for Stammering Children, United Kingdom, ages 2–6 years.
[h]Also found that the highest risk for stuttering occurs in male relatives of female probands.

studies of the family backgrounds of stutterers appears to rule out any simple Mendelian type of inheritance, such as sex-linked, autosomal dominant, or recessive. None of these is compatible with the observed distribution of stuttering relatives. This does not, however, exclude the possibility of more complex types of genetic transmission.

Andrews and Harris (1964, chap. 7), with the assistance of Roger Garside and David Kay, carried out a detailed analysis of stutterers' familial backgrounds that appeared to show that certain genetic hypotheses were tenable. This can be viewed as the first segregation analysis, in which pedigrees are used to fit familial patterns of transmission to known models of inheritance. From their data, they determined the probability of occurrence of stuttering in various categories of relatives in the immediate families of stutterers. They found that their results could be accounted for by assuming a sex-limited transmission by means of a large number of nonspecific genes. That is to say, a given amount of predisposition to stuttering might be inherited by the same type of polygenic inheritance responsible for such continuously distributed, finely graded characteristics as stature or intelligence. Accordingly, they drew the conclusion that a tendency toward stuttering might be passed down by polygenic inheritance or by a "common dominant gene with a multifactorial background." In either case, it is necessary to assume the operation of sex limitation, a mechanism by which the effects of the same genes are manifested to different degrees in males and females.

Added support for the belief that genes play a part in stuttering came subsequently from work by Kidd, Reich, and Kessler (1973, 1974) in the Department of Human Genetics at Yale University. These workers were concerned with human traits that have a high familial incidence, but show no Mendelian patterns of inheritance because they are brought about in part by environmental factors. Such traits can usually be explained genetically by either multifactorial (polygenic) or single-gene models. Kidd and his associates had shown that when a sex ratio exists and sufficient information is at hand on the incidence of the trait in relatives of affected individuals, it is possible to test the relative adequacy of these two models statistically. Looking about for human traits to which to apply their methods, they recognized that stuttering fulfilled all the requirements.

By analyzing the data of Andrews and Harris combined with other available data, Kidd, Reich, and Kessler concluded that there is probably a genetic factor in stuttering with a "single major locus." They pointed out, however, that the polygenic model also gave an adequate fit to the data and that even entirely nongenetic inheritance was not totally excluded, inasmuch as unambiguous demonstration of biological transmission can only result from adoption or genetic linkage studies. Both the monogenic and polygenic models they tested assumed that an individual's total (genetic and environmental) liability to stutter is a variable trait manifested overtly in stuttering when exceeding a certain threshold value that is lower for males than females.

Further data collected by Kidd and his associates on the families of several hundred stutterers following their first study produced similar results (Kidd, 1977; Kidd, Heimbuch, & Records, 1981). Their gene-environment interaction model predicted with considerable accuracy the proportions of stuttering fathers, mothers, sisters, and brothers in these families.

Doubt has persisted over the question of single-gene versus polygenic inheritance. Contrary to the original findings, Cox, Kramer, and Kidd (1984) determined that the multifactorial (polygenic) model offered a more satisfactory explanation for the transmission of stuttering than the monogenic model. Their results also allowed for the possibility that stuttering might be environmentally influenced in some cases. In another study, Ambrose, Yairi, and Cox (1993) found that data on the extended families of 69 young stutterers were consistent with a single-gene hypothesis.

Mellon et al. (1991) reported on a large Utah family with over 1,200 members, all descended from one adult male stutterer. Branches of the family tree differed in the transmission of stuttering, with two of eight branches showing no stuttering, five branches showing moderate transmission of stuttering, and one branch showing a very high transmission rate (approximating almost one-third of 150 descendents). The authors suggested that a monogenic autosomal dominant model with reduced penetrance best fit the patterns observed in this particular family.

The debate continues over the appropriate genetic model of transmission for stuttering. Teams in a number of locations have isolated new populations against which to test genetic models of the mode of transmission and heritability values for stuttering. In Houston, a team centered at Baylor College of Medicine (Viswanath, Lee, & Chakraborty, 2004) constructed 56 family pedigrees for adult persistent stutterers (the probands). In a methodology somewhat different from some others we report, the authors asked the relative respondents to imitate what they considered to be stuttering behaviors in themselves or others to unify judgments of stuttering by the researchers. They also considered only persistent adults to be affected; some of the other studies we report also included young children during what might be transient periods of stuttering. The team utilized complex segregation analysis. Eighty-four percent of the probands were characterized by multiplex pedigrees (families in which more than one member was reported to stutter, the condition of interest), which was higher than found in other studies in this section (ranges have been from 23 percent from Johnson and Associates [1959] and Ambrose et al. [1993]), despite the fact that participants had not been recruited for an active family history of stuttering. Results were more consistent with a Mendelian model of transmission, also favored in a report by Ambrose and Cox (1997) with best statistical fit for an autosomal dominant model. In the derived model, probability that affected females have at least one affected parent was estimated at 19 percent, while the probability that an affected male had an affected parent was extremely high, at 67 percent. After weighing the gender factor, the authors' model of choice was "an autosomal diallelic major locus model in which the penetrance of the dominant allele is mainly influenced by two covariates: sex and affection status of the parents." (p. 409). The authors specifically rejected a polygenic threshold model. In such a model, variations of many genes would contribute to the trait, but the individual is symptomatic only when the number of predisposing genes crosses over a given threshold. Such models explain and describe disorders with relatively low penetrance.

Finally, the differing results of the studies that we discuss in this section do raise the possibility that transient and persistent stuttering are behaviorally similar, but genetically different conditions (Viswanath, Lee, & Chakraborty, 2004). The authors describe a plan to use this study, best viewed as a segregation analysis, to conduct a linkage analysis, the kind of work that could eventually locate a "stuttering gene." To distinguish between these two important steps, as noted earlier, segregation analysis is a method to statistically test whether an observed pattern of behavior or performance (the phenotype) seen in families is compatible with any existing explicit models of inheritance. Once a pattern of inheritance has been ascertained, one can then progress to a much more difficult task, linkage analysis. "Linkage" is the tendency for genes to be inherited together because of their location near one another on the same chromosome. Linkage analysis is what one might call a "gene hunting" technique that traces conditions in high-risk families (families with more than one affected member), in an attempt to locate the specific causative gene by identifying genetic markers that have known chromosomal location and appear to be co-inherited with the trait of interest. The statistical estimate of whether two loci are likely to lie near each other on a chromosome and are therefore likely to be inherited together is called a LOD (logarithmic odds) score. A LOD score of 3 or more (odds 1,000 to 1) is generally taken to indicate that the two loci are linked and are close to one another. However, this assumption is based on Mendelian models of transmission, and alternative statistical measures are under development for traits that show complex inheritance patterns, such as stuttering.

Some progress has been made in narrowing down the exact locus of the gene associated with stuttering. In a study of 68 North American families, a team of University-based and NIH researchers (Shugart et al., 2004) identified a potential locus for a "stuttering gene" on chromosome 18, known to be involved in intercellular transmission. This locus was not identified in an earlier report based on analysis of stuttering in the Hutterites, a highly intermarried community in North Dakota, by the University of Illinois team (Cox, Yairi, and colleagues). That team, as reported by Shugart et al., found support for linkage on chromosomes 1, 13, and 16. A 2004 study of a multigenerational extended West African (Cameroon) family, with 106 members of whom 45 stutter as adults, produced significant evidence of linkage (LOD score >4) on chromosome 1 (Levis, Ricci, Lukong, & Drayna, 2004). A study conducted using an inbred Pakistani cohort consisting of 44 intermarried families with 144 affected members, Riaz et al. (2005), showed preliminary linkage on chromosomes 1, 5, 7, and 12. Follow-up analysis using an additional two families with 16 additional members showed that linkage on chromosome 12 was characterized by an LOD score of 3.5, which, as noted earlier, is significant indication of linkage to a specific chromosome. However, not all families showed evidence of linkage on this chromosome. Another linkage study (Suresh et al., 2006) carried out with a relatively large sample (100 American, Swedish, and Israeli families, containing 252 persistent stutterers, 45 recovered stutterers, and 19 children too young to classify) identified other potential loci, although few LOD scores met a value of 3 with the exception of chromosome 9 for those with any history of stuttering and chromosome 15 for persistent stutterers. When the set was divided by gender, chromosome 7 was identified as a potential locus for men, while chromosome 21 met accepted levels of significance for the women. It should be noted that chromosome 7 has also been identified as a potential locus for autism and specific language impairment, including other communication disorders.

It should be apparent from Table 3-6 that the studies to date have not identified a consistent chromosomal locus. As multiple sites explore segregation analyses to guide their linkage analyses, we appear to be closing in on a "stuttering gene". What it does and how its activity is moderated by experience will then need to be shown.

As noted earlier, Kidd, Heimbuch, Records, Oehlert, and Webster (1980) could find no evidence that the severity of stuttering is influenced by heredity. An interesting finding from many studies (but not from that of Ambrose, Yairi, and Cox) was that female stutterers tended to have more stuttering relatives than male stutterers. Puzzling as this may seem initially, it is readily explained on the assumption that a predisposition to stuttering is genetically transmitted. As Andrews and Harris (1964, p. 141) pointed out, the effect may occur for the same reason that tall women are more likely to have tall relatives than are tall men. Since men tend to be taller than women, a six-foot-tall woman is more exceptional (i.e., in a more extreme part of the distribution of females with regard to stature) than is a six-foot-tall man. Consequently, she is more likely to come from a family of tall individuals. The same reasoning can be applied to stuttering if we suppose that the presumed hereditary predisposition to stutter is a continuously variable trait, like human stature, and that it takes a heavier predisposition to make a girl stutter than a boy. Yet another possibility raised by some research is that there may be sex-specific loci for genetic transmission of stuttering (Suresh et al., 2006).

Social Interpretations of Familial Stuttering

Several forms of purely social inheritance have been suggested to explain the familial incidence of stuttering. The earliest of these was imitation of other stutterers in the family. Imitation is no longer regarded as an important factor by most researchers. One reason for this is that stutterers who have stuttering relatives frequently have had no personal contact with them, as Nelson (1939) showed. When they do, as in the case of parents, Kidd, Kidd, and Records (1978) found that so many no longer stuttered by the time the child was born, that of 511 cases only 12 percent had a stuttering parental model to imitate. Another reason for the widespread rejection of the imitation hypothesis is that there is so often a marked dissimilarity between the features of stuttering of a young child in the earliest phase of the disorder and those of the adult whom the child might be presumed to have imitated.

The form of nongenetic inheritance of stuttering that has been accorded most serious consideration is the social transmission from one generation to the next of a family environment that for one reason or another is conducive to the development of the disorder. Particular emphasis was given to such a concept in the thinking of Johnson and his students within the framework of his diagnosogenic

TABLE 3-6 Studies Seeking to Identify a "Stuttering" Gene

	Subjects	Identified	Locus
Ambrose and Yairi (1997, 1996)	66 stuttering children	No	Statistical evidence was presented for both a single major locus and polygenic component Data is consistent with the hypothesis that persistence is in part due to an additional genetic factor
Viswanath, Lee, and Chakraborty (2004)	56 U.S pedigrees of European origin constructed based on responses of adults with persistent developmental stuttering; 43 were verified	No	Results indicated that the transmission of persistent developmental stuttering is consistent with an autosomal diallelic major locus model in which the penetrance of the dominant allele is mainly influenced by the effect from the parents and sex covariate
Shugart et al. (2004)	68 families of European ancestry	Possible	Modest evidence of linkage to chromosome 18q (NPL(Sall) = 1.15)
Riaz et al. (2005)	46 highly inbred Pakistani families	Yes	Genomewide-significant linkage to chromosome 12q (LOD = 4.61) and suggestive evidence for linkage to chromosome 1q (LOD = 2.93)
Suresh et al. (2006)[a]	100 families of European descent ascertained in the United States, Sweden, and Israel including 252 persistent stutterers, 45 recovered and 19 too young to classify	Possible	Ever stuttered (persistent and recovered) linked to Chromosome 9 (LOD = 2.3 at 60 cM) Persistent stuttering only linked to chromosome 15 (LOD = 1.95 at 23 cM) Sex-specific linkage was significant Male only was linked to chromosome 7 (153cM) Female only was linked to chromosome 21 (33.5 cM)

[a]LOD stands for logarithm of the odds (to the base 10). An LOD score of 3 or more is generally taken to indicate that two gene loci are close to each other on the chromosome. (An LOD score of 3 means the odds are 1000:1 in favor of genetic linkage.)

theory. Johnson believed that stuttering frequently occurs in the same family because of the handing down of a "climate of anxiety" about the hesitant speech of children.

Some observations in support of this viewpoint were made by Gray (1940) in her investigation of a "stuttering" family in Iowa. Although there had been stutterers in this family for the last five generations, it appeared that there was a fairly large branch of the family living in Kansas in which there was very little stuttering. It might be argued that on the hypothesis of genetic transmission this was an improbable occurrence. Gray interviewed the living members of the Iowa branch and contacted the Kansas branch by mail. The chief result of her study was a detailed genealogy (see Figure 3-3), which showed that the last two generations of the Iowa branch stemmed from a woman whom Gray designated as III A. Not only was III A a stutterer herself, but her father and her maternal aunt and grandmother had also been stutterers. She was, moreover, the youngest of four children, all but one of whom stuttered. When these children grew up they all moved to Kansas, with the exception of III A who remained in Iowa, and there had subsequently been little contact between the two branches of the family except by occasional letter. In the last two generations of the Iowa branch (i.e., the children and grandchildren of III A), about

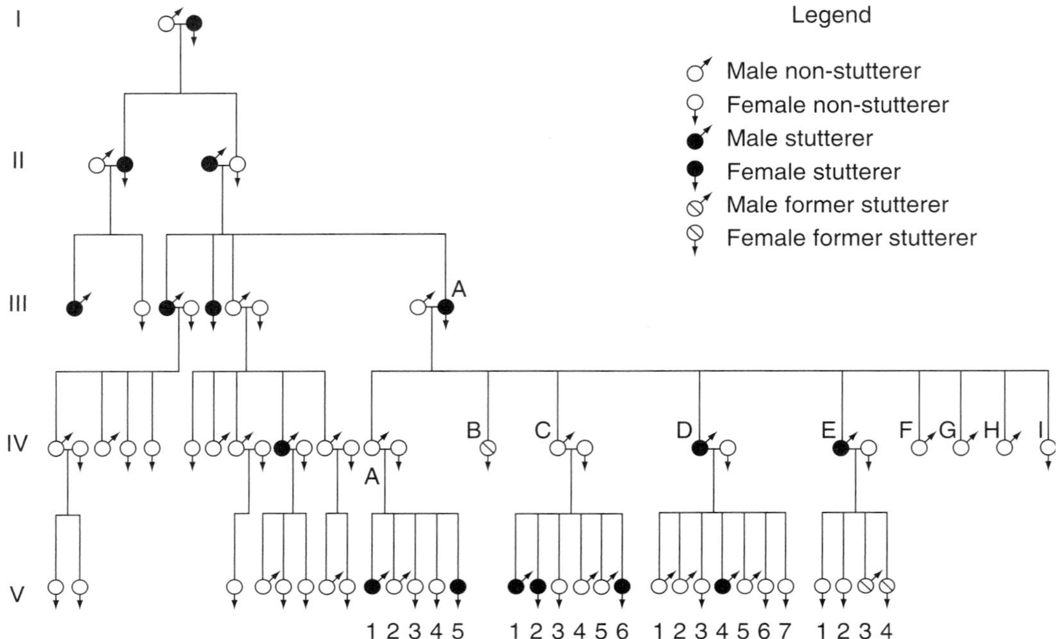

FIGURE 3-3 Five generations of a "stuttering" family. About 40 percent of the Iowa branch (the descendants of III A) were found to be or to have been stutterers. Of the seventeen living members of Kansas branch (descendants of the siblings of III A) only one was a stutterer. These findings have been used in support of an environmental explanation of the familial incidence of stuttering. Reprinted with permission from Gray, M. The X family: A clinical and laboratory study of a "stuttering" family. Journal of Speech Disorders, 5, 343–48. Copyright 1940 by the American Speech-Language-Hearing Association. All right reserved.

40 percent were stutterers, while of 17 living Kansas members, only one stuttered.

Gray offered the interpretation that the stuttering in the Iowa branch arose largely out of attitudes that were conducive to the diagnosis of more or less normal speech as stuttering. She believed that in this the "tone" was set for the Iowa group by IV E, the last of III A's five biological children, by virtue of his dominant position in the family and the severity of his stuttering. Her informants made such comments as, "We wondered whether our children would stutter like IV E," or, "I couldn't stand it if I stuttered like IV E." As a group they appeared to be "stuttering conscious." They believed that the disorder was hereditary in their family and seemed to watch their children anxiously for signs of it.

At the time that Gray did her study of this family, various members of the Iowa branch received advice and information about stuttering in the context of a diagnosogenic orientation toward the problem. Twenty years later, Johnson carried out a follow-up investigation of the family (Johnson, 1961b, pp. 83, 84; Johnson et al., 1967, pp. 265, 266). By now the fifth generation, children at the time of Gray's study, had grown up and many of them had children of their own. Johnson reported that of 44 people in the sixth generation, only one had ever been considered a stutterer. He related this decline in the number of stutterers to indications that there had been a change in the familial assumptions about stuttering and a reduction in their tendency to make an issue of childhood lapses in fluency.

Stuttering and Twinning

While interesting, Gray's research cannot really inform the relative contributions of nature and nurture, but other approaches can offer interesting perspectives. The subject of twins has been of importance for stuttering, as it has been for other traits, in relation to hypotheses about the role of heredity in its causation. A number of different questions involving twins have been considered in connection with stuttering.

Prevalence in Twins

Several studies have been done on the prevalence of stuttering in the twin population. These have consistently shown unexpectedly large proportions of stutterers, although the size of the prevalence reported has varied consideration. In fairly large groups of twin pairs, stuttering has been found in 9 percent of the individual members by Berry (1938a) and in 13 percent by Nelson, Hunter, and Walter (1945), but in only 1.9 percent by Graf (1955).

In view of the large numbers of stutterers found among twins, it is reasonable to expect the converse, a high incidence of twins among stutterers. Berry (1937b) found that 4.5 percent of 461 stuttering subjects were members of a twin pair, as against only 1.2 percent among 500 nonstutterers. Later research by Johnson and Associates (1959, p. 71) showed that among 200 stutterers, three were twins, while in a like number of nonstutterers one was a twin. When all of these findings are considered together, the weight of evidence at present seems to favor the view that there is some relationship between stuttering and twin membership, although the extent of the relationship is still far from clear.

This finding has been subject to various interpretations. West and his students held that a tendency toward twinning and a predisposition to stuttering are genetically linked in some families (West & Ansberry, 1968, p. 127). An alternative hypothesis offered by West (1958) was that the slowness of early maturation frequently associated with multiple births may contribute to a general constitutional retardation, which he believed to underlie stuttering. We do know that twins are more likely to experience intrauterine complications, and prenatal and antenatal risk factors, especially prematurity and intrauterine growth retardation (Garite, Clark, Elliott, & Thorp, 2004).

Explanations stressing environmental factors have also been offered. Schuell (1946) offered the hypothesis that when stuttering occurs in fraternal twins, it is usually to be found in the physiologically less mature member and results from pressure to keep pace with the other one. It might be that in both fraternal and identical cases, some part is played in producing stuttering by the competitive pressures that members of a twin pair often encounter as a result of the comparisons inevitably made between them, but it would appear difficult to test this hypothesis in any standardized way.

Incidence in Twinning Families

While it is reasonable to consider environmental explanations for an increased incidence of stuttering in twins, it would be difficult to account in this manner for any increased stuttering to be found in twinning families, particularly those in which the twins themselves were not stutterers. It is therefore of some significance that Berry (1938a) reported that in the immediate families of a group of 250 pairs of twins she had found that 5.5 percent of the children (i.e., the twins and their siblings) were stutterers. This large percentage was due chiefly, it is true, to the abundance of stutterers among the twins themselves. When the singleton siblings of the twins are considered alone, however, as many as 2.9 percent of them prove to be stutterers. This is far higher than would be expected.

There has yet been no definite confirmation of this finding that stuttering and twinning tend to be associated in the same families over and above their tendency to be associated in the same individuals. In a different study by Berry (1937b), the converse of the one just referred to, twins were found to be more common in the immediate families of stutterers than in the families of nonstutterers, but this difference appears to have been due essentially to the number of twins among the stutterers themselves rather than among their siblings. Johnson and his coworkers (1959, p. 72) found that of the parents of 150 stutterers, 21 mothers and 19 fathers identified twins among their relatives while of the parents of 150 nonstutterers, 28 mothers and 21 fathers reported relatives who were twins. Andrews and Harris (1964, p. 77) reported that of a group of 80 stutterers, 19 had a family history of twinning as opposed to 11 in a like number of controls, an interesting trend that was not, however, statistically significant. Unfortunately, head-counting studies are a type of research in which large numbers of subjects are often needed in order to rule out the possibility that differences are due to chance.

Concordance in Identical Twins

Because identical, or monozygotic, twins result from the cleavage of a single fertilized ovum and consequently have exactly the same heredity, they have long been of interest to scientists concerned with the relative influence of heredity and environment on human traits. It can be argued that if a trait such as stuttering is invariably found in both members of an identical twin pair and is found in both members of a fraternal pair no more often than it occurs in any two siblings, it is probably hereditary. It should be noted that this is actually quite a different question from the ones we have just discussed and would be of considerable significance even if there were no reason to believe that stuttering was rather common among twins. It is of interest, therefore, that a series of studies has been done on the concordance for stuttering in identical and fraternal twins.[11] One study by Susan Felsenfeld and colleagues (Felsenfeld et al., 2000) utilized the Australian Twin Registry and directly interviewed 91 pairs of twins in which at least one member stuttered. Of twins identified as monozygotic (MZ), 45 percent were concordant for stuttering, while only 15 percent of the dizygotic (DZ) twins were concordant. Ooki (2005) used a questionnaire to determine both zygosity and history of stuttering (both transient and persistent) in a large (N=1896 twin pairs) sample of Japanese twins.[12] Structural equation modeling results suggested that between 80–85 percent of behavioral (phenotypic) variance in stuttering (for males and females, respectively) could be attributed to a genetic component. Pair-wise concordance in the sample was 10:12 for MZ twins and only 2:19 for DZ twins. Yairi and Ambrose (2005), in the comprehensive summary of their longitudinal study of early stuttering, identified five sets of twins, two of which were identified as MZ and three as DZ. In this small sample, all twins were concordant, although, consistent with other studies that have examined the transmission of stuttering severity, symptom severity varied.

Two conclusions appear to be warranted by the evidence from these studies (see Table 3-7). One is that there is a fairly high degree of concordance for stuttering in identical twins. The other is that there are exceptions. The exceptions do not invalidate a genetic theory of inheritance of stuttering; they only show that environment plays some part. However, it will be necessary to further define what is meant by "environment."

We wish to emphasize that the use of monozygotic (identical:MZ) twins to discriminate between nature and nurture has become more complex than it had been in earlier times. A useful reference for issues surrounding this concept can be found in Wong, Gottesman, and Petronis (2005), and we will cite some of their concepts because they bear careful consideration whenever one tries to pit genetics against "the environment." As they note, for *most* heritable medical conditions, there is a certain degree of discordance between verified

[11]In addition, Howie (1981b) obtained equivocal results in investigating the similarities of stuttering frequency within identical and fraternal twin pairs. She found some evidence of a genetic influence on frequency of prolongations and "blocks," but not on frequency of sound, syllable, or word repetitions.

[12]Although one purpose of the study was to examine whether stuttering co-occurred frequently with tic disorder, this relationship was not found.

TABLE 3-7 Numbers of Identical and Fraternal Twin Pairs Concordant and Discordant for Stuttering

	Identical		Fraternal	
	Concordant	Discordant	Concordant	Discordant
Nelson, Hunter, and Walter (1945)	9	1	2	28
Graf (1955)	1	6	2	7
Luchsinger (1959)[a]	13	2	0	29
Godal, Tatarelli, and Bonanni (1976)	10	2	2	17
Howie (1981a)	10	6	3	10
Andrews, Morris-Yates, Howie, and Martin (1991)	10	40	3	82
Felsenfeld, Kirk, Zhu, Statham, Neale, and Martin (2000)[b]	SS 20 IS 17	SS 98 IS 21	SS 8 IS 8	SS 121 IS 45
Ooki (2005)	27	40	3	50
Total	43	17	9	91

[a]Observations gathered by Luchsinger from his own clinical records and those of other workers: Seeman, Brankel, Gedda, and Bruno.
[b]Screening Sample (SS) = 1,567 pairs of twins. Interview Subsample (IS) = 197 pairs of twins.

MZ twins. They note that in "virtually all complex, non-Mendelian diseases in which there is clearly some appreciable degree of heritable risk . . . a significant proportion of MZ twin pairs is discordant for the disease. . . . These differences have usually been attributed to the effects of environment . . . as a default explanation for variation that remains after genetic effects are accounted for . . . [however] there is an increasing body of experimental evidence suggesting that the generally accepted assumption—variation not attributable to genetic factors must therefore be environmental—may require revision" (p. R12).

What is this evidence? It has been difficult to carefully control "human laboratory experiments" by using populations such as twins reared apart. However, it is possible to create MZ animal twins and then control their environments. For example, in mice, one can create MZ and DZ (dizygotic, or fraternal twins); while some growth milestones, such as weight and time to achieve some developmental stages, such as eye opening, are more variable for DZ than MZ twins, there is still some variation in the MZ group. The conclusion from a number of studies that the authors discuss is that, "significant phenotypic variation, including crossing a threshold to . . . disease, can emerge from animals that have an identical, cloned genetic background" (p. R14). The authors conclude that "there exists a component of phenotypic variation whose source remains unexplained." As possibilities, they note that a substantial amount of what they call "epigenetic variability" can arise over the millions of mitotic divisions that occur early in the embryonic development of otherwise identical organisms. Thus, they suggest that MZ twins sometimes differ, not because they are exposed to different postnatal environments, but because of these embryonic developmental differences. They also caution that the evolving data from animal models may cause "major paradigmatic shifts" in how we view the debate between nature and nurture (p. R17).

More mundane prenatal influences have been noted that bear on differences in the phenotype of MZ twins, and additionally bear on some potential causes of stuttering that are discussed in greater detail in Chapter 4. As mentioned earlier, twins share a cramped and somewhat riskier uterine environment than does a singleton fetus. Many MZ twins are actually discordant for handedness, which is known to have genetic transmission, but is not apparently determined by handedness of adopting parents. This discordance in handedness has been attributed in the past to complicated and preterm birth patterns for twins, regardless of their genetic relationship, that can result in left hemisphere brain injury and deviant resulting patterns of language dominance. In a further analysis of this phenomenon, a Dutch research team (Sommer, Ramsey, Mandl, & Kahn, 2002) examined language lateralization using fMRI in 12 MZ twins and 13 DZ twins. They found that handedness discordance in MZ twins was often accompanied by discordance in their dominant hemisphere, and speculated that such a result might be caused by "relatively late time of splitting of the original embryo, which disrupts the normal development of left-right asymmetry" (p. 2710). They note that MZ twinning is in general, "more susceptible to malformations." Because cerebral lateralization atypicalities have often been targeted as a finding in people who stutter, such a finding bears directly on why MZ twins can differ for a major condition such as stuttering for "non-environmental" reasons. The authors further pose an interesting hypothesis about the origins of handedness and hemispheric patterns that differ from familial history—they note that up to 70 percent of twin pregnancies diagnosed prior to the 10th week of gestation either miscarry or convert to a single fetus: "left-handedness and right cerebral dominance in some subjects born as singletons may also be the result of a late monozygotic twinning process from which only one twin survives" (p. 2716).

To constitute more conclusive evidence of the biological inheritance of stuttering, its concordance would have to be demonstrable in identical twins that had been reared apart. Some information on this question has resulted from work by Farber (1981). Farber was concerned with essentially the entire range of physical and behavioral traits of identical twins that had been reared apart. She combed the literature from 1923 to 1973 to collect all available accounts of such cases. Her book *Identical Twins Reared Apart: A Reanalysis*, is a detailed description of 95 pairs of twins about whom there was reliable information. However, we note that this information could not have included DNA analysis, the most reliable indicator of MZ status. Many DZ twins can appear "identical" when in fact, they are not. Startling similarities of behavior emerged. The twins tended to have the same tastes in clothing, books, and music and the same mannerisms and ways of sitting, holding themselves, walking, laughing, and gesturing. In one instance, they had the same nickname. The similarities extended to the twins' speech patterns and vocal characteristics, including such features as talkativeness, high pitch, and hoarseness. The only exception among speech characteristics was stuttering. Among her 95 cases Farber identified five with stuttering. In all five cases, only one member of the pair stuttered.[13]

In a footnote, Farber mentioned an additional twin pair that was concordant for stuttering. This was a Japanese pair, reported by Yoshimasu in 1941, who had been separated at birth and reunited at age 32 years. One, Takao, had been imprisoned for theft and embezzlement and the other, Kazuo, had become a Christian minister. Both were said to stutter. They were not included in Farber's series of 95 cases, presumably because of failure to satisfy her stringent criteria for reliability.

Commenting on the twins' speech characteristics, Farber stated, "Only stuttering seems environmentally related." Most workers in the field of speech and language pathology would probably hesitate to draw so bold an inference at the present time.

Stuttering in the Families of Adopted Stutterers

There is still a further stratagem by which the issue of heredity in stuttering might be resolved, and that is by studying the familial backgrounds of stutterers who have been raised as adopted children. We know as a result of past research that, because they are stutterers, approximately one-third to two-thirds of such a group are likely to have identifiable histories of stuttering in their families. But where are these histories to be found—in the biological or

[13]The relevant data in Farber's book are on page 86 and in Table A9 in the epilogue.

the adoptive families? A clear answer to this question would go far to show whether the tendency of stuttering to recur in successive generations of the same family is mainly biological or mainly social.[14]

Investigation of the biological families of adopted children unfortunately presents practical difficulties. Much might be learned, however, by limiting our study to a sufficient number of stutterers' adoptive families on the assumption that presence or absence of stuttering would indicate the reverse in the biological families. As yet, we do not have information of this kind based on an adequate sample of adopted stutterers. A small series of such cases were reported by the first author when there were five stutterers (see Bloodstein, 1961b) grew to a final sample of 13. Among the 13 stutterers, four had a history of stuttering in the adoptive family[15] and nine did not. Nature is equivocating as usual. The resultant ambiguous trend seems to signal the now familiar message that hereditary and environmental factors make their contribution to the familial incidence of stuttering—and the etiology and development of the disorder. To these kinds of data, we need to add the evolving understanding of "epigenetic" factors, such as discussed previously. Further, the evolving field of behavioral genetics (mentioned previously) also remarks on the potential of genetically affected or genetically predisposed individuals to interact with their children (who may also have such genetic predispositions) in ways that differ from those that might occur in non-genetically affected families. Such changes in how we can view the potential contributions of "nature" and "nurture," from less of a polar choice to a more intricately braided series of contributions to eventual behavioral (phenotypic) outcomes.

Summary Remarks

The large proportion of stutterers who have stuttering relatives and the high concordance for stuttering of identical twins have long suggested to researchers that biological inheritance plays some substantive role in stuttering. With the discovery of models of genetic transmission that can account for observational data on the distribution of stuttering among stutterers' relatives, the evidence that biological inheritance plays some part in stuttering has become quite strong. It should be noted, however, that these models imply some form of interaction between heredity and environment. The same evidence therefore points as clearly to the importance of environmental factors, which in the past have been equated with cultural influences and parental child-rearing styles. This appears to be confirmed by the exceptions to the concordance of identical twins for stuttering, although more recent research in genetics demonstrates that there are a class of "epigenetic" effects on fetal development that could produce similar results. While there appears to be evidence of the influence of environment in accounts that have come to light of discordance for stuttering in identical twins that were reared apart,[16] such facts tell us little about the nature of the environmental factors that might potentially play a part. For that we must turn to other types of research that have addressed this possibility.

---

[14]Children who are brought up in adoptive homes might be more likely or less likely than others to become stutterers, but this has little bearing on the question of the distribution of stutterers in their biological and adoptive families. The possibility that adults who stutter or have stuttering relatives might be more prone or less prone to give or receive children in adoption must be considered for the sake of strict logic, but this would clearly have to be a tendency of extreme dimensions in order to affect the results of such a study.

[15]One of these four cases met reasonable criteria for inclusion in a study of this type somewhat imperfectly. This was a 12-year-old boy reared from the age of 20 months by a foster mother who told the author that he "always stuttered." The foster mother's older sister as well as her only biological child, aged 4 years, were said to be stutterers. The only member of the boy's biological family known to the foster mother was his mother who was said to be a normal speaker. Two other foster children in the adoptive family, a girl 8 years of age and a boy of 11, did not stutter.

A second case was that of an 8-year-old boy, adopted at 7 months of age, who began to stutter at age 4 or 5 years. His adoptive mother had stuttered severely as a child, and her nephew, aged 18 years, was a severe stutterer.

A third case was a 7-year-old girl who had not begun to talk at age 18 months when she and her twin brother were adopted by her present mother. She was said to have stuttered from the beginning of speech at age 2 years. The adoptive mother's younger sister and brother stuttered as children. The fourth case was a 6-year-old boy, who had stuttered severely from age 1.5 years to 5 and resumed stuttering at age 6 years after the parents adopted a second child. The adoptive mother's brother and his son had also stuttered.

[16]Environmental influence is revealed by still another observation. Using the pooled data of several studies, Andrews et al (1983) calculated that an

THE INFLUENCE OF ENVIRONMENT

The studies of the prevalence of stuttering that are relevant to environmental variables are chiefly those that have been concerned with stuttering in various cultures and socioeconomic groups. We now discuss their findings.

Prevalence in Other Cultures

Earlier in this chapter, we reviewed information on the prevalence of stuttering in the general population of the United States, England, and other countries representative of European culture. Toyoda[17] reported a prevalence of stuttering of 0.82 percent among Japanese schoolchildren, a figure that might have been found in any Western country. Nor is there any reason to expect markedly different figures from India or China on the basis of general observation. On the other hand, there has been a steady accumulation of evidence suggesting the existence in various places in the world of societies in which the prevalence of stuttering does differ quite a bit from the amount that is usual in Western nations. In many cases it is less; in a few it seems to be more.

One of the earliest studies of the cultural incidence of stuttering was reported by Adelaide Bullen (1945). For the most part, Bullen was concerned directly, not with cultures, but with anthropologists. She sent letters to such well-known workers in the field as Reo Fortune, Margaret Mead, and Clyde Kluckhohn and simply asked them to state to what extent they recalled cases of stuttering among the "primitive" people with whom they were familiar. The answers were striking in their uniformity. Fortune said, "I have not met a primitive who stuttered." He estimated that in the course of his investigations in New Guinea, he had talked with about 6,000 people among the Mundugumor, Arapesh, Tchambuli, Manus, Dobuan, New Hanover, Tabor, and Kamamentira tribes. He said he had seen leprosy, hemophilia, insanity, and "running amok," but no stuttering. Margaret Mead, referring chiefly to natives of New Guinea and parts of the South Pacific, said, "I have never seen a case of stuttering or stammering among primitive people, although I remember hearing of one among the Arapesh." Two of Bullen's informants, W. Lloyd Warner and Joseph Birdsell, had worked extensively among the aborigines of Australia. Warner had never observed stuttering among them, while Birdsell had the impression that it was "very rare." In addition, no stutterers were reported by W. Elmer Ekblaw among 250 Polar Eskimos with whom he had lived continuously for four years.

ordinary same-sexed sibling of a stutterer has an 18 percent chance of being a stutterer, whereas the risk rises to 32 percent in the case of a same-sexed fraternal co-twin, who presumably shares a more similar household environment.

[17] Cited by Van Riper (1971, p. 39).

The Bannock and Shoshone

Some of our knowledge about the cultural prevalence of stuttering has come from studies of American Indians. Bullen's information included several reports about the Navaho that suggested that stutterers might be rather rare among them, although they clearly indicated that cases of stuttering were to be found. Cultural contacts that have taken place between the Navaho and our own stuttering society, however, make it difficult to interpret these reports. Likewise, Clifford, Twitchell, and Hull (1965) counted 32 stutterers, a prevalence of 1.8 percent, among 1,799 children in several South Dakota Indian schools and believed this reflected the effects of acculturation.

This difficulty did not exist in the case of the Bannock and Shoshone, living in relative isolation on reservations in southeastern Idaho. Some years before the Bullen study, it had been reported to Wendell Johnson at the University of Iowa that the Bannock and Shoshone Indians appeared to have no word for stuttering. From 1937 to 1939, one of Johnson's students, John C. Snidecor, carried out among these American Indians what seems to have been the first anthropological investigation of stuttering (Johnson, 1944; Snidecor, 1947). Snidecor's mission was to find a stuttering Native American, if any existed. His first step was to gain an audience with the tribal council of chiefs. Since he knew no Bannock-Shoshone word for stuttering, he could only demonstrate what it was he was looking for. He reported that the chiefs were much amused by his behavior, but had never seen anything like it. For the next two years, Snidecor pursued his investigation with the help of a native guide to whom he had promised a reward for information leading to the discovery of a stuttering Indian. In this period, during which he personally interviewed 800 persons and obtained information on 1,000 more, he failed to find "one pure-blooded Indian who stuttered."

In attempting to suggest reasons for what they believed to be the absence or low incidence of stuttering among certain tribes of American Indians, Bullen, Johnson, and Snidecor appeared to be in agreement on the importance of one factor—the absence of heavy cultural pressures, including speech pressures. In these societies the children were allowed a relatively large measure of freedom, and little was expected of them in the way of adherence to culturally approved standards of behavior until adolescence. Correspondingly, children were likely to receive little criticism of the way in which they spoke. As Snidecor observed about the Bannock and Shoshone, "Ability to speak appears to be evaluated as a normal developmental process, not to be quickened by over-anxious parents for purposes of display." Even in adulthood far less seemed to depend on the ability to speak than in our culture. There was rarely the feeling of necessity to speak under pressure. It was not obligatory to talk merely to keep a conversation going. In a tribal council an opinion could be expressed by a simple yes or no. Later, Stewart (1960) found evidence that the Ute, a people of Shoshonean stock, tended to be relatively permissive with regard to nursing, toilet training, crying, and body contact with parents, allowed children to develop independence and language at their own rate, and placed little emphasis on conformity to standards of speech fluency.

In Johnson's mind, the apparent absence of a word for stuttering among the Bannock and Shoshone was of the utmost significance in view of his theory that stuttering is caused by parental mislabeling of children as stutterers. In time, however, publication of independent observations by Sven Liljeblad, an anthropologist, and Art Frank, a speech pathologist, left little doubt that the Bannock and Shoshone possessed both stutterers and words for stuttering.[18] Both men had informants who identified individuals on the reservation who stuttered. Frank interviewed two stutterers who had been living there at the time of the Snidecor study and noted characteristic symptoms as well as word and situational avoidances. Liljeblad recorded a number of Bannock-Shoshone expressions relating to stuttering. These consisted of derivations of the stem *pybya-*. Both Frank and Liljeblad stated that they had to overcome considerable reticence, embarrassment, and distrust before anyone would admit to them that they had any knowledge of stuttering on the reservation.

The Kwakiutl, Nootka, and Salish

In actuality, the notion that American Indians do not stutter was dispelled as early as 1953. In that year, Edwin M. Lemert, a social anthropologist of the University of California at Los Angeles, reported finding numerous stutterers among the Kwakiutl, Nootka, and Salish tribes of Canada. These are people who have lived from very ancient times by salmon fishing on the Pacific Northwest Coast, who carve totem poles, and who have, or had, a distinctive type of tribal organization marked by bitter interclan rivalry. They are noted for the institution of the "potlatch," a ceremonial feast at which the hosts gave away or destroyed their most treasured possessions, thereby humiliating their guests from rival clans who could then hold their heads high only by giving away or destroying even more valuable possessions at a potlatch of their own. Among these people, Lemert found an abundance of stutterers. Although he made no actual count, his personal contacts with stutterers and his informants' reports of stuttering cases left little room for doubt that the disorder is rather commonplace on the Northwest Coast.

[18] These observations, made in the 1960s, were not published until many years later. See Zimmermann, Liljeblad, Frank, and Cleeland (1983) and Zimmerman (1985).

The question that immediately arises is whether stuttering is indigenous to these people or acquired through the process of acculturation they have undergone in recent times. Lemert found three pieces of evidence that speak for the antiquity of the disorder among them. First, there are native words for stuttering as well as for other speech disorders in their language. Second, their folklore contains rituals and incantations for the treatment of stuttering. Third, in some cases living members of these tribes had memories of the stuttering of their grandfathers whose childhoods must have gone back to the 1850s, or earlier, when contact with other cultures was largely limited to sporadic fur trade.

To explain the prevalence of stuttering among the Northwest Coast Indians, Lemert pointed to their unique social competitiveness. It was a kind of competition in which the prestige of the family group and the clan was the prime concern and in which the failures or shortcomings of each individual might jeopardize the status of the entire group. This tended to have two consequences that may be of some importance in relation to the etiology of stuttering. In the first place, it led to exacting educational practices and the imposition of rigid standards of behavior at an early age. It may be significant, for example, that young children were often obliged to participate in solemn rituals, requiring knowledge of songs and dances of some complexity, under the scrutiny of adults of their own and rival clans. In the second place, it meant that the individual who was different in some way was a source of embarrassment to the group as a whole and did not generally strive to be conspicuous. The coastal Indians of the North Pacific exhibit attitudes of pity, condescension, amusement, and social rejection toward such differences as left-handedness, obesity, smallness, mental deficiency, and orthopedic disability, as well as toward a variety of speech impairments.

The Ibo and Idoma of West Africa

Observations on the incidence of stuttering in tribal societies have not been limited to American Indians, as we have already seen. A comprehensive cultural investigation of stuttering was reported in an unpublished dissertation by Morgenstern (1953) and summarized in some detail by Johnson et al (1967, p. 244 ff.). From 258 anthropologists working in the field, Morgenstern systematically obtained information about the prevalence of stuttering and of various cultural traits and attitudes in nonliterate groups all over the world. He found some 13 communities in New Guinea, British Guiana, Borneo, Malaya, and India who reportedly had no stuttering and no word for stuttering. He also discovered that the societies in which stuttering was said to be absent tended to be societies that were rated as relatively permissive in their child-training practices and relatively tolerant of personal shortcomings and deviations from the typical.

Among the most interesting of Morgenstern's findings were those relating to the Idoma and Ibo (also known as Igbo) peoples of West Africa (primarily located in what is today Nigeria and Cameroon), among whom there appeared to be an exceedingly large number of stutterers. Of the Idoma, Dr. Robert Armstrong, an American anthropologist, reported to Morgenstern, "Stammering (in the sense of spasmodic repetition of the same speech sound) is practically a mass phenomenon here. I have met many dozens of persons who stammer in some degree." Among the Ibo, 2.67 percent of a group of 5,618 schoolchildren were reported to stutter on the basis of a survey conducted by teachers and headmasters. Armstrong commented further, "Ability to speak well in public is vastly admired in West Africa, and Idoma and Ibo country is no exception to this statement. People make speeches on the slightest pretext. . . . There is strong ridicule from the stammerer's age-mates. . . ."

From other sources, one learns that the Ibo place great stress on the attainment of an education and that they have frequently been regarded by other tribes as the most competitive and economically aspiring people of West Africa. It would seem to be a particularly revealing kind of distinction that, of the young men who have gone from this part of Africa to study at European and American universities, an unusually large number appear to belong to the Ibo people. Interestingly enough, one such student to whom the author was introduced some years ago was a stutterer himself. In commenting on his childhood in Nigeria, he said that at age 5 years he was sent to live with his uncle's family because his parents, who hoped very much that he would acquire traits of leadership, feared that he would be excessively coddled at home. He recalled that his uncle would slap him whenever he stuttered, in a well-intentional effort to correct his speech. He remembered other children who stuttered, particularly among the boys who shared with him the good fortune of being able to go to school.

However, it is important to place these observations in a complementary focus. Because the high incidence of stutterers in Cameroon had been noted, there has been genetic study of an extended Cameroonian cohort showing patterns of affected family members that are quite compatible with some form of inherited transmission of stuttering (Levis, Ricci, Lukong & Drayna, 2004).

Summary Remarks: Culture and Stuttering

We have reviewed a number of studies of the cultural prevalence of stuttering. To these may be added several other observations. Lemert (1962) related the apparently low incidence of stuttering in Polynesian society and its relatively higher incidence in Japan to a difference in pressures for achievement and social nonconformity. Aron (1962) found a prevalence of stuttering of 1.26 percent among 6,581 Bantu schoolchildren of Johannesburg. Noting that Bantu languages contain words for stuttering that are thought to antedate the arrival of Western civilization in South Africa, she related the apparent similarity in prevalence of stuttering between European and Bantu urban societies to a similarity in basic social structure and attitudes toward acquisition of speech. Nwokah (1988) cited surveys yielding the unusually high prevalence figures of 5.5 percent for schoolchildren in Dakar (Senegal) and 3.5 percent for schoolchildren in Accra (Ghana). Kirk (1977) reported on the high frequency of a type of stuttering in Ghana among speakers of Ga, but this is said to be chiefly nonpathological in nature and is identified by speakers as a normal occurrence when it is pointed out to them. Platzky and Girson (1993) interviewed four indigenous healers of the Tsonga, South Sotho, Xhosa, and Zulu groups of South Africa. All had native names for stuttering. All cited factors consistent with their cultural beliefs, as well as heredity, as causes of stuttering. Most considered stuttering a handicap and a cause of lowered self-esteem.

Reflecting on all these observations, we may ask what our anthropological information on stuttering adds up to. That stuttering is absent from any society, as some have claimed, is a hypothesis that is essentially impossible to prove by any practical scientific investigation. So is the contrary, that stuttering is universal, as others have insisted. An easier question to answer, and a far more important one from the standpoint of our understanding of stuttering, is whether there are cultural differences in the incidence of the disorder. Those who have collected these data believe that it is possible that stuttering is a significant comment on the culture that produces it. To say that there are many stutterers in a given society is possibly to say that it is a rather competitive society that tends to impose high standards of achievement on the individual and to regard status and prestige as unusually desirable goals, that it is sternly intolerant of deviancy, and that, as a by-product of its distinctive set of cultural values, it in all likelihood places a high premium on conformity in speech. Alternatively, these prevalence differences may reflect differences in the culture's identification of typical and impaired speakers, or of genetic variability that can differentiate some communities (particularly those that are less likely to be mobile and thus are more genetically homogeneous) from others.

Regardless, we should not lose sight of the fact that cultural values will affect how stuttering is tolerated or how members of the community view its etiology and appropriate treatment. This has become more of a concern for researchers and practitioners in dealing with those who stutter (as evidenced by research publication trends) than the quest for cultural factors that might cause incidence and prevalence variability. We address these factors relevant to assessment and treatment in Chapter 14.

Prevalence in Relation to Socioeconomic Level

If stuttering actually does have these cultural implications, one might reasonably expect to find confirmation of this in the prevalence of the disorder in those subcultures of our own society known as socioeconomic levels. It is provocative from this point of view that public school speech pathologists who have had wide experience in a large metropolitan educational system frequently report that some schools seem to produce an unusually large caseload of stutterers and that these schools seem to be located in the "better" neighborhoods. Research findings on the question are meager, however, and may reflect referral patterns. Research by the Australian National Health Service, which included stuttering in its targeted behaviors of interest, found no evidence for socioeconomic status (SES) on the incidence of speech disorders, although its effects on language development in children are relatively well-documented (Keating, Keating, Turrell, & Ozanne, 2001). Similar lack of SES impact on stuttering incidence was found for a large cohort of Australian schoolchildren enrolled in parochial schools (McKinnon, McLeod, & Reilly, 2007).

Educational Level

One useful measure of socioeconomic status is level of educational attainment. Not only must people usually be able to pay to attend college, but they also need to have acquired the social, cultural, and economic values that make a college education desirable. It is therefore of considerable interest that in speech surveys conducted in the 1930s in five American colleges and universities as reported by Bender (1939, p. 2), the prevalence of stuttering was found to be 1.87 percent at the City College of New York, 2.60 percent at Dartmouth College, 2.70 percent at the University of Minnesota, 7.80 percent at the University of Ohio, and 2.00 percent at Queens College. These percentages vary from twice as high to perhaps more than three times as high as most prevalence figures for the grade school population of the United States.

Moreover, there is indirect evidence that these figures might have been even higher if not for the operation of some selective factors. In the first place, in a series of studies, college stutterers in the 1930s were consistently found to be distinctly higher, on the average, in measured intelligence than college nonstutterers.[19] By contrast, the general grade school population of stutterers, as will be seen later, is no more intelligent than the general population of nonstutterers. Evidently, stutterers who would otherwise have attended college frequently failed to do so in the past because of their speech problem, unless they had superior intellectual endowment to compensate in part for it.

To this selective factor, it is very possible that we must add another. Schuell (1946) found evidence that the sex ratio was markedly higher among university students than among the non-university population of the same age. The difference was 7.4:1 as compared to 3.7:1 for the 17- to 21-year age group, and 10.0:1 as contrasted with 7.6:1 in the 22- to 30-year age range. It is a reasonable inference that this difference was due to the number of female stutterers who, given the social expectations of the time, chose to stay away even though they had the superior intellect and the socioeconomic background that would normally have sent them to college.

It is plausible to hypothesize that, at the time the relevant information was being gathered, stuttering was particularly prevalent, or at least more likely to be reported, in those segments of American society contributing most heavily to the college population. If so, to what extent this has continued to be true is a pertinent question. The numbers receiving higher education, and the pressures to do so, have been rising over time so that both socioeconomic distinctions and stuttering have become less effective deterrents to college attendance. Perhaps it is for this reason that later prevalence figures from colleges and universities have been considerably lower than those reported in 1939 by Bender. Morley (1952), in a 10-year speech survey of students at

[19] See Travis (1931, p. 101), Johnson (1932), Steer (1936), and Fruewald (1936).

the University of Michigan, found a prevalence of stuttering of only 0.81 percent, with the rather ordinary sex ratio of 4.3:1. Other most recent figures are: 0.6 percent among students at Berkeley and the University of California at Los Angeles (Sheehan & Martyn, 1970), 2.1 percent at the University of Massachusetts (Porfert & Rosenfield, 1978), and 0.3 percent at the University of Alabama (Culton, 1986). We do not know of any studies that have updated these earlier reports. In any event, educational level is not the only measure that has been used in investigating the socioeconomic status of stutterers, and there are other forms of information on the subject to which we may turn.

Parental Occupational Class and Other Characteristics

The most systematic study to date of socioeconomic factors in stuttering was carried out in Scotland by Morgenstern (1956) in the course of investigations already referred to. Morgenstern was aided in his research by the fact that, in 1947, the Scottish Council for Research in Education had completed a survey that showed the proportionate distribution of a large number of schoolchildren among nine socioeconomic levels. These levels were based on the occupational status of the father and ranged from unskilled salaried farm workers to members of the professional class. Using these statistics as a standard of comparison, Morgenstern conducted a speech survey of a comparable sample of Scottish schoolchildren aimed at determining whether those children who stuttered were distributed among these occupational categories any differently from the population as a whole.

The results showed a general similarity between the two distributions, particularly—interestingly enough—on the middle and upper occupational levels. There were also, however, some differences. Disproportionately few stutterers had fathers who were on the lowest level of the scale, corresponding to unskilled industrial and agricultural workers. The outstanding finding was an unexpectedly large number of stutterers whose fathers fell into a classification relatively low on the socioeconomic scale, which was termed "semi-skilled manual weekly wage-earner" and included such occupations as truck driver or machine-tender. What was the explanation for this? Morgenstern believed that it lay in the somewhat unique upward mobility of this particular occupational class in Scottish society. He observed that, to a greater degree than appeared to be true of members of any other class, the semi-skilled workers had both the opportunity and the aspiration to rise above their origins. This being so, they could be expected to exert somewhat greater pressure on their children to improve themselves and perhaps tended to evince a somewhat finer appreciation of the advantages of such personal refinements as fluent speech in the competition for social and economic status.

Given the emerging genetic data, however, alternative explanations are also possible. Given normal intelligence, parents who themselves stutter may have experienced limitations on their actual or perceived occupational aspirations. Findings suggestive of this come from retrospective study of American students with a history of mild articulation disorders, another communication disorder now thought to have familial transmission (Felsenfeld & Broen, 1994).

Morgenstern also found a definite tendency for stuttering to be related to rate of occupancy of homes. Relatively speaking, fewer stutterers came from more crowded homes (two or more persons per room, on the average). A disproportionately large number of stutterers came from homes with the relatively low average occupancy rate of one to two persons per room, and also—but to a considerably less marked degree—from homes with a rate of less than one person per room. Morgenstern did not find the prevalence of stuttering to be related to density of population in which homes were located. This is in general accord with the data of Louttit and Halls (1936), Schindler (1955), and others showing little or no difference in the percentage of stutterers in urban as compared with rural areas. On the other hand, Brady and Hall (1976) found the prevalence of stuttering among urban schoolchildren almost twice as high as among rural schoolchildren in Illinois and Pennsylvania.

Morgenstern's survey produced the most convincing evidence we have of socioeconomic variations in the prevalence of stuttering. However, this evidence is not clearly corroborated by the results of other studies using similar measures of socioeconomic level. In a survey of over 20,000 Iowa schoolchildren, Schindler (1955) found no significant difference in mean occupational levels of parents of stutterers and nonstutterers, although about one-third of the stutterers as opposed to only one-sixth of the nonstutterers were in the upper levels. Nor is there any more corroboration in the data of Andrews and Harris (1964, p. 51) on either social class or upward mobility of the families of 80 stutterers in Newcastle Upon Tyne.[20]

Prevalence with Era

Some American speech-language pathologists with long clinical experience believe that the prevalence of stuttering is considerably less than it was some decades ago. Although there is little adequate evidence on the question, a few public school surveys cited by Van Riper (1982, p. 49) do show a marked decline between the 1940s and 1960s, at least in enrollment of stutterers for speech therapy. The very low prevalence figures of 0.3 percent and 0.35 percent obtained in the surveys of schoolchildren by Hull (1969) and Brady and Hall (1976) may also be indicative. Furthermore, the conviction of many speech-language pathologists that stutterers in their caseloads were once both more numerous and more severe is too firm and general to dismiss.[21]

If it is true, there are various possible reasons for it. Some researchers attribute it to the permissive revolution in child rearing that is often laid to Spock's popular manual on child care and appears to go back ultimately to the influence of Freud. Van Riper (1982, p. 49) believed it due primarily to a change in the attitudes of society toward stutterers resulting from the development of speech-language pathology as a profession. Others ascribe it more specifically to the wide influence of Johnson's diagnosogenic theory of stuttering in the United States. It is clear that we may be able to narrow the possibilities somewhat by comparing the impressions of American clinicians with those of speech clinicians in other countries. Referral patterns by parents and professionals also clearly vary from place to place, as do opportunities to collect and report demographic data. More standardized diagnostic criteria for classifying individuals as stutterers, particularly young children, will also facilitate comparison of incidence data.

SUMMARY REMARKS

The prevalence of stuttering in the school population in Western society at the present time is approximately 1 percent and appears to be marginally higher in Europe than in the United States. The incidence of those who will have stuttered at some time in their lives is substantially greater, at least 4 or 5 percent and perhaps indeterminately higher if early childhood episodes of brief duration are counted.

From certain points of view, stuttering may be regarded as a disorder of childhood. It begins in childhood, typically in the early years. A very large proportion of children spontaneously recover from it. In earliest childhood, mild and transient forms of stuttering appear to be very common.

Stuttering is more prevalent among males than females. The sex ratio among American schoolchildren is roughly 3:1. It is probably lower than that in preschool children and higher in adults. The sex ratio has been attributed to nature (sex-linked patterns of genetic transmission, sex differences in constitution, physical maturation) or nurture (speech and language development, differences in parental attitudes and expectations with regard to

[20] In an exhaustive study of 150 stutterers by Johnson and Associates (1959, p. 75 ff.) in which subjects were matched for socioeconomic status with their controls, a relatively large proportion were found to be in the middle and upper classes on the basis of multiple criteria, but their method of selection made it difficult to be certain that the subjects could be validly compared with the general population.

[21] Figures obtained by Dean and Brown (1977) from departments of special education of nine states for the 10 years from 1963 to 1973 show about the same number of stutterers annually, suggesting that the prevalence of stuttering may have stabilized by the 1960s.

boys and girls). The first set of factors appears to be more likely influences than the latter.

Certain features of the incidence of stuttering strongly suggest that, to a greater or lesser degree, biological heredity may be a factor in the etiology of stuttering. There is a high familial incidence, as indicated by the presence of stuttering among the relatives of roughly 50 percent of stutterers. There is also a high degree of concordance of stuttering in identical twins. Neither of these findings represents conclusive evidence that genetic transmission plays an immutable role, but genetic models of inheritance that allow for the interaction of environmental variables are capable of accounting fairly accurately for data on family backgrounds of stuttering. The possibility of such inheritance raises the challenging question of specifically what might be transmitted that would incline a child to stuttering. That is, the data may explain how an individual comes to be a stutterer, but not what the underlying "cause" of stuttering is, in physiological or other terms.

There have been efforts to explore the influence of environment in the incidence of stuttering. The incidence of stuttering appears to vary somewhat in different cultures. There is some evidence that the cultures in which there are relatively large numbers of stutterers are those characterized by outstanding competitive pressures. In addition, some believe that in our own culture, stuttering may be more common on certain socioeconomic levels, especially those marked by unusual upward mobility. In this respect, however, the evidence is decidedly less conclusive, and it should be considered that such cultures are also more likely to seek assistance for children who have developmental concerns and keep data on such referrals. This may skew reported incidence values. Moreover, it is difficult to use culturally isolated societies to test the influence of culture on stuttering incidence as such communities are likely to be genetically isolated from other groups as well.

In this chapter, we have been concerned with what has been learned about stuttering from studies of its prevalence and incidence in various populations. In addition to the populations we have discussed, there are a number of specific groups of individuals with respect to which this question has been raised—those with deafness, blindness, cerebral palsy, epilepsy, psychosis, mental deficiency, left-handedness, and bilingualism. These findings will be considered later in appropriate contexts.

Chapter 4

The Person Who Stutters: Central Neurological Findings

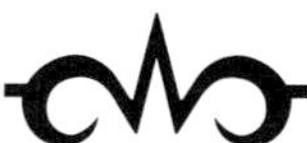

The next three chapters will be concerned with the question of whether the person who stutters uniquely differs from fluent speakers physiologically and neurologically, and whether such differences can shed light on the underlying causes of the disorder and its best treatment. A great many studies have addressed this basic question by comparing groups of stutterers with groups of nonstutterers with regard to an almost inexhaustible list of human features, behaviors, and traits.

This chapter will be devoted to research on the central neurological characteristics of people who stutter. Perhaps no other focus of this book has seen such dynamic and active research growth since its last edition. Historically, the physiological approach to discovering the basis of stuttering began with early behavioral studies of breathing, motor capacities, and heart rate. Researchers later turned to investigations of the stutterer's tissue chemistry, neuromuscular organization, handedness, and cortical function. More recently, emphasis has shifted to central psycholinguistic and neurolinguistic concepts such as auditory perception, as well as specific cortical structures and functional processing patterns for speech and language processing that might distinguish speech-language production in people who stutter from their fluent peers. Because, in the end, many potential differences between people who do and do not stutter may rest in central neurological control of motor and linguistic function, we will start with discussion of cortical functions that may distinguish stuttering and fluent speakers.

Viewed over time, much of the research has tried to "compartmentalize" possible areas of deficit or difference in people who stutter. In other words, research has presumed that stuttering might arise from peripheral motor function differences, biochemical markers, or auditory processing deficits.

However, as our methods of neuropsychological and neurophysiological investigation have evolved, it has become increasingly difficult to view areas of human functioning as isolated modules. In fact, increasing bodies of research suggest dynamic interactions among speech motor, linguistic, and cognitive systems in speech and language production, whether in typical or stuttering speakers.

It should not be surprising that more recent investigations of stuttering have focused on the cortical substrates of speech and language production, particularly as the research techniques available to neurolinguists have expanded. Researchers are now capable of appraising the time course of speech and language processing, and can image both the structural properties of the brain and its functional activities during specified tasks. As we shall see, use of these techniques has revealed numerous differences between people who stutter and fluent comparison groups. However, as these differences emerge, their interpretation becomes increasingly problematic.

We can further divide studies discussed in this chapter into those that have primarily investigated whether hemispheric specialization for manual and linguistic tasks (laterality) differs in people who stutter, and studies of cortical functioning having other primary objectives. Because the question of laterality has a long history in stuttering research, we will start with those types of studies first. However, as we address more recent studies, it is difficult to discuss hemispheric comparisons without reference to specific intra-hemispheric findings. Thus, although we will start with the broad question of dominance for speech and language in people who stutter, we will progress to more nuanced discussion of how cortical function, in terms of activated areas, level of activity, timing of activity, and change in activity following therapy may inform the underlying nature of stuttering.

LATERAL DOMINANCE

Perhaps no other aspect of the person who stutters has been investigated as persistently and resourcefully as the normal tendency of certain functions to lateralize to one side of the body. Beginning with observations on the reversal of manual dexterity in some stutterers early in the last century, this research led to investigations of handedness and other aspects of peripheral sidedness, was abandoned for a while, and is being discussed again today in studies of cerebral lateralization of language functions.

Reversal of Manual Dexterity

Although a special urgency was given to research on the laterality of stutterers by the Orton-Travis theory of cerebral dominance in the 1930s (see Chapter 2), work on the subject goes back at least as far as a systematic attempt by Ballard (1912) to verify a "frequently urged" notion that interference with handedness might cause a child to stutter. His findings added considerably to interest in the question. In a survey of school-aged children in London, Ballard found stuttering in 17 percent of the dextrosinistrals, whom he defined as congenitally left-handed children who had been forced to write with the right hand. Somewhat later, Wallin (1916) reported that, of the children who were found to stutter in a school survey in St. Louis, 9.5 percent had been shifted from left- to right-handed writing, as compared with only 2.0 percent of all pupils who had been shifted; he was careful to point out that 80 percent of the shifted stutterers had begun to stutter before receiving any instruction in writing. In 1924, Inman (cited by McAllister, 1937, p. 337) related that, in an experiment at the Lingfield Colony Special Schools in England, left-handed training was given to a group of children with "mental deficiency" and epilepsy in the hope that "additional centers in the brain might be opened up." About five months later, a number of the children who were making the most rapid progress began to stutter.

Not all of the evidence pointed in the same direction. In the early decades of the last century, an intensive campaign was begun in the public schools of Elizabeth, New Jersey, to abolish left-handedness by compelling all of the pupils to write with the right hand. Some time later, Parson (1924, p. 102) wrote, "Investigation showed that in the four years that the policy had been in effect in Elizabeth not a single case of defective speech could be traced to the reversal of manual habit."

In the late 1920s, Travis and his students became concerned with the question of confused or ambiguous lateral dominance in stutterers. One of these students, Fagan (1931), presented a series of 13 cases, in the majority of which stuttering was said to have developed within a year after right-handed training. Travis (1931, p. 140 ff) offered various bits of anecdotal evidence, including a few contributed by Bryngelson. One of these was the case of a child who, on three successive occasions between the first and sixth grades, began to stutter when forced to write with his right hand and stopped stuttering when allowed to return to the use of his left. Another boy, determined to become a "southpaw" pitcher, began to stutter while zealously training himself in left-handed skills and reverted to normal speech on giving up the attempt. Still another interesting case of Bryngelson's was that of a 58-year-old man who had been a right-handed normal speaker until an injury made it necessary to amputate his right forearm. Shortly afterward, he began to stutter.[1]

[1]To this, however, Bluemel (1933) counterposed a reference to a Professor Bestelmeyer of Munich, who described a group of 1,200 persons, each of whom had only one arm: "Among them there is not a single case of stammering." Among 20 preferred arm amputees whom Zaner (1950) contacted through state authorities in Wisconsin, 4 told of experiencing some speech difficulty following the amputation and described it in such terms as, "slight hesitancy in speaking and thinking of what to say," "stammering and failure of words," "as though my mind has gone blank for a second and failed to supply me with words." Of 19 non-preferred arm amputees, none had noted any speech difficulty.

In a letter to the author, the late Dr. Bryngelson offered the following correction of the story cited about a 58-year-old amputee: "Facts were—this patient fell in an elevator shaft and he had to have part of his fingers removed—anyway he couldn't use right hand running the elevator and other things like writing, etc. He came to me after two months of using his left hand to hold his job and had a speech defect for which he had no name—he came to me to find out what it was. It was a common kind of blocking and clonic spasm. When asked if it could be eradicated I said, there is a way of trying. I sent him to a place where prongs or hooks can be used like fingers. And this he did, and it pleased him as he said he is very awkward using his left hand—although he had his job back, but didn't like to 'stutter' to his friends, etc. I could see no emotional tie-up as he was getting on well with left hand but did not prefer it. So he went back to right and did almost as much with it as prior to accident and lo and behold (why I know not) he came over three months later and nary a sign of stuttering."

Handedness

The cerebral dominance theory gave a strong impetus to research on stutterers' handedness. This research took several forms.

Surveys of Hand Usage or Preference At first, investigators simply set out to determine whether stutterers differed from nonstutterers in the proportions of each group who were right-handed, left-handed, and ambidextrous, on the assumption that people tended to belong in three more or less distinct categories with regard to handedness. The methods used to ascertain the participant's category varied. In some investigations, people were simply asked to self-report their hand preference, while others made use of questionnaires or of tests in which hand usage could be observed. The results of this research proved to be rather remarkable. Before it had proceeded very far, an exceedingly wide disparity began to be evident among findings reported by various researchers (see Table 4-1). Estimates of left-handedness among groups of stutterers ranged from 0.9 to 21 percent. Estimates of ambidexterity varied from 0 to 61 percent. One researcher found far more ambidexterity among stutterers than among typically fluent speakers, but comparatively little left-handedness. Another found a very large proportion of left-handed stutterers. Still a third reported little difference between stutterers and nonstutterers in the proportion of either type of handedness. Even more remarkable were the reports of percentages of stutterers whose handedness had been shifted from left to right in childhood; these ranged from 5 to 73 percent.

The reason for these differences gradually became apparent. Various definitions of ambidexterity or left-handedness were possible. How many ambidextrous stutterers one found depended in part on how one inquired about or determined ambidexterity. Furthermore, handedness was not an all-or-none property, but a matter of degree. It was realized that what was needed for both clinical and research purposes was a measure of handedness that was both objective and quantitative.

TABLE 4-1 Percentage of Stutterers and Nonstutterers Found to Be Left-Handed, Ambidextrous, and Shifted in Handedness

	Stutterers				Nonstutterers			
	N	Left-handed	Ambidextrous	Shifted	*N*	Left-handed	Ambidextrous	Shifted
Wallin (1916)	683			9.5	88,373			
Bryngelson (1935)	700	0.9	61.1	73.1				
Millsen and Johnson (1936)	23			34				
McAllister (1937)	139	6.5						
Berry (1937a)	119	21.0	17.6					
Bryngelson and Rutherford (1937)	74	4.1	34.3	71.6	74	16.7	8.3	9.5
Bryngelson (1939)	78	2.0	29.0	58.0	78	8.0	0.0	1.0
Daniels (1940)	20	5.0	20.0	5.0	1,574			4.8
Spadino (1941)	70	15.7	0.0		70	10.0	1.4	
Johnson et al. (1942)	46	13.0	8.7	26.1	46	8.7	13.0	30.4
Meyer (1945)	104	11.5	7.7	16.3				
Despert (1946)	50	12.0	4.0					
Andrews and Harris (1964)	80	3.8	26.3		80	6.3	28.8	
Records, Heimbuch, and Kidd (1977)	449	12.9	4.7		356	12.1	9.3	
Accordi et al. (1983)	2,802	5.1	5.1		1,602	6.4	9.7	
Adlla et al. (1994)	37	5.4	2.7		1,842	6.5	8.0	

TABLE 4-2 Dextrality Quotients of Stutterers and Nonstutterers

	N	Stutterers	Nonstutterers
Millsen and Johnson (1936)	23, 23	0.95	0.78*
Morris (1938)	20	0.71	
Johnson and King (1942)	98, 71	0.88	0.87
Johnson et al. (1942)**	36, 46	0.89	0.94

*Normally fluent speakers whose handedness had been changed.
**Data reported In Johnson (1955a).

The Dextrality Quotient Travis's students, notably Johnson, had for some time been developing a device known as a hand-usage questionnaire. This was a questionnaire instructing subjects to indicate which hand they used to perform each of a list of manual activities such as using a pencil or throwing a ball. From the subject's answers, it was possible to compute a dextrality quotient, or D.Q., which represented essentially the proportion of right-handed responses and varied from 1.00 (perfect right-handedness) to 0.00 (complete left-handedness). The laterality questionnaire scored by means of the D.Q. appeared to offer an ideal solution to the problems that had arisen in attempts to investigate the stutterer's handedness. The results were fairly consistent in several studies in which it was used by Johnson and his coworkers (see Table 4-2). Somewhat unexpectedly, however, the stutterers did not seem to differ from the nonstutterers at all. In most cases, they turned out to be relatively right-handed, in roughly the same proportion as most other people.

Innate Lateral Dominance

The laterality questionnaire in itself did not immediately settle the handedness controversy, however. The principal reason for this was that the questionnaire was concerned almost entirely with activities highly subject to training. Proponents of the cerebral dominance theory argued that, while stutterers often seemed to be right-handed because of the influence of a right-handed society, they usually possessed an innate ambidextrous tendency that did not reveal itself on handedness inventories.

Measures of Native Laterality Clearly, what was needed was a measure of innate, also termed native or cortical, laterality. Researchers, principally under the direction of Travis, carried on a sustained effort to devise tests of sidedness relatively uninfluenced by culture. Human structure and function were scoured for covert reflections of bilateral asymmetry, and what was found was applied in studies of stutterers. These included eyedness as measured in various ways,[2] foot preference,[3] the dominant thumb (the one uppermost when the hands are clasped),[4] simultaneous bimanual writing,[5] writing or drawing in mirror vision,[6] mirror reading ability,[7] and the relative size, strength, or skill of the two hands.[8] Several neuromuscular measures of innate laterality were tried-bilateral action potentials,[9] the relative excitability of bilaterally paired muscles on electrical stimulation,[10] and differences in motor lead of the two hands in simultaneous antitropic movements.[11] In addition, signs of deviant lateral dominance were sought in the cortical potentials of stutterers (see discussion later in this chapter), and also in certain perceptual phenomena.[12] Jasper (1932) and Morris (1938) made use of many of these measures

[2]Travis (1928a).
[3]Bryngelson and Rutherford (1937).
[4]Johnson (1937).
[5]Jasper (1932), Fagan (1932), Van Riper (1934, 1935).
[6]Travis (1928a).
[7]Peters (1936).
[8]Cross (1936), Van Dusen (1937, 1939).
[9]Orton and Travis (1929), Travis and Lindsley (1933), Metfessel and Warren (1934).
[10]Jasper (1932).
[11]Travis and Herren (1929).
[12]Jasper (1932), Morris (1938).

to construct batteries of diagnostic tests of "native" sidedness.

Considerable support for the Orton-Travis theory was amassed by means of these studies. The most common procedure was to select comparison groups of right-handed, left-handed, and ambidextrous persons by means of a laterality questionnaire and to compare their performance on a given test of native dominance with that of a group of stutterers. In the main, these measures served to classify the stutterers with the ambidextrous or left-handed normal speakers. It was evident that many stutterers who were right-handed in their ordinary daily activities actually did seem to exhibit a latent ambidexterity or a mixed or confused dominance when they were given tests of this type. It would have been difficult to foresee the rather surprising conclusion to which such studies finally led.

The Critical-Angle Board Test One of the most promising of these tests made use of simultaneous writing with both hands. It was based on the observation that in writing a word or copying a number or design simultaneously with both hands it was natural for most people to produce with one hand a mirror image of what they did with the other hand. The normal tendency was to copy the figure correctly with the dominant hand and to mirror with the other. Those who showed little tendency to mirror, or mirrored first with one hand and then with the other, could be presumed to be ambidextrous. Simultaneous writing, then, seemed to afford an indication of an individual's lateral dominance that was relatively uninfluenced by training.

The chief drawback of this procedure was that its success depended on the person's cooperation in reacting quickly and spontaneously; most people failed to mirror if they exercised some care. This difficulty was effectively disposed of in a modification of the procedure, introduced by Van Riper (1934), which required the participants to write simultaneously on both sides of a vertical board. It is readily seen that mirroring is difficult to avoid under these conditions. In fact, one of the problems of the vertical board test was the very difficulty that all but the most ambidextrous persons had in drawing the figure *correctly* with both hands.

Van Riper hit upon an ingenious solution to this problem. He hinged two boards together so that they could be presented to the subject open or closed at angles of varying degrees. In giving this test, which he called the "critical-angle board test," Van Riper placed the board before the participant fully opened with instructions to draw the figure correctly (i.e., without mirroring) on both surfaces at the same time. The drawing or writing was then repeated successively with the board closed at various angles until, in its fully closed position, it duplicated the conditions of the vertical board test. It is clear that, at some point in this process, there will be a "critical angle" at which almost every participant begins to mirror with the nondominant hand. Strongly right- or left-handed people could be expected to mirror with the angle board slightly closed, while highly ambidextrous ones presumably would not do so until it was almost completely closed. This proved to be precisely the case.

Van Riper (1935) gave the critical-angle board test to a number of the most highly right-handed, left-handed, and ambidextrous people he could find among several hundred college students, selecting the subjects on the basis of their dextrality quotients on hand-usage questionnaires. He found that ambidextrous people tended to have critical angles that were markedly larger than those of the highly unilateral subjects and that indicated that they mirrored far less readily. Now there was only one question left. How would stutterers perform on this test-essentially like right-handed, left-handed, or ambidextrous people? Van Riper gave his test to a group of stutterers. The results appeared to support the cerebral dominance hypothesis in a most convincing manner. The stutterers had critical angles that were, on the average, *almost exactly like those of the ambidextrous group.*

The matter was not to end here, however. Van Riper had compared his stutterers with three groups of nonstutterers who had been very carefully chosen as representative of three different types of handedness. In doing so he had taken for granted a premise that few people would have been inclined to dispute—that, broadly speaking, the population was divisible into three categories with respect to handedness, the great majority being both innately and outwardly right-handed to some degree. Was this assumption strictly valid? There certainly seemed little enough reason to doubt it. But several years later, Daniels, who had been investigating the handedness of stuttering and nonstuttering students at Syracuse University, remarked:

> "The observational procedure . . . revealed that the popular concept of kinds of handedness (right, left, and ambidextrous) is inaccurate to a degree of becoming almost meaningless. It was shown that three distinct types of handedness groups do not exist; a concept of widely varying degrees of ambidexterity among all individuals more nearly approaches the actual situation. . . ." (Daniels, 1940)

That was a bold statement. Suppose that it were true? In that case, any group of people carefully selected for their right-handedness was certainly an unusual aggregation of persons, possessing a degree of unilaterality not at all representative of the general population. There was one way to settle the question. Johnson and King (1942) gave the Van Riper critical-angle board test to a group of 98 stutterers and compared their performance with that of a group of nonstutterers who had been selected entirely *at random* with regard to handedness. Their findings bore out Daniels' contention in a manner that was arresting. Again the stutterers made responses that were similar to those of Van Riper's ambidextrous students. *And the nonstutterers performed almost exactly like the stutterers.* On a hand usage questionnaire, both groups appeared essentially right-handed. The implications were clear. As Johnson and King pointed out, many stutterers did indeed have inborn ambidextrous tendencies, but that was simply because most people do.

Johnson and King were concerned specifically with the critical-angle board test. In the light of their findings, however, it becomes necessary to reevaluate the validity of a host of other indications of weak or confused innate lateral dominance among stutterers obtained in past studies in which available groups of stutterers were compared with comparison groups specially selected with regard to handedness. This is underscored by the results of an exhaustive study that was completed at Columbia University by Spadino (1941). Spadino studied 70 stutterers and 70 nonstutterers of elementary school age, selecting them on the same basis and without regard for handedness. On numerous tests of handedness, eyedness, footedness, simultaneous bimanual writing, and mirror reading, there were no significant differences between the two groups. In later studies of simultaneous bimanual writing, Fitzgerald, Cooke, and Greiner (1984) and Greiner, Fitzgerald, and Cooke (1986a) found that stutterers performed as well as nonstutterers with the dominant hand, wrote more poorly with the nondominant hand, and did more mirroring with the nondominant hand. Similar results were obtained by Webster (1988). These findings conflict sharply with the Travis theory of cerebral dominance.

By the 1940s, it had become apparent that stutterers as a group were not distinguished by an anomalous type of handedness. This conclusion has been confirmed by the later studies of Johnson and Associates (1959, p. 84), Andrews and Harris (1964, p. 100), Records, Heimbuch, and Kidd (1977), Accordi et al. (1983), Bishop (1986), Webster and Poulos (1987), and Ardila et al. (1994). The only recent evidence of a connection between stuttering and left handedness was provided by Geschwind and Behan (1984). These researchers adopted a unique approach. Whereas all other researchers had asked how many stutterers were left-handed, Geschwind and Behan asked how many left-handed individuals stuttered, and focused on extreme cases. They compared 440 individuals who were very highly left handed on the *Oldfield Handedness Inventory* with 652 extremely right-handed persons. By self-report, 4.5 percent of the left-handed and 0.9 percent of the right-handed participants stuttered.

CEREBRAL DOMINANCE FOR LANGUAGE AND SPEECH

Following the early work on handedness, interest in stutterers' lateral dominance lay dormant for many years. In the 1960s, however, this interest revived, and the term *cerebral dominance* began to be heard again in discussions of stuttering. Studies of individuals with brain damage or aphasia have long shown that there is a hemispheric dominance for language functions.[13] Travis and his students did not include it in the long list of innate bilateral asymmetries that they investigated for the simple reason that at the time, there was no useful clinical test for hemispheric language dominance aside from as the indirect measure of handedness itself. But we now have a wide and ever increasing variety of such tests, and over the past decades researchers have administered them to stutterers.[14]

The Wada Test

A first conclusive method that was developed for determining which half of a patient's brain is dominant for language is the injection of intracarotid sodium amytal, also known as the Wada test. The left and right carotid arteries, passing upward through the neck, provide the blood supply to the left and right cerebral hemispheres, respectively. If sodium amytal is injected into the left carotid artery and the patient temporarily loses the ability to speak, it is clear that the patient has a language center in the left hemisphere. By injecting each artery in turn, it can be determined on which side the dominance lies, or whether, as is sometimes the case, speech is represented in both hemispheres. This, in brief, is the Wada test.[15]

In 1966, R. K. Jones, a neurosurgeon, published an unusual report on a series of four of his cases. All of them, ranging in age from 13 to 50, had stuttered severely since childhood. Each one had an intracranial lesion of recent origin in the region of the presumed speech areas. In each case, routine Wada testing prior to surgery showed that speech was represented in both hemispheres. Following the removal of the lesion, the stuttering disappeared in each case, and the Wada test disclosed normal unilateral speech representation. On follow-up ranging from 15 months to 3 years, each person was still speaking normally.

Jones' report caused a stir. To former champions of the role of cerebral dominance in speech fluency, it was tempting to see it as a vindication of the Orton-Travis theory, despite some puzzling aspects. Unfortunately, attempts at verification were some time in coming, in part because the Wada test is invasive and not entirely without risk. In time, however, three volunteers came forward from the Council of Adult Stutterers,[16] a self-help organization then affiliated with the Speech and Hearing Clinic of the Catholic University of America. Their Wada tests uniformly and unequivocally showed normal left hemispheric dominance for speech; injection of each side revealed no evidence of bilateral representation (see Luessenhop, Boggs, LaBorwit, & Walle, 1973).

Walle (1971) published a brief preliminary report of these results in order to forestall needless Wada testing of stutterers by others. In the meantime, however, a group in Sydney, Australia, had tested additional stutterers who proved to have normal left-sided speech/language dominance (Andrews & Quinn, 1972; Andrews, Quinn, & Sorby, 1972). They also tested a person who had begun to stutter at age 31 years following the onset of aphasia due to a head injury. In his case, the test showed evidence of bilateral lateralization of speech/language functions.

No doubt, anyone who looked for the meaning of these results soon made the same deduction. Stuttering did not seem to have much to do with grossly reversed cerebral dominance for speech, although more subtle patterns of difference might eventually be found; brain injury might possibly be related to stuttering.

Dichotic Listening Tests

A much less invasive measure that can be used to explore lateralization of speech and language functions

[13] See Dingwall (1998) for discussion of the historical discoveries that established hemispheric dominance for language function.

[14] The reader interested in surveys of the methods that have been developed for exploring lateralization, and typical lateralization patterns may find texts by Hellige (2001) and Springer and Deutsch (1997) useful.

[15] Named for the physician who developed the procedure, Juhn Wada (see background discussion of the technique in Dingwall, 1998).

[16] Later the National Council on Stuttering.

is dichotic listening, a technique usually attributed to Doreen Kimura (1961). When normal listeners are given the task of listening to a series of words that are heard in only one ear at a time, there is generally no appreciable difference between the number of words they hear accurately with the left and right ears. The results are quite different, however, when the task is dichotic—that is, when the participant listens to different, competing words that are presented simultaneously to both ears. In that case, most right-handed people will tend to report more accurately the words heard with the right ear than with the left. This is because the auditory pathways are, for the most part, contralateral. A word presented to the right ear accesses the left hemisphere language centers more rapidly than those presented to the left ear and right hemisphere; the latter must cross the corpus callosum before reaching the language centers (see Figure 4-1). Thus, words presented to the right ear typically have an advantage and "beat" those presented to the left ear. For nonspeech sounds such as environmental noises, there is most often a left-ear advantage, because of the right hemisphere's primary role in interpreting such sounds. Dichotic word listening tasks are generally presumed to demonstrate which hemisphere is dominant for language processing, so they have been considered a safe and convenient alternative to the Wada test in describing language dominance. They also excited the interest of investigators of stuttering.

Curry and Gregory (1969) gave dichotic listening tasks to a group of stutterers and obtained two significant findings. In the first place, only 45 percent showed the usual right-ear advantage on the dichotic word test, as compared with 75 percent of their fluent peers. In addition, the difference between the scores for the left ear and right ear was more than twice as great, on the average, for the nonstutterers as for the stutterers. It is not difficult to interpret such results as support for a cerebral dominance theory of stuttering.

A series of further investigations of dichotic listening in stutterers has been carried out over the years (see Table 4-3). As in the Curry and Gregory study, these have generally explored two questions: the number of stutterers and nonstutterers who show the expected right-ear advantage, and the difference between the groups in amount of right-ear advantage as measured by the mean difference

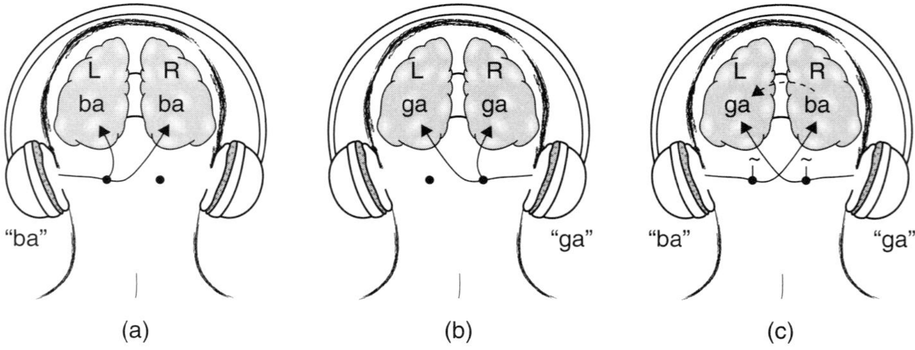

FIGURE 4-1 Kimura's model of dichotic listening in normal subjects. a) Monaural presentation to the left ear (LE) is sent to the right hemisphere (RH) by way of contralateral pathways and to the left hemishphere (LH) by ipsilateral pathways. The participant will report "ba" accurately. b) Monaural presentation to the RE is sent to the LH by way of contralateral pathways and to the RH by ways of ipsilateral pathways. The participant reports "ga" accurately. c) In dichotic presentation, ipsilateral pathways are suppressed, so "ga" goes only to the LH and "ba" to the RH. The syllable "ba" is accessible to the left (speech) hemisphere only through the corpus callosum. As a consequence, "ga" is usually reported more accurately than "ba" (a right-ear advantage). Adapted from W. Dingwall in Berko Gleason and Bernstein Ratner, 1998.

TABLE 4-3 Studies of Stutterers' Ear Preference in Dichotic Listening: Outcome in Relation to Meaningfulness of Stimuli

	Outcome[a]		
	Positive	Negative	Comments
Curry and Gregory (1969)	Words		
Mattingly (1970)	Meaningful and meaningless stimuli		10 nonstutterers were right-ear dominant, whereas 10 stutterers had no consistent pattern. No information given on difference between meaningful and meaningless stimuli.
Perrin and Elsenson (1970)	Words and nonsense syllables		Nonstutterers showed a right-ear preference. Stutterers showed no ear preference for nonsense syllables and a left-ear preference for words.
Slorach and Noehr (1973)		Digits	Subjects were 6- to 9-year-old children. A right-ear effect was observed equally in the stutterers and the nonstutterers.
Carf and Prins (1974)		CV syllables	Of 19 stutterers, 17 had a right-ear preference.
Gruber and Powell (1974)		Digits	Neither stutterers nor nonstutterers showed a right-ear advantage. Subjects were mainly children.
Brady and Berson (1975)		CVC syllables	There was no difference between groups in between-ear scores, although 6 of 35 stutterers, and no controls, showed a left-ear preference.
Dorman and Porter (1975)		CV syllables	
Sommers, Brady, and Moore (1975)	Words and digits		The stutterers had fewer right-ear responses than the controls for both the words and the digits.
Sussman and MacNeilage (1975)		CV syllables	
Quinn (1976)		CVC syllables	Updates Quinn (1972) with additional subjects.
Hall and Jerger (1978)	Words		Fewer stutterers than nonstutterers showed a right-ear advantage on the staggered spondaic word test.
Davenport (1979)	Words and digits		
Pinsky and McAdam (1980)		CV syllables	The groups did not differ in dichotic indices of laterallty. All 5 controls and 4 of 5 stutterers showed a right-ear advantage.

(continues)

TABLE 4-3 *(continued)*

	Outcome[a]		
	Positive	Negative	Comments
Rosenfield and Goodglass (1980)		CV syllables	The groups did not differ in degree of right-ear advantage. Five of 19 stutterers and 2 of 20 nonstutterers showed a left-ear advantage.
Liebetrau and Daly (1981)		CV syllables	The groups did not differ. The right-ear advantage was slight in both groups.
Cimorell-Strong, Gilbert, and Frick (1983)	CV syllables		Higher right-ear scores were found in 82% of controls and 55% of stutterers. The subjects were children aged 5, 7, and 9.
Blood (1985)	CV syllables		Subjects aged 7 to 12 showed fewer right-ear preferences than controls; those 13 to 15 did not.
Blood, Blood, and Hood (1987)	CV syllables		At age 7 to 9, 50% of stutterers and 80% of controls showed a right-ear preference. At age 10 to 12, 60% of the same stutterers and 80% of the controls did so.
Cross (1987)	CV syllables		For accuracy of identification of syllables, 58% of stutterers and 83% of controls showed a right-ear advantage. For reaction time, 75% of stutterers and 92% of controls did so.
Blood and Blood (1989a)	Words		The groups did not differ in the percent showing a right-ear advantage, but the magnitude of the difference between ears was greater for the nonstutterers.
Foundas, Corey, Hurley,[b] and Heilman (2004)	Right-handed women who stutter; Left-handed men who stutter	Right-handed men who stutter	Right-handed men who stutter matched controls and showed right-ear advantage in the non-directed attention conditon. Left-handed men and right-handed women who stutter demonstrated atypical auditory processing.

[a]Positive outcome refers to one in which a difference appeared between stutterers and controls.

[b]Left-handed men who stutter were better at shifting attention in both directions in comparison to all other groups; in contrast, right-handed women who stutter had no ear bias in the non-directed attention condition, made more perceptual errors, and had difficulty shifting attention to the left and right. Unfortunately left-handed woman were not examined in this study.

in score between the subjects' left and right ears. Table 4-3 shows conflicting positive and negative outcomes; 8 studies that found distinct differences between the groups are apparently contradicted by 10 studies that did not. It has been pointed out, however (by Moore, 1976), that stutterers have generally been found to differ from nonstutterers when investigators used meaningful verbal stimuli. The table offers considerable confirmation of this. Of 10 studies that used only nonsense syllables, all but 2 found stutterers and nonstutterers to perform essentially alike. Of the remaining eight that used words or digits, only two studies—both of which, incidentally, used children as subjects—produced negative outcomes. Thus, differences in ear advantage appear when language processing is involved.

Although we have placed the studies of Brady and Berson (1975) and Rosenfield and Goodglass (1980) in the negative column in Table 4-3, in both cases, a few stutterers showed a left-ear preference whereas no or fewer nonstutterers did so. Similar qualifications apply in the case of Blood, Blood, and Hood (1987), Cross (1987), and Blood and Blood (1989a). Moreover, Blood and Blood (1989b) showed that the outcome of dichotic listening studies may vary with the type of data analysis used. Regardless, it has long been clear that whatever anomalies of ear advantage are present among stutterers, they do not characterize all individuals. This has led to the frequent suggestion that the dichotic listening research may be revealing significant subtypes of stutterers.[17] With this in view, Blood and Blood (1986) divided 86 stutterers into those with right-ear advantage, left-ear advantage, and no ear advantage. They found no difference among the groups in number or type of disfluencies.

In another variation on dichotic listening, Rastatter and Dell (1987a) recorded stutterers' manual reaction times as they selected a picture that corresponded to a stimulus word. The word was introduced to one ear each time. The fluent participants showed a distinct right-ear advantage with either hand, consistent with a concept of left hemisphere dominance for language processing. The stutterers showed no ear advantage. Their reaction time was the same for the two ears, with either hand.

Innovative variations on the dichotic listening test have been applied to the study of cerebral dominance in stutterers. Tsunoda and Moriyama (1972) devised a test in which participants heard feedback, in the form of either a pure tone or a vowel, from their key-tapping of a simple temporal pattern. The feedback was presented to both ears, but was delayed in one ear, and the participant was told to attend to the feedback in the other. As measured by the number of errors they made while attending to each ear, 79 percent of normally fluent speakers had a right-ear advantage for vowels and a left-ear advantage for tones, whereas only 39 percent of the stutterers showed this pattern of dominance.

In a somewhat similar paradigm, Foundas, Corey, Hurley, and Heilman (2004) studied 18 adults who stutter and 28 matched peers using dichotic presentation of consonant-vowel stimuli in three attentional conditions: nondirected attention, attention directed right, and attention directed left. They also attempted to study dichotic responses by gender and handedness, although they could not locate any left-handed female stutterers to complete the comparison. Right-handed fluent and stuttering men both showed the expected right-ear advantage, while left-handed stuttering men showed an expected left-ear advantage. Right-handed women who stutter did not show any lateralized ear advantage. The authors concluded that further study into the lateralization patterns of stutterers is warranted.

Auditory Tracking

In a different type of study, Sussman and MacNeilage (1975) used an auditory tracking task requiring the participant to match the pitch of a tone heard in one ear to the varying pitch of a tone heard in the other. They found that when the pitch was controlled by movements of the tongue or jaw, most normally fluent adults did better when the varying tone was presented in the right ear. There was no lateralization effect when the hand was used to

[17]This hypothesis appears to be partially supported by the findings of Foundas et al. (2004) regarding anatomical anomalies that characterize a subgroup of stuttering adults, discussed later in this chapter.

control the pitch. By contrast with the normally fluent speakers, only 57 percent of a group of stutterers exhibited this right-ear effect on a jaw-tracking task. Sussman and MacNeilage concluded that stutterers appear to have a less distinct lateralization of a speech-related auditory sensorimotor integration.

Conflicting findings were reported by Neilson, Quinn, and Neilson (1976). They confirmed the observations of Sussman and MacNeilage for normally fluent speakers, but found no difference between normally fluent speakers and stutterers.

Nudelman, Herbrich, Hess, and Hoyt (1992) analyzed how much pitch differential was required for 20 adult stutterers and 13 matched comparison speakers to change their humming pitch to match to a tone signal. Stutterers required a statistically greater pitch change to provoke a change in hum fundamental frequency, but made changes as rapidly as did nonstutterers.

Tachistoscopic Investigations

Another way to tap hemispheric specialization for various tasks is by tachistoscopic presentation of stimuli (each eye has a separate right and left visual field, assessed individually by use of the tachistoscope; see Springer & Deutsch, 1997, for extensive discussion). Moore (1976) presented pairs of words simultaneously to different halves of the visual field, and the subjects were asked to say which word they saw first. Normally fluent speakers showed a significant preference for the right half of the visual field (left hemisphere), whereas stutterers did not. A larger proportion of stutterers than nonstutterers showed a left half-field advantage. Victor and Johannsen (1984) employed nonsense syllables as visual stimuli in a study otherwise similar to Moore's. Of 42 stutterers, 11 correctly identified more syllables in the left visual field than in the right; only 4 of a like number of typically fluent participants did so (see also Johannsen & Victor, 1986).

Hand and Haynes (1983) reached similar conclusions with a quite different procedure. They presented real words and nonwords (e.g., "*ramy*") to either the right or left visual fields of their participants. The task was to respond to real words by pressing a key (or, in a different condition, by saying /a/). The experimenters measured reaction times. As a group, the stutterers had faster reaction times when the words were presented to the left visual field (right hemisphere) than to the right. Normally fluent speakers showed no significant difference between fields, though they tended to react faster to stimuli presented to the right visual field. In a replication of the Hand and Haynes study with children aged 7 to 14 years, Hardin, Pindzola, and Haynes (1992) found no difference between stutterers and normally fluent children.

In a similar study by Wilkins, Webster, and Morgan (1984), letters and representations of faces were presented separately to participants' left and right visual fields. They were asked to respond with one button press to a target face or letter and with another button press to other stimuli. No significant difference in reaction time between visual fields for either stutterers or typically fluent speakers was found.

A series of tachistoscopic studies by Rastatter and his coworkers made use of a reaction-time format in which adults named letters or pictures or read words presented to left and right visual fields or responded with phonation of /a/ to visual presentations of words.[18] The investigations yielded some evidence of right-hemisphere dominance in stutterers, but in somewhat inconsistent and distinctly qualified ways. Rastatter, Loren, and Colcord (1987) commented, "These processes are obviously multidimensional in nature and reach beyond current themes focusing on the relative processing superiority of one hemisphere versus the other."

Szelag, Garwarska-Kolek, Herman, and Stasiek (1993) found a relationship between severity of stuttering when tachistoscopic responses of 9 severely and 11 mildly stuttering children and 48 normally fluent children were compared. While an expected left-hemisphere superiority was detected for the fluent speakers and mild stutterers, a right-hemisphere advantage was seen for the severe stutterers. The

[18] McGuire, Loren, and Rastatter (1986), Rastatter, Loren, and Colcord (1987), Rastatter and Dell (1987c, 1988), Rastatter and Loren (1988), Rastatter, McGuire, and Loren (1988).

authors suggested that lateralization of language functions might differ between mild and more severe presentations of stuttering.

Hemispheric Interference Tests

A number of studies have shown that in right-handed normally fluent speakers, verbal activity tends to reduce the rate of finger tapping with the right hand, but not with the left. This is easily seen as an interference effect resulting from the fact that the left hemisphere of the brain, which controls the right hand, is also used for speech by right-handed individuals. Such dual-task procedures presumably afford still another way of studying the cortical lateralization of speech and language, and they have been used in several studies of stutterers with somewhat equivocal results.

Sussman (1982) had subjects read aloud or count backwards by threes while tapping as fast as they could. During oral reading, right-handed normal speakers showed the expected reduction in tapping rate with the right hand, whereas stutterers showed the same amount of disruption in both hands, suggesting a lack of distinct cerebral dominance for speech. In counting backwards, however, the stutterers experienced much more interference with the right hand than the left.

In a study of stuttering children, Brutten and Trotter (1985, 1986) found that speaking tasks such as picture naming and storytelling reduced the rate of tapping in both hands. They found the same effect, however, in a nonspeech control condition in which the children were asked to imitate the sound of a siren. Consequently, they concluded that neither their results nor Sussman's could be interpreted to support a hypothesis of bilateral representation of language in people who stutter.

Replacing simple finger tapping with a task more vulnerable to interference, Greiner, Fitzgerald, and Cooke (1986b) instructed participants to tap as rapidly as possible beginning with the index finger, tapping outward to the little finger, and beginning again with the index finger. Interference by spontaneous speech, oral reading, and singing revealed no evidence of a difference between typically fluent speakers and stutterers in cerebral dominance for speech.

Webster (1990b) found evidence of right-hemisphere overactivation in stutterers in a different kind of study of rapid finger tapping in which adults tapped twice with one hand for each single tap with the other. Among normally fluent right-handed speakers, performance has been found to be better when it is the right hand that taps twice, whereas left-handers perform similarly under both conditions. Webster's comparison speakers performed accordingly, but the right-handed stutterers performed like the left-handed nonstutterers.

EVIDENCE FROM ELECTROENCEPHALOGRAPHY (EEG) AND EVENT-RELATED POTENTIALS (ERP)

Electroencephalography

The neurophysiological investigation of stuttering begun by Travis has consistently spurred a large amount of electroencephalographic research. It had been known since 1929 that the cerebral cortex was the site of a concentration of electrical activity, or "brain waves." One of these, the alpha wave, sinusoidal in form, about 10 cycles per second in frequency, and of relatively high voltage, is interesting because it is noticeably affected by varying physiological states—for example, by attention, fright, or reduced states of consciousness as in sleep, stupor, or anesthesia. The alpha rhythm has been of clinical value because it is altered by pathological conditions of the brain such as epilepsy or even, in some cases, an unsuspected proneness to epilepsy.

In view of these facts, it is not difficult to see why interest should have developed in the cortical potentials of stutterers. Since 1936, when Travis and Knott published the first of these studies, a considerable number of them have been done. The major historic studies—those that have employed quantitative methods and made systematic use of control groups—are summarized in Table 4-4 with emphasis on those findings obtained from comparisons of stutterers with normally fluent speakers. The results of these studies are difficult to compare because of

TABLE 4-4 Cortical Potentials of Stutterers and Nonstutterers

	Electrode placement	Brain area	Measures	Conditions	Results*
Travis and Knott (1936)	Bipolar	Left visual and motor	Amplitude duration	Silence Speech	Found small differences that they considered difficult to interpret. The waves during the nonstuttered speech of stutterers were larger and slower than those for the speech of normal speakers.
Travis and Knott (1937)	Bipolar	Left and right visual and motor	Synchronization and similarity of the two sides	Silence Speech	During silence the stutterers were more likely than the controls to have dissimilar potentials from the two sides, and during speech (stuttered and nonstuttered) were more likely to have perfectly matched potentials.
Travis and Malamud (1937)	Bipolar	Left motor and occipital	Frequency and amplitude	Silence Fluent Speech	The waves of stutterers during fluent speech were larger and slower than the waves during speech of nonstutterers.
Lindsley (1940)	Bipolar	Left and right occipital	Asynchronism and unilateral blocking	Silence Speech	During silence and speech 2 adult stutterers had more out-of-phase waves than did 48 right-handed and 8 left-handed children and the same percentage as did 9 ambidextrous children.
Freestone (1942)	Bipolar	Left and right frontal, motor, and occipital	Amount of alpha activity, amplitude, amplitude range, amount of wave similarity	Silence Speech	No clearly significant difference on any of the measures. Stutterers had more alpha similarity between areas, indicating a "lack of heightened foci of cerebral activity."
Douglass (1943)	Monopolar	Left and right occipital and motor	Bilateral and unilateral blocking	Silence Speech	The stutterers and nonstutterers did not differ in mean percent time of blocking of the alpha rhythm in silence. In speech the stutterers had greater bilateral blocking in the occipital areas. In silence the stutterers tended to show more blocking in the left occipital area; the nonstutterers, a greater amount of blocking in the right.
Knott and Tjossem (1943)	Monopolar	Left and right occipital and motor	Percent time alpha present	Silence	Confirmed findings of Douglass that during silence there is a tendency for stutterers and nonstutterers to differ with respect to which half of the occipital areas has more alpha activity.

Rheinberger, Karlin, and Berman (1943)	Bipolar and monopolar	Left and right frontal, central, occipital, intermastoid	Dominant frequencies above 7.5 per sec., irregular mixed activity, slow waves, bilateral asymmetry, changes under hyperventilation	Silence	Comparisons disclosed an essential similarity between the two groups.
Scarbrough (1943)	Monopolar	Left frontal, motor, and occipital	Frequency, variability of frequency, qualitatively abnormal records	Silence	The stutterers did not differ significantly from their controls in frequency or variability of frequency. Three of the stutterers and one of the nonstutterers ($N=20$ in each group) had qualitatively abnormal records.
Jones (1949)	Bipolar and monopolar	Left and right occipital	Unilateral and bilateral blocking, amount of bilateral out-of-phaseness, clinical abnormalities	Silence	There were no significant differences for any of the measures, except that stutterers exceeded nonstutterers in amount of left unilateral blocking in bipolar recordings.
Douglass (1952)	Monopolar	Left and right occipital	Wave alterations in response to stimuli	Silence Speech	Stutterers showed greater cortical reactivity in the dominant hemisphere to emotional stimuli (e.g., words, pictures).
Murphy (1953)	Monopolar	Left and right occipital	Wave alterations in response to frustration	Silence	Cortical disruption during frustration was significantly greater in stutterers when like hemispheres of the two groups were compared. Following frustration, stutterers recovered cortical equilibrium to a markedly smaller degree than did nonstutterers for both like-hemisphere comparisions.
Knott, Correll, and Shepherd (1959)	Bipolar and monopolar	Left and right occipital and occipital-parietal	Amount of voltage output at various frequencies, "driving"**	Silence	On various measures presumed to indicate "anxiety-proneness," each of two stuttering groups differed from the nonstuttering group in some way, but the two stuttering groups differed from each other more than from the nonstuttering group.
Fritzell, Petersen, and Sellden (1965)	Bipolar and monopolar	Left and right frontal, central, temporal parietal, and occipital	Incidence of atypical features	Silence	Normal EEG's were significantly more frequent among the controls. Unspecific abnormalities (increased low frequency activity) were more common among the stutterers, especially the younger ones.

(*continues*)

TABLE 4-4 *(continued)*

	Electrode placement	Brain area	Measures	Conditions	Results*
Fox (1966)	Bipolar	Left and right occipital	Prominence of a dominant frequency, interhemispheric synchronization, wave quality	Silence Speech	There were no significant differences between the two groups, either in silence or in nonstuttered speech. The only intergroup differences that appeared were between the stuttered speech of the stutterers and imitation of stuttering by the controls.
Sayles (1971)	Bipolar and monopolar	Left and right frontal, motor, parietal, occipital, anterior-temporal, midtemporal, posterior-temporal	Incidence of atypical responses to sleep, hyperventilation, and photic stimulation	Silence Speech	Abnormal or borderline wave patterns were found in 48% of the stutterers as compared with 12% of the controls. The stutterers also showed a greater cortical sensitivity to hyperventilation. The abnormalities were unrelated to speech activity or stuttering.
Okasha, Moneim, et al. (1947)	Bipolar and monopolar	Left and right frontal, central, temporal, parietal, and occipital	Incidence of atypical features	Silence	The EEG showed epileptic changes in 22% of the stutterers and none of the controls.
Zimmermann and Knott (1974)	Monopolar	Left and right interior frontal	Amplitude of shifts in slow potentials	Anticipation of speaking	Preceding normal utterances of single words most control subjects, but only 2 of the 9 stutterers, showed a greater slow potential shift in the left hemisphere than the right.
Ponsford et al. (1975)		Left and right frontal and temporal***	Averaged evoked responses	Visual presentation of the word "fire"	For nonstutterers the responses to the word "fire" in two different contexts were more different in the left hemisphere than the right. For stutterers the difference was greater in the right.
Moore and Lang (1977)	Monopolar	Left and right temporal	Percent time alpha	Between repeated oral readings	Nine of the 10 normal speakers showed greater percent time alpha over the right hemisphere, whereas 8 of the 10 stutterers showed it over the left.
Moore and Haynes (1980)	Monopolar	Left and right temporoparietal	Integrated alpha amplitude	Stimulation by pure tones and speech	The stutterers showed less alpha in the right hemisphere than the nonstutterers for both verbal and nonverbal stimuli.

Moore and Lorendo (1980)	Monopolar	Left and right temporoparietal	Integrated alpha amplitude	Auditory presentation of words	The nonstutterers had less alpha in the left than the right hemisphere; the stutterers, just the reverse.
Morgan, Cranford, and Burk (1997)	Electrodes were placed laterally on the right and left hemispheres according to the 10-20 system	Left (C3) and right (C4) hemispheres	P300 event related potentials[a]	Tonal stimuli	The two groups exhibited different patterns of interhemispheric activity. Although all 8 nonstutterers exhibited higher amplitude P300 activity in the right hemisphere for tonal stimuli[b], 5 of the 8 stutterers had higher amplitude activity over the left hemisphere. Evidence that stutterers and nonstutterers may exhibit hemispheric differences in processing of some types of nonlinguistic (tonal) stimuli.
Rastatter, Stuart, and Kalinowski (1998)	4 electrodes (T5, T6, P3, P4) placed according to the 10-20 system	Posterior portion of the left and right hemispheres	Beta band activity	Paragraph reading under three conditions: non-altered auditory feedback (NAF), delayed auditory feedback (DAF), and frequency altered auditory feedback (FAF)	NAF-stuttering participants displayed Beta band hyperactivity with right temporal parietal lobe showing the greatest activity. Under DAF and FAF, stuttering participants decreased stuttering behavior with a strong reduction in Beta activity for the posterior temporal parietal sites and the left hemisphere posterior sites showed a larger area of reactivity.
Ratcliff Baird (2001)	Monopolar recordings were collected from 19 sites in accordance with the 10-20 system of electrode placement	Homologous locations across the two hemispheres	EEG Activity	Written verbal fluency task, auditory delayed match to sample key press task and a written digit span task	Stutterers exhibited more activity than nonstutterers in frontal regions in all conditions. Increased cortical activity and increased sensitivity to stimuli supported the hypothesis that stutterers experience excess sensory stimulation while attempting motor plan assembly.

(*continues*)

TABLE 4-4 *(continued)*

	Electrode placement	Brain area	Measures	Conditions	Results*
Cuadrado and Weber-Fox (2003)	32 electrodes arranged according to the 10-20 system	Homologous locations across the two hemispheres	ERPs	Reading sentences, half containing verb-agreement violations	Behavioural and neurophysicalogical distinctions were present for online grammaticality judgments of verb agreement. These differences were accentuated by length and syntactic complexity. Results suggest that neural functions underlying visual sentence processing are altered in adults who stutter, even when no speech production is required.
Weber-Fox, Spencer, Spruill, and Smith (2004)	28 electrodes arranged according to the 10-20 system	Homologous locations across the two hemispheres	Event-related brain potentials (ERPs) and reaction times (RTs)	Rhyme judgement task for visually presented word pairs; half were congruent across words, the other half were incongruent	No major ERF differences. However, longer RTs for adults who stutter may indicate greater vulnerability to increased cognitive loads imposed by the incongruency condition. Stutterers also exhibited right hemisphere asymmetry in the rhyme judgment task.
Ozge, Toros, and Çömelekoglu (2004)[c]	19 EEG channels placed in accordance with the 10-20 system	Not specified	Visual EEG and QEEG analysis	Resting state and hyperventilation	Visual EEG revealed significantly higher parieto-occipital slow waves and slower fronto-central asynchromic waves in the stutterers than in the controls. QEEG showed significantly increased delta activity, especially in the right frontal parietal regions, and decreased alpha frequency bilaterally in the frontal regions in the stutterers.

*only those results relating to comparisons of stutterers and nonstutterers are summarized here.

**Driving occurs in response to a flashing light when the participant produces EEG rhythms at the same rate as the flashing of the light.

***The electrodes were placed over Broca's and Wernicke's areas and over the homologous points in the right hemisphere.

[a] One of the features of the ERP response is a response to unpredictable stimuli. This response (known as the P300) manifests as a positive deflection in voltage approximately 300 milliseconds after a stimulus is presented.

[b] This finding would seem to be consistent with evidence that this hemisphere is dominant for certain nonlinguistic functions, including tonal and musical perception.

[c] EEG, electroencephalography.

wide differences in procedure. In conducting this research there is, to begin with, a choice of various areas of the brain to focus on. Moreover, different features of the record may be chosen for study—for example, the amplitude, duration, or frequency of the waves; the percentage of the time they are present or "blocked"; their similarity to corresponding waves from the other hemisphere; and various other measures that may be derived from these. In addition, the participants may be studied in silence, during speech, while stuttering, and with various alterations in the experimental conditions. Finally, some researchers using EEG used monopolar leads (one electrode over the cortex and the other at the ear), while others utilized bipolar placement of leads (both electrodes over the cortex).

The earliest studies summarized in Table 4-4—most of those done through 1943—were in large part attempts to test the Orton-Travis cerebral dominance theory by determining whether stutterers differed from normally fluent speakers in the manner in which the two hemispheres seemed to be coordinated with each other. In some cases, differences were found. These tended to be unexpected and difficult to interpret, however, such as the tendency found by Travis and Knott (1937) for stutterers to have more dissimilar activity in the two halves of the brain than nonstutterers during silence, but better synchronization than nonstutterers during speech.

The investigation by Rheinberger, Karlin, and Berman (1943) appears to have been in part a straightforward attempt to analyze those aspects of the electroencephalographic (EEG) records that are significant in clinical diagnosis. The study disclosed no features distinguishing stutterers from normal typically fluent speakers. In addition, they found no unusual interhemispheric relationships.

After 1950, much of the electroencephalographic research consisted of attempts, due once more chiefly to Travis and his students, to find in the EEG patterns of stutterers correlates of such behavioral tendencies as emotional reactivity, frustration, or anxiety-proneness. This is evident in the later studies summarized in Table 4-4, as well as in a study by Shopwin (1959), in which stutterers were judged to be higher in passive-dependency as indicated by significantly higher alpha indices.

In a different programmatic approach, largely of European origin, an accumulation of EEG observations of an essentially clinical type have centered on the question of pathological indications in the EEG tracings of stutterers. Quite a few researchers reported abnormal records to be common among stutterers; others did not.[19] An interesting sidelight was thrown on the subject by Luchsinger and Landolt (1955), who found the EEG to be normal in the large majority of stutterers but abnormal, as a rule, in clutterers and in stutterers with a cluttering "component." Similar observations were made by Morávek and Langová (1962).

In view of the largely qualitative and uncontrolled nature of most of these clinically oriented observations, the studies of Andrews and Harris (1964, p. 101) and Graham (1966) are of special interest. Andrews and Harris randomized the EEG records of 30 stuttering children and their matched fluent peers and gave them to an EEG consultant for blind evaluation. The records were then rearranged in matched pairs, and the consultant was asked to judge which record in each pair was "more abnormal." In neither case was there a difference between the evaluations of the stutterers and those of the nonstutterers. Graham arranged a double-blind evaluation of adults' EEG records using three neurologists as judges and found no significant differences between stutterers and typically fluent speakers.

On the other hand, Sayles (1971), whose EEG recordings were also evaluated by an expert without knowledge of the participants' speech histories, found so many more abnormal wave patterns among the stutterers than their controls as to suggest that stutterers as a group "occupy a region

[19] Large proportions of stutterers with EEG abnormalities were reported by Segre (1951), Streifler and Gumpertz (1955), Bente, Schönhärl, and Krump (1956), Umeda (1962a), Schilling (1962), Hirschberg (1965), Cali, Pisana, and Tagliareni (1965), Schmoigl and Ladisch (1967), Sayles (1971), Okasha, Moneim, et al. (1974), Rastatter, Stuart, and Kalinowski (1998), Khedr, El-Nasser, Abdel Haleem, Bakr, and Trakhan (2000), and Özge, Toros, and Çömelekoglu (2004). Essentially normal findings in the great majority of participants were reported by Luchsinger (1954), Luchsinger and Landolt (1955), Busse and Clark (1957), Pierce and Lipcon (1959), Morávek and Langová (1962), Andrews and Harris (1964, p. 101), and Graham (1966).

somewhere between normal controls and epileptics." Sayles suggested that the negative findings of many previous studies were due to their failure to use such provocation techniques as hyperventilation and sleep, which are now routine in the clinical diagnosis of convulsive tendencies. Some evidence corroborating Sayles has been offered by Okasha, Moneim, et al. (1974).

Looking at the research on stutterers' cortical potentials as a whole, we might perhaps draw two conclusions. First, the weight of evidence from controlled, quantitative studies supports the view that, except for small differences that are difficult to account for, stutterers' brain potentials during silence tend to be normal. Second, there is a considerable body of additional work suggesting the presence of brain pathology in a large proportion of stutterers, but this has not received sufficient confirmation from adequately controlled studies, and conflicting findings exist.

Zimmermann and Knott (1974) measured the contingent negative variation[20] in brain activity as adults prepared to say each of a series of words exposed in turn on a screen. In four of five normally fluent speakers, they made the expected observation of greater changes in the brain waves over the left hemisphere than the right. Before fluent utterances of words by stutterers, this was true in only two of nine cases. This finding was not confirmed, however, by Pinsky and McAdam (1980) or by Prescott and Andrews (1984), and Prescott (1988) found few differences between stutterers and nonstutterers in the contingent negative variation.

Ponsford, Brown, Marsh, and Travis (1975) measured the brain potentials evoked by visual presentation of the word "fire" in the two phrases "fire is hot" and "fire the gun." For the nonstutterers, the different grammatical function (noun vs. verb) of the target word produced a greater difference in potentials in the left hemisphere than in the right. For the stutterers, the reverse was true.

Moore and Lang (1977) reported a suppression of alpha waves over the right hemisphere in 8 of 10 stutterers before each of several oral readings of a passage. In nonstutterers, on the other hand, they noted less alpha activity over the left hemisphere, which accords with past findings on normally fluent speakers engaged in linguistic processing. Moore and Haynes (1980) found reduced alpha in stutterers' right hemispheres whether they listened to recorded speech or pure tones. They suggested that stutterers demonstrate, not reversed cerebral dominance for speech, but right-hemisphere processing of both verbal and nonverbal stimuli. In subsequent studies, Moore and his coworkers used auditory stimulation with lists of words that the participants were told they would later be asked to recall or with reading passages about which they knew they would later be questioned.[21] Again the stutterers showed more alpha suppression in the right hemisphere than in the left; the nonstutterers showed the reverse. In a further study of alpha asymmetry, Wells and Moore (1990) found evidence of right-hemisphere activation in stutterers during speech, using a sentence repetition task.

Few replications of Moore's research have been attempted. Pinsky and McAdam (1980) found that stutterers did not differ from fluent speakers in alpha asymmetry during verbal processing tasks. Somewhat unexpectedly, Fitch and Batson (1989) discovered little difference between the two hemispheres in alpha activity during silent verbal processing for either stutterers or nonstutterers. Results obtained by Boberg, Yeudall, Schopflocher, and Bo-Lassen (1983) agreed with those of Moore and his coworkers, but the use of expressive verbal tasks (the Wechsler vocabulary test and counting backward by sevens) by Boberg's group makes it somewhat difficult to interpret their findings; events occurring during stuttering may be a cause, a result, or an aspect of stuttering. They reported the startling fact that, after three weeks of therapy during which stuttering was markedly reduced by training in the use of a slow speech rate and gentle onsets of phonation, the stutterers demonstrated a normal alpha relationship during performance of the verbal tasks. A similar observation was made by

[20]The contingent negative variation is a negative wave that appears following a warning to prepare for a signal to perform a response.

[21]Moore and Lorendo (1980), Moore, Craven, and Faber (1982), Moore (1986).

Moore (1984b) in a study of a single stutterer.[22] Citing studies showing that stress results in greater activation of the right hemisphere, Boberg et al. (1983) suggested that the finding might be due to the fact that speech tasks, even receptive ones, are threatening to stutterers as a result of past emotional conditioning.

Not many of the EEG studies have utilized children as participants. Özge, Toros, and Çömelekoglu (2004) used conventional EEG techniques and quantitative EEG (QEEG) analysis to study brain waves in 26 stuttering Turkish children and 21 comparison children. QEEG analysis showed significantly increased delta wave activity, especially in the right frontal and parietal regions and decreased alpha wave frequency bilaterally in frontal regions of stuttering children, compared to the fluent children. Delayed maturation of frontal lobe function in stuttering children was suggested.

Event-Related Potentials (ERP)

More recently, event-related potentials (ERPs) have been used extensively to explore the processing of speech and language stimuli in a wide variety of populations, including people who stutter. ERPs can be viewed as similar to EEG tracings, but reflect activity that is finely time-locked to sensory, motor, or cognitive events/processes. ERPs can provide indirect information suggestive of site and hemispheric focus of cortical activity, as well as charge (positive/negative), latency (how long it takes the brain to reflect a response to the stimulus or task), and amplitude (a reflection of response strength) associated with stimulus processing. They do not appear to be under conscious control, and so presumably can tap basic aspects of the brain's response to external stimuli and task demands. At this point, a number of typical ERP responses to varying stimuli, changes in stimuli, and aspects of linguistic processing have been identified.[23] For example, patterns have been identified for sensory processing, discrimination tasks, memory, language, and error detection. They are conventionally labeled in terms of whether the change from baseline electrical signal is positive (P) or negative (N), and the time elapsed from target signal presentation in milliseconds. Some well-investigated ERP patterns include the N400, which appears after the listener perceives a semantic anomaly (as in when the phrase, "The pizza is too hot to ____" ends with an incongruous word such as "drink").

In some cases, ERPs have been combined with EEG studies. Khedr, El-Nasser, Haleem, Bakr, and Trakhan (2000) studied a broad range of stuttering and fluent speakers, from the ages of 6–25. Tasks and measures included visual-evoked potentials, auditory-evoked potentials, event-related potentials, *Wechsler Intelligence Scale* performance, and electroencephalographic profiles. Visual- and auditory-evoked potentials differed between groups, while ERPs did not. Overall EEG rhythm was slower and more asymmetric in the stuttering participants. The stutterers' EEGs were classified as pathological in nature in 54 percent of the cases, with wave patterns consistent with epilepsy seen in over 16 percent of these cases. The authors' major conclusion was that stuttering appears to have an organic basis.

Morgan, Cranford, and Burk (1997) selected the P300 event-related potential for study. P300 is thought to reflect attention and information processing activity, and can be observed for nonlinguistic as well as linguistic stimuli. The two groups differed in ERP responses to tone sequences. Although all eight typically fluent participants exhibited P300s that were higher in amplitude over the right hemisphere, five of the eight stutterers displayed higher amplitude activity over the left hemisphere. They concluded that stutterers might differ in cortical processing of auditory signals.

Another well-explored ERP response is mismatch negativity (MMN), studied by Corbera, Corral, Escera, and Idiazábal (2005). MMN appears to reflect perception of change in an ongoing stimulus sequence and appears roughly 150–250 milliseconds following the deviant signal. The authors

[22] Similar findings have been obtained using other techniques to study plasticity of brain activation following therapy, as later sections in this chapter indicate.

[23] A tutorial on ERP recording and interpretation relevant to visual and language processing can be found in Bentin (1989).

compared the MMN to simple tone (frequency and duration) and phonetic contrasts. The stutterers' MMN responses appeared similar to those of fluent speakers when processing tones, but differed when processing phonetic (linguistic) changes. Differences in MMN responses also appeared to correlate with self-reports of stuttering severity. The authors concluded that speech sound processing and representation is atypical in stuttering.

As noted in further discussion in Chapter 8, Christine Weber-Fox and colleagues at Purdue University have conducted a series of studies that have employed ERP recordings to investigate cortical activity that accompanies linguistic processing in people who stutter. In the first study, Weber-Fox (2001) examined ERPs linked to the reading of function words, content words, and semantically anomalous words in sentence contexts. While the nine pairs of stuttering and fluent participants scored similarly on tests of their grammatical and vocabulary ability, the ERPs seen during the reading tasks differed in ways that suggested differences in functional brain organization. The stutterers' ERPs were characterized by reduced negative amplitudes expected to accompany processing of function words, content words, and semantic violations. In particular, the N280 (function word) and N350 (content word) ERPs were of lower amplitude in the stutterers, although earlier ERPs that reflect visual processing of the stimuli did not differ (see Figure 4-2 for illustrative findings from this study). Because the N400 response to semantic violations was also reduced in amplitude, Weber-Fox concluded that, "neural processes related to linguistic functioning may underlie the differences observed" between individuals who stutter and those who do not.

Next, Cuadrado and Weber-Fox (2003) used ERPs to further explore syntactic processing in nine pairs of fluent and stuttering adults. Participants read sentences, some of which contained subject-verb agreement errors (as in "the boys *is* running"), both during ERP recording (online) as well as afterward, and were required to identify grammatical and ungrammatical sentences. Some errors were in simple sentence constructions, while some violations were

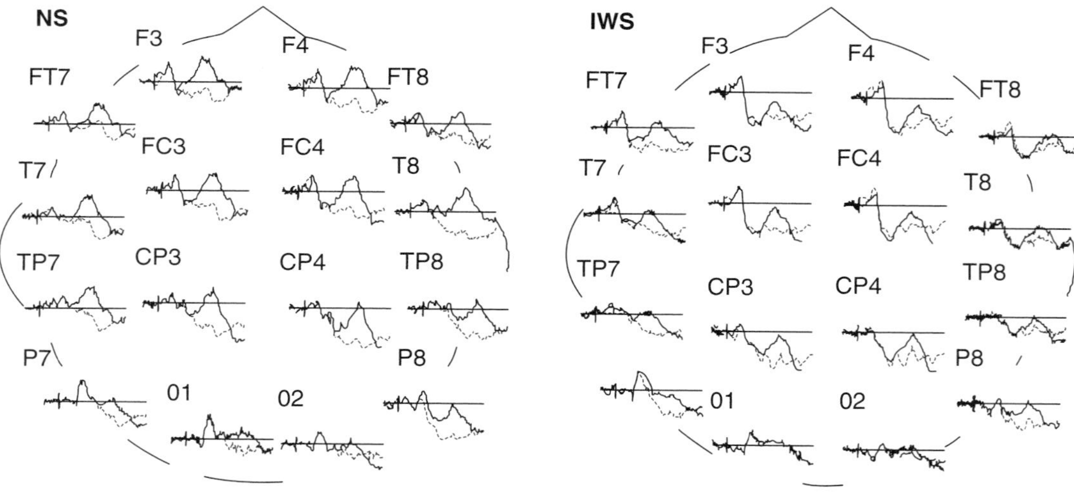

FIGURE 4-2 Grand averages of the ERPs elicited by semantic anomalies (dark) and best completions (light) for normally fluent speakers (NS) and individuals who stutter (IWS). The large negative peaks (N400) elicited by semantic anomalies are readily apparent in the ERPs of the NS and reduced in the amplitude in the ERPs of the IWS. The calibration bar (1 μV above and below 0 value) for each waveform marks the onset of the stimulus presentation. The epochs include a 100-ms baseline and 600-ms poststimulus onset. From C. Weber-Fox, *JSLHR*, 2001, p. 821.

interrupted by an embedded clause to maximize processing complexity. Fluent and stuttering speakers did not differ when completing the "offline" paper and pencil task. However, judgment accuracy during ERP recording was depressed for the stutterers, particularly for subject-verb agreement violations that occurred in the more demanding sentences. Further, while fluent participants showed a typical positive spike roughly 600 msec. following detection of an error (the P600 ERP response), those seen in stutterers were reduced in amplitude. Both the judgment data and ERP responses suggested to the authors that stutterers have atypical syntactic analysis abilities even when not required to produce spoken language.

In a later study, Weber-Fox, Spencer, Spruill, and Smith (2004) analyzed another aspect of linguistic processing (rhyme judgment) in 11 pairs of fluent and stuttering adults. For half of the stimulus word pairs, the words looked orthographically similar and did rhyme (e.g., *thrown, own*) or did not look similar and did not rhyme (e.g., *cake, own*). However, the phonologic and orthographic characteristics of the remaining word pairs were designed to make processing more difficult: these words looked similar but did not rhyme (e.g., *gown, own*) or did not look similar but rhymed (e.g., *cone, own*). In this study, no major differences were seen for the accompanying ERPs, accuracy of judgments, or reaction times. However, unlike those of normally fluent speakers, the stutterers' electrophysiological responses during rhyme judgments were characterized by a right-hemisphere asymmetry. Given their prior experimental results, the authors concluded that stuttering was unlikely to reflect a core phonological processing deficit; rather, areas of relative weakness might reside in lexical or syntactic processing, or generalized processing capacity limitations.

FUNCTIONAL IMAGING OF SPEECH-LANGUAGE FUNCTIONS

Electrophysiological measures have certain limitations, as noted by De Nil (2004). They cannot detect activity deep in the cortex or reflect activity that travels along certain planes. Thus, there is need to augment what can be found in such studies with additional methods for imaging brain function. In this regard, the techniques discussed in this section have relatively good spatial resolution of both cortical and subcortical regions, although their temporal resolution is less good than ERP, for example. There has been a relatively large number of functional imaging studies conducted with adults who stutter since the last edition of this text. In reporting what has been learned in recent years, we will first summarize findings obtained using specific techniques, such as Positron Emission Tomography (PET), Functional Magnetic Resonance Imaging (fMRI), and so on, and then integrate these findings with those from anatomical studies to provide a picture of what we have learned and what we have yet to learn about central neuropsychological and neurolinguistic functioning in people who stutter.

The reader who is more keenly interested in functional imaging studies of speech and language production in people who stutter is well-advised to ground these studies within the context of similar (and much more numerous) studies of typical speakers. To summarize the normal cortical substrates of speech and language production is beyond the scope of this text. However, most of the studies reported in this section have utilized paradigms first described by Petersen, Fox, Posner, Mintun, and Raichle (1988), which have guided much subsequent work in brain imaging. In addition, readers are referred to two influential meta-analyses of programmatic studies in this area by Levelt et al. (2000) and Indefrey and Levelt (2004). Finally, extremely thorough summaries of imaging studies in stuttering are offered by De Nil (2004) and Ingham (2004), who both provide more background and detail than is permitted in this chapter's coverage of this increasingly growing area of inquiry. De Nil notes that the imaging studies can be assigned to two primary sets of hypotheses: whether there are differences between the brain's activity during speech/language perception and production in normally fluent and stuttering speakers, and whether one can discern any cortical patterns characteristic of fluent as opposed to stuttered speech production.

Positron Emission Tomography (PET)

PET technology is based on the assumption that increased brain activity will be reflected in an increase in the metabolism of oxygen or glucose. If the patient is injected with a radioactively tagged isotope prior to the brain imaging tasks, increased blood flow in a given area of the brain will be detectible using the PET scanner's ability to track the radioisotope's concentration in given brain regions. Variations in the PET studies that we describe include the use of different tracking isotopes, as well as the speakers' tasks and differing time spans over which the scan was conducted in order to observe blood flow changes. This last was of particular concern, as it led to very poor ability to link the blood flow changes to specific behaviors in the earliest studies.

In the earliest reported study, Wood, Stump, McKeehan, Sheldon, and Proctor (1980) found that cerebral blood flow during stuttering was greater in the right hemisphere Broca's area, and the left hemisphere Wernicke's area. Pool, Devous, Freeman, Watson, and Finitzo (1991) used xenon 133 single-photon emission computed tomography and found reduced blood flow in the frontal lobes of 20 stutterers in "recognized cortical regions of speech-motor control," as well as in the left temporal lobe. They concluded that their findings "suggest that stuttering is a neurogenic disorder." In follow-up work, Watson et al. (1992) found that extreme asymmetry in blood flow in left and middle temporal regions of interest (ROIs) was associated with longer laryngeal reaction time, suggestive of a subgroup of stutterers for whom premotor processing might be impaired. In a further study, Watson et al. (1994) divided their adult stutterers into two different groups: one that achieved normally on a series of linguistic tasks and another that displayed linguistic performance deficits. Once again, cerebral blood flow asymmetries, in this case with left hemisphere showing less activity than right, were seen only for the linguistically deficited group, rather than all participants. The team concluded that their series of studies supported models of stuttering "that explicitly recognize that efficient integration of linguistic, motoric, and cognitive processes is critical to the production of oral/verbal fluency and to understanding sources of fluency failure."

In 1995, Wu et al. used [18F] deoxyglucose (FDG) to track cerebral blood flow in four stutterers as they read aloud singly and in unison to induce fluency The stutterers were also compared against typically fluent speakers. In the more disfluent condition, decreased blood flow was seen in both Broca's and Wernicke's areas, in comparison with their more fluent reading and reading in the typically fluent participants. There also appeared to be decreased blood flow in the left caudate region within the basal ganglia for the stutterers, regardless of reading condition; the caudate is believed to play a role in multiple functions, including motor control, feedback processing, attention, memory, and learning.

Most studies after this have used radioactively tagged water, because it permits better temporal resolution of scans. Fox et al. (1996) also utilized choral reading to examine more and less fluent speech production in stutterers. They found relatively widespread and right-hemisphere, rather than left, overactivation of motor system areas in both cerebrum and cerebellum. During stuttering, there was also relative deactivation of left hemisphere auditory areas. These areas are thought to support self-monitoring of speech production. Another area typically activated in speech production tasks in the frontal-temporal regions was similarly deactivated. During choral reading, which induced fluent speech production, these atypical patterns of over- and under-activation were largely eliminated. The authors speculated that stuttering results from over-activation of the speech motor system and a deficiency in self-monitoring of speech production. In a companion study, Ingham et al. (1996) could not find any obvious rest state differences between the stuttering and fluent men; this suggested that there are no gross differences in brain structure that distinguish fluent and stuttering speakers.

Braun et al. (1997) also measured regional cerebral blood flow in 18 adult stutterers and 20 typically fluent volunteers during a series of speech and language tasks designed to elicit differing degrees of fluency. During conversational speech and a structured sentence production task, the stutterers did not demonstrate the degree of left-hemisphere activation seen in the fluent participants; instead, normally expected patterns were either absent, bilateral in nature, or lateralized to the right hemisphere. These differences were seen even when the stuttering participants were perceptually fluent. When more fluent speech was compared with disfluent speech conditions, there was a high degree of anterior area activation, while posterior areas typically associated with auditory perception and processing were relatively under-activated. The authors suggested that left-hemisphere activation might play a role in precipitating stuttering, while the right hemisphere is recruited to compensate for fluency breakdown.

De Nil, Kroll, Kapur, and Houle (2000) examined the neurological correlates of single word production. Ten right-handed male stuttering adults and appropriately matched fluent speakers both orally and silently read single words that appeared on a screen one at a time. When contrasted with a baseline condition that did not involve language processing, stutterers displayed increased activation in the left anterior cingulate cortex (ACC) even during silent reading (this area had been described as relatively over-activated by Braun et al. as well; see Figure 4-3). The ACC has been hypothesized to play a role in selective attention and covert articulatory practice. Given this, the authors speculated that the stutterers were more actively planning speech to avoid anticipated fluency breakdown. As in so many studies we have discussed, the authors also found a proportionally and expected greater left-hemisphere activation in the typically fluent speakers, and a proportionally greater right-hemisphere activation in the stuttering participants.

Fox et al. (2000) studied 10 pairs of fluent and stuttering men. In particular, they were interested in the correlation between degree of disfluency and activation patterns. The frequency of stutters was negatively correlated with the right hemisphere areas (specifically, the superior and middle temporal gyrus) traditionally thought to be responsible for speech perception and auditory processing; in other words, increased stuttering appeared to be associated with deactivation of these areas. Ingham et al. (2004) replicated their paradigm with 10 pairs of female stuttering and fluent adults. The women's stutter rates were correlated with bilateral (rather

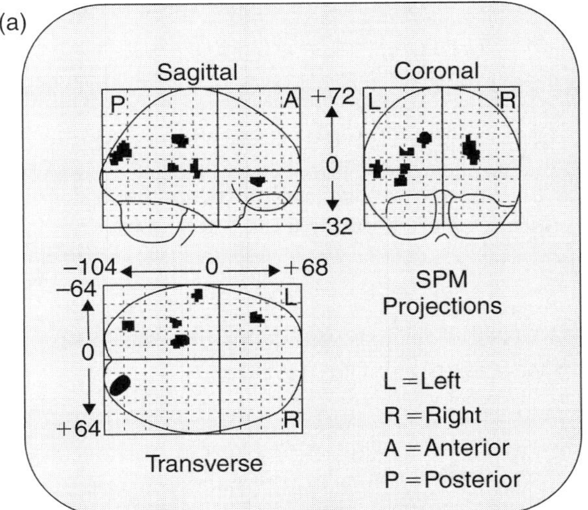

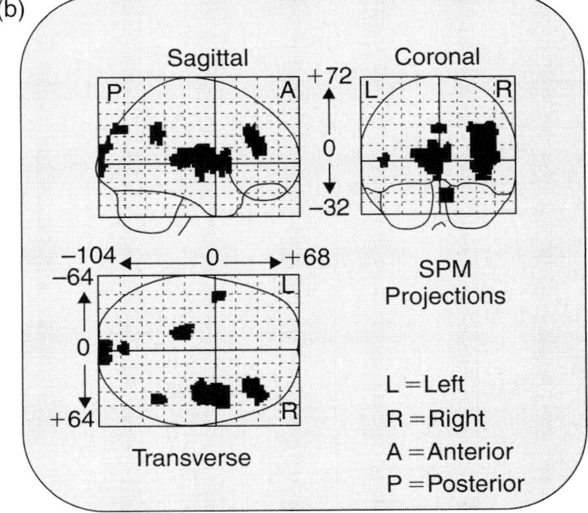

FIGURE 4-3 Statistical parametric maps of between-group comparisons for increases in regional cerebral blood flow during oral reading relative to silent reading (a) Nonstuttering versus stuttering speakers; (b) Stuttering versus nonstuttering speakers. From De Nil, Kroll, Kapur, and Houle, 2000, *JSLHR*, p. 1047.

than right-hemisphere) activation, as had been seen in the male stutterers. As in their earlier report and those by Braun et al. (1997) and De Nil and Kroll (2001), they also noted increased activation of cerebellar areas, which has been associated with motor learning demands.

De Nil, Kroll, and Houle (2001) specifically examined cerebellar activity during single word reading and the more linguistically demanding task of generating verbs to prompt. They did not identify major differences between the two conditions, and thus concluded that stuttering might be more strongly associated with motor planning and execution than with linguistic processing.

Stager, Jeffries, and Braun (2003) used PET to see whether brain activation in stutterers differed when fluency was induced by either singing or paced speech. During these tasks, increased bilateral activation of auditory association areas and motor control areas were seen in both fluent and stuttering speakers, probably as a function of task requirements in each of these conditions, which require relatively greater coordination between auditory and speech production systems than conversational speech. However, relatively higher activation in left hemisphere areas was seen for the stutterers. The authors suggested that more active recruitment of the left hemisphere might be required to produce fluent speech.

Ingham, Fox, Ingham, and Zamarripa (2000) found that brain activation appeared similar when four stutterers imagined that they were stuttering or fluent, and when they scanned during actual speech production tasks that increased and decreased fluency. There was somewhat less good correspondence between activation patterns in imagined and actual production in four matched fluent participants. As noted earlier, De Nil, Kroll, Kapur, and Houle (2000) had also noted atypical activation in the left anterior cingulate cortex that distinguished stutterers from fluent participants, even in silent reading.

Ingham (2004) notes that, while virtually every published study appears to show differences between stutterers and typically fluent speakers during speech production or comprehension, the existing PET studies of stuttering do not show any consistent areas of over- or under-activation, with the exception of the cerebellum. However, some larger patterns appear to be emerging. De Nil (2004) concurs and notes that there is an overarching pattern of atypical activity in brain regions believed to be responsible for motor planning and execution, as well as those implicated in monitoring of sensory feedback. Finally, Ingham (2004) suggests that the available research more strongly supports physiological determinants of fluency and fluency failure than affective and cognitive factors.

Limitations of PET

To understand why PET studies cannot fully answer many questions about the underlying basis of stuttering, it is important to consider its limitations as a research technique (see De Nil, 2004; Ingham, 2004, for more extensive discussion). First, because patients must be injected using radioactive isotopes, studies have been limited to adults. This inherently makes it more difficult to ascertain whether any specific differences found between stuttering and fluent participants reflect the underlying deficit in stuttering, or the speaker's accommodation to stuttering over time. Further, exposure to the radioactive isotope should be relatively limited—thus, one cannot perform innumerable scans on a single person, as one might want to do to see changes over the course of a therapeutic intervention. Finally, the actual signal produced during local activation of a cortical region, compared against baseline activity is of a relatively low level, forcing investigators to combine and average patients' responses over tasks and individuals.

Functional Magnetic Resonance Imaging (fMRI) Studies of Stuttering

While fMRI has better resolution than PET, and represents much less risk to participants because it does not require injection of radioactive isotopes, it had been significantly limited for studies requiring oral or motor responses because it is extremely vulnerable to movement artifacts. Van Borsel, Achten, Santens, Lahorte, and Voet (2003) acknowledged this problem in their pilot investigation of six pairs of fluent and stuttering adults. Participants were scanned during both oral and silent reading of both meaningful text and nonsense words. The stutterers' activation patterns were characterized by relatively more diffuse patterns and greater right-hemisphere activity.

Viswanath, Karmonik, King, Rosenfield, and Mawad (2003) also found atypical activation patterns in a single stutterer during oral reading. Over recent years, improvements in design have enabled event-related fMRI designs, which block and separate responses that require motion from rest state periods. However, many of the studies using the technique on typically fluent speakers have required only single word responses to stimuli, a task not likely to provide ample opportunity to visualize activation patterns related to stuttering. Preibisch et al. (2003a) performed a feasibility study in which they piloted imaging during the reading of short sentences. They were able to suppress movement artifacts and show activation of speech motor and language areas reported in other studies. Next, Preibisch et al. (2003b) reported an fMRI experiment using 16 adult stutterers and 16 typically fluent speakers. During oral reading, stutterers showed atypical activation in an area called the right frontal operculum (RFO). This area is anatomically connected to the anterior portion of the temporal lobe, and its activity has been associated with time estimation tasks (Coull, Vidal, Nazarian, & Macar, 2004); additionally, it appears to be selectively recruited when speech tasks become more complex (Bohland & Guenther, 2006). Some have considered this area to be the right hemisphere's equivalent of Broca's area. Thus, to the researchers, "it seem[ed] plausible that it compensates for deficient signal transmissions between Broca's area and left-sided articulatory motor representations, . . . or for a dysfunctional Broca's area, by automatically taking over its disturbed functions, as occurs during recovery from aphasia after frontal injury." Activation in this region was negatively correlated with stuttering severity; to the researchers, this suggested that its activity was compensatory—the less severe stutterers showed proportionally greater activity. As noted later in this chapter, some of these atypical patterns of activity appeared to resolve after fluency therapy.

Blomgren, Nagarajan, Lee, Li, and Alvord (2003) completed an fMRI study that required seven stutterers and nine fluent comparison speakers to silently retrieve words whose definitions were supplied auditorily. No overt speech was required. Large variations in activation were seen across participants. However, the stuttering speakers displayed a trend toward "more activation in right Broca's area homologue and along the precentral gyrus in the right hemisphere. The auditory association area (Wernicke's area) in the right hemisphere also appeared to activate to a larger degree than in the nonstuttering speakers" (see Figure 4-4). In general, while fluent speakers showed predominantly left-hemisphere speech and language area activation, patterns were more bilateral for the stutterers.

Increasingly, researchers in many disciplines are utilizing meta-analyses to combine results from a number of studies to ascertain more generalizable patterns of performance. Brown, Ingham, Ingham, Laird, and Fox (2005) performed two such meta-analyses of imaging data, one of which targeted stuttered events in stuttering participants; the other examined correlates of fluent speech in typically fluent speakers. For fluent speakers, it was possible to identify typical activation in the primary motor cortex, the premotor cortex, as well as the supplementary motor area, operculum, cerebellum, and auditory processing areas. While somewhat similar, patterns also differed somewhat in the stutterers: a number of motor areas were over-activated, such as primary motor cortex, the supplementary motor area, and regions in the cerebellum. In addition, the frontal operculum was one of three areas more right-lateralized in stutterers. Activation associated with self-monitoring of speech was extremely depressed in the stuttering group.

Limitations of fMRI

As with all techniques we report here, fMRI has both strengths and weaknesses. At this point, some readers may have themselves experienced scanning for a suspected medical condition. The most obvious

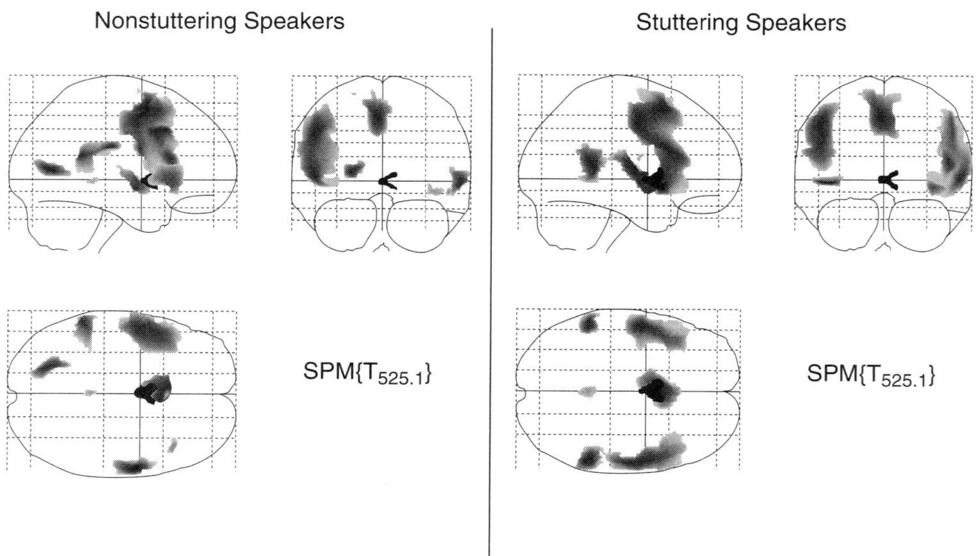

FIGURE 4-4 This figure displays three glass brain renderings for each speaker group. The left half of the figure displays the significant average activation areas for the nonstuttering speakers; the right half of the figure displays the average activation for the stuttering speakers. Within each right and left block of three figures, the upper left figure is a view toward the right hemisphere, the upper right figure is a view toward the back of the brain, and the lower left figure is a top-down view, with the occipital lobe on the left and the frontal lobe on the right. Reprinted with permission from Blomgren, M., Nagarajan, S. S., Lee, J. N., Li, T., & Alvord, L. (2003). Preliminary results of a functional MRI study of brain activation patterns in stuttering and nonstuttering speakers during a lexical access task. *Journal of Fluency Disorders*, 28, 337–57.

feature of the process is the extremely high noise level generated during the process. In addition to making it difficult to record any participant speech production and the constraints on movement we have already mentioned,[24] the background noise of the scanner may artificially induce fluency via a masking effect. Relative to ERP, fMRI also has less good temporal resolution.

Magnetoencephalography (MEG)

Magnetoencephalograpy (MEG) is one of the more recent techniques to be employed in examining speech and language processing in stutterers. As should be apparent, each imaging technique appears to have its specific strengths and weaknesses. MEG's particular advantage is its very good temporal resolution, in particular, its ability to track the sequence of brain activity across various areas of the cortex during speech and language processing. Salmelin, Schnitzler, Schmitz, and Freund (2000) recorded MEG data while 9 German stutterers and 10 fluent comparison speakers read sequences of nouns. Even in fluently produced speech, differences in the pattern of sequential activation differed: in the normally fluent speakers, cortical activity advanced from the left inferior frontal cortex, the area that subserves programming of articulatory gestures, to the left lateral central sulcus and dorsal premotor cortex, normally presumed to be the area responsible for motor preparation of these gestures. This sequence was reversed in stutterers.

Walla, Mayer, Deecke, and Thurner (2004) conducted a MEG study that contrasted recordings

[24]Very recent improvements in design, such as event-related and interleaved data acquisition techniques (see Zeffiro & Frymiare, 2006, for discussion), may overcome these limitations.

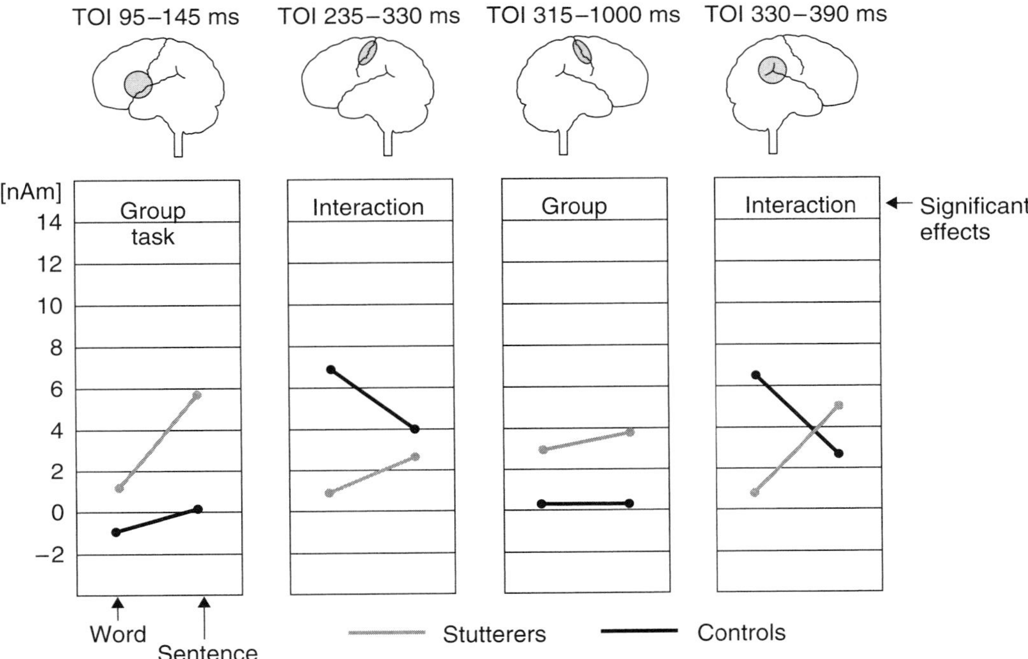

FIGURE 4-5 MEG profiles of stuttering and typically fluent adults from Biermann-Ruben, Salmelin, and Schnitzler (2005). Mean activation strengths [nAm] for ROI/TOIs (separate columns), tasks (word: left, sentence: right) and subjects (controls: black; stutterers: grey); only significant results of comparisons are shown. Effects (group, task, group-by-task interaction) are listed at the top of each box. Adapted from Bjermann-Rebuen, Salmelin, and Schnitzler, 2005.

derived under three different word reading conditions: silent reading of words, spoken reading of words, and delayed word production cued 1.3 seconds after written word presentation. The most marked differences between stutterers and normally fluent speakers was seen in the second condition, where typical speakers showed evidence of neural activity prior to speech production. The authors interpreted this signal as evidence of focused verbal anticipation. Only nonstutterers showed clear neural activity before speech onset, in a pattern linked to visual word presentation and thought to reflect focused verbal anticipation. The authors speculated that stuttering might result from impaired focused attention or anticipation during verbal tasks.

Biermann-Ruben, Salmelin, and Schnitzler (2005) recorded MEG data from 10 pairs of male stuttering adults and typical peers. There were three tasks: listening to pure tones, repeating words, and either repeating sentences or transforming active sentences into passives. While there were no differences in the simple tone perception condition, differences were observed in the other tasks, both in terms of lateralization, amount, and timing. Interestingly, areas normally associated with speech production were activated even when participants were listening to stimuli, and differences between the groups were apparent even when speaking was not required. Some results of this study are illustrated in Figure 4-5.

PLASTICITY AND CHANGE FOLLOWING THERAPY

One might reasonably question whether any of the differences we have discussed thus far are the cause or result of stuttering. Answers to this question are not quite straightforward, insofar as virtually all of the imaging techniques that have been used to date cannot be utilized with children of the typical age when stuttering first presents (usually, as we have noted, somewhere in the range between 2 and 4 years of age). This problem is not merely one of human subjects' approval, which places a much higher burden on justifying the use of these paradigms with children. The fact is that the typical toddler could not perform the tasks required to make the imaging results interpretable.

In the absence of knowing whether observed atypicalities precede or follow the onset of stuttering symptoms, another reasonable question is to ask whether they are responsive to therapeutic intervention that results in out-of-clinic fluency improvement. Such studies are now emerging, and they suggest that some differences disappear when stutterers achieve greater control over fluent speech production.

The first such study to examine differences between pre- and post-therapy imaging results was conducted by De Nil, Kroll, Lafaille, and Houle (2003). The researchers first PET-scanned 13 male adult stutterers and 10 matched comparison speakers. During baseline tasks, participants were scanned at rest, during silent single-word reading, and during oral reading of an equivalent word list. Stutterers then participated in a version of the Precision Fluency Shaping Therapy Program (Webster, 1974). Their average conversational stuttering rate declined from approximately 7 percent stuttered words to 1.6 percent immediately following therapy, although some gains were lost one year later.

Prior to therapy, stutterers' PET scans showed cortical activity that was much elevated when compared to the nonstuttering participants. In particular, areas of over-activation included the inferior frontal gyrus, precentral gyrus, and cerebellum, both areas that the researchers noted are involved in speech motor control. Most of this over-activation was right lateralized. In addition, researchers noted significant left activation in the anterior cingulate and in the right superior temporal gyrus. They speculated that activation in these areas reflected attention and auditory processing. Immediately following therapy, levels of activation decreased and became more lateralized to the left hemisphere. Previously bilateral activation in the inferior frontal cortex was replaced by a unilateral left activation. Activation in the precentral gyrus progressively moved from a right-hemisphere lateralization pattern to one that was bilateral following therapy and left-lateralized after one year. Thus, at one-year follow-up, brain activation during speech tasks was more similar to that of typically fluent speakers.

Neumann et al. (2005) conducted a similar study, using fMRI technology. Nine adult stutterers were scanned while reading sentences before and 12 weeks after participating in fluency shaping therapy. Following therapy, higher levels of activation were seen in the frontal and temporal areas of both hemispheres, and became more left-lateralized. The researchers were intrigued to observe that some post-therapy activation increases were in areas previously identified by M. Sommer et al. (2002; see discussion in the next portion of this chapter) as anatomically underdeveloped (see Figure 4-6). To

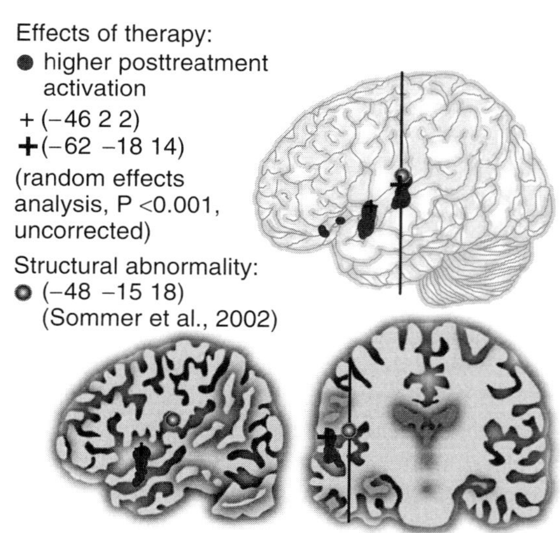

FIGURE 4-6 Left hemispheric increase of activation (random effects analysis at $p < 0.001$, uncorrected) after therapy (dark blotches). Some of them are located in the direct vicinity of the recently detected structural abnormality (light point). Vertical lines indicate the respective positions of the depicted coronal and sagittal slice. Adapted from Neumann et al., 2005.

the authors, this suggested that fluency therapy might reorganize connections for speech-language production within the left hemisphere and reduce compensatory activity of the right hemisphere.

Stager, Jeffries, and Braun (2003) took a slightly different approach to this question, asking if there were common functional imaging indices that distinguished fluency-enhancing tasks such as paced or sung speech from typical conversational performance. Higher activation during fluency-enhancing tasks were noted for both auditory processing areas and those motor regions associated with oral-motor and laryngeal movement, although they were seen in normally fluent speakers as well, suggesting it is the tasks, rather than anything unique to stuttering, that produces such activations. However, the researchers suggested that better coordination of auditory and speech-motor areas is required to produce more fluent speech.

Morphological (Anatomical) Differences

The first evidence of potential neuroanatomic differences between stutterers and typically fluent speakers was obtained by Foundas et al. (2001). These authors studied 16 pairs of participants, matched for age, gender, handedness, and general level of education, using three-dimensional magnetic resonance imaging (MRI). Planum temporale differences were noted, with atypical asymmetry of left- and right-hemisphere planum areas; left asymmetry is more typical in normal speakers. There were also differences within the perisylvian fissure region. In particular, gyrification was atypical, which might have consequences for connectivity among brain regions. In a follow-up study, Foundas, Corey, et al. (2003) examined behavioral correlates of these neuroanatomical findings. Stuttering severity was not associated with specific anatomic configurations, whereas the relatively lower language assessment results within the group of adults who stutter were associated with reduced volume in the prefrontal and occipital regions. Most recently, Foundas, Bollich, et al. (2004) examined 14 pairs of stuttering and fluent adults. A subset of the stutterers showed the atypical asymmetry reported on in their earlier work, while others did not. Stuttering severity was higher for the first group, and, in an experimental manipulation, these stutterers were more fluent under delayed auditory feedback (DAF, see Chapter 11), while those with more typical brain anatomy did not appear to benefit from the altered feedback. The authors speculated that atypical brain architecture might predispose certain speakers to stuttering, but also identified specific treatment options more appropriate for them than other stutterers.

Sommer, Koch, Paulus, Weiller, and Büchel (2002) utilized diffusion tensor imaging (DTI) and found differences in volume of gray and white matter in the area of the Rolandic operculum (see Figure 4-7). This area is close to the portion of the motor strip that controls oral tract function, as well as the arcuate fasciculus (which links Broca's and Wernicke's areas in speech production and perception processing). The authors speculated that the anatomical differences could lead to disturbed signal transmission and thus diminished sensorimotor integration during speech production. They further hypothesized that functional imaging aberrations seen in stutterers might reflect right-hemisphere compensation for this underlying structural deficit.[25]

Jäncke, Hänggi, and Steinmetz (2004) have confirmed and broadened the search for neuroanatomical markers of stuttering. They studied 10 pairs of stuttering and fluent adults matched for age, handedness, and educational history using high-resolution MRI scans. They found comparatively increased volume of white matter in the right-hemispheric structures that include the superior temporal gyrus (including the planum temporale, implicated in earlier studies), the inferior frontal gyrus (including the pars triangularis), the precentral gyrus near areas responsible for facial and mouth movement representation, and the anterior middle frontal gyrus. In addition, nonstutterers had greater white matter asymmetry favoring the left auditory cortex, while stutterers showed more symmetry in

[25]The authors have also written a concise summary of past and present research into the nature of stuttering posted to the recently developed Public Library of Science (PLoS), a free-access Internet repository for scholarly, peer-reviewed scientific work. It may be viewed at *http://biology.plosjournals.org* by searching the keyword "stutter."

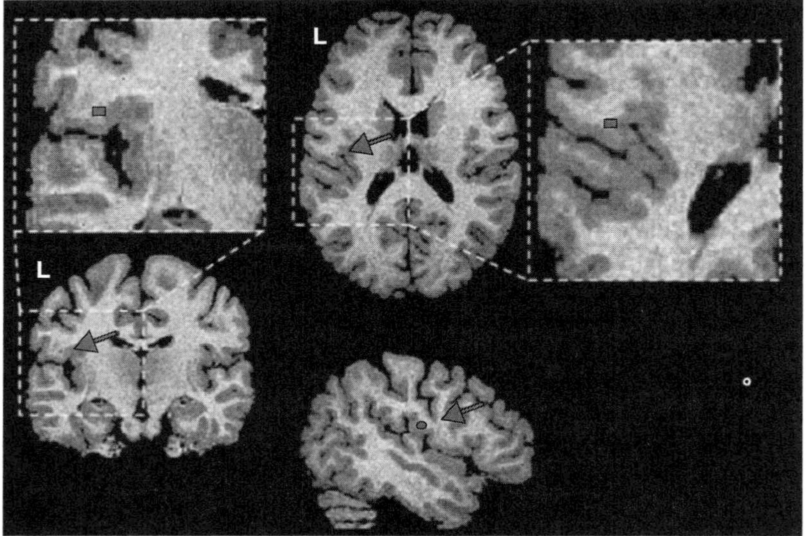

FIGURE 4-7 Diffuse tensor imaging (DTI) findings of decreased fiber coherence in the Rolandic operculum in adults who stutter. "Disconnection of speech-relevant brain areas in persistent developmental stuttering." *The Lancet*, Volume 360, Issue 9330, Pages 380–83. M. Sommer, M. Koch, W. Paulus, C. Weiller, C. Büchel.

left and right auditory cortices. The authors concluded that anatomical differences between stuttering and fluent speakers are more widespread than had been reported previously. However, whether anatomical differences cause stuttering or develop over the speaker's lifetime after stuttering onset cannot as yet be determined.[26]

PREVALENCE OF STUTTERING IN PERSONS WITH BRAIN DAMAGE

The persistent suspicion of brain abnormality among stutterers, whether or not well-founded, has received some strength from scattered reports that stuttering tends to be highly prevalent in populations with known neuropathology.

In a state hospital for persons with epilepsy, Gens (1950) identified 4.5 percent who stuttered among 1,047 patients with speech. This is at least four times the usual prevalence. Harrison (1947), in a more unusual report, stated that stuttering was 36 times as frequent among 60 institutionalized persons with epilepsy as in the general population.

Many who work with children who have cerebral palsy have the impression that stuttering is common in this group, but data on the subject are scarce. Rutherford (1938), in her description of 54 selected children with cerebral palsy and speech impairments, noted that 24 percent of them were stutterers, and this certainly suggests the possibility of an exceptional incidence. Heltman and Peacher (1943) found stuttering in 3.9 percent of a group of 102 individuals with cerebral palsy. Ingram (cited by Andrews and Harris, 1964, p. 7) reported a prevalence of stuttering of 15 percent in a survey of children with cerebral diplegia.

As we will see in Chapter 6, stuttering appears to have a very high incidence among persons with intellectual impairments, generally, whether brain-injured or not. Schlanger and Gottsleben (1957), however, found that in an institution for individuals

[26]The possibility that anatomical differences may be present relatively early in life is suggested by work in progress as this edition goes to press by Chang, Erickson & Ambrose (2005) and Chang, Erickson, Ambrose, Hasegawa-Johnson, & Ludlow (2006).

with intellectual deficiency 18 percent of those with organic etiologies stuttered as compared with 10 percent who had a record of familial deficiency.

Goodall and Brobby (1982) found 5 stutterers among 10 West African patients with sickle cells. They speculated that stuttering in West Africa may be caused by "minimal brain damage resulting from cerebral malaria modified by sickling".

Böhme (1968) found a prevalence of stuttering of 19.3 percent among 802 children and adults with brain damage dating from birth or early childhood. Diagnoses of brain damage were made on the basis of electroencephalograms, observation of fine motor function, general neuropsychiatric examination, and other tests. The majority of the group had intellectual impairment. Among the 313 cases with normal intelligence 24 percent stuttered. More recently, Table 4-5 Alm and Risberg (2007) found a subgroup of 17 out of their 32 adult stutterers who had experienced pre-onset neurological insults of a variety of types.

ACQUIRED STUTTERING

There is now an accumulating literature that reports acquired stuttering or stutter-like disfluency following brain injury or degenerative neurological conditions. Acquired or neurogenic stuttering is a relatively uncommon phenomenon having sudden onset in adulthood.

Causes of Acquired Stuttering

Although adults have been reported to acquire stuttering as a result of combat fatigue or other types of emotional stress,[27] adult-onset stuttering is generally a symptom of brain injury. Sometimes also known as cortical stuttering,[28] it may be transient or persistent. It has been observed in cases of traumatic head injury, stroke, degenerative diseases of the central nervous system, brain tumor, brain surgery, and drug-induced brain dysfunction. The frontal, parietal, or temporal lobes may be involved. The damage or lesion is usually reported to be in the left hemisphere of the brain, but sometimes in the right in right-handed individuals. Neurogenic stuttering is often associated with aphasia, apraxia of speech, or dysarthria, but may occur in the absence of any other speech or language difficulties. The majority of cases reported have been male.

The advent of modern neuroimaging techniques has permitted documentation of the wide variety of brain lesions that have been associated with more recent reports of acquired stuttering. We summarize some of these findings in Table 4-5. Further, while stuttering is the major complaint in some of these case reports, in others, the fluency disturbance is part of a much wider array of impairments in cognitive or motor domains.

Fluency Symptoms

In most instances, the fluency-related symptoms of neurogenic stuttering are described as repetitions or prolongations of initial sounds, syllables, or words without effort, secondary symptoms, or signs of anxiety. However, exceptions to this description are not uncommon. Pauses, hesitations, and "blocks" are sometimes said to occur.

In a case described by Baratz and Mesulam (1981) stuttering was accompanied by grimacing, and Rosenbek et al. (1978) cited three cases in which signs of effort, hurry, grimacing, and eye-blinking were evident. Koller (1983) noted mild

[27] See Peacher and Harris (1946), Dempsey and Granich (1978), Deal (1982), Roth, Aronson, and Davis (1989), Tippett and Siebens (1991), Mahr and Leith (1992).

[28] In addition to the cases shown in Table 4-4, past reports have included: Schiller (1947), Arend, Handzel, and Weiss (1962), Shtremel (1963), Canter (1971), Caplan (1972), Rosenfield (1972), Helm and Butler (1977), Quinn and Andrews (1977), Helm, Butler, and Benson (1978), Rosenbek, Messert, Collins, and Wertz (1978), Donnan (1979), Inglis (1979), Helm, Butler, and Canter (1980), Rosenfield, Miller, and Feltovich (1980), Baratz and Mesulam (1981), Mazzucchi, Moretti, Carpeggiani, Parma, and Paini (1981), Homer and Massey (1983), Koller (1983), Lebrun, Leleux, Rousseau, and Devreauz (1983), Lebrun, Rétif, and Kaiser (1983), Rentschler, Driver, and Callaway (1984), Lebrun and Leleux (1985), McClean and McLean (1985), Ardila and Lopez (1986), Nagafuchi and Saso (1986), Rousey, Arjunan, and Rousey (1986), Marshall and Neuburger (1987), Nowack and Stone (1987), Lebrun, Bijleveld, and Rousseau (1990), Market, Montague, Buffalo, and Drummond (1990), Meyers, Hall, and Aram (1990), Rosenfield, Viswanath, Callis-Landrum, Di Danato, and Nudelman (1991).

TABLE 4-5 Recent Cases of Neurogenic/Acquired Stuttering: Causes and Features

	Subjects	Site of lesion	Notes on symptoms
Aram, Meyers, and Ekelman (1990)	20 children with unilateral left hemisphere lesions and 13 with right lesions, compared to normally developing peers	NA	Left- and right-lesioned children provided quantitatively more and qualitatively different patterns of nonfluencies than their neurologically normal peers.
Heuer and Sataloff (1996)	Case 1: 40-year-old woman diagnosed with Moya Moya disease	Case 1: MRI showed abnormal patterns in the periventricular white matter of the frontal lobes bilaterally as well as within the left thalamus and right caudate nucleus.	Case 1: Difficulty walking, leg pain, cerebellar symptoms, severe stuttering (prolongations of all consonants and occasional sound repetitions), strained voice.
	Case 2: 53-year-old man with CVA; after one year, symptoms worsened	Case 2: By MRI, increased signal intensity to the left putamen bordering on the internal capsule: virtually the entire region of the left caudate. After one year, additionally, hypoplasia of the right anterior cerebral artery.	Case 2: Broca's aphasia, stuttering (blocks, part-word repetitions, sound repetitions, and frequent use of fillers), and right-sided weakness.
	Case 3: 55-year-old left-handed male with history of two CVAs, followed by an epileptic seizure, who later developed a glioblastoma	Case 3: Mass (glioblastoma) involving the left thalamus and medial and lateral aspects of the tip of the left temporal lobe.	Case 3: Stuttering resolved after two strokes and reappeared after the glioblastoma.
Van Borsel, Van Lierde, Van Cauwenberge, Guldemont, and Van Orshoven (1998)	69-year-old right-handed male with no history of speech or language deficits	Left supplementary motor region	Severe acquired stuttering; disfluencies were not restricted to the initial word position.
Ciabarra, Elkind, Roberts and Marshall (2000)[a]	Case study of three patients with subcortical lesions Case 1: 53-year-old right-handed male	Case 1: Left rostromedial pons, consistent with a small vessel infarction	Case 1: Episodic vertigo, ataxia, left internuclear opthalmoplegia, dysarthria, left facial droop, jaw tremor, right dysmetria, and stuttering. Speech was characterized by repetition of every syllable with intermittent aphonia.
	Case 2: 54-year-old right-handed female	Case 2: Infarction of the left putamen extending to the caudate and corona radiata	Case 2: Initial prolongations of consonants and occasional repetitions of initial syllables. Also mild right facial droop and slowness of right finger movements.

	Case 3: 63-year-old left-handed female	Case 3: Small subcortical infarct in the left corona radiata and a small left lateral putamen and subinsular infarct	Case 3: Change in vision, right-handed weakness, and word finding difficulty. Stuttering consisted of repetition of the initial syllable with occasional initial prolongations.
Franco, Casado, López Domínguez, Díaz, Blanco, and Robledo (2000)	53-year-old right-handed male	Cortical infarct on the left pre-central circumvolution	No aphasia or neurological deficits; stuttering was the only symptom and was characterized by blocks, repetitions on the first syllable of words, and improvement on automatic tasks.
Turgut, Utku, and Balci (2002)	61-year-old right handed male	Left parietal cortex	Acute right-sided weakness onset and speech disturbances for 2 days. Stuttering was described as severe, characterized by multiple monosyllabic repetitions, and blocks mainly on initial syllables. No adaptation effect noted. Language appeared normal.
Doi, Nakayasu, Soda, Shimoda, Ito, and Nakashima (2003)[b]	60-year-old male with a brainstem infarct	By MRI, lesions in the midbrain, paramedian area, and upper pons	Acute onset of vertigo, truncal and limb ataxia, paralytic pontine exotropia, dysarthria, and stuttered speech characterized by repetitions of initial syllables and occasional final syllables; no repetition of words or phrases was observed. No aphasia observed.
Van Borsel, Van Der Made, and Santens (2003)[c]	38-year-old right-handed male with no history of speech or language problems presenting with neurogenic stuttering following an ischemic lesion	Left thalamus	Stuttered severely in propositional speech but only slightly in non-propositional speech.
Balasubramanian, Max, Van Borsel, Rayca, and Richardson (2003)	57-year-old male with an ischemic lesion	Orbital surface of the right frontal lobe and the pons	No adaptation response or fluency improvement under choral, DAF, and FAF conditions.
Hamano, Hiraki, Kawamura, Hirayama, Mutoh, and Kuriyama (2005)	77-year-old right-handed female	Lesion in the corpus callosum and deep white matter	Dizziness, nausea, and speech disturbances. Speech characterized by initial syllable repetitions; adaptation effect present, but no decrease in stuttering while singing.

(continues)

TABLE 4-5 *(continued)*

	Subjects	Site of lesion	Notes on symptoms
Sahin, Krespi, Yilmaz, and Coban (2005)	Case 1: 65-year-old right-handed female Case 2: 85-year-old right-handed male Both admitted with sudden onset of speech disturbance and right-sided weakness	Case 1: Small cortical infarct in the left parietal lobe Case 2: Cortical infarct in the left posterior parietal lobe Both cases involved the supramarginal gyrus (Broadmann Area 40)	Both patients presented initially with neurogenic stuttering; however, symptoms eventually resolved. Other symptoms included right hemiparesis and right facial palsy at onset.
Yeoh, Lind, and Law (2005)	12-year-old boy with a closed head injury after falling from his skateboard	Normal CT scan	Headache, stuttering speech, and truncal and bilateral peripheral cerebellar dysfunction. All symptoms resolved within 24 hours.
Osawa, Maeshima, and Yoshimura (2006)	51-year-old right-handed male	Posterior part of the left temporal lobe to the parieto-occipital lobe	Wernicke's aphasia and acquired stuttering.
Tanaka, Nishida, Hayashi, Inzuka, and Otsuki (2006)	54-year-old right-handed woman with no history of stuttering	MRI revealed atypicalities in the right cerebellar peduncle, right temporal lobe, left occipital lobe, and corpus callosum	Diagnosed with acute disseminated encephalomyelitis. Symptoms included acquired stuttering, consciousness disturbance; later interview showed pure alexia without color naming defects, continuation of stuttering, and one-way disturbances of somesthetic transfer from the left hand to the right.

[a] Internuclear opthalmoplegia—disorder of conjugate lateral gaze causing an impairment in adduction.
[b] Paralytic pontine exotropia is an eye movement disorder.
[c] Propositional speech included conversation, monologue, confrontation naming, and word retrieval. Non-propositional speech included automatic speech sound, word and sentence repetition, and reading aloud.

annoyance or frustration as reactions to stuttering in three of six patients, though none had the ability that most stutterers possess to predict the occurrence of their blocks.

There is frequent mention of more stuttering on function words than on content words. In contrast, developmental stuttering occurs more often on content words (see Chapter 12), although difficulty on function words does occur and is very common in its early forms. Canter (1971), however, heard repetitions and prolongations on the final consonants of words in most of his cases of neurogenic stuttering—an observation rarely noted in ordinary stuttering. This was not so in any of the seven cases of Rosenbek et al. (1978), but in the single case described by Lebrun and Leleux (1985), a few repetitions occurred "in medial or final positions," and Ardila and Lopez (1986) noted repetitions in final positions in their case. In eight cases described by Rosenfield, Viswanath, Callis-Landrun, Di Danato, and Nudelman (1991), all were said to stutter on sounds in all positions in words, including final sounds.

Canter (1971) suggested, on the basis of his clinical observations, that disfluency that failed to diminish in frequency with repeated readings of the same passage (adaptation; see Chapter 11) was one of the features by which neurogenic stuttering could be differentiated from developmental stuttering. In confirmation, others have reported the absence of an adaptation effect.[29] The adaptation effect was evident, however, in the 16 cases studied by Mazzucchi et al. (1981) and in the 6 reported by Koller (1983). One of the two neurogenic stutterers presented by Quinn and Andrews (1977) exhibited both adaptation and the consistency effect. The five cases reported by Caplan (1972) adapted in repeated answers to questions, but not while reading sentences. From a questionnaire survey of 81 cases, Market, Montague, Buffalo, and Drummond (1990) concluded that about 46 percent did not exhibit the adaptation effect.

[29] Helm and Butler (1977), Helm, Butler, and Benson (1978), Ardila and Lopez (1986), Nagafuchi and Saso (1986), Nowack and Stone (1987), Rosenfield, Viswanath, Callis-Landrum, Di Danato, and Nudelman (1991).

We note that, in the case of typical developmental stuttering, individuals who do not show the adaptation effect are not uncommon, nor are those who fail to exhibit secondary symptoms or clear signs of anxiety. Very rare, however, is the person who stutters when singing, speaking in time to rhythm, speaking at a reduced rate, or when subjected to various other fluency-inducing conditions (see Chapters 10 and 11). Rosenfield (1972) reported on a patient with neurogenic stuttering whose speech difficulty did not decrease in singing or while speaking rhythmically or in unison with another person. Of the two cases described in detail by Quinn and Andrews (1977), one showed improvement with masking noise, delayed auditory feedback, and the use of a slow speaking rate, but the other did not. The patient cited by Helm and Butler (1977) stuttered more rather than less when speaking syllable by syllable with the aid of a pacing board. Koller (1983) mentioned two individuals with neurogenic stuttering who stuttered when singing. In contrast, Horner and Massey (1983) described a 62-year-old stroke patient who sang without stuttering. However, the authors preferred a diagnosis of palilalia, rather than neurogenic stuttering, for this patient inasmuch as his speech pattern was dominated by rapid rate, monotony, and more word and phrase than sound or syllable repetitions. A further counterexample was a 42-year-old man who began to stutter after being put on Dilantin for the control of seizures due to an accidental head injury (McClean & McLean, 1985); his stuttering was reduced in unison reading and when speaking at a decreased rate under delayed auditory feedback. However, the stroke patient cited by Ardila and Lopez (1986) stuttered in unison reading and metronome-timed speech. One of the two patients described by Nowack and Stone (1987) stuttered when whispering. And most of the eight patients reported by Rosenfield, Viswanath, Callis-Landrun, Di Danato, and Nudelman (1991) stuttered when singing, speaking at a slow rate, and speaking in masking noise.

A recent comprehensive discussion of the extant literature on adult-onset neurogenic stuttering is provided by De Nil, Rochon, and Jokel (2007). Consistent with the reports in this section, they also note that acquired or neurogenic stuttering has been associated with lesions in many different parts of the brain as well as some neurodegenerative conditions.

In sum, it has become increasingly clear that the stuttering seen in individuals with brain damage has features that distinguish it from the developmental variety of stuttering. Thus, the contributions of neurogenic stuttering to our understanding of the nature or cause of developmental stuttering are not yet clear.

An additional global caution in interpreting this literature is whether or not studies of such impaired populations define stuttering as we conventionally do in this book. Recent work that has examined children with language impairments (Boscolo, Bernstein Ratner, & Rescorla, 2002; Hall, 1999; Hall, Yamashita, & Aram, 1993; see review in Bernstein Ratner, 2005c) suggests that such children demonstrate atypically numerous stutter-like disfluencies in their speech, such as part- and whole-word repetitions, prolongations, revisions, and even subtle block-like behaviors. However, they lack the awareness and struggle characteristic of true stuttering. In considering the literature on stuttering in any number of exceptional conditions, including stuttering that appears to emerge after brain damage, we must consider the possibility that the disfluencies that have been documented bear a resemblance to stuttering, especially for doctors or educators relatively unfamiliar with stuttering, but are not fully consistent with the disorder as we discuss it in this book.

INTERPRETATION OF ERP AND BRAIN IMAGING STUDIES

What should we conclude from the recent and lively investigations that have capitalized on successively newer methods of "seeing inside the brain" of the person who stutters? (De Nil, 2004; Ingham, 2001, 2003, 2004). While numerous differences have been observed between the brain activation patterns of adults who stutter and fluent comparison speakers, their interpretation is not at all straightforward. Different areas appear to show under- and over-activation across different studies. Whether differences that are seen represent the underlying problem that leads to stuttering or reflect the speakers' attempts to compensate for the deficit is also as yet unclear.

It is also important to note that ERP and brain imaging studies differ from previous attempts to locate the "source" of stuttering in brain function not only in the use of more sophisticated techniques, but in the types of tasks employed with participants during study. Most, but not all, such studies are done while participants listen to or produce language, which makes their findings relevant not only to this chapter, but to our discussions of potential psycholinguistic differences between people who do and do not stutter, as we examine in Chapter 8. Thus, as in many other parts of this text, we will discover that it is increasingly difficult to "compartmentalize" our research questions and findings into simple dichotomies such as contrasting linguistic vs. motor systems, brain anatomy vs. brain physiology, or even basic questions of nature vs. nurture/experience. Some of the more recent models of stuttering that we discuss in Chapter 2 are now careful to specify such multifactorial and dynamic interactions in attempts to explain the cause and development of the disorder.

SUMMARY REMARKS

Left-handedness and reversal of manual dexterity had been associated with stuttering by scattered observations since the early years of the twentieth century. In the late 1920s, an additional emphasis on ambidexterity arose as a result of the Orton-Travis theory, and a very large amount of research was subsequently done on both the peripheral handedness of stutterers and supposed indicators of "native" laterality. By the 1940s, good evidence had accumulated that stutterers did not differ from nonstutterers in their handedness. This conclusion has been confirmed by such later research as has been done, for example, by Johnson and Associates (1959, p. 84), Andrews and Harris (1964, p. 100), and Records, Heimbuch, and Kidd (1977).

As for the inference that a change of handedness may cause a child to stutter, the fact that in the end no unusual tendency toward native left-handedness seemed to characterize stutterers may indirectly cast some doubt on it. The practice of forcing left-handed children to write with the right hand has not been favored in schools for many years. With its demise, the opportunity to study its effects on speech is gone, although there is no evidence that stuttering rates have declined since the practice was discontinued. In the vast majority of cases, it has clearly never been an important etiological factor. That it was once thought capable of contributing significantly to the etiology of stuttering may ultimately go down as one of the curious superstitions of our time.

In recent years, interest in research on the lateral dominance of stutterers has been revived by the increasingly broader availability of tests of cerebral dominance for language and speech processing. On the intracarotid sodium amytal (Wada) test, a total of six typical stutterers have shown normal lateralization of speech and language functions The results of a large number of dichotic listening tests have been conflicting, although there is compelling evidence that when meaningful stimuli are used in place of nonsense syllables, many stutterers show less right-ear advantage than nonstutterers. A few tachistoscopic studies have found that at least some stutterers differ from most nonstutterers in preferring the left half of the visual field in processing visual verbal stimuli.

A very large number of electrophysiological studies suggest evidence of atypical right-hemisphere processing of speech by stutterers, as well as slowed and reduced electrophysiological responses. Moreover, there is now an accumulating body of evidence obtained in brain imaging studies to suggest that processing of speech and language is somewhat atypical in adults who stutter, although relatively few consistent patterns of activity have been found from study to study. Atypicality is seen whether or not the stutterers are required to produce speech or language responses or merely listen to stimuli. The general pattern appears to be relative over-activation of cortical areas, as well as more bilateral or reversed hemispheric activity. Whether these patterns are a consequence of or adaptation to stuttering, or reflect the underlying basis of the disorder is as yet unclear, although in some cases, over-activation has been observed to be greater in more fluent stutterers, suggesting that it reflects compensation for some as yet unknown underlying deficit. Studies of children will certainly add to our ability to interpret existing studies.

Finally, most recently, a few studies have begun to identify subtle morphological (structural) differences in brain composition between fluent and stuttering adults. These findings make it more likely, although far from certain, that the functional differences seen in brain imaging may reflect preexisting limitations on speech-language and/or speech-motor function that lead to stuttering, rather than reflecting broadly compensatory or adaptive responses to it. The most certain statement that we can make is that there will be much more research in this topic area in the years to come.

Chapter 5

The Person Who Stutters: Motor Abilities

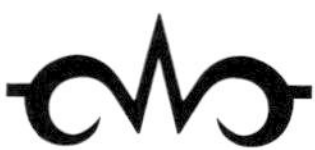

GROSS AND FINE MOTOR COORDINATION

It is not surprising that a number of early researchers sought to explain stuttering by reference to aspects of motor function and coordination. In the earliest work to examine motor coordination in people who stutter, Arps (cited by Strother & Kriegman, 1943) found stutterers to be poorer than nonstutterers in gymnastic exercises involving rhythm and coordination, and Kiehn (1935) reported slightly poorer performance in a test requiring subjects to carry a full glass of water. Bilto (1941) carried out a more detailed investigation of a group of stutterers using several standardized tests of motor ability concerned with bodily strength, agility, balance, and control. Although his stutterers tended to perform slightly below the test norms, on the average, the disparities were so small that it is difficult, for the most part, to rule out the possibility that they were due to chance factors operating in the selection of participants. Furthermore, the stutterers did as well, on the whole, as a group of children with articulation disorders to whom the same tests were given.

In view of Bilto's observations, the findings reported by Helene Kopp (1946) were rather unexpected. Kopp administered the *Oseretsky Tests of Motor Proficiency* to a group of 50 stuttering children and discovered that, on the basis of test norms, all but three of the subjects were delayed in motor development by amounts ranging from 2 to 9 years; 46 percent performed more than five years below their age levels. The *Oseretsky Tests*, standardized on 5,000 Russian children in the early 1920s, is an instrument of broad scope, with stress on general physical activities requiring coordination, balance, and speed. Kopp concluded that her findings revealed a "marked disturbance of the motor function" in stutterers. Like so many other investigations of stuttering that made use of standardized tests, however, this study did not employ a comparison group. The omission was particularly serious in this case, because the *Oseretsky Tests* as then formulated often allowed considerable latitude to the examiner's discretion in both the administration and scoring of items. Finkelstein and Weisberger (1954) administered the tests to 15 stuttering children and a comparison group of 15 nonstutterers matched for age, sex, and laterality. They found no statistically significant differences between the two groups. However, comparison with the test norms showed an average delay of three and a half months for the stutterers.

Further work using the *Oseretsky-Gollnitz Tests* with German children was reported by Schilling and Kruger (1960). They found that 100 stutterers performed more poorly than 100 typically fluent children, but better than 100 children with articulation disorders. For example, 18 percent of the stutterers, 5 percent of the typically developing children, and 41 percent of the children with articulation difficulties were classified as "severely retarded" in motor development.

The findings on gross physical abilities are conflicting. While we have not had conclusive evidence that differences between stutterers and nonstutterers exist, the possibility has not been ruled out.

Manual Skills

Investigations of stutterers' manual abilities have concerned themselves with strength, steadiness, speed and regularity of repetitive movement, hand-eye coordination, and various types of psychomotor serial discrimination tasks (see Table 5-1).

Individuals who stutter seem relatively normal in manual strength, regularity, and accuracy in reproducing rhythmical patterns. Several other areas of research, however, have produced conflicting results. In particular, some researchers found stutterers to perform slightly more poorly in tests of manual diadochokinesis (chiefly rapid finger tapping), in tests of hand-eye coordination as in accurate aiming or tracing, and in serial discrimination tasks as in rapid sorting of cards into slots. In other studies of essentially the same abilities, no differences were found. We will discuss reaction time studies later in this chapter. In reaction time, some differences have been noted.

Findings as inconclusive as these leave us with considerable freedom to speculate that stutterers tend to have a mild neuromuscular disorder, or to conclude that no atypical function has yet to be identified. We might also infer, as did Hill (1944b) and Rotter (1955), that stutterers may exhibit some motor evidence of anxiety. We might view the last as suggesting that any atypical performance reflects the speaker's adaptation to stuttering and responses to it under conditions of demand.

Perseveration As a result of Eisenson's perseverative theory of stuttering (see Chapter 2), some interest developed in the stutterer's proficiency at making rapid shifts in motor set. This kind of ability is usually tested by first giving the subject practice in each of two motor tasks independently—for example, the writing of AAAA, followed by BBBB, then observing the number of errors the participant makes when instructed to alternate the tasks, as in writing ABAB. It was in a variation of this task taken from the *Mahler-Elkin Attention Test* that Eisenson and Pastel (1936) first noted excessive perseverative behavior in a group of adult stutterers. Eisenson hypothesized that there was a constitutional tendency to perseverate in a substantial proportion of stutterers. King (1961) found distinct corroboration of Eisenson's earlier observations in giving a series of such alternating-activity tests to adult stutterers, but was inclined to believe that this could be adequately explained as the effect of greater anxiety-tension on the part of the stutterers. Some support may be lent to this interpretation by the fact that Martin (1962) was able to find no differences in the performance of such tasks when he administered them to stuttering and nonstuttering children. Samson and Cooper (1980) replicated King's study with adult speakers and also found no differences between stutterers and normal speakers.

TABLE 5-1 Studies of Manual Abilities of Stutterers and Nonstutterers Classified with Regard to Whether the Stutterers Were Found to Be of Poorer (Positive Outcome) or Equal (Negative Outcome) Ability

	Outcome	
Manual ability	**Positive***	**Negative**
Strength		McDowell (1928) Westphal (1933)
Steadiness	Kiehn (1935) Snyder (1968)	Westphal (1933) Jones, White, Lawson, and Anderson (2002)
Speed of repetitive movement	West and Nusbaum (1929) Cross (1936) Snyder (1958) Borden (1983) Doyton et al. (1998) Max, Caruso, and Gracco (2003) Smits-Bandstra, De Nil, and Saint-Cyr (2006)	Strother and Kriegman (1943) Chworowsky (1952) Rotter (1955)
Regularity of repetitive movement	Seth (1958) Cooper and Allen (1977)	Blackburn (1931)
Accuracy of reproduction of temporal patterns	Zaleski (1965)	Wulff (1935), Cross (1936), Strother and Kriegman (1943) Max and Yudman (2003) Smits-Bandstra, De Nil, and Saint-Cyr (2006)
Hand–eye coordination	Bilto (1941) Carlson (1946) Snyder (1958)	Westphal (1933) Cross (1936)
Psychomotor serial discrimination	Bills (1934) Simon (1945) Rotter (1955)	Cross (1936) Lightfoot (1948) Ross (1955) Postma and Kolk (1991)

*Studies with more than one outcome for a given ability are classified as "positive" if any outcome was positive.

Complex and Dual-Task Performance More recent research on stutterers' manual skills has tended to emphasize relatively complex tasks. Williams and Bishop (1992) timed participants as they lifted a finger from one key to press another, then touched a box and pressed another key as rapidly as possible. Stutterers proved to be slower than both normal speakers and speakers with disordered articulation. Vaughn and Webster (1989) found that more stutterers than nonstutterers showed anomalies in the way they performed tasks that required synchronous movement of the two hands, such as threading a string through a needle's eye.

On the premise that stuttering might be due to an underlying difficulty in organizing sequential motor activities in general, Webster (1985, 1986b, 1989b) had adults tap with four fingers in various sequences. The stutterers did make more errors than the matched fluent speakers. Webster found the premise somewhat insufficient, however. He initiated a research program on the guiding hypothesis that stutterers' left-hemisphere mechanisms are especially subject to interference from an overactive right hemisphere. While participants tapped out sequential patterns with the fingers of one hand, they engaged in knob turning or button pressing with the other (Webster, 1986a, 1989a). True to the hypothesis, when participants tapped with the right hand, the concurrent activity with the left hand created more interference for the stutterers than for their typically fluent peers; when they tapped with the left hand, concurrent activity with the right affected both groups equally.

Forster and Webster (1991) carried out a critical test of the theory of an interfering right hemisphere. Participants engaged in sequential finger tapping as before, but in place of a concurrent activity with the other hand, they activated a pedal with a foot. According to the hypothesis, the stutterers should have shown more interference than the nonstutterers when using the contralateral foot, but no greater interference when using the ipsilateral foot. This did not prove to be the case. The groups did not differ, both showing more interference with the ipsilateral than the contralateral foot. Forster and Webster concluded that there may be a "generally greater susceptibility to interference of left-hemisphere mechanisms in stutterers from any ongoing neural activity regardless of hemisphere."

In an earlier study, Webster (1987) had obtained results that suggested that the interference might indeed be more general. The procedure of that study required participants to transcribe sequences of letters that were presented aurally faster than they could write them down, so that participants had to monitor and respond concurrently. Under those conditions, the stutterers made more errors than the nonstutterers. The result seemed to point to an interference effect that was present regardless of whether one or both hemispheres were involved. However, Webster questioned whether there was an interference effect at all. In a further study of letter transcription (Webster, 1990a), he therefore had participants listen to the letter sequence first and write down any that they could remember afterward. This did not result in any improvement of the stutterers' performance. The nature of the stutterers' letter transcription deficit—and of stuttering itself—remained obscure.[1]

In the past decade, relatively few studies have examined motor abilities in people who stutter other than speech-motor or oral-motor tasks. Zelaznik, Smith, Franz, and Ho (1997) utilized a bimanual movement task with 15 pairs of adults who were required to flex and extend index fingers in tandem with a metronome beat that was gradually increased. Stutterers paced as well as fluent adults, but their movements had less amplitude and peak velocity.

Visual-Motor Skills

Jones, White, Lawson, and Anderson (2002) found evidence of relatively poorer visual-motor function (including ballistic movement, steadiness, and ability to track) in 12 pairs of stuttering and typically fluent adults. Differences were found for reaction time, tracking accuracy, and dynamic visual perception. Stuttering severity was also correlated with reaction time and dynamic perception. The authors found their results to be compatible with evidence of an overactive dopamine system in people who stutter, a concept explored more fully in discussion of pharmacological treatments (Chapter 14).

SPEECH AND ORAL MOTOR ABILITY

Many researchers have considered the possibility that stuttering results from a deficit of some type that is unique to the neuromotor systems that support speech production (for recent discussion of this viewpoint, see Ludlow and Loucks, 2003). The question is perfectly reasonable, but it is a curious one in that there would appear to be no technically feasible means of answering it. If the deficit is unique to speech, we may fail to observe the relevant aspects of it by studying nonspeech activity. Nor can we do it by making observations during the occurrence of stuttering; researchers recognized

[1]There is some possibility that short-term memory (STM) limitations may play a role in such findings; subtle STM limitations have been found for verbal materials in individuals who stutter (see Chapter 8).

long ago that such observations may reflect the effort, arousal, and compensatory motor actions that result from stuttering if they are not merely observations of stuttering itself. Thus, a number of researchers have conducted investigations of the stutterer's perceptually "fluent" speech.[2]

THE "FLUENT" SPEECH OF STUTTERERS

Pursuing this line of research, investigators have become increasingly concerned about the possible existence of various types of abnormalities (be they acoustic or neurophysiological) in intervals of speech that are presumed to be free from stuttering. The studies that have resulted have differed somewhat in their purposes as well as in some of their basic assumptions.

Listener Perception of the Fluent Speech of People Who Stutter

A question that was immediately raised is whether listeners can distinguish the recorded speech of stutterers from that of nonstutterers if all identifiable instances of disfluency are removed. Wendahl and Cole (1961) reported that listeners could in fact do this, and that they judged stutterers' edited samples of oral reading to contain more force and strain and to be less normal in rate and rhythm than samples of nonstutterers' speech. In a replication of this study using a different type of analysis, however, Young (1964) found that listeners were not able to pick out the stuttering speakers reliably. Young also pointed out that the outcome of such research must depend to a large degree on such factors as the participants' stuttering severity and the experimenter's definition of disfluency. Such judgments may also depend upon the listener's experience in listening to the speech of people who stutter (Brundage, Bothe, Lengeling, & Evans, 2006).

Love and Jeffress (1971) used an electronic speech-pause counting device to study the occurrence of brief pauses in the oral reading of stutterers who were ostensibly fluent while reading aloud. The stutterers were discovered to have significantly more brief pauses in the 150- to 250-millisecond range than did a group of normally fluent speakers, although a trained listener was unable to differentiate the stutterers from the nonstutterers. A treatment shown to improve fluency, reduction of short phonation intervals, which is discussed in Chapter 14, prompted Godinho, Ingham, Davidow, and Cotton (2006) to see if such atypically short phonated segments (those less than 150 msec. in duration) were more typical in the speech of adults who stutter than typically fluent speakers. No difference in the relative frequency of such short segments was detected in a matched sample of 13 pairs of stutterers and nonstutterers.

Few and Lingwall (1972) obtained somewhat inconclusive results in a study of stutterers' 10-second spontaneous speech samples, all of which were judged to be fluent by three trained observers. There was a consistent tendency for people who stutter to be rated slower in speaking rate by listeners, to articulate more slowly in terms of number of phonemes per second, and to have more pause time than nonstutterers, but none of these differences reached statistical significance. Few and Lingwall also reported that listeners could not distinguish the stutterers' samples from those of the nonstutterers. Applying an alternative type of analysis of their data, however, Young (1984) showed that the listeners were able to make the differentiation to an extent exceeding chance.

Krikorian and Runyan (1983) used perceptually fluent samples of young children aged 4 to 6 years. They found that sophisticated judges did not correctly identify stutterers and nonstutterers often enough to rule out chance with confidence. Also working with young children aged 4 to 9 years, Colcord and Gregory (1987) found that listeners had considerable difficulty identifying children who stutter from those who had perceptually fluent

[2] However, these precautions are increasingly being recognized as potentially futile because, as Bloodstein (1981) and Armson and Kalinowski (1994) have pointed out, there is no way to be sure that unusual events recorded during these "fluent" utterances are not caused by the anticipation of stuttering or are not imperceptible stutterings themselves. How, then, are we to study the stutterer's motor speech control? It will be interesting to see if this dilemma can be resolved.

speech. By contrast, when the speech samples were produced by adolescents aged 12 to 16 years, judges discriminated well between stutterers and normally fluent speakers in most cases (Brown & Colcord, 1987).

Howell and Wingfield (1990) extracted perceptually fluent segments from the speech of stutterers. They found that listeners could reliably distinguish segments that were adjacent to stuttered words from those that were not. Spectrographic examination showed a decrease in rate and intensity in segments judged to be near stutterings.

Phonation during "Fluency"

As noted, the first few efforts to examine the fluent speech of people who stutter had been prompted by the question whether stuttering is confined to discrete "moments," as has commonly been assumed, or whether it is a broader abnormality in a person's way of speaking of which the discernible moments are only a part. In the mid-1970s, a somewhat different reason arose for conducting such investigations. As we have seen in Chapter 1, it became apparent that the laryngeal musculature functions abnormally during stuttering. Some researchers believed that this abnormal functioning might be the immediate cause of the stuttering block. If so, this possibility could be verified by observing the activity of the larynx during intervals of nonstuttered speech produced by people who stutter.

Raising the question whether the larynx is "responsible for the disfluencies observed in stuttering," Gautheron, Liorzou, Even, and Vallancien (1973) studied samples of the conversational speech of four stutterers by glottography. They came to the conclusion that people who stutter do not use the larynx correctly, even when not stuttering. In producing sequences such as "sha," in which a voiceless consonant is followed by a vowel, the stuttering speakers frequently appeared to preset the laryngeal musculature with so much tension that phonation was possible only with strong airflow; consequently, the transition to the vowel was often delayed and initiated with a glottal catch.

Voice Onset Time (VOT) in Fluent Speech

Voice onset time (VOT) is the time (typically measured in milliseconds) between a supra-laryngeal articulatory gesture and the onset of phonation. Differences in VOT are typically perceived categorically by a listener; however, subtle differences in VOT may indicate differences in control over the voicing process (Berko Gleason & Bernstein Ratner, 1998). In an early study, Shaffer (1940) found that the interval between initiation of jaw movement and phonation was longer for stutterers than for nonstutterers. Agnello (1975) reported that spectrograms of stutterers' fluent utterances of nonsense syllables such as /pa/ and /ap/ showed that they tend to take longer than nonstutterers in both initiating and terminating phonation.[3] This observation was confirmed by Hillman and Gilbert (1977), who found that, during what was perceived as fluent oral reading, stutterers' VOTs following voiceless stop consonants were on the average nine milliseconds longer than those of fluent peers.

Subsequent findings on VOT during stutterers' fluent speech have been conflicting. No differences between stutterers and nonstutterers were reported by Watson and Alfonso (1982), Borden, Baer, and Kenney (1985), Borden, Kim, and Spiegler (1987), and Jäncke (1994). In fluent utterances of single words, Janssen, Wieneke, and Vaane (1983) found that the time interval between voice onset and electromyographic activity in the articulatory muscles was the same for stutterers and nonstutterers. Metz, Conture, and Caruso (1979), observing longer VOTs for stutterers on about one-third of the sounds they studied, considered their findings equivocal. Healey and Gutkin (1984) studied fluent production of words and syllables beginning with stop consonants in people who do and do not stutter, and found that stutterers had longer VOTs than nonstutterers for voiced stops. Healey and Ramig (1986) found longer VOTs for stutterers and

[3] One offshoot of this finding—a long series of studies of voice initiation time (VIT)—has involved stutterers saying words, nonsense syllables, or simple phonated syllables such as /a/ as quickly as possible on signal. Almost without exception, the studies have agreed that stutterers on the average have longer voice initiation times than nonstutterers, even when no stuttering is perceived.

reported as a major result of their study that the difference was greater for utterances extracted from a reading passage than for a short nonsense phrase. All of these observations were made on adults.

Metz, Samar, and Sacco (1983) found a significant positive relationship between frequency of a subject's stuttering and the amount of silence in the voiced stop consonant intervocalic interval during fluent speech. In a later study, Samar, Metz, and Sacco (1986) found a positive correlation between release of the consonant and peak air flow.

Two studies of school-age children both produced negative findings (McKnight & Cullinan, 1987; De Nil & Brutten, 1991b). In preschool children, positive findings were reported by Seebach and Caruso (1979) and Adams (1987), while negative findings were reported by Zebrowski, Conture, and Cudahy (1985) and Molt (1991).

Other Acoustic Features of the Fluent Speech of People Who Stutter

Klich and May (1982) reported that formant frequencies were more centralized in the spectrograms of stutterers' vowels than in those of nonstutterers. They interpreted the finding to mean that stutterers "use restricted articulatory adjustments to control their speech." Prosek, Montgomery, Walden, and Hawkins (1987) failed to find any greater vowel centralization in stutterers' than nonstutterers' fluent speech, but they observed a trend for the second formant frequencies of stutterers' front vowels to be lower than those of nonstutterers.

In contrast to the many studies that appear to find slower articulatory movement in people who stutter, Robb and Blomgren (1997) found that second formant (F_2) transitions, which are the acoustic traces of vowel-consonant articulatory transitions, were actually more rapid in their sample of stutterers than the fluent comparison group. Wingate (1982) noted that whereas amplitude tracings of normal speakers' stress patterns showed distinct peaks corresponding to stressed syllables, in stutterers' fluent speech, the stressed syllables were less clearly identifiable.

Pitch in Fluent Speech Stutterers' pitch levels have not been found to differ from nonstutterers' during fluent speech.[4] Healey (1982) reported a more limited range of pitch variation in stutterers' fluent production of sentences. In subsequent studies of pitch variation during fluency, however, Healey (1984), Healey and Gutkin (1984), and Sacco and Metz (1989) obtained largely negative results. Likewise, Ramig, Krieger, and Adams (1982) failed to find any difference between stutterers and nonstutterers in pitch variation or vocal intensity during fluent speech.

Newman, Harris, and Hilton (1989) observed more shimmer (cycle-to-cycle variations in amplitude) in stutterers than nonstutterers when speakers were instructed to sustain a vowel, and they suggested that stutterers had "less stable neuromuscular control" of phonation. Hall and Yairi (1992) reported the same observation with regard to vowels selected from the spontaneous speech of preschool children.

In an electroglottographic study of preschool children, Conture, Rothenberg, and Molitar (1986) measured the proportion of the vibratory cycle in which the vocal folds were in contact during their fluent utterances. During consonant-vowel and vowel-consonant transitions, all eight stutterers, as compared with four of the eight nonstutterers, showed what the experimenters defined as atypical patterns of glottal activity. Electroglottographic observations by Peters and Boves (1988) showed abrupt voice onsets to occur more often in stutterers than typically fluent peers in perceptually fluent utterances of single words.

By means of a transducer inserted in the trachea through the nose and glottis, Peters and Boves (1987, 1988) observed patterns of subglottal air pressure build-up during adult stutterers' fluent productions of single words. Stutterers more frequently exhibited disruptions in the typically smooth and continuous increase in pressure and more often began phonation at least 100 msec. after pressure had reached a maximum. Peters and Boves interpreted

[4] Ramig, Krieger, and Adams (1982), Healey (1984), Healey and Gutkin (1984), Bergmann (1986), Hall and Yairi (1992).

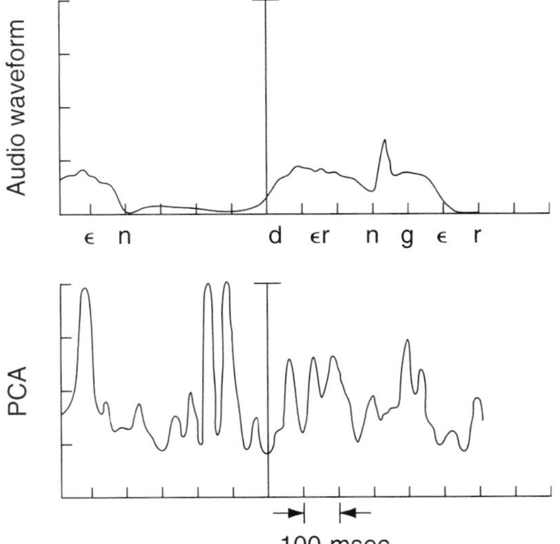

FIGURE 5-1 Abnormal abductor (posterior cricoarytenoid muscle) activity before and during a perceptually fluent utterance. Because the word "danger" is voiced throughout, there should be no abductor activity. Reproduced by permission of the publisher of "An electromyographic analysis of the fluent and dysfluent utterances of several types of stutterers," by Arnold Shapiro, *Journal of Fluency Disorders*, 5, 203–31. Copyright 1980 by Elsevier Science Publishing Co., Inc.

these findings to mean that "covert stuttering" can occur in perceptually fluent speech. Shapiro (1980) observed the same abnormally high levels of electromyographic activity in the supraglottal musculatures of stutterers during "acoustically fluent" utterances of words that were usually present in the recordings of stuttered words (see Figure 5-1).

Articulatory Rate and Coordination during Fluency

Segment Duration Various other abnormal characteristics have been observed in what is judged to be the fluent speech of stutterers, especially with regard to aspects of duration and rate. Di Simoni (1974) found longer durations of both consonants and vowels in production of nonsense words. Colcord and Adams (1979) found longer voicing durations in oral reading. Starkweather and Myers (1979) reported longer vowel-consonant-vowel segments in connected speech; the lengthening usually occurred in the transitional segments rather than the steady-state portions. On the other hand, during a study in which both school-age and adult speakers produced consecutive fluent utterances of the same sentences, Healey and Adams (1981) observed no consistent differences between stutterers and nonstutterers with respect to duration of consonants, vowels, pauses, or utterances. Healey and Adams speculated that the repetitions of the utterances may have had a "normalizing effect" on the stutterers' speech.

McMillan and Pindzola (1986) measured the duration of the first vowel in a vowel-consonant-vowel nonsense word embedded in a carrier phrase. Stutterers and participants with articulation disorder both produced longer steady-state portions of the vowel than did typically functioning peers. The stutterers also had shorter vowel-to-consonant transitions than the typically fluent speakers (see also Pindzola, 1987). In fluent utterances of the word "two" in a series of numbers, Borden, Kim, and Spiegler (1987) found that the stop gap and vowel durations of severe stutterers were longer than those of fluent speakers. Jäncke (1994) had speakers continuously repeat a three-syllable nonsense word. Stutterers did not differ from normally fluent speakers in the duration of the first vowel, but demonstrated more intrasubject variability.

Bosshardt, Sappock, Knipschild, and Hölscher (1997) found increased syllable durations in responses of stutterers asked to imitate questions having different stress and rate patterns. In a study by Viswanath (1989, 1991), stutterers read a passage aloud five times. Analysis showed that words stuttered in the first reading were significantly lengthened when they were uttered without perceptible stuttering in subsequent readings. Viswanath also observed a lengthening of words preceding stuttering and a lengthening of the last word in a clause preceding one in which stuttering occurred.

Janssen, Wieneke, and Vaane (1983) found that in successive fluent repetitions of a word, the durations of the stutterers' words varied more than those of nonstutterers. The same within-subject variability was found with regard to repeated sentences by Janssen and Wieneke (1987) and Wieneke and Janssen (1987, 1991). Cooper and Allen (1977) found stutterers more irregular than nonstutterers in the duration of repeated fluent utterances of the same sentence, paragraph, or nursery rhyme.

Similar studies of younger stutterers have yielded more equivocal results. Reimann (1976) found shorter vowels in the speech of three adolescent stutterers than in that of three typically fluent speakers. Both Winkler and Ramig (1986) and McKnight and Cullinan (1987) found no differences in vowel or consonant durations of school-age stutterers and nonstutterers. Adams (1987) recorded longer vowel and consonant durations in the speech of preschool stutterers and interpreted these lags as "inherent features of their speech-timing control." This was in sharp contrast to the findings of Zebrowski, Conture, and Cudahy (1985), who found no differences between 3- to 6-year-old stutterers and nonstutterers in either vowel and consonant duration or duration of transitions between sounds in fluent utterances.

Speech Rate In keeping with most of the reports on the duration of stutterers' speech sounds has been the repeated finding that stutterers tend to have slower speech rate, even when measuring their fluent speech. In an early study, Bloodstein (1944) found that stutterers had a slower average rate of oral reading (in words per minute), even when the total duration of observed stuttering was subtracted from the total reading time. Slower rates of fluent utterances have been reported in a series of more recent studies of adult stutterers.[5]

Meyers and Freeman (1985c) found slower rates of fluent speech in preschool stutterers. Hall, Amir, and Yairi (1999) found no differences in articulatory rate (as measured by syllables per second) among fluent preschoolers, those who recovered from early stuttering, and those whose stuttering persisted. However, when rate was measured in phones per second, both groups differed from preschoolers with no history of stuttering.

Indices of Speech and Nonspeech Motor Coordination

In addition to the analyses described, indices of difference in the motor coordination abilities of people who stutter have come from an array of study designs. For example, considerable early evidence of articulatory slowness in stutterers came from a computer analysis of a cinefluorographic film of movements of the lip and jaw of six stutterers and seven normal speakers by Zimmermann (1980b). In what were judged to be fluent utterances of the syllables /bab/, /pap/, and /mam/, the stutterers had longer transitions, longer steady state positions, longer time intervals between the onset and peak velocity of movement, and longer latency of onset of movement. Zimmermann also found less coordination between lip and jaw movements in the case of the stutterers.

However, Caruso, Abbs, and Gracco (1988) found patterns that were not consistent with these findings. In fluent productions of the utterance "sapapple," they found that stutterers were not deficient in the range and velocities of lip and jaw movements. Instead, the stutterers deviated from the usual order of onset of speech movements: upper lip, then lower lip, then jaw. This sequence was followed by all of the six fluent speakers, but only one of the six stutterers. McClean, Kroll, and Loftus (1990) reported a further replication of this study with the addition of a group of stutterers who had recently undergone speech therapy that focused on rate reduction. This group exhibited abnormal movement durations. There was little difference between the other stutterers and the normally fluent speakers. As for the sequence of activation of the lips and jaw, 7 of the 10 untreated stutterers used the supposedly normal sequence and 4 of the 10 nonstutterers did not. In a later analysis of their results, McClean,

[5]Adams, Runyan, and Mallard (1975), Ramig, Krieger, and Adams (1982), Borden (1983), Schäferskūpper and Dames (1987), Bosshardt and Nandyal (1988), Van Lieshout, Hulstijn, and Peters (1991). In conflict was a report by Gronhovd (1977). Pindzola (1986) found no difference between stutterers and nonstutterers in the velocity of transitions from vowel to consonant and consonant to vowel in nonsense words.

Kroll, and Loftus (1991) found that the more severe stutterers had a slower lip closure on the first "p" in "sapapple." Ward (1997) found phase differences in lip and jaw movement between five stutterers and comparison speakers. Jäncke, Bauer, Kaiser, and Kalveram (1997) found subtle differences in jaw movement during nonsense word production at varying speech rates between stutterers and nonstutterers, but attributed them to compensatory strategies that stutterers used to achieve fluent production of the target.

In a study by Guitar, Guitar, Nelson, O'Dwyer, and Andrews (1988), stutterers repeated the words "peek," "puck," and "pack" until their utterances were fluent. Activation of two lip muscles for the initial "p" was studied. In 50 percent of the fluent utterances, the depressor labii inferior was activated before the depressor anguli oris. This was the reverse of the nonstutterers' pattern, but was similar to 82 percent of the stuttered utterances. Van Lieshout, Peters, Starkweather, and Hulstijn (1993) recorded electromyographic potentials during lip rounding for Dutch /o/ in initial position in stutterers' fluent syllables, words, and sentences. The stutterers had higher levels of activity than their fluent peers and a longer delay between the beginning of electromyographic rise and the onset of speech.

Smith and Kleinow (2000) specifically examined stability of motor gestures for speech under varying rates of speech (fast, habitual, and slow) in a sample of 14 pairs of stuttering and nonstuttering adults, using an index of spatio-temporal stability (STI). While most stutterers appeared to show motor stability in the slow speech condition, some appeared unstable even at habitual rate. Because the stutterers performed particularly less well at non-habitual rates, the authors speculated that they are more susceptible to destabilization of motor performance when demand is increased. Continuation studies that examined effects of linguistic demand on motor ability are discussed in Chapter 8.

The proposal that atypical oro-facial movement may reflect adaptation to stuttering or less efficient motor control strategies for speech is supported by the findings of Kelly and Smith (1995). In their study of electromyographic (EMG) activity in nine pairs of stuttering and typically fluent children, only the oldest children showed evidence of tremor behavior.

Temporal Synchrony Many of the studies discussed here make it clear that typically fluent speech is characterized by certain regulatories in the timing of articulatory events. (For example, the latency of onset of the stop consonant in a vowel-consonant-vowel sequence is always a constant fraction of the interval between the onset of the two vowels.) In contrast to studies finding atypical indices of coordination or regularity in the fluent speech of stutterers, Prosek, Montgomery, and Walden (1988) studied four such ratios in the fluent reading of 15 stutterers and found them comparable to those of 15 normal speakers. Similarly, Molt (1991) found that the timing of velopharyngeal movement for nasal consonant production in the fluent speech of five stutterers aged 5 to 6 years was very similar to that of five nonstuttering children. Conture, Colton, and Gleason (1988) recorded the onsets, offsets, and durations of activity of the rib cage, abdomen, larynx, and lips during single word production by preschool children. They concluded that there was no appreciable difference between the speech coordination of stutterers and nonstutterers during fluent speech.

Van Lieshout, Hulstijn, and Peters (1996) asked stuttering and typically fluent adults to name pictures and words. Words varied in the number of syllables and complexity of syllable onsets. The authors measured reaction times, word durations, and relative timing of motor activity in the respiratory, phonatory, and articulatory subsystems. Stutterers showed longer speech reaction times that did not interact with word size, but word durations were longer for persons who stutter and did interact with word size. Both findings were related to longer delays for stutterers in the onset of upper lip and respiratory activity and to the order of upper and lower lip activity in word production. The authors suggested their stuttering participants were compensating for some unspecified deficit in verbal motor skill.

Max and Yudman (2003) suggest that evidence of durational differences alone is not sufficient evidence of miscoordination in the speech timing control of people who stutter. They also note that miscoordination could be within speech gestures, across speech gestures, or in integrating gestures into the rhythmic pattern of the speaker's language.

One way to distinguish among these possibilities is to require the speaker to shadow or track an external stimulus such as a metronome by producing syllables or finger taps. As Max and Yudman (2003) observe in their review of work in this area, studies comparing adults who stutter to those who do not have produced conflicting results: some have found stutterers to be more variable than fluent peers when producing syllables synchronized with an isochronous metronome (Boutsen, Brutten, & Watts, 2000), but others have shown no differences between the groups in rate and variability of finger tapping synchronized with a metronome whose rate varied unpredictably (Zelaznik, Smith, & Franz, 1994). Some studies have required their participants to continue a rhythm after being synchronized to an external stimulus that is discontinued. A similar set of conflicting results emerges from these studies. One group reported increased variability when children who stutter were required to continue a set of nonspeech lip movements (Howell, Au-Yeung, & Rustin, 1997) whereas no differences were found either for the synchronization or continuation phases by Hulstijn, Summers, van Lieshout, and Peters (1992).

In a study representative of this area of inquiry, Max and Yudman (2003) asked 10 pairs of stuttering and nonstuttering adults to synchronize speech, nonspeech oral, and finger movements to a series of tones. They were also instructed to continue their response for 10 movements past termination of the stimulus. The selected speech response was the syllable /pa/, the nonspeech response was a lip-popping movement, and the motor response was approximating the index finger to the thumb. No differences either in synchronization or continuation of rhythmic patterning were found. They concluded that if stuttering represents a disorder of timing of motor movements, it is one that goes beyond simple ability to replicate and generalize rhythmic sequences, either speech motor or more generally.

In companion work that performed kinematic analyses of more complex speech, oral motor, and finger movements, Max, Caruso, and Gracco (2003) did observe differences between stutterers and fluent speakers across a number of gestures involving all of these tasks that were embedded in responses varying in length.[6] The authors interpreted their findings to suggest that stutterers may have deficits in the execution of goal-directed movements across a number of unrelated motor systems.

McClean, Tasko, and Runyan (2004) were not able to fully replicate these findings, nor their team's earlier finding that ratios linking lip and tongue speed to jaw speed increase with stuttering severity (McClean & Runyan, 2000). Forty-three typically fluent adult speakers and 37 who stutter were recorded while producing a nonsense phrase and a sentence. Only perceptually fluent productions were measured to movement speeds, durations, and ratios of lip and tongue speed to jaw speed. In addition to comparisons between fluent and stuttering speakers, analyses were also run to compare more and less severe stutterers. Relatively shorter durations of lower lip and jaw closing as well as jaw closing speed were seen in the group of stutterers as a whole. However, in the sentence tasks, more and less severe stutterers demonstrated distinct patterns, suggesting the possibility of subgroups within the stuttering population. Speed ratio measures did not distinguish any of the groups.

The same team (Tasko, McClean, & Runyan, 2007) examined respiratory, orofacial kinematic, and acoustic measures in 35 stutterers before and at completion of a one-month intensive treatment program that emphasized fluency shaping (see Chapter 14). Simultaneous with fluency improvement, participants "increased the amplitude and duration of speech breaths, reduced the rate of lung

[6]An ancillary post hoc observation was that neither motor instability nor stuttering were increased over length of response required, a finding that the authors noted was inconsistent with many of the reported associations among length and complexity of spoken utterances and disfluency (see Chapter 8).

volume change during inspiration, reduced the amplitude and speed of lip movements early in the test utterance, increased lip and jaw movement durations, and reduced syllable rate." Changes in respiratory measures and one orofacial kinematic measure accounted for much of statistical improvement in fluency.[7]

Summary: Stutterers

In summary, the weight of evidence strongly suggests that, on careful study, what observers consider to be the fluent speech of stutterers frequently reveals features that are not to be found, at least to the same degree, in the speech of nonstutterers. Although the precise extent of these differences is not yet fully clear, most of them appear to entail aspects of slowness or limitation of movement, lateness of response, or incoordination of the articulators and larynx. Many of the abnormal features of stutterers' "fluency" appear to bear a broad resemblance to those of overt stuttering. And there are hints in the literature we have cited that these disturbances may be more likely to occur in the near vicinity of overt stuttering than when subjects are free from any tendency to stutter.

What these observations mean involves difficulties of interpretation not often recognized. If we discover that stutterers exhibit a "mismanagement" of their speech during what we take to be intervals of fluency, one possible inference is that this mismanagement is a reason why they stutter. An alternative interpretation is that it reflects the reduced spontaneity and excessive caution of a person who expects to have difficulty with speech. The abnormalities in the stutterer's fluent speech, then, may be a cause or a result of the stuttering. There is, however, yet another possibility. It would be just as reasonable to conclude that we were mistaken about the fluency. What appeared to us to be fluent intervals of speech may perhaps have contained instances of stuttering so minimal that we only perceive them, with the aid of refined techniques of measurement, as subtle forms of slowness, incoordination, and the like. It is not, after all, so farfetched to suppose that, just as identifiable stutterings may range from very severe to extremely mild, the mild ones may merge by fine degrees with many more that are imperceptible. This view was aptly expressed by Adams and Runyan (1981) when they suggested that stuttering and fluency are "events along a continuum, so that as speech flows forward there is a drift, sometimes gradual, sometimes rapid, toward stuttering."

We have not yet arrived at the main difficulty, however. At first glance, the question of whether such imperceptible disfluencies as brief pauses or delayed voice onsets are stuttering may seem to be a sensible question. But further reflection will show that there are no logically imaginable observations that will serve to answer it. Observation will reveal only that the delayed voice onsets and other deviations are there. What we ought to call them is only a question of definition of terms. We can define stuttering in any way that we agree on, but the question of whether anything is "really" stuttering or "really" fluency is unanswerable. Who is to say that slowness, uncoordination, and brief pauses are not stuttering, whether they result from anticipation of difficulty in speaking, from neurological impairment, or from anything else? We must conclude that many of the questions raised about the so-called fluent speech of stutterers are not meaningful questions. There are, however, certain meaningful questions we can ask about the nonspeech activities of the stutterer's vocal tract that relate to the issue of whether some of the abnormalities we have been discussing are symptoms or causes of stuttering. We now turn to these questions.

SPECIFIC SPEECH MOTOR ABILITIES

If people who stutter have a neuromuscular abnormality or weakness of some kind, then, regardless of its precise nature or the parts of the body whose functioning it affects, its presence should be recognizable in atypical functioning of the component systems in speech production if it is to be regarded as a cause of stuttering. It is a matter of common

[7] However, there was a tendency for the stutterers showing greatest reductions in stuttering frequency to be rated as sounding more unnatural on discharge from the program.

observation that most stutterers, unlike so many persons who have speech impairments due to cerebral palsy, are able to use speech mechanism without difficulty in such nonspeech activities as eating. This would imply that there is nothing wrong with the speech motor systems of people who stutter. There is an answer to this argument, however. The muscular adjustments involved in chewing, biting, sucking, swallowing, and the like are relatively gross ones. It may be possible to harbor a neuromuscular weakness so subtle that it reveals itself only in the rapid, fine coordinations required for speech. This explanation is plausible enough, but a crucial test of its validity immediately suggests itself. Do stutterers tend to be less able than nonstutterers to produce rapid, fine adjustments of the articulators in nonspeech activities? So effectively does this question appear to roll up into a ball the whole issue of motor factors in the etiology of stuttering, that it has received a considerable amount of attention (see Table 5-2).

Diadochokinetic Abilities

The earliest study of rapid repetitive movement, or diadochokinesis, in people who stutter was reported by West and Nusbaum (1929). Using a measure consisting of the combined rate of movement of the jaw and eyebrow for each subject, they found that stutterers tended to achieve poorer scores than nonstutterers. Cross (1936) reported slower rates of movement of the tongue, jaw, and diaphragm among stutterers than among right-handed typically fluent speakers. Spriestersbach (1940), however, found no differences between stutterers and nonstutterers in speed of movement of the tongue, jaw, brow, and lips. Similarly, Strother and Kriegman (1943) found no significant differences in the diadochokinetic rates of the tongue, jaw, and lips of stutterers and nonstutterers matched for age, sex, dextrality quotient, and rhythm discrimination. Strother and Kriegman discovered, moreover, that when comparable data from previous conflicting studies were pooled, they revealed, in the aggregate, essentially no differences between stutterers and normal speakers. Finally, Chworowski (1952) showed that stutterers performed as well as nonstutterers in the rapid repetitive articulation of isolated speech sounds and did so under both presumed emotional stress and normal conditions.

Temporal Patterning Abilities

Comparable studies, with conflicting findings, have been done on stutterers' ability to move their oral structures rhythmically or to use them in reproducing temporal patterns accurately. We will describe some of these studies in addition to the large number of those summarized in Table 5-2. A study by Zaleski (1965) found stutterers less able to reproduce rhythmic patterns with the syllables "pa," "ta," and "ka." Barrett and Stoeckel (1979) and Newman, Channell, and Palmer (1986) also reported stutterers to be less able to wink with just one eye. Mallard, Hicks, and Riggs (1982) could find no difference between stutterers and normal speakers in the ability to produce the vowel /a/ with a gentle onset of phonation.

Caruso, Gracco, and Abbs (1987) introduced a load on the lower lip of adult speakers as they said the /p/ in /apa/. Stutterers responded with the same compensatory adjustments as controls, but with longer latencies and smaller changes in magnitude of movement. Brown, Zimmermann, Linville, and Hegmann (1990) found stutterers slower than nonstutterers when instructed to tap with a finger, move the jaw, and say "ah" repeatedly at a comfortable rate. Riley and Riley (1991) administered their *Oral Motor Assessment Scale* to children ages 4 to 8 years. The stutterers' performance was comparable to that of children with articulation disorders, but poorer than that of normal speakers. Viewed as a whole, the research on the nonspeech activities of the stutterer's speech mechanism does not lend itself to any straightforward conclusions.

Reaction Time Studies

In our discussion of motor abilities so far, we have made no mention of a very large number of investigations of stutterers' reaction times. Following an early period of inconclusive effort, research on

TABLE 5-2 Studies of Motor Proficiency of the Speech Musculature of Stutterers and Nonstuttereers Classified with Regard to Whether the Stutters Were Found to Be of Poorer (Positive Outcomes) or Equal (Negative Outcomes) Ability

Manual	Tongue		Lips		Jaw		Diaphragm	
ability	Positive[a]	Negative	Positive[a]	Negative	Positive[a]	Negative	Positive[a]	Negative
Strength		Palmer and Osborn (1940)						
Speed of repetitive movement	McClean and Runyan (2000), McCLean and Tasko (2004)	Cross (1936), Spriestersbach (1940), Strother and Kriegman (1943)	McLean and Runyan (2000), Max, Caruso, and Gracco (2003),[b] McLean and Tasko 2004,[c] Namasivayam and Van Lieshout (2004)	Cross (1936), Spriestersbach (1940), Strother and Kriegman (1943)	West and Nusbaum (1929),[d] Bauer, Kaiser, and Kalveram (1997), McLean and Runyan (2000) Max, Caruso, and Gracco (2003)[e]	Cross (1936), Spriestersbach (1940),[f] Strother and Kriegman (1943)	Cross (1936)	Friedman (1955)
Regularity of repetitive movement	Blackburn (1931)		Blackburn (1931)	Seth (1934)	Blackburn (1931), and Loucks and De Nil (2006)	Seth (1934)	Blackburn (1931), Seth (1934)	
Accuracy of reproduction of temporal patterns	Hunsley (1937)	Wulff (1935), Strother and Kriegman (1944)	Hunsley (1937)	Wulfl (1935), Strother and Kriegman (1944)	Hunsley (1937)	Wulfi (1935), Strother and Kriegman (1944)	Hunsley (1937)	

[a] Studies with more than one outcome in a given category are classified as "positive" if any outcome was positive.
[b] Lip closing, not opening.
[c] Lower lip only.
[d] Combined jaw and brow rate.
[e] Jaw closing, not opening.
[f] Found no difference for either separate or combined jaw and brow rates.

the motor performance of stutterers dwindled for a time. When it was resumed with enthusiasm in the 1970s, it was mainly in response to questions about stutterers' reaction time, particularly in relation to the functioning of the larynx.

Voice Initiation and Termination Time As noted earlier in this chapter, vocal abnormalities are a well-documented feature of stuttering behavior and are clearly apparent to an alert observer. It is not surprising that at widely separated times in the history of thinking about stuttering, the larynx has been suspected of being the primary source of the problem.[8] A renewed flurry of interest in this hypothesis was caused in part by the electromyographic studies of Freeman and Ushijima (1975, 1978), which vividly depicted the abnormal state of the intrinsic muscles of the larynx during stuttering. One result of this interest has been an extensive series of investigations of the phonatory reaction times of stutterers (see Table 5-3). In studies of this type, speakers have been instructed to produce voice in various forms as quickly as possible in response to a signal. With few exceptions, the results have shown stutterers to be slower on the average than nonstutterers in initiating phonation. Tests of stutterers' ability to terminate phonation have produced similar results. Stutterers have been found to differ from nonstutterers by an average order of magnitude ranging from well under one-tenth to about three-tenths of a second.

In some of these studies, speakers were asked to respond with words or nonsense syllables. Only those utterances judged by the experimenters to be fluent were retained for analysis. As we noted earlier, the trouble with such observations is that they lead to the unanswerable question of whether the observed delay in phonation is a cause, a result, or a minimal form of stuttering. In search of less ambiguous data, most investigators have therefore resorted to the use of isolated vowels such as /a/ or /ə/. Although stutterers rarely appear to have difficulty with isolated speech sounds, it is arguable that because even saying vowels is a form of speech activity, the task is not totally free from the possible influence of stuttering. For this reason, a few studies have elicited nonlinguistic phonatory responses such as throat clearing and phonation on inspiration. In two of these studies, the stutterers were found to be slower than nonstutterers; in a third the difference approached significance.[9] On the other hand, Yoshiyuki (1984) found stutterers as fast as typically fluent comparison speakers in changing the pitch of the voice.

Some researchers have regarded these findings as evidence that stuttering results from laryngeal dysfunction. A different interpretation was advanced by Cullinan and Springer (1980). Pointing out that many stutterers have difficulties in their early speech development (a subject we will come to in Chapter 8), they divided 20 stuttering children into a group of 11 who had mild to moderate language or articulation problems or learning disabilities and a group of 9 who did not. The stutterers with the speech or language problems had significantly slower voice initiation and termination times than nonstutterers; in the case of the other stuttering children, the difference was smaller and not significant. Cullinan and Springer concluded that the poorer performance of stutterers in such tasks seemed to be related to the frequency of language and articulation difficulties among them. McKnight and Cullinan (1987) found that stuttering children receiving special education services, chiefly for learning disabilities, had longer voice initiation and termination times, whereas stutterers without such problems differed from nonstutterers only in having longer voice termination times.

Cullinan and Springer also noted that the relative slowness of phonatory reactions of the stutterers was considerably more pronounced in the older children than in the younger ones, suggesting that it may develop as a reaction to stuttering. Their study children ranged in age from 5 to 11 years. In a study of 4- to 6-year-old children who were free from disorders of articulation or language, Murphy and

[8] See Rieber and Wollock (1977), Kenyon (1942).

[9] Adler and Starkweather (1979), Reich, Till, and Goldsmith (1981), Till, Reich, Dickey, and Sieber (1983).

Baumgartner (1981) found no difference between stutterers and nonstutterers in vocal initiation or termination time. Cross and Luper (1979) reported slower voice reaction times in 5- and 9-year-old stutterers unselected with regard to language or articulation difficulties. Till, Reich, Dickey, and Sieber (1983) found evidence of phonatory slowness in stutterers aged 8 to 12 years who had normal language and articulation. Bishop, Williams, and Cooper (1991a, 1991b) found that both stuttering children and children with articulation disorders in the age range of 3 to 10 years had longer vocal and manual reaction times than children with age-appropriate speech. The issues raised by Cullinan and Springer are as yet unresolved.

Initiating voice as fast as possible in response to a signal is a complex act involving, among other things, a preparatory set to respond, the perception of a stimulus, and the activation of both respiratory and laryngeal muscles. Where in this chain of events do stutterers lag? Because most studies have employed a tone as the stimulus, a few studies have used both visual and auditory cues to rule out the possibility that the delay is in the auditory perception rather than in the vocal response. The effect is the same. Watson and Alfonso (1982) thought the delay might be in stutterers' readiness to respond and gave participants a warning signal before presenting the cue to respond; they found no significant difference between stutterers and fluent speakers. Their subsequent replication of the study (Watson & Alfonso, 1983), however, did find differences between severe stutterers and nonstutterers despite the preparatory warning period.

A question that remains is whether the lag is in the stutterer's laryngeal or respiratory adjustments. Both Venkatagiri (1981, 1982c) and Watson and Alfonso (1982) attempted to address this question by asking participants to respond with voiced and whispered utterances of the same sounds. Unfortunately, their results were inconclusive because a difference between the stutterers and nonstutterers did not emerge for either voiced or voiceless sounds. It is noteworthy that in normally fluent speakers, laryngeal and respiratory reaction times are by no means the same. In a study of normally fluent speakers, Shipp, Izdebski, and Morrissey (1984) timed both the occurrence of increased subglottal breath pressure and the appearance of changes in the action potentials from three intrinsic laryngeal muscles. They found respiratory response slower than laryngeal muscle response, suggesting that "it is not laryngeal adjustment time that principally determines vocal reaction time, but rather it is the temporal interval for activation of the respiratory system." Indirect support for the assumption that stutterers' slow vocal reactions may actually reflect slow respiratory reactions has come from some research by Prosek, Montgomery, Walden, and Schwartz (1979). They timed participants' reactions by two measures: the start of electromyographic activity at the larynx and the actual onset of voicing. The stutterers' laryngeal responses were as fast as those of the typically fluent comparison speakers, but their reaction times on the acoustic measures were longer. Prosek and his coworkers suggested that "the initial gesture may occur with normal latency, but the release of the gesture or the onset of airflow may be abnormally long." In two severe stutterers, Watson and Alfonso (1987) found indications of a delay in both respiratory and laryngeal activity.

Bakker and Brutten (1989) made a similar division. They reasoned that stutterers' increased phonatory reaction times must be due either to a lag in premotor activity (i.e., perceiving the signal and programming the response) or to slow laryngeal adjustment (posturing the larynx for phonation). After instructing adults to say the vowel /a/ as quickly as possible in response to a signal, they measured the time interval from the onset of the signal to the point where an electroglottograph showed the first low frequency changes that marked the start of laryngeal adjustment. The beginning of vocal fold vibration gave the total laryngeal reaction time. Subtracting the premotor interval from the total reaction time then gave the laryngeal adjustment time. Analysis of the results showed that the stuttering speakers exceeded the typically fluent speakers in both premotor and laryngeal adjustment times. In short, they took more time both in planning the response (or perceiving the signal) and in preparing the larynx for voice production.

TABLE 5-3 Studies of Phonatory, Oral, and Manual Reaction Times of Stutterers and Nonstutterers

	Subjects	Cue	Response	Results
Adams and Hayden (1976)	Adults	Tone	Initiation and termination of /a/	Stutterers were slower in both initiation and termination
Kerr (1976)	Adults	Light	Change from one sound to another	Stutterers were slower in changing from a voiceless to a voiced sound
Starkweather, Hirschman, and Tannenbaum (1976)	Adults	Illumination of screen	Nonsense syllables and words	Stutterers were slower
Cross (1978)	Children aged 5 and 9; adults	Tone	Finger press	Stutterers were slower at each age level
McFarlane and Prins (1978)	Adults	Offset of light or tone	Lip closure, /pæ/, /bæ/	Stutterers were slower (difference was significant only for tone)
Adler and Starkweather (1979)		Visual	Oral, laryngeal, linguistic, nonlinguistic	Stutterers were slower under all conditions
Cross and Cooke (1979)	Adults	Visual or auditory	/a/ or switch press	Stutterers were slower in both vocal and manual responses, whether to visual or auditory stimulus
Cross and Luper (1979)	Children aged 5 and 9, adults	Tone	/ʌ/	Stutterers were slower at each age level. Not all had long reaction times
Cross, Shadden, and Luper (1979)	Adults	Tone	/ʌ/	Stutterers were slower, regardless of which ear received the tone
Lewis, Ingham, and Gervens (1979)		Visual or auditory	Initiation and termination of phonation	Stutterers were slower in response to both visual and auditory cues
Prosek, Montgomery, Walden, and Schwartz (1979)	Adults	Tone, light, or, VC word	Button press or VC word	No significant differences were found
Webster (1979b)		Visual stimulus	Syllables	Stutterers were slower
Cullinan and Springer (1980)	Children aged 5 to 11	Tone	/a/	Stutterers with additional speech or language problems were slower; those below age 8 did not differ from controls

McFarlane and Shilpey (1981)	Adults	Offset of light or tone	/bæ/, /pæ/	Stutterers were slower in response to auditory but not visual cues
Murphy and Baumgartner (1981)	Children aged 4 to 6	Tone	Initiation and termination of /a/	There were no significant differences between groups in either initiation or termination
Reich, Till, and Goldsmith (1981)	Adults	Offset of tone	Button press, throat clearing, inspiratory phonation, /ʌ/, "upper"	Stutterers were significantly slower only in the speech responses, though their reaction times were longer on all tasks. In throat clearing the difference approached significance
Venkatagiri (1981)	Adults	Tone	Voiced and whispered /a/	Stutterers did not differ from nonstutterers in either response
Hayden, Adams, and Jordahl (1982)	Adults	Tone	Oral reading of sentences beginning with /a/	Stutterers were slower in initiating sentences
Venkatagiri (1982c)	Adults	Tone	/s/ and /z/	Stutterers did not differ from nonstutterers in either response
Watson and Alfonso (1982)	Adults	Offset of tone or light	Voiced and whispered /a/, nonsense-syllable phrase	No differences between stutterers and nonstutterers were found
Borden (1983)	Adults	Tone	Finger counting and speech counting	Stutterers were slower than nonstutterers in the execution but not in the initiation of the tasks
Cross and Luper (1983)	Children aged 5 and 9; adults	Tone	Key press	Stutterers were slower at each age level
Hand and Haynes (1983)	Adults	Exposure of stimulus word	Key press or /a/ if stimulus was real word	Stutterers were slower in both manual and vocal reaction time
Till, Reich, Dickey, and Sieber (1983)	Children aged 8 to 12	Offset of tone	Button press, throat, clearing, inspiratory phonation, /?ʌ/, "upper"	Stutterers were significantly slower in throat clearing and "upper"
Watson and Alfonso (1983)	Adults	Offset of /a/	/a/	Severe stutterers were slower
Starkweather, Franklin, and Smigo (1984)	Adults	Offset of tone	Button press, /ʌ/	Stutterers were slower in both manual and vocal responses
Wilkins, Webster, and Morgan (1984)	Adults	Exposure of letters or representation of faces	Button press on appearance of target face or letter	Stutterers were slower in reacting to faces

(*continues*)

TABLE 5-3 *(continued)*

	Subjects	Cue	Response	Results
Yoshiyuki (1984)	Adults	Tone	Initiation and termination of /i/	Stutterers were slower in voice initiation, but not in termination or in shadowing tone as it changed in pitch
Hurford and Webster (1985)	Adults	Visual display of XXX	Button release	Stufferers did not differ significantly from nonstutterers and were faster after therapy
Long and Pindzola (1985)	Children aged 4 to 8	Commands based on Token Test	Manual execution of commands	Stutterers did not differ significantly from nonstutterers
Bakker and Brutten (1987)	Adults	Light, tone, electric shock	/a/ or /pa/	Stutterers were slower in voice initiation, but not in lip reaction in saying /pa/
Cross and Olson (1987b)	Adults	Tone	/^/	Stutterers' voice and jaw reaction times were longer than controls' but not significantly
McKnight and Cullinan (1987)	Children aged 6 to 12	Light, tone	/a/	Stutterers with learning disabilities had longer voice initiation times than controls and other stutterers; stutterers without other problems had longer voice termination times than controls
Peters and Hulstijn (1987)	Adults	Tone	Words and sentences	Stutterers had longer laryngeal, lip, and masseter muscle reaction times
Stromsta (1987)	Adults	Light	/ə/	Five stutterers with prolongations and tonic blocks were slower than controls; five with repetitions were not
Lees (1988)	Adults	Offset of tone	/a/	Stutterers were slower than controls, and the difference approached statistical significance
Bakker and Brutten (1989)	Adults	Light, tone, electric shock	/a/	Stutterers were slower than controls
Peters, Hulstijn, and Starkweather (1989)	Adults	Tone	Words and sentences	Stutterers were slower than controls, and the difference increased with increasing complexity of the response
Bishop, Williams, and Copper (1991a, 1991b)	Children aged 3 to 10	Light	/a/, words, finger movements	Both stutterers and children with defective articulation were slower than controls in vocal and manual responses; the difference increased with task complexity

Dembrowski and Watson (1991b)	Adults	Light	/a/, VCV syllables	Stutterers were slower than controls, severe stutterers more so than mild ones; only partial support was found for the response complexity effect
Ferrand, Gilbert, and Blood (1991)	Adults	Tone	/a/	Stutterers and controls did not differ in vocal reaction time
Webster and Ryan (1991)	Adults	LED	Hand movement	Stutterers were slower than controls; increasing the complexity of the task did not change the difference
Wijnen and Boers (1994)	Adults	Visual presentation of a cue word	Words	There was no difference between stutterers and controls in reaction time
Jones et al. (2002)	12 moderate to severe stutterers, matched to a group of typically fluent adults	Randomly timed (3–7 sec latency) stimuli	Fastest possible arm movement in response to non-target stimulus (no accuracy required)	Stutterers were shown to have slower reaction times

A few additional observations remain to be noted. Borden (1983) and Cross and Luper (1979, 1983) both highlighted a distinct overlap in voice initiation time between groups; some stutterers had faster reaction times than some nonstutterers. In three studies, a severity effect was observed—the more severe stutterers tended to have slower reaction times.[10] In two other investigations, however, no such relationship was found.[11]

Cross and Olson (1987a) restricted adults' jaw movement by means of a bite block on the theory that stutterers' longer vocal reaction times might result from abnormal movements of the upper articulators. The effect of the bite block proved to be variable; some stutterers increased vocal reaction time, others decreased it. Finally, some provocative reports have indicated that speakers tend to initiate voice faster under conditions known to reduce stuttering markedly. Webster (1979b) noted this as an effect of masking noise. Hayden, Adams, and Jordahl (1982) and Hayden, Jordahl, and Adams (1982) were not able to confirm this phenomenon, but found that stutterers' voice initiation times were faster when they spoke in time to rhythm.

Logan (2003) studied speech initiation time (SIT) and whether it was differentially affected by linguistic demand in 11 pairs of stuttering and normally fluent adults. Adults who stutter were slower in most conditions, but neither group showed effects of linguistic complexity on SIT.

Oral and Manual Reaction Times Inevitably, the results obtained on the vocal reaction times of stutterers have led to questions about their other reaction times, specifically in oral and manual activities (see Table 5-3). With reference to oral responses, McFarlane and Prins (1978) found consistently longer reaction times for stutterers in a lip closure task, regardless of whether the participant was producing a syllable such as /pæ/ or a simple movement of the lips. Likewise, Adler and Starkweather (1979) reported stutterers to be as slow in comparison with nonstutterers on an oral task as on a laryngeal one, whether the task was linguistic or nonlinguistic.

Considerably more research has been done on manual reaction times, generally by having the participant press a button with a finger. The results have been conflicting. Over the years, some studies have recorded slower finger reaction times in stutterers, while numerous others have not. Those failing to show any difference included a study in which stutterers were slower in the execution of finger counting tasks,[12] but not in their initiation (Borden, 1983). Another involved such complex commands as "Touch the little red circle and the big green square" (Long & Pindzola, 1985). Cross and Luper (1983) found that stutterers' voice and finger reaction times were highly correlated, but Starkweather, Franklin, and Smigo (1984) did not. Curiously, both Wilkins, Webster, and Morgan (1984) and Hurford and Webster (1985) reported that stutterers' manual reaction times were faster after speech therapy than before.

Motor Encoding and Motor Learning

If stuttering reflects some inherent difficulty in realizing motor targets, it might conceivably be aggravated by the presumed difficulty of the motor gestures to be realized. Indeed, stuttering has been observed to be exacerbated when speech targets are longer or more complex (as measured by various linguistic indices, see Chapter 8). However, at the level of latency for word or stimulus naming, no differences were found between adults who do and do not stutter on targets varying in word length (van Lieshout & Hulstijn, 1996). This finding prompted the authors to reject the notion that stutterers have difficulty in assembling motor plans. However, integrated electromyographic signals taken from the participants' upper lip and lower lip (IEMG peak latency) did reveal differences between the groups of speakers. The authors speculated that stutterers may use slower speech movement speeds as a control strategy in maintaining fluency.

[10] Venkatagiri (1982c), Borden (1983), Watson and Alfonso (1983).

[11] Murphy and Baumgartner (1981), McFarlane and Lavorato (1983).

[12] Counting by touching the thumb to the index, middle, ring, and little finger and beginning again with the index finger.

Smits-Bandstra, De Nil, and Rochon (2006) asked 12 pairs of fluent and stuttering adults to finger-tap sequences under single and then dual task conditions. Stutterers' performance in the single task was as slow and variable as that of fluent speakers under the dual task condition. The results suggested that, while fluent speakers can achieve quick, accurate, and increasingly automatic performance after practice with a motor task, people who stutter cannot.

Some recent investigations have also examined non-word repetition in people who stutter (see Anderson, Wagovich, & Hall, 2006; Hakim & Bernstein Ratner, 2004; see additional discussion in Chapter 8). This type of task requires participants to repeat nonsense words that gradually vary in phonetic complexity. Although not strictly a motor learning task, the relatively poorer performance that has been shown for people who stutter may relate to more generalized deficits in implementing novel motor sequences.

Proprioceptive Ability

Loucks and De Nil (2006) tested the hypothesis that stuttering involves a deficiency in oral kinesthesia. Seventeen pairs of stuttering and typically fluent adults were cued to perform jaw opening movements, both when guided or unaided by feedback provided by a computer display, and when self-paced and timed. Stutterers were less accurate and more variable when they did not have access to visual feedback, but particularly so under time pressure. The authors suggested that stuttering may involve an oral kinesthetic deficiency.

CONCLUSIONS

The hypothesis that laryngeal dysfunction plays a primary part in the stuttering block has lent unusual interest to the observation that people who stutter tend to have longer voice reaction times than nonstutterers. That observation has now been repeatedly confirmed and even appears to extend to nonspeech activities such as throat clearing. For a number of reasons, however, the implications of this fact are far from clear.

In the first place, a vocal response, even throat clearing, is obviously not a function of the larynx alone, but also of the respiratory mechanism, and when speakers are asked to produce an identifiable vowel, the oral structures are involved as well. Although the reaction times measured in these studies have sometimes been referred to as "laryngeal," there is consequently little reason to assume that these reaction times have an exclusive connection with the larynx.

Moreover, speech is so dependent on the interrelated activity of the respiratory, laryngeal, and oral musculatures that it is difficult to imagine by what observations we might determine that one part of this activity is more "important" or "necessary" for speech fluency than the others, or what meaning such words might have in this context. That the larynx participates in stuttering is certain. If we did not have other evidence of it, we would have only to note how we involuntarily constrict the glottis when we say a sound such as /b/ with extra effort. It would be futile, however, to try to establish whether it was the closure of the glottis or the pressure of our lips that was the "primary" aspect of our behavior.

Moreover, the vocal tract does not function independently of central control at cortical and subcortical levels (see Chapter 4). As such, discovery of motor atypicalities does not tell us how or where they arise in the speech production system.

We are led to conclude that there is little evidence that abnormal functioning of the larynx has any sort of primacy in stuttering behavior, nor is it clear what form such evidence could take. For instance, it is difficult to reconcile a concept of such primacy with well-confirmed reports that some people who stutter continue to do so with esophageal speech, with a surgically constructed neoglottis, or with an electrolarynx following surgical removal of the larynx,[13] although such a view is consistent with limited efficacy reports for Botox injections in the

[13] Doms and Lissens (1973), Tuck (1979), Wingate (1981a), Rosenfield and Freeman (1983).

control of stuttering (Rosen & Ludlow, 1990; Brin, Stewart, Blitzer, & Diamond, 1994). Descriptions of stutterlike reactions in the manual communication of the deaf by Silverman and Silverman (1971) and Montgomery and Fitch (1988) tend to raise the question whether it is necessary to use the speech mechanism at all, let alone the larynx, in order to stutter.

The delay that characterizes some stutterers' vocal reaction times is very small, but the regularity with which researchers have obtained this finding is nevertheless impressive, and we are challenged for an explanation. Some adopt the view that it reflects some type of overall neuromotor deficit in stutterers. Investigations of manual reaction time may tell us more about this possibility, but the studies that have been published to date have been so inconsistent in their outcomes that it already seems clear that if any lag in manual reaction time exists, it is not comparable to the delay in vocal reaction time.

Another hypothesis that some researchers find congenial at the present time is that the stutterer's slower voice initiation is due to a specific impairment of cortical mechanisms responsible for motor speech control. As noted in the previous chapter, Watson, Pool, Devous, Freeman, and Finitzo (1992) reported that stutterers with reduced blood flow to regions of the brain that support speech motor control had longer reaction times for words and sentences.

Alternatives to central processing deficit explanations have also been considered, however. Bakker and Brutten (1989) suggested that reaction time delays may reflect a "learned strategy . . . to slow down to reduce the risk of fluency failure." As noted previously, Armson and Kalinowski (1994), in a critique of the use of findings on the perceptually fluent speech of stutterers to support organic theories of stuttering, have expressed the belief that even the "fluent" productions of isolated vowels that have generally been used in vocal reaction time studies may be contaminated by stuttering or stuttering-related events that are not evident perceptually. We concur with them that the question of whether such contamination has occurred in a given case may not even be answerable.

Chapter 6

The Person Who Stutters: Other Physical Findings

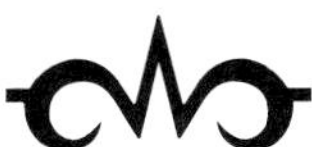

PHYSIOLOGICAL PROCESSES

In Chapter 3, we saw that there is evidence of genetic influences on stuttering, and for some researchers, this aspect of its etiology has loomed larger than any other. There has been continual pursuit of a clue to an inherited predisposing abnormality underlying the disorder. We have seen that physiological studies have been done—for different purposes and with different implications—during stuttering, during what is judged to be the stutterer's "free" speech, or during silence. Most physiological measures are responsive to muscular effort and autonomic arousal, both of which may reflect responses to stuttering rather than its root cause. Consequently, if convincing evidence of an etiological factor is desired, it must be obtained during silence, preferably under basal conditions and when the participants have not been engaged in speech for several hours. In addition, it is imperative to compare the measures obtained in this way with those of a comparison group of typically fluent speakers on the identical task rather than to make use of so-called textbook norms for this purpose. The failure to adhere to these principles has sometimes resulted in disagreement and confusion in this area of research. In this discussion, we will for the most part omit mention of uncontrolled studies or casual observations where better information exists.

Breathing Patterns

Because of their conspicuous disturbance during stuttering, breathing movements were the first physiological phenomena to arouse the interest of researchers, and they had been studied in Europe by the end of the nineteenth century. When Travis established one of the first American laboratories for the study of speech disorders at the University of Iowa in 1927, this was among the topics to which he immediately gave his attention. By this time, any serious prior belief that respiratory abnormalities were a cause of stuttering had largely fallen into disrepute, however, and the detailed pneumographic investigations of Travis and his students were undertaken primarily as studies of symptomatology (see Chapter 1).

The broad conclusions of these and other studies of the breathing movements of stutterers may be briefly stated. During moments of stuttering, one can observe anomalies of a number of different kinds, which were described in Chapter 1.[1] In general, however, these anomalies are not present during silence, and therefore may reflect the speaker's attempts to manage speech or stuttering rather than an underlying causal factor in stuttering. In fact, as discussed in Chapter 14, many studies have reported normalization of respiratory patterns following successful treatment for stuttering (Hasbrouck & Lowry, 1989; Murdoch, Killin, & McCaul, 1989; Story, Alfonso, & Harris, 1996). Furthermore, many of the patterns seen in the speech breathing behaviors of stutterers are also to be found in the breathing of normally fluent speakers during speech production, although not to the same degree.

In studies of stuttering children and adolescents that did not employ typically fluent comparison speakers, Schilling (1960, 1962) observed abnormal diaphragmatic movements during silent breathing. Both Moore (1938) and Kurshev (1968b), however, found that, during silence, stutterers and nonstutterers did not differ in measures of breathing movement. Using measurements of respiratory high-frequency oscillations to appraise metabolic respiratory control in fluent and stuttering adults, Denny and Smith (2000) found evidence that a subset of stutterers showed atypical patterns of respiratory control, but that these differences were not linked to stuttering severity and seemed unlikely to serve as speech fluency disruptors.

As noted, it is relatively easy to observe respiratory differences between fluent and stuttering speakers during speech tasks. Williams and Brutten (1994) are among those who have observed atypical patterns of respiration in pre-speech and speech production by people who stutter: they found atypical timing relationships between respiratory and laryngeal movements, as well as atypical rib cage and abdominal activity when compared to patterns observed in normally fluent speakers. Johnston, Watkin, and Macklem (1993) found similar maladaptive respiratory patterns when comparing fluent speakers and people who stutter. However, it is not clear that these behaviors reflect a root cause of stuttering rather than reflect maladaptive responses to it. In a sense, in the adult who stutters, atypical respiratory postures or sets may in fact precipitate moments of stuttering, even if they were not present at stuttering onset and did not cause its emergence.

Cardiovascular Factors and Basal Metabolic Rate

Heart rate was another object of early laboratory investigation. In 1914, Fletcher observed an acceleration of the stutterer's pulse rate during speech, "in the period anticipatory of speaking and, in general, under those conditions that are calculated to produce stuttering." McDowell (1928) compared stutterers and nonstutterers in average heart rate and blood pressure and found no difference. Travis, Tuttle, and Cowan (1936) observed faster heart rates than normal in stuttering adults before and during speech and, like Fletcher, attributed this chiefly to the emotional reactions and respiratory abnormalities associated with stuttering.

It seemed clear that the cardiovascular changes that had been observed during stuttering were merely symptoms of the disorder. But several years later, studies by Palmer and Gillette (1938, 1939) appeared to indicate that stutterers had both faster

[1] See references in Chapter 1, footnote 12. Although such aberrations are not typically observed at rest, they may occur during expectancy of stuttering (Van Riper, 1936) and possibly also during silent reading and reasoning (Murray, 1932).

heart rates and more sinus arrhythmia[2] than normally fluent speakers even in silence and under basal conditions. Furthermore, unlike typically fluent speakers, among whom there is a sex difference with respect to these factors, the male and female stutterers seemed to have cardiac rates and rhythms that were much alike. Palmer and Gillette speculated that there was a "sex-linked, neurophysiological, metabolic mechanism for stuttering."

Ritzman (1943) replicated this research with refinements in technique. He found no differences between adult male stutterers and fluent comparison speakers in heart rate, sinus arrhythmia, blood pressure, and basal metabolic rate (BMR). Among four female stutterers, however, he found less marked sinus arrhythmia and higher pulse pressure and basal metabolic rate than in the fluent comparison speakers and a definite tendency for them to resemble the male stutterers in these measures, in general corroboration of the observations made by Palmer and Gillette. Ritzman interpreted this as a reflection of more intense sensitivity to stuttering on the part of the female stutterers. McCroskey (1957) found no differences between stutterers and nonstutterers in BMR, but did not report separately on the three female subjects in his group. Golub (1953), whose experimental group was made up solely of males, confirmed Ritzman's finding that their heart rates do not differ from those of nonstuttering males, as did Walker and Walker (1973). But Brunner and Frank (1976) found higher resting pulse rates in both stutterers and successfully treated stutterers than in fluent comparison speakers. The stutterers also had greater fluctuations in pulse rate, as well as sharper increases after work.

Most recently, Alm (2004b) reviewed past work on heart rate in people who stutter and concluded that some individuals show paradoxical slowing of rate limited to stressful speaking situations, probably reflecting past negative speech experiences. However, such patterns do not appear to be universal.

[2] Sinus arrhythmia refers to normal variations in heart rate occurring regularly in the course of the respiratory cycle.

Other Measures of Autonomic Arousal

In addition to heart rate, one may use skin conductance measures to explore whether the person who stutters is more easily aroused, particularly in stressful situations such as speaking. Peters and Hulstijn (1984) could not identify differences in such measures between fluent and stuttering adults, while Baumgartner and Brutten (1983) and Kraaimaat, Janssen, and Brutten (1988) were able to find positive correlations between stutterers' fluency and increased skin conductance.

Biochemical Factors

For a brief period, it appeared that clues to the etiology of stuttering might be found in the chemical makeup of the stutterer's body. This line of inquiry, while not as popular recently as in earlier years, still attracts periodic attention.

Alveolar Carbon Dioxide, Salivary pH and Salivary Cortisol Biochemical research on stuttering owed its beginnings to a belief of Edwin B. Twitmyer of the University of Pennsylvania that the large majority of stutterers were shallow breathers suffering from fatigue or lethargy brought on by insufficient aeration of their blood, and that the rest—a comparatively small number—were for the most part "hyperexcitable psychopaths" who tended to the opposite extreme. Twitmyer had a colleague, Henry E. Starr, who was interested in salivary pH[3] as a measure of states of emotion or excitement. Starr saw an opportunity to test both his own and Twitmyer's assumptions. He reasoned that Twitmyer's lethargic, "subbreathing" stutterers should have a low salivary pH as a consequence of their carbon dioxide (CO_2) excess, and that the "hyperexcitable psychopath" stutterers should have low alveolar CO_2 and high salivary pH. In controlled studies of both types of stutterers, who were

[3] pH is an index of the hydrogen ion concentration: the lower the pH of a solution, the higher the hydrogen ion concentration and the greater the acidity. Salivary pH is believed to be influenced by alveolar CO_2.

presumably selected and classified with Twitmyer's guidance, this is exactly what he found.[4]

Corroborative findings came shortly from a study of the blood cells of stutterers done by one of Twitmyer's students, Max A. Trumper.[5] Trumper based his study on the knowledge that oxygen deficit in the arterial blood results in a compensatory increase in the number and hemoglobin content of the red blood cells. Among a series of 101 cases of stuttering, he identified one-third as shallow breathers. In blood studies of this group he found that, judged by standard medical norms, there was an increased red blood cell count and relatively high hemoglobin.

With regard to salivary pH, there was some further corroboration of Starr's results in findings by Kelly (1932) of pH values that he considered "below the normal range" in a small group of stutterers. Some time later, however, Hafford (1941) obtained findings in direct conflict with those of Starr. She found no difference between stutterers and normally fluent speakers in the distribution of salivary pH values, either under basal conditions or after a period of speech. In addition, she cited unpublished results from the doctoral dissertation of George A. Kopp, completed in 1933, which showed no difference between stutterers and normally fluent speakers in alveolar CO_2, a finding that was confirmed further by Johnson, Young, Sahs, and Bedell (1959). As Hill (1944a) summed it up after an exhaustive review, " . . . that stutterers as a class are in a condition of CO_2 excess is very questionable."

More recently, Blood and Blood (1994) examined baseline salivary cortisol levels and responses to self-selected stressful conditions, such as taking a final college examination, for 11 pairs of typically fluent and stuttering men. Following a stressful situation, stutterers' cortisol levels were significantly higher than those of persons who do not stuffer. However, cortisol responses were similar during the baseline and low-stress conditions to those of persons who do not stutter. This suggests that perceived high stress in persons who stutter can lead to higher cortisol responses. In turn, such hormonal changes may be linked in a bi-directional fashion with higher states of anxiety and panic. This assumption was supported in a follow-up analysis (Blood & Blood, 1997) in which elevation in salivary cortisol levels was correlated with scores on an assessment of communication apprehension: those individuals who showed the highest degree of communication apprehension showed the highest increases in salivary cortisol following imposition of stress.

Chemical Composition of the Blood A second line of biochemical inquiry concerned with blood constituents received its major impetus from the theory advanced by West and his students at the University of Wisconsin that stuttering was the symptom of a metabolic disorder, evidence of which might be found in abnormalities of tissue chemistry. The first general blood analyses of stutterers, however, were reported by Johnson, Stearns, and Warweg (1933) and had a somewhat different theoretical basis. These researchers were concerned with testing the hypothesis that stuttering was due to a form of latent tetany, and their principal objective was consequently to determine whether there was a deficiency of calcium in stutterers' blood. Taking samples from 15 adult male stutterers, they established that, judged by clinical norms, these men were normal in amount of serum calcium as well as such other blood constituents as inorganic phosphorus, potassium, and blood sugar.

In the same year, Kopp (1934) was bringing to completion his extensive biochemical study of stutterers at the University of Wisconsin. Kopp, too, found that the blood chemistry of stutterers was essentially normal by accepted medical standards. But when he compared his stuttering participants with a control group of nonstutterers, he discovered a variety of differences. The stutterers appeared to be not lower, but higher, in serum calcium. They were also higher in inorganic phosphorus and blood sugar and lower in potassium, total protein, albumin, and globulin, and they seemed to differ as well in the degree of relationship between some of these

[4] See Starr (1922, 1928).

[5] Trumper's unpublished study, completed as a doctoral dissertation in 1928, was summarized in detail by Twitmyer (1930).

components. Kopp concluded that stuttering was a manifestation of a disturbed metabolism and suggested that it might one day be possible to control it by dietary means. Somewhat later, however, a study of Karlin and Sobel (1940) disclosed essentially no differences between stutterers and nonstutterers in chemical composition of the blood and failed to confirm the correlations between constituents found by Kopp.[6]

Since 1940, studies of stutterers' tissue chemistry have been comparatively few. Anderson and Whealdon (1941) found that stutterers did not appear to differ from the general population in distribution of blood types and therefore in the proteins controlling agglutination. Lovett Doust (1956) reported stutterers to show more marked changes than normal speakers in oxygen saturation of capillary blood in response to the stress of breath-holding and interpreted this as a sign of less stable oxidative metabolism in the stutterer. Girone and Bruno (1957) found evidence of a possible disturbance of glucose regulation. Galamon, Szulc-Kuberska, and Tronczyńska (1969) reported an increased level of urinary histidine in some school-age children with "hereditary" stuttering. Laczkowski (1965) reported results that appear to contradict this. Finally, Podolskaya and Shklovsky (1973) obtained findings that seemed to point to a heparin deficit in the blood of stutterers and laid the blame for it on "constant and protracted emotional stress."

It is of interest that, after an interval of 25 years, Johnson, Young, Sahs, and Bedell (1959) returned to the hypothesis of latent tetany that had led to the first study of blood constituents and found a convincing refutation of it in the failure of stuttering to increase following hyperventilation. More recently, Sayles (1971) observed that overbreathing produced a decrease in stuttering in many of his subjects, possibly as a result of distraction. Laštovka (1978) found no clinical manifestations of tetany in a group of 28 stutterers.

Rastatter and Harr (1988) measured neurotransmitter and amino acid blood levels in five stutterers and compared them with norms. A consistent abnormal finding was high levels of glutamine in all five subjects.

Although investigations of blood chemistry have been infrequent over recent years, pešák and Opavský (2000) reported decreased serum copper levels in 16 male stutterers that might potentially relate to neuromuscular irritability; copper concentrations showed a negative correlation with stuttering severity. Alm (2005) replicated this study with 16 additional adult stutterers and comparison speakers and found no significant group differences in plasma copper levels or copper-binding protein. Nor did stuttering severity show a negative correlation with plasma copper; in fact, an inverse positive correlation between high plasma copper levels and superfluous motor activity during stuttered events was observed.

Neurotransmitter Levels

In Chapter 4, we discussed a number of studies that have found differences in cortical activity between people who stutter and normally fluent speakers. A few studies have specifically investigated whether dopamine and other neurotransmitter levels are different or differently distributed in stuttering. In addition to providing some explanation for cortical activity differences between groups of speakers, these studies have great relevance to attempts to develop effective pharmacological treatments for stuttering, as discussed in Chapter 14. Both Rastatter and Harr (1988) and Wu et al. (1997) found increased levels of dopamine activity in people who stutter that might affect the activities of brain regions responsible for speech and language formulation. Such findings have had ramifications for the experimental treatment of stuttering using particular classes of drugs known to affect dopamine activity, as we note in Chapter 14.

[6] Among the 22 blood constituents tested, Karlin and Sobel actually found one statistically significant difference: stutterers were lower in potassium. They attached no importance to it, however. By definition, 5 percent of the differences in a large series of correlations of this sort will prove to be significant at $p = 0.05$ simply by chance. Consequently, in current statistical treatments of such large numbers of comparisons, it is typical to use an adjusted and lower p level that is divided either by the number of comparisons or the number of principled hypotheses (also called the Bonferroni correction).

Peripheral Neurophysiological Findings

Neurophysiological investigation of stuttering was pioneered by Lee E. Travis at the University of Iowa. In an intensive research program that occupied the period from about 1927 to 1937, he and his students produced a steady output of laboratory findings. The major focus for this work was provided by the theory, which Travis developed together with Samuel T. Orton, that stuttering resulted from an underlying condition in which the bilaterally paired muscle systems of the vocal tract tended to work independently of each other because of the lack of a sufficient margin of cerebral dominance.

Action Potentials from the Paired Speech Musculatures The Orton-Travis concept led to research in which the bilateral neuromuscular organization of stutterers was studied in various ways. Rigorous test of the hypothesis was afforded by the development of the electromyograph. From a recording of action potentials from the muscles on the two sides of the speech structures, it should be evident whether these muscles are starting their contractions at different times or are acting dyssynchronously in any way. Accordingly, in what was thought to be a crucial test of the cerebral dominance theory, Travis (1934) recorded electrical potentials from the left and right masseter muscles of stutterers and nonstutterers while they were speaking. He found that the recordings from the two sides were essentially identical for almost all of the nonstutterers, as well as for the stutterers when they were speaking normally. During stuttering, however, there were striking differences in the latency of onset of the potentials as well as other bilateral dissimilarities in the patterns in the majority of cases.

Events observed only during the act of stuttering, of course, always tend to raise the troublesome question of whether they are a cause or an effect. Nevertheless, these findings stood as a last support of the cerebral dominance theory long after the research on the laterality of stutterers had created serious objections to it and Travis himself had become absorbed in other etiological concepts. Finally, Williams (1955) replicated Travis's study with some additional aspects of procedure. He found many of the same action potential anomalies that Travis had observed. These anomalies, however, occurred to the same extent in the speech of the nonstutterers when they were "faking" stuttering. Furthermore, he found that they could be produced in silence in both stutterers and nonstutterers by instructing them to perform specific jaw movements.

Reflex Responses Various autonomic reflexes have been tested in stutterers during silence. For many years, Seeman and certain other European writers have commented on evidences of lability, sensitivity, or irritability of the autonomic nervous system in stutterers.[7] Confirmation from controlled studies has been essentially lacking, however. Sovăk (1935) reported normal oculocardiac and positive solar plexus reflexes in the majority of a group of stuttering children and adults. Jacoby (1947) investigated the carotid sinus reflex in stutterers and found it to be normal. Walker and Walker (1973) tested stutterers' autonomic reactivity to stress by measuring the increase in their heart rates following bursts of noise. On the average, their heart rates did not differ from those of nonstutterers in response to the stimulus.

Schilling (1959, 1962) reported electronystagmographic abnormalities in 47 percent of a group of stuttering children. Bruno, Camarda, and Curi (1965) found such abnormalities in 29 of 50 stutterers. Castellini, Salami, and Ottoboni (1972) observed them in 14 of 30 cases. In none of these studies was a control group used. Široký, Langová, Morávek, and Šváb (1978), using a comparison group, found a considerably greater number of saddle-shaped nystagmic jerks in the records of stutterers, whether in silence or speech. In a further study, however, these researchers failed to confirm previous findings of abnormality (Langová, Široký, Šváb, & Morávek, 1979).

Laštovka (1979c) recorded longer durations of the electrically evoked innervation pause[8] in stutterers

[7] See Hogewind (1940), Sedláčková (1963).

[8] A pause that may be induced in the voluntary contraction of skeletal muscle by electrical stimulation of the nerve.

than in nonstutterers. This finding was interpreted as indirect evidence of deviations in the central feedback function of the extrapyramidal system and the cerebellum.

Neilson, Andrews, Guitar, and Quinn (1979) found no differences between four stutterers and six normal speakers in stretch reflexes of the jaw-closing muscles. Stutterers did not differ from fluent speakers in reflex changes in biting force in response to loud noise and tactile stimulation of the lip, tongue, and teeth in research by Smith and colleagues: Smith and Luschei (1983) and McFarland, Smith, Moore, and Weber (1986). Nor were any differences found by McClean (1987) in reflexes of the orbicularis oris inferior and depressor labii inferior muscles in response to cutaneous stimulation.

McLean-Muse, Larson, and Gregory (1988) studied reflex changes in the fundamental frequency of the voice in response to auditory click stimuli (a brain stem reflex) as speakers sustained a tone at a constant pitch and intensity. There were no differences between stutterers and nonstutterers. However, more recently, Guitar (2003) investigated acoustic startle responses in 14 pairs of stuttering and fluent speakers in an attempt to relate reactivity or temperament to stuttering. When startled by white noise bursts, stutterers demonstrated larger magnitude startle responses across the series of repeated stimuli. While a temperament scale (the *Taylor-Johnson Temperament Analysis*) administered to both groups did not distinguish the groups, one subtest (the Nervous subscale) did; however, the startle response better differentiated the participants. Guitar concluded that results were supportive of the hypothesis that "individuals who stutter, as a group, may have a more reactive temperament than nonstutterers" (p. 238). Such findings have been used to develop more recent models of stuttering that include temperament as a factor in its development, as discussed in Chapter 2.

Alm (2006) has investigated acoustic startle within a differing theoretical framework. Because there have been proposals that stuttering represents increased gain in brain stem auditory reflexes (Zimmermann, 1980c), a normal inhibitory function in acoustic startle responses was assessed in 22 pairs of stuttering and normally fluent adults. Approximately 90 msec. before presentation of the normal noise burst that elicits a startle response, a weaker noise was presented; this should diminish the startle response in normal listeners (a function called prepulse inhibition, PPI). PPI was not found to differ between stutterers and fluent adults. Alm and Risberg (2007) continued to explore acoustic startle and its relationship to other potential variables. For 32 pairs of stuttering and fluent adults, no significant group differences were found for startle responses. Nor was startle significantly correlated with trait anxiety. However, the stutterers obtained significantly higher scores for anxiety (as well as childhood attention deficit hyperactivity disorder [ADHD]). In fact, two subgroups emerged, one of which appeared to have family predisposition to develop stuttering while the other did not, but showed evidence of brain trauma in childhood prior to any onset of stuttering symptoms. Alm and Risberg concluded that excessive reactivity was not characteristic of stuttering and that anxiety levels observed in this and other studies are more likely to reflect the speaker's experiences as a person who stutters.

Tremor Herren (1932) studied the occurrence of tremors in the voluntary hand movements of stutterers and normally fluent speakers. He found that during silence as well as speech, a relatively rapid tremor, at the rate of 40 to 75 per second, occurred more frequently in the records of the stutterers. Herren offered no hypothesis to account for this finding. Hill (1944b) suggested that they might be traced in part to increased adrenaline output during stuttering.

McFarland, Smith, Moore, and Weber (1986) found no differences in amplitude of tremor of the jaw-closing muscles as speakers exerted a constant force on a bite block inserted between upper and lower teeth. In a more recent investigation of tremor activity in stuttering, Laštovka (1995) found atypical subclinical tremor in the hand muscles of stutterers during isometric contractions, and concluded that it was due to "reflection tremor, resulting from changes in the function of structures that establish motor feedback, especially in the extrapyramidal and cerebellar field" (p. 322).

Muscular Tension Several different methods have been used to study muscular tonus in stutterers. Travis and Fagan (1928) measured the resistance of the pendant hand to 40-ounce blows. They found that more resistance was offered by stutterers than by normally fluent speakers during silence. This might conceivably have resulted from either situational or chronic "nervous" hypertension among the stutterers. Another inference, however, that was considered by Shackson (1936) is latent tetany. Shackson measured the time intervals between the appearance of action potentials and the beginning of muscle thickening and voluntary movement in various muscles of stutterers and fluent comparison speakers. There was a tendency toward faster muscle contraction in the stutterers during silence, which Shackson interpreted as evidence of chronic latent tetany.

Brown and Shulman (1940) measured muscular tension by determining the pressure needed to inject a minute amount of saline solution into the body of the biceps muscle. Unlike the earlier investigators, they found no evidence that stutterers were more tense than nonstutterers. Body tension as a factor in the etiology of stuttering has not been explored in recent research.

SENSORY AND PERCEPTUAL PROCESSES

Audition

The normal performance of speech activity depends in part on sensory, perceptual, and integrative skills. Is stuttering perhaps basically a receptive disorder? Some have speculated as much, inspired chiefly by the theory that stuttering is analogous to the breakdown of speech under delayed auditory feedback in typically fluent speakers (see Chapter 2).

Auditory Threshold There is an early report by Harms and Malone (1939) that each of 62 stutterers examined by pure-tone audiometry had an impairment of hearing, but a succession of further studies failed to disclose any significant loss.[9] Tomatis (cited by Van Riper, 1982, p. 379) stated that 90 percent of his stutterers had a hearing loss in one ear and related it to a theory involving both auditory feedback and cerebral dominance. Neither Hugo (1972) nor Aimard, Plantier, and Wittling (1966) could find any difference in sensitivity between the left and right ears of stutterers, though Hugo found that the right ears of his stutterers were poorer, on the average, than the right ears of his typically fluent listeners. MacCulloch and Eaton (1971) reported a lowered auditory pain threshold for pure tones in a comparison of 44 stutterers with a group of fluent speakers.

Phase Disparities A literal interpretation of the analogy between stuttering and the delayed auditory feedback (DAF) effect in normal speakers would seem to imply that there is some sort of "built-in" delay in the stutterer's auditory monitoring system. Evidence suggesting that such an aberration might actually exist was obtained by Stromsta (1957). His method made use of the fact that two pure tones of equal frequency and amplitude and diametrically (i.e., 180 degrees) out of phase cancel each other out. Stutterers and normally fluent speakers listened to an air-conducted tone and to a bone-conducted tone of the same frequency simultaneously introduced at the teeth. The participants then varied the phase and amplitude of the air-conducted tone until a critical adjustment was achieved at which no sound was audible to them. Using this procedure at frequencies of 500, 1,000, and 2,000 Hz, Stromsta found that at 2,000 Hz, there was a difference between stutterers and nonstutterers in the average relative phase angle of the air- and bone-conducted sounds as indicated by the amount of adjustment they made.

Later, by the use of a similar method, Stromsta (1972) found an unusual phase disparity between stutterers' left and right ears. His participants adjusted the amplitude and phase of two air-conducted tones heard at either ear until they cancelled an identical

[9] See Bullen (1945), Sternberg (1946), Aimard, Plantier, and Wittling (1966), Asp (1968), St. Louis and Hinzman (1988), among others.

bone-conducted tone. At the point of cancellation, the air-conducted tones at the two ears had a phase disparity at several frequencies about twice as wide, on the average, for the stutterers as for the nonstutterers. Mangan (cited by Gregory & Mangan, 1982) replicated Stromsta's earlier study and failed to find a difference between stutterers and nonstutterers in the phase and amplitude adjustments of air- and bone-conducted sound needed to obtain a null.

Effect of Auditory Feedback on Nonspeech Oral Activity A unique approach to the investigation of the stutterer's auditory feedback mechanism was devised by Stark and Pierce (1970). It is possible to reason that, if stuttering is due to the misinformation that speakers get about their speech movements from a feedback system with an inherent delay, then the same delay should also create problems in their nonspeech activities if we ply them with auditory information about their performance. The rationale that Stark and Pierce gave for their study was not precisely this, but it was closely related to it. They argued that "if abnormal delays were present in the stutterer's speech feedback system, his responses to time delays artificially introduced in the auditory feedback loop would also be abnormal." The essential purpose of their study was to see if stutterers would produce deviant responses under delayed auditory feedback in a simple oral activity such as lip closure. They trained stutterers and nonstutterers to reproduce a sequential pattern of lip closures—silent repetitions of the syllable "muh"—with their lips positioned around an apparatus that generated an audible click with every lip closure. The subjects then performed these temporal patterns under normal, or synchronous, auditory feedback (NAF; sometimes called side-tone), delayed auditory feedback (DAF), and a combination of DAF by air conduction and NAF by bone conduction.

For both the stutterers and the nonstutterers, the delayed feedback conditions produced disturbances in the pattern such as errors, prolonged lip closures, and prolongations of the pattern. In general, however, the effect of DAF was about the same for both groups of speakers. It was only under NAF that any difference appeared—the stutterers tended to have longer lip closures. In addition, a study of individual scores showed that a third of the stutterers made unusually frequent errors under NAF, both in the training period and during the experiment. This is interesting, since it is under synchronous feedback—from the point of view of an outside observer—that stutterers ordinarily have difficulty with their speech. As Stark and Pierce observed, the results were inconclusive, but the method appeared to have promise.

We will return to the issue of auditory feedback and stuttering in Chapters 11 and 14. Perturbed auditory feedback has been used in the treatment of stuttering, and most "devices" sold to ameliorate stuttering operate on the principles of delayed auditory feedback and/or frequency-altered feedback.

Other Evidence of Deviant Auditory Feedback A different kind of evidence of delay in stutterers' auditory feedback systems was sought by Dinnan, McGuiness, and Perrin (1970). By pairing pure tones with electric shock, they conditioned their volunteers to emit a psychogalvanic skin response (GSR) to the auditory stimulus. They then measured the time between the pure-tone signal and the peak GSR response. On the average, it was 0.95 seconds longer for the stutterers than for the nonstutterers. This is several times longer than the most effective delay time for producing artificial stuttering in normally fluent speakers, but the finding is interesting nonetheless.

Neilson and Neilson (1979) found that stutterers had an excessive phase lag between stimulus and response in an auditory pursuit task in which participants had to control the pitch of one tone to match the varying pitch of another by movements of the jaw or hand. In a visual tracking task, by contrast, the performance of the stutterers and fluent volunteers was comparable. Nudelman, Herbrich, Hoyt, and Rosenfield (1987) had four stutterers match the pitch of a tone that varied periodically in frequency by humming. The stutterers' tracking was more out of phase with the signal than that of three nonstutterers.

Fukawa, Yoshioka, Ozawa, and Yoshida (1988) reported that stutterers were more susceptible than nonstutterers to delayed auditory feedback as shown by the effect on their reading rates. Similarly, Jäncke (1991) found a greater lengthening of the stressed vowel of a nonsense word by stutterers under delayed auditory feedback, and also a greater shortening of the vowel when "feedback" was delivered in advance of the utterance. Jäncke suggested that there may be a greater dependence of phonation on hearing in stutterers.

As noted in Chapter 4, Foundas, Bollich, et al. (2004) found atypical asymmetry of the planum temporale (PT) in a number of people who stutter. These people also had uniquely significant responses to delayed auditory feedback: their fluency greatly improved, while stutterers with more typical patterns of PT symmetry did not experience fluency enhancement under DAF.

Tests of Central Auditory Function At an early date, theories linking stuttering to delayed auditory feedback focused the attention of researchers on the clinical integrity of the stutterer's central auditory system. The available diagnostic tests were soon put to use. Rousey, Goetzinger, and Dirks (1959) reported that stuttering children did not perform as well as nonstutterers in making median plane sound localization responses. In a broader study of central auditory function, however, Gregory (1964) found that adult stutterers did not differ for the most part from nonstutterers on tests of sound localization, binaural loudness balance, and discrimination of speech distorted by frequency filtering. Sound localization findings by Kamiyama (1964) and Asp (1968) were in agreement with those of Gregory, although Asp observed some differences on tests of loudness balance and Herndon (1967) found differences in the ability to discriminate between different durations of tone.

These initial efforts, then, produced largely negative results. Since the 1960s, however, a number of more sensitive clinical procedures for evaluating central auditory function have come into use through the work of Jerger and others. Hall and Jerger (1978) compared the performance of stutterers and nonstutterers on a battery of seven such tests. On most of these, the stutterers' responses were normal. There were small differences between the groups, however, on three tests that are especially sensitive: the acoustic reflex amplitude function, synthetic sentence identification with ipsilateral competing message (SSI-ICM), and the staggered spondaic word (SSW) test devised by Katz (1962).[10] Although emphasizing that the overall pattern of the stutterers' test findings failed to suggest "substantial central auditory disorders," Hall and Jerger stated that the pattern was suggestive of subtle central auditory disorder at the level of the brain stem.

A study by Toscher and Rupp (1978), using identification of synthetic sentences with ipsilateral competing message (SSI-ICM), corroborated the findings of Hall and Jerger. Molt and Guilford (1979) also obtained findings essentially identical to those of Hall and Jerger on the synthetic sentence identification test: with a contralateral competing message, the stutterers and nonstutterers did not differ, but with an ipsilateral competing message, stutterers scored lower than nonstutterers, though within the normal range and considerably higher than individuals with known brain stem pathology. Interestingly, Wynne and Boehmler (1982) and Nuck, Blood, and Blood (1987) found that even normally fluent speakers who exhibited some part-word repetitions in their speech had lower scores on the SSI-ICM than those who did not. Only Hannley and Dorman (1982) and Kramer, Green, and Guitar (1987) found no difference on this test.

On the staggered spondaic word (SSW) test, results conflicting with those of Hall and Jerger were reported by Karr (1977), who found no difference between stutterers and nonstutterers. On the other hand, Barrett, Keith, Agnello, and Weiler (1979), although obtaining no differences with central auditory processing tests employing frequency-filtered and time-compressed speech, found a significant difference on the SSW Test. In a study of central auditory function in 8- to 11-year-old stutterers,

[10]The other tests were: the acoustic reflex threshold, performance-intensity functions for monosyllabic (PB) word lists (PI-PB), performance-intensity functions for synthetic sentences (PI-SSI), and synthetic sentence identification with contralateral competing message (SSI-CCM). The tests are described by Jerger (1973, 1975).

G. W. Blood and I. Blood (1984) found no significant difference from nonstutterers on the SSW Test, the *Pitch Pattern Sequencing Test*, the *Competing Environmental Sounds Test*, or on tests involving time-compressed speech, dichotic synthetic syllables, or auditory localization. There was a subgroup of stutterers, however, who performed poorly on the SSW Test and the *Competing Environmental Sounds Test*.

As a result of these conflicting but provocative findings, central auditory function in stutterers has become a well worked area of research with a variety of testing methods. On a sound fusion task, Bonin, Ramig, and Prescott (1985) found that stutterers appeared to require a longer time interval between sounds before they heard them as two sounds; the difference approached statistical significance. In a study by Cohen and Hanson (1975), stutterers performed more poorly than nonstutterers on a test of auditory-visual integration in which listeners were presented with an irregular series of taps and had to select a series of dots having the same pattern.

In a study by Kramer, Green, and Guitar (1987), stutterers performed more poorly than typically fluent speakers on the masking level difference task, a test of brain stem function. Liebetrau and Daly (1981) reported similar results for a subgroup of "organic" stutterers who had positive signs on the *Michigan Neuropsychological Test Battery*. In a series of studies, Howell and colleagues (Howell, Rosen, Hannigan, & Rustin, 2000; Howell & Williams, 2004; Howell, Davis, & Williams, 2006) have found some evidence of poorer auditory performance under various listening conditions, including backward masking for children who stutter and for persistently stuttering children compared to children who spontaneously recovered from stuttering.

Anderson, Hood, and Sellers (1988) obtained negative results with the *Phonemic Synthesis Test*, which evaluates a subject's ability to fuse separate phonemes into words, and on the *Binaural Fusion Test*, in which high and low frequency components of a spondaic word are presented simultaneously to different ears. In a study by Hageman and Greene (1989), there was no significant difference between groups on the *Revised Token Test*, but the stutterers performed more poorly on a competing message task derived from the test. Meyers, Hughes, and Schoeny (1989) found that stutterers did not differ from comparison speakers in judging which ear received the stimulus first when syllables were presented in pairs to both ears with different degrees of asynchronization between ears. Harris, Fucci, and Petrosino (1991) found that in scaling the magnitude of tones of different intensity, stutterers tended to use a restricted range of numerical values.

Finally, some research has been done on stutterers' speech discrimination and listening ability. A study by Bright (1948) appeared to show that stutterers had some difficulty on tests of listening ability involving discrimination between vowels and comprehension of paragraph material. On the other hand, Welch (1961) found stutterers to be normal in listening proficiency. Hugo (1972) likewise found no differences in speech discrimination ability except that, unlike Spielberger (1956), he found that stutterers seemed to have lower perceptual thresholds for some of their previously stuttered words.

Auditory Evoked Potentials In a study of slow cortical auditory evoked responses, Molt and Luper (1983) found that stutterers had faster average peak latencies than normally fluent speakers. Finitzo, Pool, Freeman, Devous, and Watson (1991) observed lower amplitudes in stutterers for all of the three major components of the auditory evoked potential. More research has been done on the early latency potentials known as the auditory brain stem response (ABR), with conflicting results. Neither Decker, Healey, and Howe (1982) nor Newman, Bunderson, and Brey (1985) observed any notable differences. I. M. Blood and G. Blood (1984) recorded longer Wave III and Wave V latencies for stutterers and abnormal interpeak latencies for five of eight stutterers. Stager (1990) found that stutterers as a group did not differ from comparison speakers on any of the latency and amplitude measures of brain stem auditory pathway intactness, but 5 of the 10 stutterers were abnormal on at least one of these measures. Smith, Blood, and Blood (1990) found no differences in latencies, but greater amplitude of Wave I for stutterers.

Middle Ear Muscle Activity Research on stutterers' middle ear muscle function has yielded relatively little. As we have seen, Hall and Jerger (1978) found a small difference between stutterers and typically fluent speakers in the acoustic reflex amplitude function. They found no difference in the acoustic reflex threshold. Neither did Delaney (1979) in a study of 4- to 14-year-old children. In Delaney's study, little if any difference appeared in the latency of onset and the rise time of the reflex. The stutterers did, however, show greater amounts and rates of middle ear muscle contraction. Hannley and Dorman (1982) observed no difference in the latency or amplitude of the reflex. Mangan (cited by Gregory & Mangan, 1982) found no significant difference between stutterers and nonstutterers in the relaxation and adaptation of the acoustic reflex.

Horovitz et al. (1978) found that the threshold of reflex response of the middle ear muscles to sound was significantly lowered by induced anxiety in stutterers, but not in normally fluent speakers. Since studies have shown that these muscles contract just prior to speech, the authors speculated that a relationship may exist between anxiety and subtle distortions of auditory feedback in stutterers. Howell, Marchbanks, and El-Yaniv (1986) found no difference between stutterers and normally fluent speakers in middle ear muscle activity during vocalization.

Lombard Sign Panconcelli-Calzia (1955) found the Lombard sign in only 27 percent of a group of 80 stutterers, as compared with 78 percent of a group with typical voice and speech. This is in conflict with a considerable amount of research showing that most stutterers do increase the loudness of their voices under masking noise.[11]

Prevalence of Stuttering among Deaf Persons In connection with the subject of audition in stutterers, it is of interest that there appeared to be an unusually low prevalence of stuttering in oral schools for deaf children in two independent surveys by Harms and Malone (1939) and Backus (1938). While some stuttering was evidently to be found, it seemed particularly rare among the pupils who had little residual hearing. Montgomery and Fitch (1988) reported a prevalence of stuttering of only 0.12 percent from a questionnaire survey of schools for the deaf. Of the 12 stutterers identified, 6 were said to stutter only in signing.[12]

Varying interpretations have been offered. Shane (1955) suggested that the parent of a deaf child is relatively unlikely to become concerned about the child's fluency. Others have related this finding to the absence of auditory feedback in persons without hearing, and this has served to raise the question whether it is necessary to have some ability to monitor the sounds of one's speech in order to become a stutterer. Since both stuttering and congenital hearing impairment are now known to have genetic influences, it is also possible that these two relatively rare conditions do not typically co-occur for reasons that have little to do with the role of audition in stuttering.

Vision

Stutterers as a group appear to have normal visual acuity.[13] In a comprehensive visual study, Hamilton (1940) found that they were also normal in phoria, binocular perception, and color vision.

Visual Perseveration Eisenson and Winslow (1938) noted a tendency toward visual perseveration in adults who stutter. In recording colors successively exposed by means of a tachistoscope, they more often than nonstutterers erroneously named colors that had been shown earlier in the series. Goldsand (1944) also obtained evidence of visual perseveration in the adaptation that stutterers made to a bright light. On the other hand, neither Sheets

---

[11] Adams and Moore (1972), Adams and Hutchinson (1974), Conture (1974), Dewar, Dewar, and Anthony (1976), Yairi (1976), Brayton and Conture (1978), Mallard and Webb (1980), Martin, Siegel, Johnson, and Haroldson (1984).

[12] The manual stuttering was variously described as easy, effortless repetitions; repetitions of the first syllable, perseverations, blocking, and choppy manipulations; beginning a sign, then stopping and repeating the sign.

[13] McDowell (1928), Hamilton (1940), Schindler (1955).

(1941) nor King (1961) found definite confirmation of such a tendency. While the results may appear quite inconsistent, it should be noted that essentially none of these studies was an exact replication of others, and in most cases widely differing tests were used. Research on perseveration in human behavior has cast doubt on the assumption that such a thing as sensory perseveration as a general factor exists; the various tests that have been devised for the purpose of studying it do not seem to measure the same thing.[14]

One of the measures that King used in evaluating sensory perseveration in stutterers was the critical flicker frequency threshold. This is the lowest rate at which a flickering light appears steady or continuous. The lower the threshold, the more lasting the after-image and the greater the presumed perseveration. Lovett Doust and Coleman (1955) reported that stutterers were lower than nonstutterers in critical flicker fusion threshold. No differences were found by King (1961) or Kamiyama (1964). Subsequently, Sayles (1971) again found a lower flicker fusion point in stutterers, which West interpreted as evidence of muscular hypertonicity (West & Ansberry, 1968, p. 124).

Perception of Visual Symbols Kelly (1932) found that stutterers had far greater difficulty than comparison speakers in a test of "visual aphasia," in which two pairs of digits were exposed successively and the participant was required to find in the second pair the digit that did not appear in the first pair. Spadino (1941), however, found no differences in errors of visual perception when volunteers said or wrote words or numbers flashed on cards. Furthermore, stutterers compared favorably with nonstutterers in speed and comprehension of silent reading in a study by Hamilton (1940) and have generally been found to have normal levels of reading achievement, as is seen in Chapter 9.

Prevalence among Blind Persons Finally, we may note that in a survey of schools for blind and partially sighted children, Weinberg (1964) found a prevalence of stuttering essentially within the range of expected values for the general population.

Touch and Kinesthesis

Schilling and Biener (1959) reported that in many stutterers, there seemed to be a marked difference between the thresholds of vibratory sensation in the left and the right extremities, while this difference appeared very rarely in their observations of nonstutterers. Fucci, Petrosino, Gorman, and Harris (1985) had participants adjust the magnitudes of a vibrotactile stimulus to the hand and tongue to correspond to a scale of six random numbers. Stutterers and nonstutterers performed the task similarly for the hand. For the tongue, however, the stutterers used a narrower range of intensity adjustments, which the experimenters interpreted as a more "conservative" scaling behavior. Harris, Fucci, and Petrosino (1991) again reported that stutterers used a more restricted range of responses and lower vibrotactile magnitude values for the tongue. In addition, Petrosino, Fucci, Gorman, and Harris (1987) reported that stutterers showed slightly higher thresholds of sensation at three tongue sites, but gave no data.

A study of the oral sensory and perceptual abilities of stutterers and nonstutterers by Jensen, Sheehan, Williams, and LaPointe (1975) showed no differences in intra-oral two-point discrimination, weight discrimination, or interdental thickness discrimination. In subsequent studies of oral recognition of forms, Martin, Lawrence, Haroldson, and Gunderson (1981) found that stutterers made more errors; Zsilavecz (1981) reported the same, but presented no data; and Stewart, Evans, and Fitch (1985) obtained somewhat equivocal findings. Carpenter and Sommers (1987) found that stutterers discriminated forms both orally and manually as well as nonstutterers, except while hearing words to be written down.

In a study of the kinesthetic acuity of stutterers, De Nil and Abbs (1991) instructed participants to make the smallest possible movements of the jaw, lower lip, tongue, and index finger. Without visual

[14] See discussions of this question by King (1961) and Martin (1962).

feedback, the stutterers made larger minimal displacements of the oral structures, but not the finger, than the nonstutterers.

SUMMARY REMARKS

We have now reached the end of three chapters that discuss the many studies that have contrasted stutterers and typically fluent speakers on an almost innumerable list of physical features and behaviors. Young (1994) once lamented the limitations of an exceedingly common type of research design in which the question is whether an average difference exists between groups of individuals. The studies we have reviewed in this chapter have been based almost exclusively on this design. No doubt, this goes far to explain why this research has been plagued from the beginning by conflicting and inconclusive findings. Yet despite the frustrating inconsistency of evidence concerning the stutterer's physical constitution, some of it has gathered so much weight that it urges us toward a number of broad negative and positive conclusions.

During silence, stutterers appear to be essentially similar to normally fluent speakers with regard to various respiratory, cardiovascular, biochemical, and neurophysiological measures, despite isolated and unconfirmed reports of certain differences. With regard to most types of motor ability, including gross physical, manual, and oral skills, the results have been inconclusive. A notable exception, as discussed in the last chapter, is phonatory initiation time, in which stutterers, on the average, have repeatedly been observed to lag behind nonstutterers. Why they do, and whether the lag is related to an overall slowness in reaction time, is as yet undetermined.

On the average, stutterers appear to achieve poorer scores on certain sensitive tests of central auditory function, and they have tended to exhibit less expected right-ear advantage on dichotic listening tests employing meaningful linguistic stimuli (see p. 122). It is also possible that many stutterers are atypical in cerebral dominance for language as evidenced by their cortical potentials during speech processing. How such traits might be related to stutterers' slower vocal initiation, and how any of them might be related to stuttering, are questions that we have hardly begun to speculate about.

As we grope for meaning in these findings, it is important to keep in mind the overlap existing between stutterers and nonstutterers whenever physical differences between them have appeared. In other words, despite group trends to the contrary, some stutterers exhibit faster vocal reaction times, greater right-ear advantage in dichotic listening tests, and the like, than some nonstutterers. This fact precludes any simple explanation of the group differences.

The overlap between stutterers and nonstutterers has been interpreted occasionally to imply the existence of subgroups of stutterers with different etiologies. On this basis, for example, investigators sometimes attempt to distinguish between "organic" and "functional" stutterers. A simpler, more parsimonious way of thinking about the overlap is to relate it to the most fundamental question we can ask regarding the etiology of a disorder: What are the conditions both necessary and sufficient to bring it about? Imagine a physical trait, say slow reaction time, in which stutterers as a group differ on the average from normal speakers as a group. Clearly, any overlap in the trait between the groups rules out the trait as a sufficient condition; if the trait, or a given amount of it, were sufficient to produce stuttering, no nonstutterers would have it in that amount. Likewise, the overlap rules out the trait as a necessary condition; if the trait were necessary to produce stuttering, no stutterer would lack it.

It follows that none of the possible or probable differences we have glimpsed between stutterers and nonstutterers represents a necessary or sufficient condition for stuttering. If the differences are not caused by stuttering, or by something else that causes stuttering as well, they may be factors that often contribute, along with others, to the etiology of the disorder in ways that will be better understood when the necessary and sufficient conditions are known. For all that the evidence has told us so far, the necessary and sufficient conditions for stuttering may yet be found in a realm far removed from those we have explored in these chapters.

Chapter 7

The Person Who Stutters: Personality

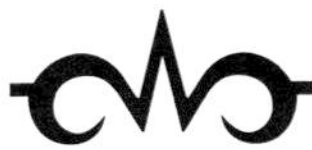

Sometime during the 1930s, a sweeping wave of interest in personality, emotional adjustment, and the psychological aspects of human illness that had been gathering momentum since the beginning of the twentieth century broke on the scientific investigation of stuttering, and from then on for a period of about 25 years, much of the search for a common distinguishing feature of the person who stutters centered on factors of personality makeup. As we shall see, the popularity of this line of research has declined over more recent years, although it has left a lasting legacy that impacts how stuttering is viewed by some disciplines.

ADJUSTMENT

The basic question motivating most of the research on the stutterer's personality was whether the average stutterer is to be regarded as a neurotic or severely maladjusted person on the basis of the criteria typically used to make such a determination. This might not appear to be such a difficult question, but the answer was notably elusive for more than 50 years and, even now that we can look back on enough research to make some judgments possible, they are not made with complete assurance.

In 1928, there appeared what was apparently the first published study of the emotional adjustment of stutterers.[1] This was part of an investigation

[1]An earlier study by Marion McKenzie Font, done under the direction of John M. Fletcher in 1924, was published in 1955 as Chapter 34 in Johnson and Leutenegger (eds.), *Stuttering in children and adults*. It was an administration of the *Kent-Rosanoff Word Association Test* to 9 stutterers and to 49 nonstuttering University of Iowa students. No sharp distinction appeared. Anderson (1923) made use of 40 words from the *Kent-Rosanoff Test* in an early exploration of certain perceptual, psychomotor, and other abilities of stutterers. In a study by Travis (1928b), stutterers were given a word and asked to write word associations as quickly as possible. The stutterers performed faster alone than in a group, just the opposite of Gordon Allport's findings on nonstutterers.

by Elizabeth McDowell that made use of several devices for measuring emotional adjustment, including the *Kent-Rosanoff Word Association Test* and two early personality inventories, the *Woodworth-Matthews* and *Woodworth-Cady* questionnaires. The questionnaires contained such items as, "Does it make you uneasy to cross a bridge over water?" "Do you talk in your sleep?" "Are you bashful?" Administering these tests to stuttering and nonstuttering children in the New York City public schools, McDowell found essentially no difference in degree of adjustment between the two groups. These conclusions were substantiated by Johnson (1932) in a study of stutterers among University of Iowa students. Johnson found that on the *Woodworth-House Mental Hygiene Inventory*, the stutterers scored as well as House's normal subjects, on the average, and tended to have distinctly more favorable scores than a group with a diagnosis of psychoneurosis whom House had tested.

In 1939, however, Bender reported results in marked disagreement. In a study of City College students with the use of the *Bernreuter Personality Inventory*, he found that stutterers tended to be more neurotic, more introverted, less dominant, less self-confident, and less sociable than nonstuttering students. Bender's findings were difficult to ignore. He had tested a very large number of stutterers, he had employed a control group of his own in place of the risky practice of comparing participants' scores with published test norms, and he had availed himself of what was then one of the newest and most highly regarded of adjustment inventories. Yet, despite all this, detailed inspection of his results reveals that an exceedingly important qualification must probably be attached to his conclusions. The stutterers' poorer performance on the *Bernreuter Inventory* was due largely to their responses to 16 test items on which the two groups of people differed significantly. Of these items the great majority put a considerable premium on adequate speech or penalized subjects in some way for being stutterers. The following are some examples:

- Do you find it difficult to speak in public?
- If you are dining out do you prefer someone else to order dinner for you?
- Do you consider yourself a rather nervous person?
- Are you often in a state of excitement?
- Can you usually express yourself better in speech than in writing?

The *Bernreuter Inventory*, of course, did not lie about the stutterer's adjustment. In a very real sense a person whose capacity for speech is impaired is maladjusted by virtue of that problem. This was not, however, what most research workers wanted to know. When Brown and Hull (1942) tested stutterers with the *Minnesota Personality Scale* three years later, they confirmed the view that stutterers tend to be poor in social adjustment as opposed to most other areas of emotional health (e.g., "morale," "family relations," "emotionality"), and the same pattern has continued to show itself in greater or lesser degree in successive research studies whenever the test used has permitted distinctions of this kind to be made.

During the 1940s the scientific study of the stutterer's personality gained ground rapidly. Further research was done with adjustment inventories of improved design (see Table 7-1) as well as with so-called projective techniques, which will be discussed shortly. Work on the stutterer's adjustment was dominated by the *California Test of Personality*. In three separate studies, the stutterers consistently fell below the test norms. The *California Test* analyzed a subject's performance on the basis of 12 categories of self-adjustment and social adjustment. Although there were disparities among the findings, all three agreed in marking stutterers low in the categories of self-reliance, freedom from nervous symptoms (of which stuttering was counted as one), and social skills.

Personality research on stuttering reached a peak in the 1950s. An outstanding development was the use of the *Minnesota Multiphasic Personality Inventory (MMPI)*. Unlike earlier personality inventories whose content was largely determined by professional judgment, the *MMPI* consisted of items empirically derived in research on psychoneurotic subjects, and it was standardized with careful attention to factors of reliability and validity. Furthermore, the studies in

TABLE 7-1 Adjustments of Stutterers and Nonstutterers as Measured by Personality Inventories

	N			
	Stutterers	Controls	Test	Results
McDowell (1928)	46	46	Woodworth-Matthews, Woodworth-Cady	No clearly significant differences were found.
Johnson (1932)	50		Woodworth-House	The stutterers did not differ from the test norms and were superior in adjustment to House's phsychoneurotic group.
Fagan (1932)	33		Woodworth-House	Mild degrees of maladjustment were found in the majority.
Bender (1939)	249	303	Bernreuter Personality Inventory	The stutterers gave significant indications of maladjustment in nearly all areas tested. In particular, they had more fears, worries and tensions, were less communicative, and were more dependent and hesitant in decision.
Brown and Hull (1942)	59		Minnesota Personality Scale	The stutterers had low scores in the area of social adjustment, but not in morale, family relations, emotionally, or economic conservatism.
Perkins (1947)	75		California Test of Personality	The stutterers revealed problems that appeared to fall consistently within the areas of self-reliance, feelings of personal worth, nervousness, social skills and social standards.
Schultz (1947)	20		California Test of Personality	The stutterers fell below the test norms, on the average, in total adjustment. They scored poorly in self-reliance, freedom from withdrawing tendencies, nervous symptoms, and social skills.
Cypreansen (1948)	14		California Test of Personality	The median of the group fell below the norm in each part of the test except one: sense of personal freedom. The greatest differences were in self-reliance, freedom from nervous symptoms, social skills, school or occupational relationships, and community relationships.
Horlick and Miller (1960)	26	30	California Test of Personality	The stutterers had slightly but not significantly lower adjustment scores than the normally fluent speakers.
Prins (1972)	66	23	California Test of Personality	The stutterers appeared to have better adjustment, on the whole, than the control group which consisted of subjects with other disorders of speech. They tended to score low in social skills, but high in social standards. There was no relationship between adjustment and either severity of stuttering or age.
Silverman and Zimmer (1979)	10	10	California Test of Personality	Female stutterers were compared with normally fluent females; their scores were found to be similar. Male stutterers gave evidence of lower self-esteem than female stutterers.

(*continues*)

TABLE 7-1 (*continued*)

	N			
	Stutterers	Controls	Test	Results
Richardson (1944)	30	30	Guilford Inventory of Factors STDCR	The stutterers were more socially introvertive, more depressed, and had fewer happy-go-lucky tendencies (rhathymia). There were no differences in thinking introversion and cycloid tendencies.
Shames (1951)	53		Guilford Inventory of Factors STDCR	The stutterers differed significantly from the norms only on "T" (thinking introversion).
Duncan (1949)	62	62	Bell Adjustment Inventory (Home Adjustment Items)	Of the 35 home adjustment items, 5 significantly differentiated a group of stutterers from a group of persons with articulation impairments. The stutterers indicated the feelings, among others, that their parents did not understand them, were disappointed in them, and treated them as children.
Bearss (1951)	23	23	Adams Personal Audit, Rotter Incomplete Sentences Blank	No differences were found between the stutterers and nonstutterers on either test.
Brutten (1951)	16	16	Maslow Test of Insecurity	No significant differences were found.
Thorn (1949)	21		Minnesota Multiphasic Personality Inventory (MMPI)	The scores fell within the normal range, and the composite MMPI profile revealed no evidence of neuroticism. There was no common "personality type" when the profiles were analyzed for "pattern" or any substantial difference in composite profile for the most severe and least severe stutterers.
Pizzat (1951)	53	1,400	Minnesota Multiphasic Personality Inventory (MMPI)	The stutterers had poorer scores on all clinical scales except Psychopathic Deviate, but the scores fell within the normal range.
Dahlstrom and Craven (1952)	100	100	Minnesota Multiphasic Personality Inventory (MMPI)	The stutterers were less well adjusted than a group of 100 college freshmen, but were not as severely disturbed as a group of psychiatric patients and most closely resembled a group of college students who had sought counselling because of personal problems.
Boland (1953)	24	24	Minnesota Multiphasic Personality Inventory (MMPI)	Degree of neuroticism as measured by the Neuroticism Index failed to differentiate stutterers from nonstutterers. Stutterers were higher in measures of anxiety.
Walnut (1954)	38	52	Minnesota Multiphasic Personality Inventory (MMPI)	On all 10 clinical scales the stutterers were well within the normal range as measured by the MMPI norms. On 2 scales, Depression and Paranoia, the stutterers had significantly poorer scores than the normally fluent speakers.

Lanyon, Goldsworthy, and Lanyon (1978)	69		Minnesota Multiphasic Personality Inventory (MMPI)	Stutterers' scores showed no relationships to measure of overt stuttering behavior or attitudes toward stuttering of anxiety or avoidance.
Sermas and Cox (1982)	19		Minnesota Multiphasic Personality Inventory (MMPI)	Although 14 subjects had an elevated score on at least one MMPI scale, no significant elevation was found when the scores were averaged for the group.
Darley (1955)	28	18	Rogers Test of Personality Adjustment	More of the stuttering children had scores indicative of maladjustment, especially in the categories of social maladjustment and daydreaming. Note of the differences in mean scores was statistically significant.
Sergeant (1962)*	60		Bell and Bernreuter Inventories	The stutterers had poorer social adjustment, less self-confidence, and greater emotional instability than normally fluent speakers. This was also true in large measure of the other speech groups with speech problems studied, however.
Wingate (1962b)	70		Edwards Personal Preference Schedule	Mild to moderate maladjustment was found in the area of social relationships.
Anderson (1967)*	50	50	Guilford-Zimmerman Temperament Survey and Gordon Personal Profile	The stutterers did not differ from the controls in general emotional stability. The stutterers, however, tended to be more shy, less self-assured, friendlier, and more respectful toward others.
Hegde (1972)	106		Eysenck Personality Inventory	The stutterers scored high on introversion, close to the anxiety group. On neuroticism they scored within normal limits, though 4 points higher than the norm, on the average.
Thomas (1976)	8	8	Eysenck Personality Inventory	The stutterers were higher in neuroticism and lower in extraversion, though both groups scored within normal limits.
Okasha, Bishry, et al. (1974)	50**	50	Junior Eysenck Personality Inventory	The stutterers, aged 8 to 12 years, were more introverted than their controls, but there was no difference in neuroticism.
Cohen, Thompson, et al. (1975)	36	46	Rathus Assertiveness Schedule	The stutterers scored significantly lower in assertiveness than the fluent comparison group.
Sermas and Cox (1982)	19		Revised Hopkins Symptom Checklist (SCL-90-R)	When compared with a group of nonpsychotic psychiatric patients, the stutterers had poorer scores on the Interpersonal Sensitivity Scale.
Greiner, Fitzgerald, et al. (1985)	41	41	Revised Willoughby Personality Schedule	The stutterers scored higher in social anxiety and sensitivity, though there was considerable overlap between the groups.

*Cited by Bloch and Goodstein (1971).
**Values of *N* are approximate.

which it was administered to stutterers for the most part made use of comparison groups, a practice not often followed before. The results of these investigations produced a very satisfactory measure of agreement (see Table 7-1). By and large, stutterers showed a consistent tendency toward slightly less favorable adjustment than nonstutterers, but their scores, on the average, fell well within what is regarded as the normal range. This was demonstrated in a particularly clarifying manner by Dahlstrom and Craven (1952), who found that college stutterers were less maladjusted as a group than psychiatric patients, were not significantly more maladjusted than ordinary college freshmen, and performed most similarly to college students who had applied for counseling with personal problems.

Various other "pencil and paper" tests have been employed in the investigation of the stutterer's adjustment, as is evident in Table 7-1. Rarely, if ever, have these studies revealed in stutterers as a group the recognized patterns of psychoneurotic disturbance that belong to such relatively well-defined nosological categories as anxiety, depression, obsessive-compulsiveness, or the like. On the other hand, signs of mild social maladjustment have been found frequently.

PROJECTIVE TEST FINDINGS

The study of adjustment as defined by a questionnaire yields a rather limited view of personality. For many years psychologists had been attempting to construct tests that would achieve more penetrating insights into the nature of individual character structure. Generally speaking, such attempts have proceeded on the assumption that our observable behavior must almost always contain important clues to our personality makeup, provided we are in a situation in which essentially no conventional or socially conforming responses are possible. Such "projective" tests have frequently proved to be of value to clinical workers who are skilled in their interpretation, particularly in the context of the clinical setting with the opportunities it affords for verification of test findings by means of interviews, personal observation, and other tests.

The chief disadvantage of the projective tests is that it has been difficult to develop them technically for the purpose of obtaining scientifically objective, valid, and reliable measures. In short, when subjects show a given pattern of responses on such a test, there is unfortunately not always sufficient assurance that they would show them again on future occasions, or that another clinical worker would agree on the interpretation of the responses, or that the responses actually mean what they are said to mean. As a result, projective tests in their present form have been the subject of considerable controversy, and generalizations about stutterers based on such tests must be viewed with some degree of caution.

Rorschach Research

Of all projective techniques of studying personality the most extensively developed is the well-known *Rorschach Test*. This consists of a series of ink blots, some in color, that are presented to the subject with the question, "What might this be?" From a variety of features of the subject's perceptions, inferences are drawn about such specific personality traits as capacity for abstract thinking, habitual concern with details, egocentricity, spontaneity, emotional stability, and so forth. This widely used test has been administered to stutterers repeatedly with findings that are conflicting and generally inconclusive.

Perhaps the earliest of these studies that could be considered a scientific investigation in any accepted sense of the term was reported by Meltzer (1934). Meltzer analyzed the *Rorschach* responses of 56 stuttering children and found little that was indicative of serious emotional disturbance. He wrote, "Unlike the problem children reported by Beck they are not repressed and do not lead restricted inner lives. To the small extent that neuroticism is suggested it takes what may be called an 'expressive' rather than repressive form." By contrast, Ingebregtsen (1936) found substantial evidence of neuroticism in a *Rorschach* study of adult stutterers.

Both of these studies were essentially clinical in nature and did not employ comparison groups. In 1944, however, Meltzer compared 50 stuttering children with 50 nonstutterers of like age, sex, and IQ on the basis of over 20 different commonly used scores or indicators of various types derived from their *Rorschach* records. There was essentially no distinction between the two groups with regard to the great majority of these indicators. In three instances, however, a significant difference did appear. One of these could be interpreted to mean that the stutterers exercised somewhat poorer "control of intellectual functioning," and the other two suggested that they had somewhat greater capacity for abstract thinking. Since the two groups had been carefully matched with respect to intelligence, Meltzer concluded that the poorer intellectual control of the stutterers was of an emotional origin and that the indications of increased capacity for abstract thinking actually represented compulsive behavior to compensate for their insecurity. He pointed out that the stutterers exceeded the nonstutterers in almost every measure usually indicative of emotional instability, but these differences were for the most part very small and not significant in any statistical sense.

In the same year that Meltzer's findings appeared Richardson (1944) reported a study that tended to corroborate Meltzer's essential finding that there were very few differences in the *Rorschach* responses of stutterers and nonstutterers. Richardson, in fact, failed to find even the three differences that Meltzer had noted. She did discover, however, that in her group of 30 adult stutterers, 7 made no use of movement or color in their responses while this was true of only 2 of the 30 nonstutterers, and she concluded that the stutterers showed a tendency not to "recognize their inner promptings" or to "respond impulsively to their outside environment."

Two years later, Krugman (1946) came to conclusions that went considerably beyond those of Meltzer and Richardson. He compared 50 stuttering children with 50 children who had behavior problems, and his basic finding was that the two groups did not differ significantly on most scores. In addition, on the basis of a qualitative evaluation of the stutterers' records, he reported that most of them were "seriously disturbed," that they tended to be emotionally immature and repressed, that they showed many signs of "neurotic involvement," and that one of their outstanding characteristics was their "obsessive-compulsive make-up."

Sheehan and Zussman (1951) found that stutterers exceeded nonstutterers in such tendencies as drive toward achievement, overemphasis on suppressive control, and intellectual defenses against anxiety as expressed in Rorschach responses. In related *Rorschach* and *Thematic Apperception Test (TAT)* studies at the University of Southern California, D. M. Wilson (1950) and Christensen (1952) obtained few findings that appear to lend themselves readily to the interpretation that stuttering children were basically neurotic or markedly different from the siblings with whom they were compared. By contrast, Moller (cited by Bloch & Goodstein, 1971) found many more signs of maladjustment among stuttering boys than among predelinquent boys, including lower self-awareness and empathic ability, poorer interpersonal relationships, and higher anxiety.

It is clear from these studies and observations that a large amount of disagreement is permitted either by the *Rorschach Test* or by the manner in which it has been used in research with stutterers. In reviewing these studies, Goodstein (1958) pointed out instances in which diametrically opposite findings were used by different workers to reach the same conclusions. In another review, Sheehan (1958b) commented that for many researchers "the *Rorschach* has seemed to offer an amorphous flux from which any desired interpretation could be pulled."

Feinberg, Griffin, and Levey (2000) suggested that one reason for the lack of clear findings from *Rorschach* testing could be the assumption of homogeneity of stutterers' profiles. They subgrouped 30 stutterers into tonic and clonic subtypes, and observed some significant differences on Rorschach sub-scores between the two groups, suggesting that clonic stutterers have relatively lower object relational capacities, diminished reality testing, and increased indicators of somatization.[2] They interpreted their findings to suggest that therapy prognosis

[2] Tonic stutterers also outscored clonic stutterers in verbal IQ, as measured by the *WAIS-R*.

might be better for tonic than for clonic stutterers, who they felt were more psychologically ready for the therapy process. Additionally, because tonic stutterers' profiles were characteristic of relatively obsessive-compulsive personality characteristics on their test battery, Feinberg et al. speculated that these speakers might benefit more from pharmaceutical treatments based on selective serotonin reuptake inhibitors.

TAT Studies

The *Thematic Apperception Test (TAT)* is another well-known projective technique that consists of a series of pictures around each of which the subject is asked to make up a story indicating what is happening, the events that led up to it, the thoughts and feelings of the characters, and the outcome. The interpretation of the test is concerned essentially with the basic needs, strivings, and attitudes revealed in the subject's productions. In a *TAT* study of adult stutterers, Richardson (1944) found no significant differences between stutterers and normally fluent speakers in proportions of needs, reactions to frustrations, attitudes toward environment, adequacy of the central character, and unsatisfactory endings. In one of the few personality studies that have been done on preschool stutterers, however, Porterfield (1969) found that on the *Children's Apperception Test (CAT)* adaptive mechanisms of repression-denial, symbolization, and projection-introjection differentiated stutterers from normal controls, but not from a group of maladjusted children. Wyatt (1958, 1969) used pictures from the *TAT* and *CAT*, as well as a story completion test, with a group of 5- to 9-year-old stutterers and their controls; blind evaluations of the records by three judges disclosed significant distance anxiety in the stutterers—that is, fear of separation from their mothers. Following on Wyatt's construct, Klaniczay (2000) used interview data from children who stutter and their mothers to suggest that stuttering emerged from the children's frustrated need to cling to their mothers.

In other investigations the *TAT* has been used chiefly for the purpose of testing hypotheses about specific character traits of stutterers. The findings of these and other projective studies will be more appropriately considered in the sections that follow.

After a period of broad exploration of the stutterer's personality and adjustment, the emphasis gradually shifted to studies of more specific personality dimensions. Although we will attempt to treat these dimensions individually, it will be understood that many of the findings with which we are concerned in the remaining discussion of the stutterer's personality are in various ways interrelated and overlapping, and the logic we impose on them in this way is somewhat arbitrary.

Much of this research represented efforts to verify the psychoanalytic postulates of such writers as Coriat, Fenichel, and Glauber (see Chapter 2). It was therefore concerned in large part with the constructs of sex and aggression and consisted in essence of attempts to identify in the stutterer's personality the classic symptoms of early psychosexual fixation (i.e., covert expressions of infantile libidinous, dependent, and aggressive needs, and their guilty repression).

Oral and Anal Eroticism

Among the most direct attempts to study repressed pregenital sexuality in stutterers have been those that made use of the *Blacky Pictures Test*. This test, originally designed as an aid in the objective testing of psychoanalytic hypotheses, consists of a series of cartoons depicting events of psychosexual interest in the life of a dog named Blacky. The subject is asked to tell a story about each cartoon and to answer such questions as, "What was Blacky's main reason for defecating there?" "How will Blacky feel about eating when he grows older?" In a study by Dickson (1954), stutterers significantly exceeded nonstutterers in scores indicative of anal fixation on the *Blacky Pictures Test*, and a tendency toward oral fixation approached significance. Merchant (cited by Blum & Hunt, 1952) found that stutterers showed evidence of disturbance in such *Blacky* dimensions as oral eroticism, oral sadism, castration anxiety, and penis envy, and concluded that their performance was in agreement with psychoanalytic theory. In a similar investigation, Carp (1962) obtained equivocal findings.

On the *TAT*, Lowinger (1952) found no difference in orality between stutterers and controls. Christensen (1952), however, noted that stutterers gave more projections involving nursing at the breast.

Passive-Dependency

Shopwin (1959) found that adult male stutterers did not differ from nonstutterers in responses to the *Kessler PD Scale*, a questionnaire designed to reveal passive-dependency. Katz (1966) investigated dependency and immaturity in 50 young stuttering children and 50 typically fluent peers by means of the *Structured Doll Play Test*. By means of mother, father, and child figures, the children were presented with a series of situations in which they had to make choices on behalf of an ego doll between bed and crib, glass and bottle, toilet and potty, and also between father and mother for purposes of feeding the ego doll, putting it to sleep, coming to its bed after a nightmare, and the like. Katz found no evidence of greater dependency or immaturity among the stutterers. The only difference she observed was that the stutterers made somewhat more father choices than the nonstutterers in dependency situations.

Obsessive-Compulsive Character Traits

Anal-sadistic fixation, most frequently mentioned in psychoanalytic writings as the basis of stuttering, is characterized by manifestations ranging from "anal" character traits (excessive orderliness, stinginess, punctuality, acquisitiveness, moral rectitude) to the symptoms of obsessive-compulsive neurosis.

Rapaport (1946, p. 443 ff.) described a series of distinctive features of the *TAT* stories of persons with obsessive-compulsive character makeup. These include concern with unessential detail, expressions of doubt or uncertainty, incorrect or ostentatious use of imposing words, criticism of the picture, psychological pseudo-insights into the behavior of the characters, and various others. Using Rapaport's descriptions, Bloodstein and Schreiber (1957) drew up a checklist of obsessive-compulsive characteristics. Transcripts of the *TAT* stories of adult stutterers and nonstutterers were then evaluated and scored independently on the basis of the checklist by three untrained judges, two of whom had no clue to the identity of the stories as belonging to stutterers or nonstutterers. The stutterers showed no greater tendency toward obsessive-compulsive behavior than the nonstutterers.

In a study of anal fixation by Keisman (1958), adult stutterers and normally fluent speakers rated themselves on a checklist of personality characteristics that included anal traits. In addition, Keisman used an *Anal Interest Picture Test* on which the criterion was the length of time the subject looked at pictures containing anal interest (e.g., a man counting bags of money) as opposed to neutral pictures. The findings were largely negative. The only qualified support for the psychoanalytic hypothesis was in the finding that the stutterers took more time to rate themselves on all traits, anal as well as others. In another study of anal fixation in stutterers, Fisher (1970) obtained somewhat equivocal results. On the semantic differential, word stimuli were rated similarly by stutterers and nonstutterers on dimensions with anal reference, such as clean-dirty. As predicted, however, the two groups assigned significantly different meanings to pictures representing anal scenes.

Hostility and Aggression

In Freudian theory, a fundamental consequence of anal-sadistic fixation is the storing up of latent hostility and the distortion of hostile expressions by guilt and anxiety. From this point of view, there is unusual interest in a series of investigations of stutterers employing the *Rosenzweig Picture-Frustration Study*. This test is made up of a series of cartoons in each of which a person is depicted making a verbal response in a frustrating situation—for example, being splashed with mud by a passing car. The response is supplied by the person taking the test. Interpretation is concerned with the manner in which the subject appears to be in the habit of coping with his or her own hostile impulses—for example, with whether aggression is turned outward, is turned inward, or is unexpressed or denied.

Using the norms of the *Rosenzweig P-F Study* for purposes of comparison, Madison and Norman (1952) found that 25 stutterers performed precisely as many psychoanalysts would have predicted. As a group, their responses revealed less tendency to cope directly with frustrating obstacles, greater inclination to turn aggressive reactions against themselves, and greater tendency to be preoccupied in a compulsive way with the solution of the problem creating the frustration. Madison and Norman concluded, "These findings seem to correspond to the psychoanalytic contention that stuttering is essentially compulsive in nature, with anal-sadistic tendencies resulting in a turning inwards of aggression." On the other hand, a study by Murphy (1953) using a control group produced almost diametrically opposed findings. Murphy's stutterers seemed to show more direct aggression outward against the frustrating person or agent and to show more self-defensive responses. Finally, Lowinger (1952) and Quarrington (1953) found that groups of stutterers showed no departure at all from the test norms, while both Seaman (1956) and Emerick (cited by Bloch & Goodstein, 1971) failed to find any differences between stutterers and normally fluent individuals.

There is clearly little in the results of these studies to indicate that stutterers as a group tend to have neurotic conflicts involving aggression. Research using the *TAT* has also produced equivocal findings. D. M. Wilson (1950) found that stuttering children appeared to be extremely aggressive and to have more inverted hostility than their nonstuttering siblings, as judged by *TAT* projections. But Lowinger (1952) found no significant difference between stuttering and nonstuttering children in intensity of unconscious aggressive drives. Solomon (cited by Bloch & Goodstein, 1971) found that adult stutterers did not differ from fluent adults on the *TAT* with respect to broad categories of aggression, but that they did express more themes involving subtler, less violent aggression. Porterfield (1969), on the other hand, failed to find any difference in aggression between preschool stutterers and nonstutterers on the *CAT*. McHale (1967) did not use the *TAT* pictures, but analyzed the written stories of stuttering and nonstuttering children for the needs expressed; he found no support for explanations of stuttering in terms of aggression.

On the *Blacky Pictures Test*, Eastman (cited by Bloch & Goodstein, 1971) obtained only partial confirmation of the hypothesis that stuttering children would show repressed hostility. On the *Rorschach Test*, however, Santostefano (1960) found clear evidence of unusual degrees of hostility in adult stutterers. The instrument he used was Elizur's *Rorschach Content Test (RCT)*, a validated method of diagnosing anxiety and hostility from the content of a speaker's responses to the ink blots. Hostility is revealed by such responses as "two men fighting," "a tiger leaping on its prey," "gun," "teeth," and other explicit expressions or cultural symbolisms of aggression. Adult stutterers demonstrated distinctly higher scores for hostility on the *RCT* than did adult nonstutterers.

Santostefano did not ascribe the difference to psychosexual fixation. Like Abbott (1947), he hypothesized that the stutterer tends to accumulate anger as a result of the frustrations of being a stutterer. The facts will support either explanation. But there is, in principle, a type of further investigation that might serve to tip the balance in favor of one or the other. The psychoanalytic hypothesis requires that the stutterer's hostility exist to a large degree in repressed form; the other does not require this as an inevitable development, even though it takes into account a normal tendency for aggression to be repressed. Criminals and delinquents tend to "act out" their aggressions; they are persons who tend to exercise too little rather than too much repressive control over their hostility. Consequently, it appears unlikely that many such persons would be stutterers if stuttering is primarily the symptom of anal-sadistic repression. The information we have on this question is meager, but suggests that there is little if any difference in the prevalence of stuttering between the criminal and noncriminal population.[3] It is true that in a study of over 2,000 case histories

[3] Fleischman (1946), Gildston (1959).

of children with behavior difficulties Schroeder and Ackerson (1931) found that stuttering appeared to be more characteristic of the shy, sensitive, inadequate child than of the child with aggressive conduct traits. On the other hand, fighting and overaggressive behavior ranks high in frequency among the findings of several studies of symptoms of maladjustment in stuttering children, as we will see later in this chapter.

Although little work has been carried out over the past half century to pursue the possibility that stuttering is associated with anal-sadistic tendencies, Plankers (1999) used a case study of a single socially withdrawn German adult male stutterer to suggest that such a fixation was at the root of his patient's fluency problem. After psychoanalysis, the patient was reportedly more fluent (although no data are provided), and was even reported to have an improved sperm count. However, the author notes that there is no obvious reason in his or other historical cases (e.g., Freud, Fenichel) why only some documented anal-sadistic conflicts result in stuttering.

Guilt

The presence or absence of guilt has been directly implied in most of the findings we have already discussed under the heading of psychosexual fixation. To a small extent, guilt has been investigated independently of other factors as a relatively persistent feature of the stutterer's personality. Lowinger (1952) found no significant difference between stuttering and nonstuttering children in projections of guilt on the *TAT*, although there appeared to be a tendency for the stutterers to be more guilt-burdened. Adams and Dietze (1965) studied stutterers' reaction times in giving written associations to words suggesting five different kinds of emotion. The stutterers reacted more slowly than the nonstutterers to all categories, including neutral words and those connoting joy. But the category that proved to be a major source of the stutterers' greater slowness were the words pertaining to guilt (i.e., "guilty," "sinner," "blamed," "misdeed").

Murphy (1999) observes that many chronic disorders engender feelings of both guilt and shame in patients and their families. He suggests that such emotions are normal consequences of living with stuttering and may require attention in counseling and treatment programs.

Somatization

As we will note in our discussion of theories of stuttering in Chapter 2, the fact that stuttering has an onset in childhood and is sometimes seen to follow some form of disruption in the child's typical daily lifestyle has raised the possibility for some professionals that stuttering might be an extreme form of somatization to trauma, a conversion reaction.

There is no doubt that hysterical conversion reactions exist, and some have been linked to stuttering onset. However, all published case studies, including those by Roth, Aronson, and Davis (1989) and Mahr and Leith (1992) involve sudden onset of stuttering in adults, while, as noted in Chapter 3, the vast majority of stuttering emerges in childhood, primarily between the ages of 2 and 4 years. Moreover, the fluency symptoms in adult psychogenic cases are not consistent with developmental stuttering and typically involve stereotypical repetition of only initial or stressed syllables, which is not ameliorated by conditions known to improve fluency in developmental stuttering, such as choral reading, altered feedback, or repeated trials (the adaptation effect). Mahr and Leith (1992) also observed that secondary (accessory) stuttering behaviors are usually absent in such cases. Hurwitz (2004) notes that in the majority of conversion cases (whether the patient develops blindness, motor weakness, seizures, or any variety of symptoms) that it is precisely because physical symptoms are inconsistent with the typical organically based condition that one can diagnose a psychogenic component.

Can preschool children experience conversion reactions? The published consensus appears to be no. In 1981, Goodyer noted that hysterical conversion reactions do not present prior to 5 years of age (and are more common in girls, the reverse gender distribution of stuttering). In a comprehensive review and series of case reports, Zeharia et al. (1999) confirm this gender bias and suggest that conversion is unlikely to appear before late childhood or adolescence. Consistent with the findings in Roth et al. and Mahr and Leith, most conversion patients have accompanying symptoms of major affective illness (e.g., depression), which is uncommonly diagnosed in toddlers. Whether or not children who stutter have had more traumatic or "trying" experiences than those who do not stutter has never been systematically investigated, but a small study by Hill (1999) showed that matched pairs of recent-onset child stutterers and fluent peers did not differ on a measure specifically designed to measure potential childhood stressors.

CHILDHOOD TEMPERAMENT

Lewis and Golberg (1997) found little support for some stereotypical views of stuttering children as temperamentally vulnerable after administering the *Parent Childhood Temperament Questionnaire for 3–7-Year-Olds* to parents of 11 stuttering children and gender- and age-matched comparison children. A discriminant analysis significantly discriminated the groups, resulting in correct classification of 86.36 percent of the 22 children. However, on the discriminating dimensions, the profile was indicative of more positive temperament for at-risk children than for their fluent peers.

In contrast, Anderson, Pellowski, Conture, and Kelly (2003) found statistically significant differences in parental ratings of 31 pairs of stuttering and fluent children between the ages of 3 and 5 years.[4] In this study, the authors used the *Behavioral Style Questionnaire* (McDevitt & Carey, 1978). Children who stutter were judged by parents to exhibit temperamental profiles more typically consistent with hypervigilance (i.e., less distractibility), nonadaptability to change, and irregular biological functions. The authors cautioned that such profiles could exacerbate stuttering or maintain it, but did not posit a role for these attributes in the etiology of stuttering behaviors. In contrast, Schwenk, Conture, and Walden (2007) found stuttering children to be more distractible in a laboratory situation and less able to adapt to change in the environment, both qualities that might also impact their ability to maintain fluency in challenging situations.

[4] The authors also summarize a number of unrefereed conference papers that additionally suggest differences between children who do and do not stutter, as well as measures of temperament and their associated outcomes in typically developing children.

SELF-PERCEPTIONS

Self-Concept

An important development in the study of personality is that concerned in various ways with images, perceptions, and evaluations of the self. In the numerous applications that have been made to stuttering, few theories of etiology have been put to any critical test. Fiedler and Wepman (1951), who conducted the earliest self-concept research on stutterers, were in fact concerned with the hypothesis that stutterers have a characteristic view of themselves because of the social handicap of stuttering.

Most of the self-concept studies employed a unique device known as the Q-technique. The subject is presented with a set of cards on each of which is a different statement describing a personality trait—for example "I feel bored," "I am always alert," or "I believe in fate." The procedure followed is best described by quoting from Fiedler and Wepman's instructions to their subjects:

> *Here are 76 statements which people have used to describe themselves. Please sort them into eight categories consisting of 1, 5, 12, 20, 12, 5 and 1 statements. Place the statement which describes you best in the first pile, the five next most descriptive statements into the second pile, and so on until you come to the one statement which is least applicable to you. Be sure each category contains exactly the right number of statements.*

If the statements, having been forced into a normal distribution, are now given scores corresponding to their categories, the entire sort may be appropriately correlated with the sort of any other subject. Furthermore, the array of intercorrelations among a whole group of subjects, or between the subjects of two different groups, may be computed and averaged to yield measures of the congruence of their self-concepts.

By this method, Fiedler and Wepman determined that the self-concepts of a group of stutterers, based on a set of 76 descriptions of personality traits by Murray, could not be differentiated from those of a group of nonstutterers. In addition, the stutterers' self-concepts were found to resemble those of a group of clinical psychologists, a "theoretically well-adjusted" group, more closely than they resembled those of a group of mental hygiene clinic patients.

The Q-technique has considerable versatility. The participant's sort may be correlated not only with those of others, but also to good advantage with further sorts by the same person. In one of the most frequent applications of this procedure, individuals arrange the statements once in accordance with their "actual" self-concept and again with reference to how well the statements describe how they would like to be. The amount of correlation between their "actual" and "ideal" self-concepts is then taken as a measure of their "self-acceptance" and contributes to an evaluation of their emotional adjustment. The studies of Wallen (1960) and Gildston (1967) have shown adolescent stutterers to be lower in self-acceptance than nonstutterers in this way, while Rahman (1956) found a tendency toward less self-acceptance in college stutterers that did not reach significance. It would appear that stutterers' concepts of themselves may not correspond as well with their ideals, generally speaking, as do those of nonstutterers when investigated by the Q-technique. Using conventional inventory methods of measuring self-acceptance, Berger (1952) obtained somewhat equivocal results, while Redwine (1959) found no evidence of less favorable self-concepts in stuttering children. Zelen, Sheehan, and Bugental (1954) found that stutterers undergoing group therapy expressed more positive feelings about themselves than did nonstutterers in a study employing the W-A-Y (Who are you?) technique.

Carrying applications of the Q-technique a step further, Wallen (1960) also had his subjects perform a "how I think others see me" sort and correlated this with their "actual" self-concepts. There was more disparity between the two in the case of the stutterers.

A different kind of study of the stutterer's self-concept, making use of the semantic differential and a type of repertory grid, was reported by Fransella (1968). Her essential findings were that stutterers typically see themselves differently from the way they see other stutterers. They tend to view other stutterers much as nonstutterers do, but tend to view themselves as unique individuals.

A study of 91 members of a national stutterers' self-help organization by Kalinowski, Lerman, and Watt (1987) employed a semantic differential devised by Woods and Williams (1976). The stutterers' self-perceptions did not differ significantly from those of a normally fluent comparison group.

In an extension of Fransella's work and the construct of self-concept, DiLollo, Manning, and Neimeyer (2005) examined the "meaningfulness" of fluent and disfluent speaker roles in a group of 29 adult stutterers. The authors used textual analysis to examine the complexity of the participants' cognitive constructs of what is involved in the role of a fluent speaker as opposed to one who stutters. The goal of this study was not to contrast the self-concepts of people who do and do not stutter. However, the authors suggest that therapy to enhance self-concept as a fluent speaker might be a useful addition to more traditional therapies in achieving carryover of fluency behaviors.[5]

Level of Aspiration and Achievement Drive

One way of studying a person's self-concept is to determine how realistic it is by comparing it with the actuality. In a sense, this is done in microcosm in level of aspiration tests. These consist of a series of trials in a test of skill, after each of which participants are asked to predict their score on the next trial. The average discrepancy between their prediction and their last performance is taken as a measure of their aspiration level. Research by Sheehan and Zelen (1955) using the *Rotter Level of Aspiration Board* and by Mast (1952) using the *Carl Hollow Square* suggested that, in general, the stutterers were less inclined than the nonstutterers to attempt what they were not sure they could do. Their attitudes, in short, tended to be somewhat overly cautious or

[5]A summary of research relevant to identity construction in the context of stuttering is provided by Daniels and Gabel (2004).

defeatist, presumably to defend against the threat of failure. On the other hand, Emerick (cited by Bloch & Goodstein, 1971) found that they did not differ from nonstutterers in goal-setting behavior as measured by the *Cassel Group Level of Aspiration Test.* Moreover, Kaiser (cited by Keese & Fischer, 1976) found no difference between stutterers and controls in a level of aspiration test based on Heckhausen's labyrinth task.

These findings are inconsistent, but more than 20 years after his study using the *Rotter Board*, Sheehan (1979) replicated it with a group of female stutterers with the same results: The subjects showed higher levels of aspiration than female stutterers had evinced in the earlier study, but they still set lower goals than typically fluent women. Stutterers also appeared to have lower levels of aspiration on a goal attitude inventory compiled by Trombly (1965).

If stutterers do have a tendency toward low levels of aspiration, this hardly seems consistent with the high achievement drives that are sometimes attributed to them on the basis of general observation or theory. Other data on this question are conflicting. Sheehan and Zussman (1951) found indications of a greater drive toward achievement in stutterers on the *Rorschach Test*. But in a study by Goodstein, Martire, and Spielberger (cited by Goodstein, 1958) stutterers did not differ from nonstutterers on two independent indices of motivation for achievement on the *TAT*. In another application of the *TAT* by Braun (1974), stuttering schoolchildren scored higher in hope for success and did not differ from control subjects in fear of failure. Luper and Chambers (1962) found adult stutterers to be overly sensitive to criticism and fearful of failure on a projective test in which subjects were required to identify "liked" and "disliked" photographs of people. Stutterers also showed greater failure anxiety than nonstutterers on the *Achievement Motivation Test* in a study by Peters and Hulstijn (1984).

Body Image

Since its introduction for this purpose by Machover in 1949, the drawing of the human figure has been widely used as a projective personality test. Its usefulness is based in part on the assumption that when individuals respond to the request to draw a person, they tend to draw a picture of themselves and that the drawing consequently contains expressions of their body needs and conflicts.

In a comparison of the figure drawings of stuttering, maladjusted, and normal adolescent boys by R. G. Wilson (1950), the stutterers' drawings, like those of the maladjusted group, contained omissions and conflict indicators and tended to be poor in movement, likeness to human beings, and detail. Putney (1955) found few differences in the self-drawings of stutterers and nonstutterers, while Fitzpatrick (1960) was concerned mainly with the distorted self-image of stutterers when asked to depict themselves in a speaking role. DePlatero (1969) found that, in comparison with normally fluent children, stuttering children tended to produce heavy body outlines "as a defense against the menacing exterior."

Glassmann (1967) submitted the figure drawings of stuttering and fluent children to three clinical psychologists for their independent, blind evaluation. The judges, each of whom employed the draw-a-person technique routinely in diagnostic work in the children's unit of a mental hospital, used a five-point scale to rate each drawing for anxiety, hostility, compulsivity, dependency, and self-concept inferiority. No significant differences were found between the two groups of drawings. The only difference approaching statistical significance was a slight tendency for the stutterers' drawings to be rated lower in compulsivity than those of the nonstutterers.

In a study of five stutterers aged 5 to 10 years, Devore, Nandur, and Manning (1984) employed the *House-Tree-Person Technique* and elicited drawings depicting both self speaking and a person of the opposite sex. The stutterers' tendency to draw smaller figures than those drawn by fluent children was interpreted as suggesting feelings of inadequacy. Their placement of the figures off-center toward the left of the page was said to suggest a tendency to withdraw or shun new experiences. These differences did not appear on retesting after 12 weeks of treatment for stuttering.

Chapter 1 illustrates some more recent studies of drawings made by stuttering children and adults.

However, such work, including Stewart and Brosh (1997) and Lev-Wiesel, Shabat, and Tsur (2005), has tended to focus on the insight such drawings provide regarding the affective and cognitive consequences of stuttering rather than on the basic personality attributes that such drawings might reveal. As in Devore, Nandur, and Manning's study, Stewart and Brosh (1997) noted changes in self-drawings following therapy that appeared to reflect positive changes in affect and cognition regarding themselves and the challenges of speaking.

Body image may be studied by other means than figure drawing. Pienaar (1968) scored the *Rorschach Test* responses of stutterers for awareness of body boundary and awareness of body interior. The stuttering children tended to score higher on the body boundary index than either children with articulation difficulties or those who spoke normally. Pienaar thought that either the stutterers' speech impairment tended to increase their concern about their body or more basic factors might be involved.

Role Perception

Buscaglia (1963) found that adolescent stutterers had difficulty perceiving their own life roles as well as the roles of others on the *Sarbin-Hardyck Role Perception Test*. However, in a study by Sheehan and Lyon (1974), there were no differences between stutterers and nonstutterers on this test. Broida (1963) made use of a number of projective techniques as well as a questionnaire administered to parents and teachers to investigate the sex role preferences of stuttering children. She reported several apparent deviations from the expected, including evidence of some ambivalence in sex role identification.

EXPRESSIVE BEHAVIOR

It is a familiar observation that people are often identifiable by their speech or handwriting or by the way they walk, laugh, or gesture. From this observation has grown an approach to psychological diagnosis that contrasts with both structured tests and projective devices, the study of so-called expressive behavior.

One of the best-known examples of this approach is the *Bender Visual-Motor Gestalt Test*, which approaches personality from the standpoint of the individual's perception and organization of visual stimuli as revealed in their copying of patterns. On this test, which is sensitive to both emotional disturbance and brain damage, Burleson (1951) found no significant differences between stuttering and normally fluent children. Likewise, Porterfield (1969) found that preschool stutterers did not differ from typically fluent preschoolers, but did differ significantly from a maladjusted group. R. G. Wilson (1950), however, reported that stutterers resembled maladjusted nonstutterers in "a certain motor ineptness" on the *Bender-Gestalt Test*, in figure drawing, and on Mira's *Myokinetic Psychodiagnosis* (a test of expressive movement involving the drawing of lines while blindfolded).

Handwriting Analysis

There has long been some serious interest in handwriting as an example of expressive motor behavior, although conflicting opinions have been expressed about its usefulness in the study of personality. On the basis of clinical observation, Roman (1960) suggested that stutterers' handwriting tends to be untidy, clumsy, obstructed in fluency and continuity, and marked by interruptions and repetitions. This view was not supported by a study of the quality of stutterers' handwriting by Spadino (1941), however. Eisenson (1937) found a tendency, too small for statistical significance, for stutterers to cross out more words than nonstutterers in written composition.

Painting

Laczkowska (1965) compared the watercolor paintings of stuttering and nonstuttering boys of the same elementary school grades and observed that in 80 percent of the cases, the stutterers preferred cool colors such as blue, green, brown, black, or purple, while the nonstutterers tended to prefer warm colors. She interpreted this to signify a tendency on the part of the stutterers to repress their inner feelings.

Language Style

In a broad sense, the highly personal ways in which people use language may be regarded as kinds of expressive behavior. Felstein (1950) found evidence of anxiety and poor social adjustment in the type-token ratios (number of different words in relation to total number of words) and verb-adjective ratios derived from language samples of stutterers and nonstutterers. Knabe, Nelson, and Williams (1966), however, were not able to observe any differences in similar measures of language behavior. Krause (1982) reported smaller type-token ratios for stutterers than nonstutterers in conversational speech, but suggested that their more restricted repertoires of words might have been a strategy for coping with stuttering.[6]

Other linguistic measures applied in research on the stutterer's personality have been concerned with the meanings and affective connotations of words as perceived by the speaker. Spriestersbach (1951) found indications of mild degrees of social maladjustment among stutterers whom he compared with normal and psychotic individuals with respect to the ratings they assigned to pictures as appropriate illustrations of evaluative words such as "good," "funny," "interesting," and the like. Fransella (1965) made use of the semantic differential, a technique developed by Osgood in which the subject is presented with a series of words and instructed to rate each of them on various evaluative scales, indicating, for example, the extent to which the thing referred to by the word is interesting or boring, difficult or easy, true or false, and so forth. Fransella reported that stutterers used the extreme positions of the scales more often than normally fluent speakers, a tendency that had also been observed in persons designated as psychotic or neurotic, as well as in intelligent, anxious individuals. This is consistent with the finding of Peterson, Rieck, and Hoff (1969) that stutterers assigned higher semantic differential ratings than did nonstutterers. In a study of conversational behavior, Krause (1982) found stutterers reluctant to use words indicating "even a rather moderate emotional involvement."

[6] Chapter 8 also raises the possibility that such profiles might reflect subtle depression of expressive language skills.

SOME BASIC RESPONSE TENDENCIES

Anxiety

Various attempts have been made to study anxiety in stutterers as a characteristic feature of behavior, independently of its arousal in speaking situations, and various kinds of evidence of what appears to be anxiety have been found. The findings have not been conclusive, but the methods employed have differed so widely that in all probability several unrelated things have been measured.

Anxiety Questionnaires Some researchers have tried to assess the stutterer's chronic anxiety level by means of questionnaires, with generally negative results. Boland (1953) succeeded in finding evidence of a higher level of general anxiety in stutterers than in nonstutterers by making use of two indices derived from the *MMPI*, *Welsh's Anxiety Index*, and the *Taylor Manifest Anxiety Scale*. Negative findings were obtained by Berlinsky (1955) on the *Saslow Screening Test*, by Agnello (1962) and Cox, Seider, and Kidd (1984) on the *Taylor Manifest Anxiety Scale*, by Molt and Guilford (1979) and Miller and Watson (1992) on the *State-Trait Anxiety Inventory (STAI)*, and by Peters and Hulstijn (1984) on the neuroticism scale and the neurotic somatic complaints scale of the *Amsterdam Biographical Questionnaire*.

These were all studies of adults. Andrews and Harris (1964, p. 78) found no difference between stuttering children and their controls on *Sarason's General Anxiety Scale for Children*, but in another study of stuttering children, Pukačová (1973) reported increased anxiety on the *Taylor Manifest Anxiety Scale*.

On the *Likert Social Anxiety Schedule*, stutterers scored higher in social anxiety than a normally fluent comparison group, but significantly lower than a group of "social phobics" in a study by Kraaimaat, Janssen, and van Dam-Boggen (1991). Mahr and Torosian (1999) utilized three separate measures of anxiety to appraise characteristics of 22 adults who stutter and comparison speakers; they found the stutterers to be significantly more anxious, but not to the degree that would be characteristic of social phobics.

Interview Findings Stein, Baird, and Walker (1996) used results from structured interviews to suggest that a number of stutterers suffer from social anxiety. Craig, Hancock, Tran, and Craig (2003) randomly surveyed over 4,500 Australian households to identify people who stutter, and verify their speech status by interview. Once identified, the trait anxiety subscale of the *State-Trait Anxiety Inventory* was administered by telephone interview. Trait anxiety was significantly higher for those who stutter than fluent comparison speakers. Treatment history affected anxiety scores: those who had a history of treatment scored higher on trait anxiety. However, severity of stuttering was not related to trait anxiety scores. The authors interpreted findings to suggest that chronic stuttering may lead to higher levels of anxiety.

Projective Measures Santostefano (1960) obtained indications of higher general anxiety in stutterers by means of a projective technique, the *Rorschach Content Test*. Anxiety is measured on the RCT by the frequency of such responses to the blots as "a fearful monster," "a little girl running in terror," "snakes," or "blood." Moller (cited by Bloch & Goodstein, 1971) also reported greater anxiety among stutterers in a Rorschach study.

Physiological Measures In a different kind of study, Berlinsky (1955) obtained physiological measures of evoked anxiety. The subjects performed a pursuit task in which they were required to manipulate a moving spot of light within a circumscribed area under threat of electric shock, while records were made of skin conductance, pulse rate, and amplitude of respiration. Under the conditions of the experiment, the stutterers proved to have lower pulse rates, but higher respiratory rate and amplitude than the nonstutterers as well as a different pattern of relationships among the measures. For the most part, the measures were not significantly related to each other. The results clearly served to call attention to some of the problems involved in defining anxiety.

Gray and Karmen (1967), using a colorimetric index of palmar sweating, found no evidence that stutterers responded with excessive anxiety in a nonverbal situation. Their study did not attempt to introduce unusual stress. Horovitz et al. (1978) induced anxiety by having participants imagine themselves in a stressful situation such as an oral examination in which questions were being asked very rapidly. Galvanic skin response (GSR) measures showed that this was effective in evoking anxiety, but stutterers and nonstutterers did not differ in mean GSR.

Peters and Hulstijn (1984) recorded adults' heart rates, pulse volumes, and skin conductance in anticipation of and during nonverbal tasks (mirror writing and items from the *Raven Intelligence Test*). Stutterers and fluent comparison speakers did not differ.

Behavioral Measures Santostefano (1960) investigated anxiety evoked by laboratory stress using disruption of a previously learned response as a measure of anxiety. Subjects first learned a series of digit-symbol associations. They were then required to respond with a written word association to each of a list of words consisting in part of such "threatening" stimuli as "penis" and "intercourse." The assumption was that these would arouse anxiety and hostility. Following each word association, one of the digits was presented and a measurement was made of the amount of time the subject took to respond with the appropriate symbol. There was a general tendency in both stutterers and nonstutterers for the threat words to result in reduced efficiency of the learned responses, but this effect proved to be greater in the stutterers.

Santostefano interpreted these findings to mean that the stutterers were made more anxious and hostile by the stressful conditions. This use of both terms is important and clarifying. It would be possible to add "guilty," and perhaps others. The point to be emphasized is that physiological or behavioral measures in themselves do not permit us to make such distinctions. The distinctions can only be inferred from the experimental conditions or from study participants' reports. Such measures of "anxiety" are perhaps better referred to as measures of autonomic arousal. Brutten and Shoemaker (1967, p. 53) reviewed literature that supports a thesis of genetic differences among individuals in threshold of autonomic response to stress and discussed this in relation to stuttering from a theoretical point of view. It is within the realm of possibility that in Santostefano's work, and perhaps in some findings of Boland and Berlinsky, there is a clue to a tendency toward higher levels of autonomic reactivity in many stutterers.

Conditionability There is evidence that anxious individuals are more readily conditioned than others and that anxiety, autonomic reactivity, and conditionability are related.[7] Moore (1938) conditioned adults to expect an electric shock following a recorded nonsense syllable and studied the effect on their breathing movements. He noted that the stutterers were not differentiated from their fluent peers by conditionability. On the other hand, Thomas (1976) compared the conditioning of the galvanic skin response in stutterers and nonstutterers in a nonspeech situation and found the stutterers to be more conditionable.

Defense Preference Prins and Beaudet (1980) studied the defense mechanisms of 16 stutterers as revealed by the *Defense Preference Inquiry* for the *Blacky* pictures. For each picture, the stutterers rank-ordered five statements representing alternative possible reactions of the dog Blacky to threatening psychosexual stimuli. The five statements in each class represented the defense mechanisms of regression, projection, intellectualization, reaction formation, and avoidance. Prins and Beaudet found that the stutterers' mean profile of preference for the five defensive styles was identical to the profile reported for American college students.

Rigidity We have already touched tangentially upon certain types of rigidity in discussing motor perseveration and obsessive-compulsive character traits. The tendency to retain habit patterns may be measured in various ways. In a study of rigidity by Solomon (1952), stutterers apparently did not differ from nonstutterers in the solution of problems requiring flexibility of attitudinal set, except in an oral test (hidden word puzzles) in which they showed more rigid behavior. Kapos and Standlee (1958) found no differences between stutterers and nonstutterers in an index of behavioral stereotypes in successive operations of a complex multiple-choice electromaze. In his study of perseveration in stutterers, King (1961) employed three tests of dispositional rigidity. Stutterers did not differ significantly from the nonstutterers on any of the tests. A representative example of these tasks was the working of simple addition, subtraction, multiplication, and division problems in which the mathematical symbols had assigned meanings different from their common ones.

It is evident that rigidity is a term to which a number of different meanings may be given. Schaie (cited by Wingate, 1966a) developed a test of behavioral rigidity based on three major dimensions of the trait, which he isolated by means of factor analysis. One of these, which he termed motor-cognitive, is seen in adjustments to shifts in familiar patterns and continuously changing situational demands. An example is a test in which the subject writes antonyms for each of a series of words, then synonyms, and finally antonyms for words printed in lowercase and synonyms for words printed in capitals. A second factor is tested by relatively simple psychomotor tasks, while a third is tested by means of a questionnaire containing such items as, "Do you feel strongly inclined to finish what you are doing in spite of being tired of it?" Schaie's *Test of Behavioral Rigidity* was administered to stutterers by Wingate (1966a), who found that they were distinctly more rigid than nonstutterers in the motor-cognitive area. His findings appear to be in conflict with the results of King's dispositional rigidity tests and with findings on motor perseveration in adult stutterers discussed in Chapter 5.

Suggestibility The information we have on the suggestibility of stutterers is scanty, but interesting. It comes chiefly from an investigation by Kelly (1935),

[7] See the discussion of such evidence by Brutten and Shoemaker (1967, pp. 52, 53).

who administered the *Otis Suggestibility Test* and the *Hull Postural Sway Test* to 42 stuttering schoolchildren and 42 matched typically fluent children. On both tests, the stutterers scored markedly higher in suggestibility. Ingebregtsen (1936), too, reported low resistance to suggestion as an experimental finding in a study of a group of stutterers, but did not describe the procedures used to measure it and did not employ a control group.

Locus of Control A trait that has acquired importance in the assessment of personality is the extent to which an individual perceives the satisfaction of needs to be under his or her personal control. Tests of this attribute measure the degree to which people believe that "reinforcements" depend upon their own behavior or powers as opposed to external agents such as chance or the action of others. Craig, Franklin, and Andrews (1984) found that stutterers scored slightly less favorably than comparison groups of nurses and university students on the *Locus of Behavior Scale (LBS)*, but distinctly more favorably than a group of diagnosed neurotic patients. In a study of 119 adults who stutter, Ginsberg (2000) found that in participants who completed the *LBS*,[8] the locus of control was not related to scores on the *Perceptions of Stuttering Inventory* (*PSI*, Woolf, 1967), although shame and self-consciousness were. McDonough and Quesal (1988) administered the *Norwicki-Strickland (ANS-IE) Scale* to stutterers and normally fluent speakers and reported no difference. Madison, Budd, and Itzkowitz (1986) also obtained negative results in a study of 6- to 16-year-old children with the children's form of the *Norwicki-Strickland* test.[9]

Self-Monitoring Ability

Burley and Morely (1987) tested stutterers with Snyder's *Self-Monitoring Scale*, which evaluates individuals' concern for the appropriateness of their social behavior and the ability to modify self-presentation appropriately for a particular social situation. The stutterers scored less favorably than the fluent comparison speakers.

SUMMARY REMARKS

It is evident that there is considerable inconsistency in the findings resulting from research on the stutterer's personality. Yet these studies, done in such number and for so long that their account comes close to being a brief survey of personality testing itself, have made certain broad conclusions inescapable.

First, the weight of accumulated evidence does not appear to indicate that the average stutterer is a distinctly neurotic or severely maladjusted individual in the usual meanings of these terms. The evidence that most stutterers perform well within the norms on adjustment inventories is too strong to support such a view. Nor do their responses on projective tests seem to point to marked deviation from the normal or to coincide in any consistent way with the patterns of the classifiable neuroses as they are recognized on these tests.

Second, there is little conclusive evidence of any specific kind of character structure or broad-set of basic personality traits that is typical of stutterers as a group.

Third, there appears to be extreme overlap between stuttering and nonstuttering groups with respect to adequacy of adjustment; the more adequately adjusted stutterers are in far more satisfactory emotional health than the more poorly adjusted nonstutterers.

Fourth, there would seem to be some justification for the inference that stutterers on the average are not quite as well adjusted as are typically fluent speakers. By and large, this appears to be a matter of social adjustment to a greater degree than it affects other identifiable categories of emotional health. In addition, there appears to be evidence of tendencies on the part of many stutterers to be rather low in self-esteem and willingness to risk failure. Several explanations of the somewhat poorer average adjustment of stutterers are possible. It may be due, as has so frequently been suggested, to the eventual influence

[8]As well as the *Internalized Shame Scale* (Cook & Cook, 1987), the *Self-Consciousness Scale (Revised)* (Scheier & Carver, 1985), and the *Perceptions of Stuttering Inventory* (Woolf, 1967).

[9]The relevance of locus of control measures to assessment and treatment outcomes is discussed in Chapter 14.

of the stuttering itself. Personality test findings on young stuttering children have not yielded conclusive evidence on this point, although a number of studies reported in Chapter 1 have now identified changes in attitudes toward speech and speaking conditions in ever younger cohorts of stuttering children that might logically impact such test findings. Or it may be due to the fact that certain environmental influences contributing to the development of stuttering are of a type that may also sometimes contribute to insecurity and maladjustment.

That stutterers tend to be distinguished by specific attitudes and assumptions with regard to various features of the speech process is fairly certain. That they may often be socially maladjusted to the extent that they avoid contact that would require them to speak with others is true by definition. They are also more likely than other people to be somewhat insecure generally, and it is possible that such insecurity as they have may have contributed in some manner to the development of stuttering. But that stuttering is in essence the symptom of a basic personality disorder, in the sense that a fear of crowds or a hand-washing compulsion is considered to be such a symptom, is an assumption lacking adequate scientific support.

Notably, one of the diagnostic features of those relatively rare cases of adult-onset stuttering that do appear to have psychogenic origin, discussed both in this chapter and Chapter 4, is that it resolves easily, almost by therapeutic suggestion, which is inconsistent with the chronic nature of stuttering that begins in childhood. If most cases of developmental stuttering were in fact psychogenic, it would seem as though they would be more tractable to intervention than they appear to be. Also, psychological and/or psychiatric treatment, so effective in conversion reactions and other psychological disorders, is not recognized as effective in treating stuttering; as noted in Chapters 2 and 14, these types of therapies are not among treatments documented as effective when viewed against therapy effectiveness criteria.

In sum, the theory that stuttering reflects a deep-lying neurotic abnormality necessitating an essentially psychiatric method of treatment has been all but abandoned by professional workers who are knowledgeable about the disorder. In this regard, it is notable that, as we write this edition (2007), the impact of outdated assumptions about the stutterer's personality can still be seen in how stuttering is classified in the *International Classification of Disease (ICD-9)*. In this taxonomy, utilized for caseload and billing purposes in most American medical settings, stuttering is classified in a section together with a number of presumed "psychogenic" and "personality" disorders, including anorexia and sleep disorders. A related taxonomy developed by the American Psychological Association, the *Diagnostic and Statistical Manual of Mental Disorders, Fourth Edition (DSM-IV)*, places stuttering among a similar grouping of conditions. Thus, a relatively short-lived period of concentrated research into personality and stuttering that failed to discover a role for this construct in the emergence or persistence of stuttering has left a lasting mark that has spread well beyond the discipline of speech-language pathology and appears difficult to update.

Chapter 8

The Person Who Stutters: Cognitive and Linguistic Abilities

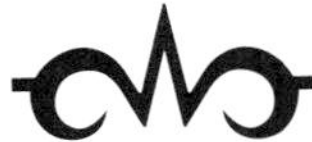

COGNITIVE SKILLS

Cognition is a broad construct, and aspects of stutterers' abilities to perform a wide variety of tasks are considered throughout many chapters of this text. However, a few specific abilities bear consideration here.

Attention

Heitmann, Asbjørnsen, and Helland (2004) studied nine matched pairs of stuttering and fluent adults (as well as eight persons diagnosed as clutterers) on the *Posner Test of Covert Attention Shifts*. The stutterers took significantly longer than the other two groups, leading the authors to speculate that these participants had impairments in the ability to focus attention.

Subramanian and Yairi (2006) studied responses of individuals who stutter, high-risk family members, and fluent speakers on a motor learning (tapping) task, as well as the classic Stroop Test. "Strooping" requires speakers to name the font color of words labeling color terms (e.g., when shown the word "red" in blue ink, the person is required to say "blue"), a notoriously harder task than reading the word itself. Stutterers were poorer at the tapping task, but not significantly different in Stroop reaction times, often viewed as a measure of attention.

Dynamic Learning

A number of tasks that have been employed to measure speech-motor capabilities of stutterers have required participants to learn novel sequences of motor gestures, and we address them primarily in that context in Chapter 5. However, results of a selected number of dynamic learning tasks are presented here, as potential cognitive processing indices.

Ardila, Rosselli, Bateman, and Guzmán (2000) contrasted the performance of three stuttering 7–12 year olds with that of the rest of their academic cohort. These boys outperformed fluent peers on a finger-tapping test and the Quantitative Concepts subscale from the *Woodcock Psychoeducational Battery*.

In contrast, using an experimental task, Smits-Bandstra, De Nil, and Saint-Cyr (2006) compared the speech and motor sequence skill learning of nine pairs of appropriately matched stuttering and fluent adults when required to learn nonsense syllable and finger-tapping sequences. They measured performance curves for accuracy, reaction time, and sequence duration, as well as retention and transfer. Poorer performance of the stutterers suggested that they have impaired abilities in sequence skill learning. In a companion study that employed 12 pairs of participants, Smits-Bandstra, De Nil, and Rochon (2006) examined finger-tapping ability under single- and dual-task conditions. Stutterers were consistently slow and variable under both conditions, while fluent adults' performance only suffered under dual-task conditions.

Time Estimation

Barasch, Guitar, McCauley, and Absher (2000) found some correlations between time judgments made by 20 pairs of stuttering and normally fluent adults and their individual measures of speech fluency. There was a negative correlation between both normal and stuttered disfluency and the ability to distinguish the relative lengths of brief tones. The authors suggested that their findings supported both the Continuity Hypothesis (Bloodstein, 1995) as well as proposals made by Kent (1984) that stuttering reflected, at some level, a disorder of speech timing. Ezrati-Vinacour and Levin (2001) found that stutterers estimated time less accurately on oral verbal tasks, particularly in a conversational task. These authors also reported an association between severity of stuttering and poorer accuracy in time estimation.

Dual-Task Demands

Although not an experimental test of dual-task demands, Mayberry, Jaques, and DeDe (1998) noted that gesture cessation during moments of stuttering (as well as normal disfluency) implies an ongoing demand on cognitive resources presumably devoted to sentence production.

Bosshardt (1999) employed a word-repetition task, in which sequences of three unrelated three-syllable nouns had to be repeated continuously. A dual-task condition required a mental addition task to be performed concurrently. Fluctuations in fluency across the components of the task suggested a drain on central executive functions that led to stuttering under increased cognitive load. In a related follow-up study, Bosshardt (2002) found that stuttered disfluency significantly increased during word repetition when similar words had to be read or memorized concurrently. Disfluencies of normally fluent speakers were not affected under these conditions. Bosshardt concluded that the speech of persons who stutter is more sensitive to interference from concurrently performed cognitive processing than that of nonstuttering persons, perhaps because the "phonological and articulatory systems of persons who stutter are protected less efficiently from interference by attention-demanding processing within the central executive system." Vasić and Wijnen (2005) found the opposite effect: stuttering was reduced when participants were required to speak while concurrently playing a computer game requiring sustained attention.

Interpretation Many studies find diminished performance, longer latencies, decreased motor stability (e.g., Kleinow & Smith, 2000), and increased stuttering (e.g., Caruso, Chodzko-Zajko, Bidinger, & Sommers, 1994; but see Vasić & Wijnen, 2005) under experimental conditions that place stutterers under increased cognitive or linguistic loading that requires them to differentially focus on one task despite conflicting or added task demands. These data must be reconciled with the body of data suggesting fluency-enhancing properties of distorted auditory feedback, which, in theory, might sap resources needed for fluent speech production.

LANGUAGE ABILITY

As we note in Chapter 9, the observed lateness of some stutterers in acquiring language has led to a series of comparisons between stutterers and nonstutterers on broad measures of language ability. Results have been equivocal. However, the age ranges of participants and nature of tasks have varied broadly. In addition, there has been almost complete reliance on the use of standardized measures designed to diagnose frank language impairment rather than subtle delays or differences (Bernstein Ratner, 1997). Studies that have employed experimental techniques have tended to identify more differences between stutterers and appropriately matched comparison groups.

A number of investigations have examined preschoolers who stutter, and significant differences have appeared in most of them. In a study by Murray and Reed (1977), preschool stutterers scored lower than their peers on the *Peabody Picture Vocabulary Test*, the *Northwestern Syntax Screening Test*, and the verbal abilities scale of the *Zimmerman Pre-School Language Scale*. Ryan (1992) found small but significant differences between 2- to 5-year-old stutterers and nonstutterers on the *Peabody Picture Vocabulary Test* and the *Test of Language Development (TOLD)*. Kline and Starkweather (1979) found that stutterers aged 3 to 6 years had a lower mean length of utterance (MLU) than nonstutterers and lower scores on the *Carrow Test for Auditory Comprehension of Language*. A group of 4- to 5-year-old stutterers did not differ from controls in MLU in a study by Meyers and Freeman (1985a), although this measure is not a sensitive index of language proficiency at such ages. Wall (1980) carried out a constituent syntactic analysis of the speech of four stutterers and four typically fluent peers aged 5 to 6 years and found that the stutterers tended to use simpler, less mature language.

In a series of studies, a cohort of young children within three months of stuttering onset performed more poorly than a comparison group of age-, socioeconomic status-(SES), and gender-matched peers on all standardized articulation and language measures (*Goldman-Fristoe Test of Articulation, Expressive One-Word Vocabulary Test, Peabody Picture Vocabulary Test*, and subtests of the *Clinical Evaluation of Language Functions—Preschool*), as well as with regard to many aspects of their spontaneous language usage, such as lexical diversity (Bernstein Ratner & Silverman,[1] 2000; Miles & Bernstein Ratner, 2001; Silverman & Bernstein Ratner, 2002). Though some differences approached statistical significance, none could be considered indicative of clinical impairment, and most stuttering children scored well above average for age. In comparing preschool children who did and did not stutter, Anderson and Conture (2000) and Anderson, Pellowski, and Conture (2005) found similar evidence of comparatively depressed language scores in young stuttering children and larger discrepancies between expressive and receptive scores. There have been reports of more obvious language differences at stuttering onset: 36 percent of 50 young children referred for suspected stuttering were found to have clinically relevant concomitant speech and language delays, as did 47 percent of the 17 eventually diagnosed as stuttering by Wevrick and Mervyn (1999).

In contrast to many other reports, the Illinois project (see summary in Watkins, 2005) did not find any noticeable patterns of language delay in the stuttering children that they followed. Most scored at or above average on spontaneous language measures or on their performance on the *Preschool Language Scale*. Similar findings have been reported by researchers tracking a cohort of young German children who stutter (Häge, 2001; Rommel, Häge, Kalehne & Johanssen, 2000).

A series of secondary analyses did not find differences between persistent or recovered Illinois project children on most measures. The single exception in their cohort, noted by Häge (2001) as well, was that *recovered* children's longitudinal profiles of expressive language development (growth curves showing increasingly complex language use) appeared to *decelerate* over time, becoming more

[1] After 2005, publishing as Wagovich.

typical, while persistent children's profiles continued to display more developmentally advanced than expected values for syntax and lexical diversity.[2]

In a study of kindergarten and first-grade children, E.-M. Silverman and Williams (1968) found a slight tendency for the stutterers to score more poorly than nonstutterers on such measures as mean length of response, mean of the five longest responses, and structural complexity of their utterances, but the groups differed significantly only in the number of one-word responses. In a later study of kindergarten and first-grade children by Westby (1979), stutterers scored more poorly than normally fluent children in frequency of grammatical errors, in receptive vocabulary on the *Peabody Picture Vocabulary Test*, and in correct responses on semantic tasks selected from the *Torrance Test of Creative Thinking*. There was no significant difference in *Developmental Sentence Analysis* scores computed on their conversational language samples.

Other studies have used elementary school children as participants. Peters (1968), employing the same measures that had been used by E.-M. Silverman and Williams (1968) as well as the type-token ratio (TTR), found no differences between stutterers and nonstutterers of elementary school age. Perozzi and Kunze (1969) found no differences between second-grade and third-grade stutterers and normally fluent peers on the *Van Alstyne Picture Vocabulary Test* and other measures of verbal output and structural complexity. In a study by Pitluk (1982), four stutterers aged 9 to 11 years performed adequately and as well as their fluent peers on the *Reporter's Test*, devised by DeRenzi and Ferrari to detect minimal expressive language impairments in persons with aphasia.

Bernstein Ratner and Sih (1987) found that 4- to 8-year-old stutterers had sentence repetition skills similar to age- and gender-matched peers on an experimentally designed set of stimuli. Sentences to be repeated were ordered in 10 steps to reflect developmental changes in language complexity. Increases in stuttering were highly predicted by increases in syntactic complexity of the probes, and somewhat less well by increases in their length (as measured in syllables).

Kadi-Hanifi and Howell (1992) reported no difference between fluent and stuttering groups in mean length of utterance (MLU) among children who ranged in age from 2;7 to 12;6 years. However, two studies produced evidence of a language deficit in school-age stutterers. St. Louis and Hinzman (1988) reported a lower average MLU in stutterers in grades one to twelve. However, MLU can be poorly sensitive to language differences, particularly when used as a sole measure of language proficiency (Eisenberg, Fersko, & Lundgren, 2001). Byrd and Cooper (1989b) found that the performance of 5- to 9-year-old stutterers compared unfavorably with test norms on the *Test of Language Development*, but not on the *Test of Auditory Comprehension of Language (TACL-R)*.

In terms of broader language use in discourse, Weiss and Zebrowski (1994) found 5- to 11-year-old stutterers equal to nonstutterers in narrative ability. Nippold, Schwarz, and Jescheniak (1991) also found 6- to 11-year-old stutterers equal to nonstutterers in narrative ability as well as in performance on the *Clinical Evaluation of Language Fundamentals*.

In studies that have used older participants, adolescents who stutter did not score appreciably lower on a sentence imitation task than their fluent peers (Silverman & Bernstein Ratner, 1997). In a study of high-level linguistic production and comprehension processes in adults, 11 of 19 stutterers, and no nonstutterers, were judged to be linguistically impaired (as measured by a nonstandardized series of language tasks) by Watson, Freeman, Chapman, Miller, Finitzo, Pool, and Devous (1991).

Finally, in this section we note the large body of data that has accumulated over the past decade to suggest that language *processing*, as distinguished from language *ability*, appears to be atypical in individuals who stutter. These studies have employed an array of brain-imaging methods, as well as study of event-related potentials (ERPs). They have primarily used adult participants, although a few ERP studies have been completed on children who

[2]A similar report has appeared regarding pre- and post-intervention profiles of children treated with the Lidcombe program (see Chapter 14; Bonelli, Dixon, Bernstein Ratner, & Onslow, 2000).

stutter. These studies are addressed in greater detail in Chapter 4, although relevant results that address specific language findings are included here.

Specific Language-Related Abilities

Lexical Skills Many studies have examined more narrowly defined linguistic skills of stutterers. A few have dealt with word-finding ability. A limited number of these studies have been done with children. Many studies of children's lexical skills have used standardized assessment measures, but a few, as noted, have employed experimental psycholinguistic techniques.

Both Weuffen (1961) and Okasha, Bishry, et al. (1974) reported lower scores for stuttering than for nonstuttering children in a task of finding words beginning with a given letter.[3] Boysen and Cullinan (1971) found no group differences for 7- to 10-year-old children in reaction time on an experimental picture-naming task. On the other hand, Telser (1971) obtained slower average latencies for 5- to 12-year-old stutterers on a similar task.

Pellowski and Conture (2005) examined an aspect of lexical retrieval, priming effects, in a relatively large cohort of 23 pairs of stuttering and fluent preschoolers 3 to 6 years of age. Normally, picture naming is facilitated by presentation of a semantically related "prime" just prior to picture presentation. This effect was seen for the children who did not stutter but was absent in the stuttering children, suggesting differential or less efficient organization of the mental lexicon in this group. A follow-up study by Hartfield and Conture (2006) contrasted functional and categorical priming in 13 pairs of preschoolers. A categorical prime was considered to be semantically related by family or category membership (e.g., use of *lemon* to prime *apple*), while functional priming used verbs typically associated with the target (e.g., use of *bite* to prime *apple*). Stuttering children were slower overall in ability to name the limited set of stimuli, and appeared to benefit best from functional priming, thought to be a less mature associative set than categorical organization of lexical items.[4]

There are some known phonological factors that influence speed of lexical encoding, such as neighborhood density (how many other words of the language are phonologically similar to the target), as well as the relative frequency of those words. Arnold, Conture, and Ohde (2005) did not observe any differential impact of these factors on naming latencies in a large cohort of young stuttering and fluent children. In similar work using an extended set of targets and adult participants, Newman and Bernstein Ratner (2007) also found similar patterns of naming latency, but lowered accuracy of naming by the stutterers.

Van Lieshout, Hulstjin, and Peters (1991) reported slower reaction times for stutterers in single-word reading. Prins, Main, and Wampler (1997) found a larger-than-expected word frequency effect as well as specifically elevated latencies for verb production in adults who stutter. A relative deficit in verb processing had been suggested in earlier work showing stuttering children's tendency to stutter on the initial components of verb phrases during sentence description tasks (Bernstein, 1981). Newman and Bernstein Ratner (2007) found no differences in latencies, but a significant difference in accuracy in adult stutterers' noun and verb production from that of fluent adults on a speeded picture-naming task. However, no group differences were observed in the profiles of noun and verb generation, specifically. De Nil, Kroll, and Houle (2001) did note differences in cortical activation for nouns and verbs across pre- and post-therapy fMRI scans in adults who stutter.

Stuttering children aged 9 to 12 years did not differ from normally fluent children in the number of words they could write after visual presentation

[3] Sometimes called a "word fluency" task in psychoeducational testing, although the focus is on speed of retrieval as measured by a number of different words produced in a limited time frame rather than on fluency as defined in this book.

[4] Although not mentioned by the authors, this distinction would seem to parallel that between paradigmatic (within category) word associations, seen in older children and adults, and syntagmatic (phrasal) word associations, seen more typically in younger children (see Ervin, 1961, among many others, for this word association shift over development).

in a study by Knura (1970). But Bosshardt (1993) found adult stutterers inferior in the recall of consonant-vowel-consonant syllables that had been presented visually.

Taylor, Lore, and Waldman (1970) found that stutterers did not have longer latencies of response than nonstutterers on a "cloze" test requiring them to supply words omitted from sentences. Rastatter and Dell (1987b) studied stutterers' reaction times under two conditions. One was simple phonation of /a/ in response to a flash of light. In the other, the participant phonated /a/ if a visually presented word was a real word as opposed to a nonsense word. The difference between the two reaction times was taken to be the lexical decision time. Stutterers were slower than fluent peers in lexical decision time.

Crowe and Kroll (1991) administered a word association test in which participants responded to the stimulus word with a beeper as soon as they had the response word in mind, after which they wrote the word. Measuring the time interval from presentation of the word to the beep, the experimenters determined that the stutterers had made word associations as rapidly as their typically fluent peers. In contrast, Bosshardt and Fransen (1996) found depressed profiles of monitoring for semantically related words in their study of stuttering adults. In psycholinguistic monitoring studies, the participant is told in advance what word or sound to respond to as quickly as detected. In this study, in addition to monitoring for the exact target, participants were also cued to find the target. For example, in German, participants would respond to *birne* (pear) by being primed to find words that were phonologically similar (rhymed), such as *gestirne* (stars), or semantically similar (members of the same category), such as "a fruit." While both groups were generally similar in monitoring, adults who stutter were slower in responding when given a category cue. Their findings suggested that adults who stutter retrieve semantic information more slowly than do typically fluent speakers.

Primarily on the basis of the distribution of stuttering observed in spontaneous language tasks across a wide age range and a number of languages, Howell and colleagues[5] have proposed that a number of lexical variables may predict fluency breakdown. These include phonological complexity and thus potential motoric encoding demand, as well as grammatical word class.[6] As we will note in Chapter 12, there is an obvious trend for young children to stutter on closed/function words, while in later years this pattern reverses, showing higher adult stuttering rates on open/content words. However, Dayalu et al. (2002) have suggested that word class effects on the frequency of stuttering may reflect word frequency, rather than grammatical, effects.

In a silent naming task, Blomgren et al. (2003) found atypical patterns of bilateral cortical activation in stutterers, using functional magnetic resonance imaging (fMRI). Similarly, Weber-Fox (2001) found significant reductions in the typical negative amplitudes seen on Event-Related Potential (ERP) recording while processing both open (lexical) and closed class (grammatical) words during silent reading in adults who stutter, suggestive of atypical sentence processing skills or strategies. Salmelin, Schnitzler, Schmidt, and Freund (2000) also found activation patterns seen in stuttering and nonstuttering adults during single word naming to be different, using magnetoencephalography (MEG).

In sum, many studies have shown some subtle differences between stutterers and fluent speakers in lexical encoding skills or their presumed cortical processing indices. Based on the fact that stuttering was seen during a nonsense word (non-word) reading task in adults, Onslow and Packman (2002) argued against the view that stuttering reflects impaired lexical encoding, specifically. However, Au-Yeung and Howell (2002) note that non-words may be processed using lexical encoding strategies. Non-word encoding has also been investigated using repetition tasks (discussed later in this section), and may reflect phonological encoding and motor planning abilities as well.

[5]Au-Yeung and Howell (1998a, 1998b), Howell, Au-Yeung, and Pilgrim (1999), Howell, Au-Yeung, and Sackin (1999), Dworzynski, Howell, and Natke (2003), Au-Yeung, Gomez, and Howell (2003), Dworzynski and Howell (2004).

[6]Although terminology varies, words are typically classified dichotomously as either open/content/lexical as opposed to closed/function/grammatical.

Syntactic Ability A number of studies have contrasted stutterers' and nonstutterers' grammatical or sentence processing skills. Postma, Kolk, and Povel (1990) reported that stutterers were slower in reproducing sentences silently, forming mental auditory images of the sounds. They inferred that stutterers used more speech planning time than nonstutterers. In a specific investigation of the effects of syntactic complexity on sentence initiation times (SIT), Logan (2003) found adult stutterers to be slower in sentence initiation time but not differentially affected by variations in syntactic complexity. In contrast, Smith and colleagues (Kleinow & Smith, 2000) found atypical destabilization of motor responses in adults who stutter when baseline utterances were manipulated to increase their syntactic complexity.

Cuadrado and Weber-Fox (2003) found less accurate "online" judgments of grammaticality in adults who stutter during an Event-Related Potential (ERP) investigation that also revealed atypical electrophysiological responses by stutterers during the task. However, untimed performance did not discriminate between stuttering and fluent participants. The authors suggested that stutterers might have weaknesses in the mechanisms required for sentence processing, even when overt production was not required.

Anderson and Conture (2004) used a syntactic priming paradigm to investigate sentence-encoding skills in young children who stutter. As noted earlier, there is a very well-known reduction in reaction time to a stimulus if it is preceded by a semantically or phonologically similar word (called the "prime"). In other words, normally, ability to name a picture of "bread" will be primed by a preceding picture of *butter*. While both groups of children benefited from syntactic priming, the authors observed a greater facilitation after priming in children who stuttered than seen in children who did not stutter, and suggested that stuttering might emerge from weaknesses in planning or retrieving sentential units. Bajaj, Hodson, and Schommer-Aikins (2004) found children who stutter to be poorer at making sentence grammaticality judgments than typically fluent children.

A number of studies have shown that children's stuttering is very likely to occur on utterances or clauses that are relatively longer and more complex, as measured by developmental psycholinguistic indices (Bernstein Ratner & Sih, 1987; Logan & La Salle, 1999; Logan & Conture, 1997; Zackheim & Conture, 2003). Following an analysis of stuttering in young children's conversational utterances, Yaruss (1999) concluded that increases in both sentence length and syntactic complexity were significantly correlated with increases in stuttering, although individual children's patterns were less well predicted than that of the group. He concluded that neither length nor complexity was sufficient to fully account for stuttering in children's conversational language. Maske-Cash and Curlee (1995) found that both utterance length and meaningfulness contributed to the disfluency rates of young children who stutter, and were more likely to affect children with concomitant speech and language problems.

We note that utterance length has been measured in different ways across investigations of language and stuttering. Brundage and Bernstein Ratner (1989) found differences in the degree to which different indices of length correlated with stuttering frequency in eight children ages 4–8. Mean Length of Utterance (MLU) was the highest predictor, followed by length in syllables (a possible motoric complexity measure), with length in words less well correlated with stuttering rate.

Auditory Processing Ability Conflicting findings have been reported on various auditory processing skills and other abilities thought to be related to speech and language. On the *Illinois Test of Psycholinguistic Abilities (ITPA)*, the stuttering children investigated by Perozzi and Kunze (1969) performed more poorly than typically fluent children only on the Visual Motor Sequencing subtest, which requires the participant to reproduce a series of pictures or designs in correct order after they have been removed. On the other hand, Stocker and Parker (1977) found that stutterers, aged 4 to 11 years, scored lower than nonstutterers on the Sequential Memory subtest of the *ITPA* and on the Auditory Attention Span for Related Syllables subtest of the *Detroit Tests of Learning Aptitude*. Williams and Marks (1972) set out to study the *ITPA* profiles of stutterers rather than to compare them with others. In relation to their total performance on the test, the stutterers, aged 5 to 9, tended to do somewhat poorly in auditory vocal sequencing. By contrast, Manning and Riensche (1976) found no differences between 5- to 10-year-old stutterers and nonstutterers in an auditory processing task in which the children had to synthesize words and nonsense syllables from discrete serial presentations of their constituent sounds.

Moore, Craven, and Faber (1982) and Moore (1986) found that stutterers had poor recognition and recall of words on auditory presentation. Carpenter and Sommers (1987), on the other hand, found stutterers and normal speakers equal in auditory memory for words.

In a reaction time study by Rastatter and Dell (1985), participants touched either of two pictures, depending on the name they heard in their headset. In one condition, they knew which name they would hear; in the other they did not. The difference in the reaction times between the two conditions was considered the time required for auditory phonemic processing. The stutterers were found to be slower in auditory processing.

Postma and Kolk (1992) found that stutterers did not differ from nonstutterers in identifying phonemic errors as they recited a string of nonsense syllables, but detected fewer errors than typically fluent participants when they monitored a tape recording of other speakers reciting the syllables.

Phonological Processing and Awareness Tiffany (1963) devised three tests to measure a special kind of skill that he called phonetic ability or sound-mindedness. One of them, the Slurvian translations test, consists of a series of apparently meaningless "slurvs" such as "scene owe weevil," or "yearn ever told tool urn," which are correctly translated as "see no evil" and "you're never too old to learn." Wingate (1967a) found that adult stutterers gave significantly fewer correct translations than a group of adult nonstutterers. This was true both when the slurvs were received visually and by ear.

Tiffany's Backward Speech test requires the participant to reverse the sounds of a spoken word so as to produce, for example, "talk" from "caught." His Phonetic Anagrams test requires the construction of a word or words from a jumbled series of spoken sounds, for example the rearrangement of /p/, /k/, and /i/ to make "keep" and "peek." Wingate (1971) reported the performance of nonstutterers to be clearly better than that of stutterers on both tests.

All of these results were obtained from the same group of subjects. A study by Perozzi (1970) produced equivocal findings. Perozzi gave the Backward Speech test to elementary school–aged children. The stutterers tended to do more poorly than the normally fluent children, but the difference was not statistically significant. Newman, Fawcett, and Russon (1986) found adult stutterers significantly inferior on this task. As in essentially all studies in which differences between stutterers and nonstutterers have been reported, there was considerable overlapping between the groups.

As Wingate (1971) pointed out, these tests seem to demand an internalized manipulation of sounds to achieve a restructuring of their pattern. His results are curiously reminiscent of an all-but-forgotten report by Kelly (1932) that stutterers made far more errors than normally fluent speakers when instructed to respond to recorded presentations of three-digit numbers by writing the number with the first two digits reversed.

Over the past two decades, phonological awareness tasks have been associated with reading readiness and proficiency in children. Bajaj, Hodson, and Schommer-Aikins (2004) did not find any significant differences in performance between stuttering and fluent children on two common tasks measuring aspects of phonological awareness, the Lindamood *Auditory Conceptualization Test* and a phoneme reversal task.

Ability to repeat nonsense words that gradually increase in complexity (non-word repetition) has been increasingly targeted as an underlying weakness in children with specific language impairment, and has generated a large body of research that positions it as one of the most sensitive measures of language impairment in children (see Bishop, North, &

Donlan, 1996). Some studies of adults and children who stutter have reported relative weakness in this ability as well. Ludlow, Siren, and Zikria (1997) and Smits-Bandstra, De Nil, and Saint-Cyr (2006) found adults who stutter to be poorer at performing this task, while Hakim and Bernstein Ratner (2004) and Anderson, Wagovich, and Hall (2006) reported relatively depressed performance on this task in children who stutter.

Burger and Wijnen (1999) found adults who stutter to be slower, but not differentially affected by phonological priming (a way to facilitate naming speed by preceding the target with a phonologically similar word), in a study that examined production of cued word responses. Melnick, Conture, and Ohde (2003) found that both stuttering and nonstuttering preschoolers decreased speech reaction times (SRTs) following a phonological prime; however, a relationship between faster SRTs and more proficient articulation skills seen in fluent children was not apparent in the responses of the children who stuttered.

While stutterers were generally similar on an experimental phonological decoding task to typically fluent adults, Weber-Fox, Spencer, Spruill, and Smith (2004) found increased reaction times for adults who stutter, as well as atypical right hemisphere Event-Related Potential (ERP) asymmetry, when task complexity was increased, as in determining whether or not two words with similar orthography but different pronunciation (e.g., *gown* vs. *own*) rhymed. Stutterers have also been shown to be significantly slower on phoneme monitoring tasks than a group of fluent adults (Sasisekaran, De Nil, Smyth, & Johnson, 2006). In a phoneme-monitoring task, participants are simply asked to press a button whenever a target sound is heard in a set of words or sentences. Phoneme-monitoring tasks are often used to measure speed of lexical processing because there is substantial evidence that adults cannot simply monitor for the sound without accessing the word it is in (see Berko Gleason & Bernstein Ratner, 1998, for discussion).

Self-Monitoring of Speech Relatively little research has addressed stutterers' self-monitoring of speech, which may be considered surprising given the rather large literature that has examined stutterers' responses to delayed auditory feedback (DAF) of their speech (see Chapters 6 and 10). Bernstein Ratner (1998) and Bernstein Ratner and Wijnen (2007) note that the struggle behaviors seen early in some young child stutterers may reflect atypically advanced self-monitoring skills. Most toddlers do not respond to perturbations in auditory feedback of their speech, and in fact most children seen clinically for language and articulation problems do not appear acutely aware of their expressive errors. However, when eight children within three months of stuttering onset were matched with peers on a single word reading task under side-tone and DAF, stuttering children significantly lengthened their speech segments, indicating awareness, while their fluent peers did not (Bernstein Ratner, 1998). Vasić and Wijnen (2005) found what they viewed as supporting evidence for the view that stutterers excessively monitor their speech: when asked to converse while playing a difficult computer game, stuttering rate diminished when compared to baseline. The authors interpreted this to suggest that diverting the monitor's attention through dual-task demand facilitated fluency.

As noted, this area has not yet attracted a great deal of research, but appears promising, insofar as it may provide an explanation for the fact that young stuttering children often react with struggle and awareness to their disfluencies. This behavior is not generally seen in expressive speech or language errors made by other groups of children.

Linguistic vs. Capacity Limitations In considering the basis of stuttering as well as childhood and adult language disorders, it has been argued that diminished performance on linguistic tasks may reflect more general processing limitations rather than language-specific impairment. This proposal is consistent with findings in many of the studies reported in this section, and explains differential performance by individuals who stutter that appears to be more evident when task complexity is manipulated (Bosshardt, Ballmer, & De Nil, 2002; Weber-Fox, Spencer, Spruill, & Smith, 2004; Bosshardt, 2006).

Prevalence of Stuttering among Bilingual Speakers Before we leave the subject of language, let us briefly note in passing that, in a group of 4,827 children about half of whom were bilingual, Travis, Johnson, and Shover (1937) found 2.8 percent of the bilinguals to be stutterers as against 1.8 percent of those who spoke only English. Surprisingly, tri-linguals actually stuttered less (at 2.4%).[7] Stern (1948) studied 1,861 children in four schools in Johannesburg. Of those who had been bilingual prior to age 6 years, 2.16 percent stuttered, while only 1.66 percent of the monolinguals stuttered. Furthermore, among the stutterers, Stern judged three times as many bilinguals as monolinguals to be severe. Bilingualism, of course, may be confounded with so many other factors that we cannot be sure of the relevance of these interesting findings to the subject we have been discussing. The most recent large-scale study of the prevalence of stuttering in bilinguals was conducted by Au-Yeung, Howell, Davis, Charles, and Sackin (summarized in Van Borsel, Maes, & Foulon, 2001), and found no obvious differences between monolinguals and bilinguals in terms of stuttering risk in a self-report Internet-based survey. We note that there are barely a handful of published papers on this topic, which has ramifications for intervention with the many of the world's speakers who are multilingual. These reports, together with a small number of unpublished conference presentations, are discussed by Van Borsel (2001), Shenker (2004), Bernstein Ratner (2004) and Roberts and Shenker (2007). Clearly, more work is needed in this area. Finally, we note that the more obvious assumption, that bilingualism is a risk factor for language delay or impairment, has not yet been substantiated (see De Houwer, 1999).

Summary Remarks

Across a wide variety of studies, both children and adults who stutter appear to demonstrate subtle weaknesses in language performance. These differences from typically fluent speakers appear primarily when experimental tasks are used, rather than clinical tests normally used to identify frank language disorder. In addition to these weaknesses, more recent methodologies have identified atypical patterns of cortical processing for speech and language tasks, even when overt speech production is not required.

Further, as Chapter 12 will show, there is an apparent relationship between language formulation and the pattern of stuttering often seen at its onset in young children. The fact that stuttered events do not appear to be randomly distributed in the earliest stages of stuttering, but gravitate to points that may reflect the encoding of sentence constituents, further strengthens the possibility that stuttering emerges at least in part because of subtle underlying weaknesses in language ability in children who stutter.

Experimental psycholinguistic paradigms are emerging that may permit a more nuanced appreciation of whether or not people who stutter are atypical in language ability, and where potential weaknesses may lie. If so, future investigations will also need to explore the stage at which such weaknesses lead to fluency breakdown—for instance, are the weaknesses best characterized as phonological, lexical, or grammatical?

For children at the onset of stuttering, there also appears to be a need to link standardized appraisal of language ability with the child's typical attempts to communicate. A few studies suggest that there may be a mismatch between what the child is easily able to say (as inferred from standardized test scores), and what the child attempts to say (as measured by indices of developmental complexity of expressive language).

In sum, we believe there is much of interest in past research on the language abilities of people who stutter. Further, we believe that there are many questions yet to be asked in this area that have the potential to shed light on the underlying deficit that leads to stuttering.

[7] I am grateful to Kathryn Kohnert for pointing this out. She also noted the foreign monolingual children stuttered at a rate of 7.4%.

Chapter 9

The Person Who Stutters: Developmental History and Home Environment

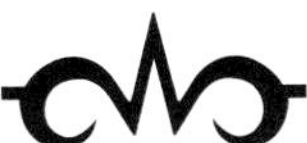

We will devote this chapter to the kinds of data that are to be obtained from case histories, medical and school records, routine physical examinations, clinical interviews, and diagnostic tests and to research findings relating to the early histories of children who stutter. We begin with a description of three major longitudinal studies that have made major contributions to this area of inquiry.

THE IOWA, NEWCASTLE, AND ILLINOIS STUDIES

Information on stutterers' early histories has been gathered in many studies, but by far the most thorough and carefully executed of these have been three extensive investigations to which we will refer throughout the remainder of this chapter as the Iowa, Newcastle, and Illinois studies.

The Iowa studies were conducted by Johnson and his coworkers at the University of Iowa over a period of more than 20 years on a total of 246 children and a comparison group of typically fluent children, and consisted of three separate investigations that Johnson and Associates (1959) referred to as Studies I, II, and III. Study I, which we have already cited as Johnson et al. (1942) and Johnson (1955a), was done between 1934 and 1940 with 46 stutterers and 46 nonstutterers. Study II was done by Darley (1955) between 1948 and 1952 with 50 stutterers and 50 control subjects. Study III was conducted from 1952 to 1957 with 150 children in each group and was reported by Johnson and Associates (1959) together with summaries of the findings of Studies I and II.

The Newcastle study was done by Andrews and Harris (1964, chaps. 4, 5, 6).[1] The experimental group consisted of 80 stutterers, most of whom were identified in a survey of all the children in the last two grades of primary school in Newcastle-upon-Tyne. For purposes of control in interpreting findings, stutterers were paired with normally fluent children of the same sex and similar age from their own class at school.

The Illinois Stuttering Research Project was conducted by Ehud Yairi and colleagues and first reported findings from its initial cohort of children in Yairi and Ambrose (1992a, 1992b; see full summary, and a full listing of study publications in Yairi & Ambrose, 2005, pp. 23–44). Three groups of children were eventually followed over time: 146 children originally referred within one year of stuttering onset, 17 additional children seen more than one year after onset, and 59 fluent comparison children.

In all three studies, the procedure, in addition to certain tests and objective measurements, involved systematic interviewing of the parents, by means of which detailed information was collected about the birth conditions, diseases, early physical development, educational and home adjustment, family background, parental attitudes, and child training policies as well as other aspects of development and home environment. Broadly speaking and with a relatively small number of exceptions, the studies have shown that there is little in the case history of the typical stutterer that could be regarded as unusual, and this agrees in general with most other investigations. The exceptions, as we will see, are in the areas of speech and language development.

MEDICAL HISTORY

Birth Conditions

Attempts to determine the extent to which stutterers might have atypical birth history factors such as gestational age, length of labor, manner of presentation of the fetus, use of instruments, injury to the infant, and other prenatal and postnatal complications have produced largely negative or ambiguous results. Berry (1938b) found no difference in complication rate in comparing the medical records of 227 stutterers and 232 comparison children. In the Iowa studies, mean duration of labor was significantly longer in the case of the stutterers than for the nonstutterers in Study III, but there was a marked difference in the opposite direction in Study I. The Newcastle study showed a tendency, just short of statistical significance, for the stutterers to have experienced more abnormal birth conditions. There were also somewhat inconclusive hints of this in studies by Milisen and Johnson (1936) and Boland (1951). No differences in conditions of birth or pregnancy were found by Accordi and his coworkers (1983), who compared the medical records of 2,802 stutterers seen over a 25-year period at the Medical-Surgical Center for Phoniatrics in Padua with data obtained by questionnaire on 1,602 schoolchildren. Cox, Seider, and Kidd (1984) also found no differences in birth and prenatal conditions between 37 stutterers and 54 of their nonstuttering relatives in interviews with the mothers. Similar results were reported for 50 children who stutter and a comparison group by Wevrick and Mervyn (1999).

Stutterers have been found not to differ essentially from nonstutterers with respect to birth weight,[2] month or season of birth,[3] and parental age at birth.[4] Allen (1948) investigated the Rh factor in mothers of stutterers with inconclusive results.

Diseases, Injuries, and Allergies

Findings with regard to disease history have also been largely negative. Berry (1938c), after analyzing the medical records of 430 stuttering and 462 nonstuttering children entering hospital clinics for general pediatric care or preventive medicine, reported that the stutterers were more prone to have such diseases of the respiratory system as tonsillitis, bronchitis, and rheumatic fever, as well as certain disorders

[1]This should not be confused with the 1,000-family Newcastle-upon-Tyne survey cited in Chapter 3, whose findings, as they relate to speech disorders, were reported by Andrews and Harris (1964, chap. 3) and Morley (1957).

[2]Berry (1938b), Johnson and Associates (1959, p. 50).

[3]Bryngelson and Brown (1939), Boland (1950).

[4]Everhart (1949), Morgenstern (1956), Johnson and Associates (1959, p. 75), Andrews and Harris (1964, p. 52).

of the nervous system—encephalitis, epilepsy, and convulsions—which were the "accepted sequelae" of these at the time. Berry interpreted this to mean that a genetic link existed between a constitutional predisposition to stuttering and a constitutional susceptibility to respiratory disease. Further research has failed to provide confirmation of Berry's findings, however. Both the Iowa and Newcastle studies showed a comparable incidence of diseases for stutterers and nonstutterers. In addition, the Iowa studies disclosed no difference in the incidence of injuries, surgical operations, or asthma. Cox, Seider, and Kidd (1984) reported no differences with respect to diseases and injuries in a comparison of 40 adult stutterers and their nonstuttering relatives. In contrast, health histories did distinguish the small cohort of young children who stutter reported by Wevrick and Mervyn (1999).

The Iowa finding with regard to asthma is of some importance because the observations of Kennedy and Williams (1938) and Gordon (1942) and intradermal tests by Card (1939) suggested that there may be an unusual amount of allergies among stutterers. The possibility has been of special interest because of the relationship often thought to exist between allergies and emotional factors, as well as more recent investigations of relationships between allergies and autoimmune disorders. As a research question, it is complicated considerably by difficulties in the diagnosis and ambiguities in the definition of allergy, and by the fact that allergies may be heritable, as is stuttering.

Physical Examination

The Iowa and Newcastle studies showed stutterers to be comparable to nonstutterers in height and weight and with regard to the information about their general health that was supplied by the parents. In a series of studies that included essentially routine physical or neurological examinations, stutterers have consistently been found to be in grossly normal physical health.[5] But Greene and Small (1944), Meyer (1945), and Despert (1946) all concurred in noting hyperactive deep tendon reflexes, perspiration and cyanosis of the hands and feet, vasomotor instability, and fine tremors of the outstretched hands, which Meyer termed the "classical manifestations of anxiety."

Finally, in a study of physical habitus by Travis, Malamud, and Thayer (1934), stutterers were found to differ markedly from nonstutterers in distribution of body types on the basis of Kretschmer's system of classification, a much larger percentage falling into the leptosome category. Bullen (1945) noted a similar distribution in a small group of stutterers and typically fluent speakers. The implications of such findings are not transparently clear.

PHYSICAL AND SOCIAL DEVELOPMENT

In general, controlled studies have shown that the early development of stutterers compares favorably with that of nonstutterers with respect to the ages at which they teethe, are weaned, feed and dress themselves, acquire bowel and bladder control, sit, creep, stand, and walk, and with regard to the frequency with which difficulties are reported in connection with feeding, sleeping, or toilet training.[6] The exceptions to this have been isolated and relatively minor. For example, Wevrick and Mervyn (1999) found some indications of delayed toilet training and gross motor development in a small cohort of 17 3-year-olds referred for stuttering. On the *Vineland Social Maturity Scale*, McHale (1967) found that stutterers aged 7 to 15 years did not differ from nonstutterers in mean social quotient.

Relevant to theories of stuttering that posit its origins in oral fixation, Berry (1938b) found that stutterers tended to have been breast-fed significantly longer, on the average, than nonstutterers, while in the Iowa studies the reverse proved to be true. A study by Sewell and Mussen (1952) appeared to yield little evidence that stuttering is likely to be associated in any direct way with bottle feeding, scheduled feeding as opposed to demand feeding, or abrupt weaning. However, Yairi and Ambrose

[5] McDowell (1928), Greene and Small (1944), Meyer (1945), Despert (1946), Graham (1966).

[6] See Milisen and Johnson (1936), Berry (1938b), the Iowa and Newcastle studies, Accordi et al. (1983), Cox, Seider, and Kidd (1984).

(2005) noted that stressors such as weaning, toilet training, and other changes in developmental routine were reported near onset of stuttering for 36 percent of children. It is of course the case that most American toddlers, at least, will be undergoing toilet training or welcoming an infant sibling into their lives at roughly the same time that stuttering is most typically diagnosed. Hill (1999) used the *Hayes Social Adjustment Scales* to compare a small cohort of children near stuttering onset with fluent age-mates and found such stressors to be no more common in the backgrounds of children who stutter and those who do not.

ABNORMAL BEHAVIOR SYMPTOMS

There is a relatively long list of behavior problems and symptoms of "nervousness" and maladjustment in children that may be indicative of varying degrees of emotional ill health, and a few of which may in some cases be symptomatic of developmental delay or disorder. These include exaggerated fears, sleep disturbances, hyperactivity, enuresis, sibling jealousy, temper tantrums, excessive thumb sucking or nail biting, lying or stealing, compulsive orderliness, difficulties in playing with other children, and a score or more of others. Stuttering and nonstuttering children have been compared with regard to these behavioral symptoms in several investigations. If we were to try to speculate about the probable outcome of such studies on the assumption that it would be consistent with the results of other research on the stutterer's personality reviewed in Chapter 7, we would be likely to predict that stuttering children as a group would not be severely affected by these problems, but might tend to have more of them, on the average, than comparable nonstutterers. This, in fact, appears to be essentially the case.

The Newcastle study found no indication of a difference between the stuttering and comparison groups on such variables, or even of a tendency toward a difference approaching significance. In the Iowa studies, however, as well as in an investigation by Moncur (1955), stutterers displayed somewhat more frequent symptoms of maladjustment than did nonstutterers. In Iowa Study III, both parents were asked to apply ratings with regard to more than 100 items pertaining to the emotional adjustment or social behavior of the child. In the case of 35 of these items, significantly more comparison group children than stuttering children were rated favorably by one or both of the parents. The reverse was true on only one item. When Iowa Studies II and III and Moncur's study are compared with regard to specific behavior symptoms, there is agreement among all three only for the more frequent evaluation of the stutterers by their parents as "nervous." Two of the three studies agreed that stutterers more often exhibited fears of some kind, nightmares or sleep disturbances, compulsive orderliness, perfectionism, and fighting or overly aggressive behavior.

Fowlie and Cooper (1978) had mothers of 6- to 11-year-old stutterers and nonstutterers rate their children on a checklist of personality traits that had previously been selected by speech clinicians in characterizing stutterers. The stuttering children were perceived by their mothers as more insecure, sensitive, anxious, withdrawn, fearful, and introverted than were the nonstutterers. Fowlie and Cooper suggested that such judgments may in part reflect a general stereotype with regard to the stutterer's personality. Riley (1983) reported high self-expectations in 3- to 6-year-old stutterers compared with children with age-appropriate speech or with articulation difficulties. Cox, Seider, and Kidd (1984), in interviews with mothers of 37 stutterers and 54 genetically related normally fluent children, found no differences in the incidence of unusual fears or problems with feeding, sleeping, or bladder and bowel management. Accordi et al. (1983) found no difference in the occurrence of enuresis or tics in their comparison of 2,802 stuttering and 1,602 comparison children referred to earlier. Using a somewhat different approach, Karrass et al. (2006) surveyed parents of 65 stuttering preschoolers and a matched cohort. They used the *Behavior Style Questionnaire* to measure parental perceptions of their children's temperament. Stuttering children were rated as significantly more reactive, less able to regulate their emotions, and less able to regulate attention.

SPEECH AND LANGUAGE HISTORY

There continues to be active investigation of the degree to which stuttering children are delayed in speech and language development or display depressed performance on standardized speech and language measures or spontaneous language analyses. This chapter will explore trajectories of speech and language development and profiles seen at initial diagnosis, while in Chapter 8, we explored cognitive and linguistic abilities that have been studied cross-sectionally, by standardized testing, language sampling, and experimental tasks.

Phonological Development

The Illinois project (see summary in Paden, 2005) scrutinized the articulation development of its stuttering children and examined the relationship of phonological acquisition to stuttering persistence and recovery in their sample. In general, when seen soon after onset, children who stutter tended to lag somewhat behind fluent comparison peers, and children whose stuttering persisted tended to demonstrate slower development than children who spontaneously recovered. No differences in profile of phonological development (order of mastery of phonemic targets or word formation strategies) were apparent among persistent, recovered, and fluent children, and phonological profile alone was insufficient to distinguish statistically between either stuttering from fluent children, or persistent from recovered children.

Language Acquisition

Historically, researchers have long believed that stutterers tend to be slow in developing language. The support for this view, though not unqualified, has now become considerable (see Table 9-1), and is strengthened by findings from experimental studies discussed in Chapter 8. Berry (1938b) found very marked differences between stutterers and nonstutterers. The Newcastle study again produced distinct evidence of slower speech development in stutterers, corroborating Berry's findings as well as other past observations by Morley (1957, p. 411) and Milisen and Johnson (1936). Only the Iowa studies showed slight or no differences. In Study III, the last and most extensive of the Iowa studies, it was found that the stutterers had been regarded as late talkers by their parents substantially more often than had the nonstutterers, but the ages at which the parents reported the children as having said their first words

TABLE 9-1 Mean or Median Number of Months of Delay of Stutterers When Compared with Nonstutterers in the Use of First Words, Phrases, Sentences, and Speech Intelligibility Outside the Immediate Family

	N					
	Stutterers	Nonstutterers	Words	Phrases	Sentences	Intelligible Speech
Berry (1938b)	243, 140	252, 154*	7.42			12.03
Iowa Studies						
I. Johnson et al. (1942)	46	46	0.0		0.0	
II. Darley (1955)	50	50	0.97	0.80	2.07	
III. Johnson and Associates (1959)	137, 136*	131	0.1		0.8	
Morley (1957)	29	111	2.7	4.9		11.2
Andrews and Harris (1964)**	78	76		4.0		

*The two values of *N* given are for the two items of information respectively.
**Referred to in the text as the "Newcastle study."

and sentences proved to be much the same, suggesting that the difference was principally in the parents' evaluations of what they had observed rather than in the actualities.

We cannot be certain about the reason for the difference between the Iowa findings and those of other studies. There was, however, a difference in the nature of the populations sampled, as Andrews and Harris (1964, p. 35) pointed out. The Iowa groups tended to be representative of the higher socioeconomic levels of Midwestern society, while the Newcastle subjects were a broad sample of the population of an English industrial city. Berry's data were obtained from Chicago hospital clinics and social welfare agencies. A hypothesis to be considered is that the relatively high socioeconomic status of the Iowa families served to obscure to some extent any difference in language development that might have appeared between stutterers and nonstutterers.

In a survey of a very large number of children, Accordi et al. (1983) found delayed language development in 28 percent of stutterers as opposed to 8.7 percent of a control group. In contrast, while Bernstein Ratner and Silverman (2000) found that mothers and fathers rated children near the onset of stuttering as less advanced in their language skills than did parents of typically fluent matched peers, the stuttering children's parents were actually more accurate in their judgments when ratings were correlated with the children's performance on standardized speech and language measures—the children did, in fact, perform more poorly on most of the speech-language assessments used in the study.

A unique study of the relationship between language development and stuttering was undertaken by Kloth, Janssen, Kraaimaat, and Brutten (1995a, 1995b, 1998). The authors tracked 93 children at risk to develop stuttering because one or both of their parents stuttered. While none of the children stuttered when first seen, a year later 26 were indeed showing stuttering symptoms. These children did not differ from the nonstuttering children on speech-language measures made prior to stuttering onset (the Dutch version of the *Reynell Language Scales, Peabody Picture Vocabulary Test*, and Mean Length of Utterance), although they spoke more rapidly. The authors concluded that slowed speech rate protected against stuttering development.

Articulatory and Phonological Difficulties

There is a rather pronounced tendency of stutterers to have functional difficulties of articulation (now more typically termed "articulation disorders of unknown etiology"), "immature" speech, and the like (see Table 9-2). In addition to the findings summarized in the table, Berry (1938b) noted frequent "infantile perseveration," "very indistinct speech," and "lisping" in a survey of medical records of stutterers, and similar observations were reported by Bloodstein (1958) in a clinical study of 108 young stutterers. Kent and Williams (1963) observed that former stutterers in second grade were more likely to have a history of articulatory difficulties than children with no history of stuttering. McDowell (1928), whose data are not in a form permitting inclusion in Table 9-2, found no significant differences in the number of school-age stutterers and nonstutterers making errors on various categories of sounds in a test of articulation, though the 33 stutterers she tested made significantly more total errors than 33 nonstutterers. Ryan (1992) likewise found no difference between 20 preschool stutterers and normally fluent peers on the *Arizona Articulation Proficiency Scale*, but reported that 25 percent of the stutterers later required treatment for frontal lisping or difficulty with /r/.

St. Louis (1991) found severe stutterers more likely to have delayed or disordered articulation than mild or moderate stutterers, but Wolk, Edwards, and Conture (1993) reported that seven preschool stutterers with disordered phonology did not differ in severity of stuttering from seven with normal phonology. A similar lack of association between phonological skill and stuttering severity was found for a sample of 28 children near stuttering onset reported by Gregg and Yairi (2007). Moreover, as a general rule, studies have not yet shown significantly higher rates of stuttering on mispronounced words or those target sounds or words that should be difficult for the children to produce, as measured

TABLE 9-2 Percentage of Stutterers and Nonstutterers Having Other Speech Disorders, Chiefly Articulatory Difficulties, or Having a History of Such Disorders

	N				
	Stutterers	Nonstutterers	Source of information	% Stutterers	% Nonstutterers
Schindler (1955)	126	252	Speech examination	49	15
Darley (1955)	50	50	Reports of parents	26	4
Morley (1957)	37	113	Speech examination	50	31
Johnson and Associates (1959)	150	150	Reports of parents	15.3	7.3
Andrews and Harris (1964)	77	78	Reports of parents	29.9	10.3
Williams and Silverman (1968)	115	115	Speech examination	23.5	8.7
Blood and Seider (1981)	1,060		Reports of clinicians	27	
Franke (1983)	336		Speech examination	44	
Accordi et al. (1983)	2,802	1,602	Medical records*	27.8	6.5
Louko, Edwards, and Conture (1990)	30	30	Speech examination	40	7
St. Louis, Murray, and Ashworth (1991)	24		Speech examination	42	

*The comparison data were obtained by questionnaires distributed in schools.

by developmental expectations (Throneburg, Yairi, & Paden, 1994; Wolk, Blomgren, & Smith, 2000).

Co-Morbidity of Stuttering and Other Communication Disorders

Some studies have commented on the overall likelihood of stuttering associated with a range of co-morbid or concomitant communication disorders. Blood and Seider (1981) found that 68 percent of stuttering children could be described as having concomitant problems requiring clinical attention. Both Arndt and Healey (2001) and Blood, Ridenour, Qualls, and Hammer (2003) have conducted relatively recent surveys of practicing speech-language pathologists' caseloads. In the Arndt and Healey study, almost 500 stuttering children were identified on caseloads across 10 states. Of these, 44 percent were reported to have concomitant language or articulation/phonology problems. Blood, Ridenour, et al. (2003) identified 2,628 stuttering children on school caseloads. Over 45 percent of them were reported to have either articulation or phonological problems. Roughly one-third of the children were diagnosed with receptive and/or expressive language problems in syntax, semantics, or pragmatics (the study noted that many children were diagnosed with more than one additional concomitant disorder). An additional 6 percent were noted to have Specific Language Impairment. More than a third of the children had nonspeech/language concomitant disorders, although some of these (literacy problems) might have been reasonably associated with some degree of language delay or impairment. The diagnostic categories in this study allow for some breadth of interpretation and overlap, but there is a clear trend for children who stutter to be classified as needing additional services for speech, language, or other educationally relevant conditions. Healey and Reid (2003) also noted that an increasingly larger number of children who stutter are being diagnosed with attention deficit hyperactivity disorder (ADHD), consistent with rising trends to label this disorder in many countries.[7] Such findings have serious ramifications for research into the putative language processing skills of individuals who stutter: failure to determine the overall speech and language profiles of study participants may collapse potential subgroups of stutterers, while those that exclude them may describe only a portion of the total population. Moreover, since at least 20 percent of children who stutter will become adults who stutter, it is notable that relatively few studies of adult stutterers have appraised their language proficiency.

Interpretations

It seems evident that concomitant speech and language delay or difficulty occurs with unusual frequency in stuttering children. We note that the diagnosis of other speech or language disorders often carries with it elevated risk for additional communicative impairments (Shriberg, Tomblin, & McSweeny, 1999), although reported numbers have not been as high as those reported for stuttering children. Aside from hypothesis, we have little to go on in speculating about the meaning of this fact. One assumption, held by Bloodstein (1975) among others, on the basis of clinical observation, is that children with communication disorders are more likely to acquire a sense of failure as speakers and to learn to struggle with their speech attempts. Horowitz (1965) attempted to verify this in her clinical examination of a series of children with faulty articulation. She reported that approximately 44 percent of these children "exhibited some degree of prolongations, repetitions, blockings, etc., listed by Van Riper as elements of stuttering behavior." The presence of such behavior, however, did not seem to have much to do with whether the parents had attempted to correct the child's articulation, despite the fact that the children who had been corrected were more often reluctant to speak and were more often seen to place their articulators in a deliberate way when producing certain sounds.

Comas (1974) reported on 1,050 cases of young children in whom stuttering was observed to appear while they were being treated for articulation problems. He was also struck by the appearance of stuttering among a group of children undergoing speech therapy after cleft palate operations, though in some cases the stuttering was noted some months before speech treatment (Comas, 1975). It is not known whether or not such stuttering persisted over time.

Another reasonable way to explain the high association between stuttering and other speech and language problems is to assume that they are caused to some extent by the same thing. This point of view was broached, for example, by West, Kennedy, and Carr (1947, p. 93), who suggested that stuttering and speech delays often tend to appear in the same individuals because they have inherited a common predisposition to both conditions. Bloodstein (1958, p. 30) could find no indication of such a relationship in a group of 70 young stutterers. About half the group had a history of slow or abnormal speech development and half had a family background of stuttering, but there was essentially no tendency for the two to be related. This was supported by Seider, Gladstien, and Kidd (1982), who found no difference in the incidence of articulation and language problems between stutterers with and without a family history of stuttering. On the other hand, in both this investigation and that of Cox, Seider, and Kidd (1984), stutterers did not differ from their nonstuttering relatives in the incidence of such problems, a finding perhaps indicating that relatives of stutterers are at a higher than normal risk for speech and language disorder. Homzie, Lindsay, Simpson, and Hasenstab (1988) surveyed stutterers in self-help groups by questionnaire. Not only did large numbers report personal histories of delayed

---

[7] Ratcliff-Baird (2001) notes EEG profiles in a group of adult stutterers that are consistent with those seen in ADHD. However, Abwender et al. (1998) noted fewer attentional deficits in their population of 22 stutterers, noting them to have more in common with individuals with Tourette Syndrome, including a relatively high incidence of Obsessive-Compulsive Disorder (OCD).

language and articulation disorder, but 25 percent of 111 responses mentioned articulation problems in relatives as well.

Observations by Yoss and Darley (1974) hint that in some children articulation problems and stuttering might both be manifestations of developmental apraxia. Among 30 children with articulation problems, 16 performed poorly on a test of oral apraxia. These children had more repetitions and prolongations in their speech than did the others. On Blakeley's *Screening Test for Developmental Apraxia of Speech*, Byrd and Cooper (1989a) found that the mean score of stuttering children fell between those of typically fluent and developmentally apraxic children. The performance profiles of the stutterers and apraxics appeared more similar to each other than to the profile of the normally fluent speakers.

SCHOOL HISTORY

Grade Placement

Historically, evidence has been found that stutterers, on the whole, are poorer in educational adjustment than normal speakers. Historically, the usual criterion has been amount of delay in grade placement at school. This type of measure may be used either by comparing a child's grade placement with that of others of the same age or by comparing a child's chronological age with that of others in the same grade. Schindler (1955) found that significantly fewer stutterers were accelerated and significantly more were delayed in grade placement when compared with nonstutterers of like age. On average, the stutterers were delayed by about one-half year, and the comparison group by slightly less than one-quarter year. This is in general agreement with the results of previous studies. McAllister (1937, p. 11) reported that stutterers in Dunbartonshire were delayed by 9.7 months, on the average. A survey of schoolchildren in six American cities by Conradi (1912) showed that in every grade the mean age of the stutterers was higher than that of all children in the grade, by seven or eight months in most grades. Comparable findings were obtained in early studies by Root, Wallin, and others (cited by Johnson, 1932). Darley (1955) found that, of 50 stuttering children and their controls, 15 stutterers and only 4 fluent peers had repeated at least half of a grade.

Placement criteria for school-aged children have evolved greatly over the years since these types of studies were conducted. Even when first published, it seemed generally agreed that the relatively poorer educational adjustments are due directly to the difficulty of speaking in a classroom situation. The oral recitation problems of stutterers and some of their effects on academic performance were documented by Knudsen (1939). There have been no more recent studies to suggest that children who have stuttering as their only single diagnosis are promoted at a rate distinguishable from that of children who do not stutter.

Educational Achievement The average historical delay of stutterers in grade placement may be compared with their performance on standard tests of academic achievement. McDowell (1928) found that stutterers' overall scores on the *Stanford Achievement Tests* were comparable to those of nonstutterers. Schindler (1955) obtained similar findings, on the whole, using the *Iowa Basic Skills Tests*, but her stutterers were seven months delayed, on the average, in basic language skills[8] on the elementary level and four months behind in basic arithmetic skills at the advanced level. Williams, Melrose, and Woods (1969) found stutterers consistently behind nonstutterers on all aspects of the *Iowa Tests*, although there was evidence that, in the area of language skills, the stutterers tended to catch up by eighth grade. On a test of computational ability, Schulz (1977) found no significant difference between stuttering and nonstuttering children in Germany.

In eight studies, the silent reading ability of stutterers was found normal or not significantly below that of nonstutterers by all except those of Murray, Bosshardt, and Nandyal.[9] Hamilton (1940)

---

[8]The test of language skills is comprised of subtests on spelling, capitalization, punctuation, and usage.

[9]See McDowell (1928), Murray (1932), Hamilton (1940), Schindler (1955), Andrews and Harris (1964, p. 99), Conture and van Naerssen (1977), Janssen, Kraaimaat, and van der Meulen (1983), Bosshardt and Nandyal (1988), Bosshardt (1990).

found also that stutterers did not differ from normal speakers in frequency of fixations and regressions or in span of fixation during silent reading. Roland (1972) observed more regressions in his group of stutterers, as did Brutten and Janssen (1979) and Brutten, Bakker, Janssen, and van der Meulen (1984). In a questionnaire survey of college students in Bogota, Colombia, by Ardila et al. (1994), 27 percent of stutterers and 15.9 percent of nonstutterers indicated that they had dyslexia.

Educational Adjustment Somewhat unexpectedly, Cox, Seider, and Kidd (1984) reported no group difference in the school adjustment of stutterers and nonstutterers. Their experimental group was limited to families in which at least five members stuttered. Information was derived from interviews with stutterers and parents regarding such items as satisfaction with school achievement; attention difficulty in school; learning disability; the child's perception of teachers as unfair; adequacy in math, reading, and writing; and being difficult to control. Ota and Nagasawa (2005) examined adjustment in a cohort of 124 third- through sixth-grade children. They found relatively good indices of adjustment and self-esteem, which related in part to the child's overall academic competence and the degree to which parents discussed the stuttering with the child.

INTELLIGENCE (IQ)

In this section, we will address intelligence as defined by intelligence quotient (IQ) and similar psychoeducational measures. Other more specific and more general cognitive abilities have been studied in people who stutter, and these are addressed in the next chapter.

It has been asserted repeatedly that the average intelligence of stutterers does not differ from that of nonstutterers, but reports of careful investigations compel us to reexamine this assumption critically. It is true that, if comparable data from control groups are ignored, estimates of the average IQ of stutterers in various studies fall unremarkably in the general region of 100, the theoretical average for the population at large. In the past, when small departures from this theoretical average were found they were tacitly assumed to have resulted from random sampling errors or from the manner in which subjects were obtained for study. Ultimately, however, Schindler (1955) and Andrews and Harris (1964, p. 97) drew samples of schoolchildren from large populations representing a broad range of socioeconomic backgrounds and compared their intelligence with that of similarly selected normally fluent children using appropriate tests of statistical inference. The results in both studies show an average IQ of about 95 for the stutterers as against about 100 for the nonstutterers (see Table 9-3). Comparable findings were reported by Okasha, Bishry, et al. (1974). In each instance, the difference was statistically significant.

Although an average difference of several IQ points is more important theoretically than practically, the striking agreement among these three studies compels us to consider seriously that there may be a small difference between stutterers and nonstutterers as groups that needs to be explained. When we examine the other findings summarized in Table 9-3 for a clue to the reason for which such a possibility might not have been apparent before, we see that in most cases there was no comparison group. In the only other controlled study, that by Johnson et al. (1942), the subjects were chosen from a relatively limited social, economic, and educational milieu. Darley's sample also represents higher socioeconomic levels, having been chosen largely from children brought to the University of Iowa Speech Clinic by their parents. Darley gives no mean or median IQ for his 50 stutterers, but reports that when their scores were grouped in three categories roughly representative of superior, normal, and below normal intelligence, the distribution of frequencies did not differ significantly by chi-square test from that reported by Wechsler for the general population.

By contrast with those of other studies, Schindler's subjects represented a broad cross section of the city, village, and rural population of Iowa, while those of Andrews and Harris consisted of the stutterers found in a survey of all of the children in the last two years of primary school in the city

TABLE 9-3 Intelligence Quotients of Stutterers and Nonstutterers

			Stutterers		Nonstutterers	
	*N**	Population sampled	Mean or median IQ	Range	Mean or median	Range
Scripture and Kittredge (1923)	62	Vanderbilt Medical Clinic	92	56–130		
McDowell (1928)	61	New York City schools	99.1	63–156		
West (1931)	4,059	U.S. public schools	96.5			
Berry (1937a)	166	Chicago Hospital clinics	99.2			
Johnson et al. (1942)	46 / 46	University of Iowa Outpatient Speech Clinic**	114	80–159	116	95–158
Carlson (1946)	50	Speech improvement classes, New York City public schools	109			
Darley (1955)	50	University of Iowa Outpatient Speech Clinic**		54–162		
Schlinder (1955)	108 / 23,326	Iowa urban and rural schools	94.9***	55–124	99.5	50–140
Andrews and Harris (1964)	80 / 80	Newcastle Upon Tyne schools	94.7***		101.8	
Hartz (1970)	126	Westphalia schoolchildren	112			
Okasha, Bishry, et al. (1974)	79 / 80	Egyptian schoolchildren	94***		101	
Pukačová (1974)	74	Czech children	95.4			
Heinzel and Ubricht (1983)	31	West German schoolchildren	112			

*Represents Stutterers/Non stutterers.
**In both the Johnson and Darley studies, most of the subjects were referred by their parents. The experimental groups were representative of upper socioeconomic levels. The control groups were chosen to be comparable in socioeconomic status.
***Significantly different from the mean of the nonstuttering group.

of Newcastle-upon-Tyne, who were matched for age and sex with control subjects from their own class at school. It is noteworthy that an average IQ of 96.5, only slightly higher than those obtained in the Schindler and Newcastle studies, was reported by West (1931) for a very large group of stutterers in the 1930 White House Conference survey of schoolchildren in 43 American towns and cities.

The very small amount of work that has been done on the subtest profiles and test scatter of stutterers has been sufficient to produce considerable disagreement. Scripture and Kittredge (1923) found that the majority of a group of stutterers tended to have an abnormally uneven scatter of scores on the subtests of the *Stanford-Binet*, suggesting the possibility of brain damage or emotional instability. Furthermore, many of the stutterers tended to have particularly low scores on the vocabulary subtest, leading Scripture and Kittredge to conclude that they appeared to have a "word disability." On the other hand, an analysis by Carlson (1946) seemed to show that stutterers, as compared with children having behavior problems, performed especially poorly on the motor coordination items of the *Stanford-Binet*. Andrews and Harris (1964, p. 98) found essentially no differences in subtest profiles for their two groups on the *Wechsler Intelligence Scale for Children*. Stuttering children tested by Heinzel and Ubricht (1983) had significantly higher performance than verbal IQs.

In search of evidence of brain dysfunction in stutterers, Cox (1982) employed a neurophysiological test battery consisting of the *Wechsler Adult Intelligence Scale* and various other tests. He found little indication of significant cerebral dysfunction.

Stuttering among Persons with Intellectual Disabilities[10]

If, as the findings we have reviewed suggest, stuttering is slightly more common in the less intelligent of the normal population, we might expect it to be especially prevalent among persons with mental retardation. There is ample evidence that it is (see Table 9-4).[11] Although the prevalence figures that have been reported vary widely, almost all of them are far higher than the 1 percent that is usual in an ordinary population. Stansfield (1990) found a modestly elevated prevalence of 6.3 percent of "idiopathic disfluency" (stuttering and cluttering) in sample of almost 800 adults with intellectual disability. Similarly, Van Borsel et al. (2006) found the prevalence of stuttering in special needs classrooms in Belgium to be four times that seen in the general school population (roughly 0.6 percent vs 2.3 percent). Stuttering, apparently of all degrees of severity and complexity, would seem to occur more frequently in this population than in any other single identifiable group of people.

A question often raised is whether the stuttering of persons with intellectual disability is the same disorder as is generally called by that name, especially since in many cases it is described as lacking much of the secondary symptomatology of ordinary stuttering. In a group of adults with intellectual disability whose speech problem had been diagnosed as stuttering, Bonfanti and Culatta (1977) found few secondary features. The subjects tended to be aware of their disfluency but not concerned about it, and there was little evidence of avoidance, frustration, or anxiety. It must be kept in mind, however, that a considerable amount of "ordinary" stuttering in its early stages also exhibits few associated or reactive features (see Chapter 1). Lerman, Powers, and Rigrodsky (1965) presented evidence that much of the stuttering of school-age children with intellectual disability is comparable to the early stuttering of children who have normal intelligence. They also pointed out that fears, avoidances, and secondary stuttering symptoms can and do occur in persons with intellectual disability. Schlanger and Gottsleben (1957) found such reactions in 26 percent of their stutterers with intellectual disability. This should not be surprising if we recall that they may occur in developmentally normal 3- or even 2-year-olds.

[10] In 2006, the American Association on Mental Retardation changed its name and recommended teminology to the American Association on Intellectual and Developmental Disabilities.

[11] See also Keane (1972) for a review that includes some unpublished studies.

TABLE 9-4 A Prevalence of Stuttering among Persons with Intellectual Disability

	N*	Population	Percentage of stutterers
Ballard (1912)	944	Special schools for "mentally defective children"	2.4
Louttit and Halls (1936)	620	Ungraded classes for "subnormals"	3.22
Wohl (1951)	145	Special schools for "mentally and physically handicapped"	5.5
Karlin and Strazzulla (1952)	50	Outpatient hospital clinic for "retarded children"	2.0
Schlanger (1953)	74	Institution for "mentally retarded"	20.3
Schlanger and Gottsleben (1957)	516	Institution for "mentally retarded"	17.0
Stark (1963)**		Educationally "subnormal children"	10.0
Schaeffer, and Shearer (1968)	4,307	Institution for "mentally retarded"	7.6
Sheehan, Martyn, and Kilburn (1968)	216	Institution for "mentally retarded"	0.8
Martyn, Sheehan, and Slutz (1969)	346	Institution for "mentally retarded"	1.0
Chapman and Cooper (1973)	1,467	Institution for "mentally retarded"	3.0
Brady and Hall (1976)	3,057	Educable "mentally retarded"	1.6
Brady and Hall (1976)	457	"Trainable mentally retarded" in schools	3.08
Boberg et al. (1978)	840	Classes for "educable mentally retarded"	1.43
Boberg et al. (1978)	439	Classes for "trainable mentally retarded"	2.51
Brindle and Dunster (1984)	351	Institution for "mentally retarded"	6.55

*Where data were obtained in institutions, *N* refers to the total number in the survey population who had speech.
**Cited by Andrews and Harris (1964, p. 7).

In an effort to find out how similar such stuttering is to that of intellectually normal subjects, Shearer and Baud (1970) investigated the adaptation effect, and Chapman and Cooper (1973) studied adaptation, consistency, and expectancy (see Chapter 10) in stutterers with intellectual disability. All of these phenomena were found, though not to quite the degree that is characteristic of most stutterers. Of 18 individuals with intellectual disability that were tested by Chapman and Cooper, only 5 indicated any expectation of stuttering, but these 5 stuttered on all words on which they had anticipated doing so.

Prevalence in Down Syndrome Among the special classifications of developmental disability, stuttering has been reported to be unusually common in Down syndrome. A prevalence of 33 percent, based on the independent judgments of three speech pathologists, was recorded by Gottsleben (1955) for a group of 36 individuals, 45 percent by Schlanger and Gottsleben (1957) for 44 cases, and 21 percent by Lubman (1955) for 48 children with that syndrome. Rohovsky, with the help of 10 other judges who listened to tape recordings, identified 48 percent as stutterers in a group of 27 (cited by Schlanger, 1973, p. 19). Similarly, Devenny and Silverman (1990) classified 42 percent of 31 adults with Down syndrome as stutterers. In two other unpublished studies cited by Van Riper (1982, p. 41), Edson found a 39 percent and Schubert a 15 percent prevalence. The only apparent exception to the general trend was the study of Martyn, Sheehan, and Slutz (1969), in which only 1 stutterer turned up among 42 subjects with Down syndrome.

The second most common identifiable cause of intellectual disability after Down syndrome, Fragile X syndrome, is also characterized by apparently elevated levels of stutter-like disfluency, although no large-scale estimates of its prevalence are available (Abbeduto & Hagerman, 1997).

In view of this remarkable prevalence of stuttering in Down syndrome and other forms of developmental disability, an inevitable question is whether what we are observing here is stuttering at all, in the usual sense. Cabañas (1954) noted an exceptional amount of speech interruption in a group of 50 children with Down syndrome, but regarded it as cluttering rather than as true stuttering, since he found no evidence of anticipations, substitutions, or other avoidance devices or memory of past blocking. On the other hand, Rohovsky, in the study previously referred to, found that of 13 persons with Down syndrome who appeared to stutter, 5 displayed observable reactions to their disfluency. Farmer and Brayton (1979) noted that disfluent subjects with Down syndrome achieved poorer ratings of intelligibility in conversational speech than fluent ones, and suggested that their disfluency was therefore more characteristic of cluttering than stuttering.

The most detailed examination of disfluency in Down syndrome to date was carried out by Preus (1972) on a sample of 47 individuals selected only for fairly intelligible speech. Preus studied chiefly the frequency of whole-word repetitions, part-word repetitions, and prolongations in the subjects' speech. He found a high frequency of each of these symptoms in the group as a whole. Using an arbitrary criterion of 5 instances of such disfluency per 100 words, he classified 46.8 percent of the sample as stutterers. Using the same cut-off point and excluding whole-word repetitions, he classified 34 percent as stutterers. (Institutional personnel judged 53 percent to be stutterers.) Unexpectedly, Preus found in 29.8 percent of the cases secondary symptoms consisting of associated bodily movements or of devices such as avoidance and postponement. With the aid of judges' ratings, he also classified 31.9 percent of the same sample as clear or pronounced clutterers, but there was no correlation between stuttering and cluttering. Preus concluded that the disfluencies found in Down syndrome may be classified as "genuine stuttering."

Otto and Yairi (1975) analyzed the speech of subjects with Down syndrome who were judged not to be stutterers and found that it contained more part-word repetitions, word repetitions, "tensions," and other disfluencies than did the speech of individuals of normal intelligence. Their rate of speech also tended to be more rapid.

FAMILY HISTORY

Birth Order and Sibling Relationship

There is considerable evidence that the various ordinal positions in the family are represented in about the expected proportions among stutterers.[12] Whether an only child is more likely to stutter, however, is a question that has produced conflicting findings. Among large groups of stutterers, Rotter (1939) and the Iowa studies found an unusual proportion of only children—18 or 20 percent as compared with only 10 or 12 percent among nonstutterers. Boland (1950) also found a higher percentage of only children among 262 stutterers than among a large sample of the general population, but noted that these were stutterers who had applied for treatment. In the Newcastle study, 8 of the 80 stutterers and 3 of the fluent cases were only children, not a statistically significant difference. Morgenstern (1956) observed no departure from the expected number of only children among 355 stutterers. Likewise, Accordi and his associates (1983) found that the same percentage of a large number of stutterers and nonstutterers were only children. Rotter and Morgenstern agreed in the finding that the average stutterer was separated from the sibling closest in age by a larger number of years than was the average nonstutterer, but this difference appeared in neither the Newcastle data nor the findings of Gladstien, Seider, and Kidd (1981).

A more recent study suggests that the mother's age at birth of her first child is associated with

[12] Morgenstern (1956), Johnson and Associates (1959, p. 72), Andrews and Harris (1964, p. 54), Gladstien, Seider, and Kidd (1981).

an interaction of the dopamine D1 gene (DRD1) with obsessive-compulsive behaviors and with stuttering (Comings & MacMurray, 2006). This is intriguing given the increasing interest in dopamine metabolism and stuttering (see Chapter 14). However, at this point, it is difficult to reconcile the existing disparities in research findings. If there is in fact any relationship between stuttering and status as an only child, perhaps it is due to the increased parental concern that the only child is accorded, as Johnson and Associates (1959, p. 225) suggested.

Familial Background

The literature contains occasional references to the incidence of such factors as left-handedness, twinning, allergies, and neurological and psychiatric disorders in the families of stutterers, rather than the stutterers themselves (as discussed in Chapters 3 and 4), but little careful investigation has been done. Bryngelson and Rutherford (1937) and Bryngelson (1939) reported findings on left-handedness that were not significant. In the Iowa and Newcastle studies, there were no differences with regard to either left-handedness or twinning in the two groups of families, though there appeared to be a trend toward significantly more twins among the stutterers' relatives in the Newcastle group. The Iowa studies showed no significant difference in the incidence of either epilepsy or diabetes among the relatives of the two groups, although there were 21 cases of diabetes in the stutterers' families as against 12 in the nonstutterers'. In the families of 2,802 stutterers and a comparison group of 1,602 typically fluent speakers, Accordi and his coworkers (1983) found no differences in diseases, neurologic disorders, cluttering, delayed language development, or parental consanguinity.

Only with regard to the familial incidence of allergies have some findings been positive. Both Kennedy and Williams (1938) and Card (1939) found that almost all of their stuttering subjects had family histories of allergies, as compared with roughly one-third to three-fifths of their control groups. On the other hand, no indication of a difference appeared in the Iowa studies, in which about half of both groups reported some type of allergy in their families. The family backgrounds of stutterers, of course, contain several times as many stuttering relatives as do the family backgrounds of nonstutterers (see Chapter 3).

Parents: Characteristics and Behaviors

From the point of view of any theory that regards stuttering as due chiefly or in part to environmental influences, the attitudes, child training practices, and personality makeup of the stutterer's parents are of profound interest. In the course of the development of theories of stuttering that accord some role to parenting behaviors, two major conceptions of the parents have emerged. In one, they are viewed as basically neurotic persons whose contacts with their children are in some measure rejecting, overprotective, dominating, ambivalent, or in other ways warped by anxiety, hostility, dependence, or guilt. In the other, which is due chiefly to the work of Johnson, the parents are portrayed as largely anxious, perfectionistic, and demanding, particularly with regard to the child's speech.

Parental Adjustment These two descriptions are clearly overlapping to some extent. One of the main differences between them lies in the degree of emotional disturbance that the parents are assumed to exhibit. Johnson regarded most of them as essentially ordinary persons whose behavior simply reflects the competitive pressures of our culture to a somewhat unusual degree. On this issue, the research findings are fairly clear. Although occasional observations have seemed to suggest that stutterers' parents differ from others in typical personality makeup, the results of a series of controlled investigations in which the emotional adjustment of stutterers' parents have been systematically compared with that of parents of nonstutterers by means of personality tests have provided little support for this assumption (see Table 9-5).

Parental Child Training Attitudes Despite this failure to discover distinct personality deviations

TABLE 9-5 Personality and Adjustment of Parents of Stutterers and Nonstutterers

	N					
	Experimental		Control			
	M	F	M	F	Test	Findings
Darley (1955)	48	49	43	43	Guilford Inventory of Factors STDCR	Differences between the experimental and control parents were not statistically significant for any of the five factors.
Grossman (1952)	21	21	21	21	Minnesota Multiphasic Personality Inventory (MMPI)	There was a significant difference on only one of 13 scales of the test, the parents of the stutterers having a higher average F score. (The F score is one of the four validity scales of the MMPI. A high F score is usually interpreted to mean that subjects are trying to place themselves in an unfavorable light.)
Goodstein and Dahlstrom (1956)	100	100	100	100	Minnesota Multiphasic Personality Inventory (MMPI)	The scores of the parents of stutterers closely resembled those of both their matched controls and the original standardization group of normal adults, although there were a few small differences, of which the most notable was a slight tendency, within the normal range, to be more anxious.
Goodstein (1956)	50	50	100	100*	Minnesota Multiphasic Personality Inventory (MMPI)	In a follow-up investigation the parents of 50 additional stutterers did not differ significantly from the experimental and control groups of the Goodstein and Dahlstrom study, except for a few small differences in a less abnormal direction.
LaFollette (1956)	85	85	50	50**	California Test of Personality	There was no difference in adjustment between the experimental and control groups as a whole, mothers or fathers. The fathers of older stutterers, aged 19–30, had poorer adjustment than the fathers in the control group.
					Psycho-Somatic Inventory of McFarland and Seitz	The fathers of the stutterers exhibited poorer mental health than the fathers of the control group. There was no difference between the two groups of mothers.

					Allport Ascendance-Submission Reaction Study	The parents of the stutterers were more submissive than those of the control group, due essentially to a difference between the two groups of fathers.
Andrews and Harris (1964)	71		79		Maudsley Personality Inventory	The mothers of the stutterers did not differ from those of the nonstutterers on either side of the two scales of the test (extraversion and neuroticism).
	49		62		Cattell 16 Personality Factor Inventory	No significant differences between the two groups of mothers appeared on any of the 16 factors.
Feldman (1976)	32	32	32	32	Jourard Self-Disclosure Questionnaire	Parents of stutterers and nonstutterers did not differ with respect to how much of their attitudes and concerns they confided to their spouses, friends, and children. Stutterers' parents, however, more often indicated items about which they would decline to disclose information.
Flügel (1979)	124		97		Maudsley Personality Inventory and Maudsley Medical Questionnaire	Mothers of stutterers scored higher on a combined measure of neuroticism and extraversion.
Zenner et al. (1978)	7	7	14	14	State-Trait Anxiety Inventory	Parents of stutterers revealed more anxiety as a personality trait than did parents of children with articulatory difficulties and parents of normal-speaking children.

*The comparison group was identical with that of Goodstein and Dahlstrom (1956).

**The size of both the experimental and comparison groups varied somewhat from these figures from test to test.

in most parents of stutterers, there is considerable evidence of differences in their attitudes and behavior toward their children. Some of this evidence, notably that of Kinstler (1961), is most readily interpreted as supporting a theory of stuttering as a neurotic disorder. Kinstler compared the responses of mothers of young stutterers and nonstutterers on a questionnaire designed to measure overt and covert maternal acceptance and rejection by means of ratings of agreement with such statements as, "I'd prefer not to have any more children," "A mother should sacrifice her own desires for what is best for her children," and "I do not permit my child to climb tall trees." He found that, although the mothers of stutterers appeared to be superficially accepting of their children, they seemed to reject their children in subtle, hidden ways to a greater extent than did the comparison mothers.

An appreciable body of other evidence seems to support Johnson's view of stutterers' parents. Of more than 800 questions asked of mothers and fathers of stuttering and typically fluent children in the Iowa studies, a large proportion dealt with the home environment, disciplinary practices, and parental attitudes and adjustments as they related directly or indirectly to the children. The results showed that, while the similarities between the two groups of parents appeared to be greater than the differences, a comparatively larger number of parents of stutterers tended to impose somewhat high standards of behavior on their children or to reveal in one form or another a tendency to be critical, anxious, or perfectionistic. For example, the stutterers underwent coercive toilet training somewhat more often and were weaned somewhat sooner than the nonstutterers, and their parents expected children to walk and talk earlier and expressed more discontentment with their spouse, their children, and their socioeconomic circumstances than did the parents of the nonstutterers.

Other questionnaire data that seemed to corroborate these conclusions were obtained by Moncur (1952), who found that parents of stutterers tended to dominate, over-supervise, and be more critical of their children. This was observed also to a somewhat lesser extent by Bloom (1959).

A study by Zenner and his coworkers (1978) was concerned specifically with the factor of parental anxiety. After viewing a videotape recording of his or her own child at play with two other children, each of a group of parents of stutterers completed the A-State portion of the *State-Trait Anxiety Inventory* with respect to the anxiety they had experienced while watching the tape. The parents of stutterers indicated more anxiety in the situation than did parents of children with typically fluent speech or disorders of articulation. They also revealed more anxiety as a personality trait on the A-Trait portion of the inventory.

It must be cautioned that any unqualified concept of stutterers' parents as dominating and demanding is not consistent either with clinical observation, which reveals many exceptions, or even with the results of the studies themselves. Quarrington (1974), in fact, reinterpreted the literature we have just reviewed in an attempt to show that much of it supports a view of stutterers' parents as excessively passive and permissive with respect to control of the child's behavior.

It is of course probable that any inherent differences between stuttering and nonstuttering children in terms of temperament or other personality features (see Chapter 7 for discussion) would influence parental perceptions and behaviors, since there are mutual influences on such characteristics.[13] For example, Karrass et al. (2006) found that parents characterized 65 preschool children who stutter as more reactive, significantly less able to regulate their emotions, and having significantly poorer attention regulation on the *Behavior Style Questionnaire (BSQ)*. At this point, it is difficult to know which characteristics of parents and of their children might interact to create profiles that exert causal or maintaining influences on stuttering.

Conflicting Evidence from the Newcastle Study The literature suggests that some parents of stutterers may impose high standards of behavior of

[13] See Elgar et al. (2004) for discussion of how maternal and child distress exert mutual influences.

all kinds, not speech fluency alone. However, before we adopt it as a broadly valid concept of the stutterer's parental environment, we must take note of some sharply conflicting evidence. From the Newcastle study, which included intensive interviewing and testing of the subjects' mothers, there emerges a remarkably different picture containing little hint of perfectionism or high standards.

Like the Iowa parents, the mothers of the Newcastle stutterers were very similar to their fluent peers with regard to most features of their personal histories, and there appeared to be about the same amount of neuroticism among them. They differed from mothers of nonstutterers, however, in several respects. They more frequently exhibited low intelligence. They tended to have poor records of school achievement. More of them had poor work histories as indicated by frequent job changes. And finally, they more frequently failed to provide an adequate home environment, as evidenced by a greater incidence of poor housing, as well as some tendency toward less unified family life and less contact with relatives outside the home. In short, the mothers of the stutterers seemed to be distinguished by a general inclination to fail—at school, at work, and in the home—and this inability to "cope" seemed to be related to low innate capacity rather than to poor emotional adjustment. Among these mothers, low intelligence was significantly correlated with such factors as low intelligence and late or poor talking in the child and with abnormal personality of the husband as evidenced by psychiatric or conduct problems destructive of family functioning.[14] Clearly, the parents of the Iowa and Newcastle stutterers seem to represent two quite different groups of people.

That these two hypothetical groups may actually exist is suggested by further evidence from the Newcastle study. Andrews and Harris (1964, p. 114 ff.) carried out a factor analysis in order to determine whether they could identify subgroups of cases with respect to the array of items on which they had gathered information. Among their 80 stutterers they discovered a small delegation, as it were, from the Iowa group. Though not differentiable from the rest in any sharp or categorical way, these children tended to be marked by high social class and upward mobility, by intelligent mothers with "neurotic traits, particularly of an obsessional kind," and by good intelligence, a mild stutter, and symptoms of anxiety, aggression and disobedience, irritability, and overactivity.

The possibility that the Iowa and Newcastle findings are applicable respectively to two more or less differentiable groups of stutterers may serve to raise the question of which group is more representative of stutterers "in general." The answer is not as simple as it may at first appear. The Iowa stutterers, to be sure, are from certain points of view a highly selected group. On the other hand, it is only with certain qualifications that the Newcastle subjects are to be regarded as broadly representative of whatever we mean by "the population." Andrews and Harris caution that in the Newcastle-upon-Tyne group "geographical isolation and the harsh realities of the environment" have produced a people with a distinctive culture and that the results of their study may not be strictly comparable with those from other communities (1964, p. 36).

In their own ways, both the Iowa and Newcastle groups, and all other individual studies of parents of stuttering children must be seen as poor representatives of the whole range of cultural variations. It must be considered that if what we have in mind as "the population" is to be defined in terms of numbers, it is possibly best represented by people who live by the hand plow, whose likes have rarely been seen in all of England or the United States outside the pages of *National Geographic*, and who can ill afford the luxury of being concerned about their children's stuttering. Thus, we cannot yet know the nature and extent of the possible role that parents play in the emergence or persistence of their children's stuttering.

[14] Fourteen of the 80 fathers of stutterers, as compared with 9 in the comparison group, were judged to have such problems on the basis of the information obtained from the mothers. Evidently, it would have been of some interest to interview the fathers of this group. This was not possible because, as Andrews and Harris (1964, p. 39) state, "In this community, not only are children thought to be the concern of mothers alone, but the prevailing unemployment meant that few fathers were prepared to risk their jobs by taking time off to attend hospital."

Stutterers' Perceptions of Parental Behavior In an investigation by Gildston (1967) of adolescent stutterers by means of the Q-technique, the subjects were asked to sort the cards on the basis of how each parent "sees you and feels you really are" and on the basis of how each parent "wants you to be." The correlations between the parental actual and parental ideal sorts yielded measures of parental acceptance as perceived by the subjects. Gildston found that perceived parental acceptance was lower among the stutterers than among the nonstutterers.

On the *Children's Report of Parental Behavior Inventory*, Bourdon and Silber (1970) found no differences between stuttering and nonstuttering adolescents in ratings of parental acceptance, rejection, control, possessiveness, tendency to instill anxiety, and the like. Using the same inventory in a study of 11- to 13-year-old children, Yairi and Williams (1971) obtained somewhat unexpected findings. The stutterers appeared to view their parents as behaving with less control and hostility and with more love and autonomy than did the nonstutterers.

Parental Level of Aspiration A unique approach to the question of parental standards of behavior was taken by Goldman and Shames (1964a, 1964b). Employing a modified *Rotter Level of Aspiration Board* procedure that enabled them to control the amount of failure and success experienced by the subject, they found that parents of stutterers did not appear to set higher goals for themselves in a motor task than did parents of nonstutterers. With a similar procedure, they then studied the goals that parents of stutterers set for their children. The parents were asked to predict the child's scores in operating the *Rotter Board* and also to predict the number of words on which the child would have difficulty in telling a story. Goldman and Shames found that the fathers of the stutterers, on the whole, appeared to exhibit unrealistic goal-setting behavior. On the speech task, their estimates of the amount of difficulty their children would have was lower, despite the fact that the children were stutterers, than those of the fathers of the control group. Furthermore, on both the motor and speech tasks, the fathers of the stutterers tended to persist in relatively high estimates of their children's success, in spite of failures, to a greater extent than did the fathers of the nonstutterers when confronted with their children's failures. The two groups of mothers did not differ, although the mothers of the stutterers showed a tendency to make higher initial estimates of their children's success on the *Rotter Board*.

Further work has failed to confirm some of these findings, however. Quarrington, Seligman, and Kosower (1969) replicated the portion of Shames' and Goldman's experiment that dealt with the goals the parents set for their children on the *Rotter Board* and found that the mothers of the stutterers tended to set lower goals, while the two groups of fathers did not differ.

Parents' Interactions with Children For many years, speech clinicians have advised parents of young stutterers to cultivate a warm, accepting relationship with the child, to decrease their speaking rate, and to avoid interrupting the child or bombarding the child with questions. In attempts to test the underlying assumptions of this widely accepted practice,[15] a number of investigators have videotaped the interactions of young stuttering children and their parents in play situations. The results have been conflicting. In addition, mothers are much more often the focus of study than are fathers, a general problem in studying children's communicative development (Perlmann & Berko Gleason, 1993).

Kaprisin-Burrelli, Egolf, and Shames (1972) recorded the conversation between school-age children and their parents and evaluated the statements of the parents as positive or negative. Positive statements were those that encouraged verbalization, indicated understanding, gave praise, accepted feelings, demonstrated interest, and the like. Negative statements were critical, dictatorial, threatening, interrupting, lacking appropriate understanding or

[15] See Bernstein Ratner (2004) and Chapter 14 for discussion of the evidence-based practice ramifications of this body of research.

recognition of feeling, and so forth. The parents of stutterers were consistently found to converse with their children in a more negative manner than the parents of nonstutterers. Fifty-eight percent of their statements were classified as negative as compared with 22 percent of those made by the control group.

In a study by Meyers and Freeman (1985a), mothers of 4- to 5-year-old stutterers and nonstutterers interacted in a free play situation with their own and others' children. No differences appeared between the two groups of mothers in numbers of positive or negative statements, initiations or terminations of interactions, questions, comments, total words or utterances, or in mean length of utterances. Meyers and Freeman (1985b) found that the mothers did not differ in the frequency of interruptions of their children. Mothers of stutterers did talk faster on the average than mothers of nonstutterers, however, when speaking to both stutterers and nonstutterers (Meyers & Freeman, 1985c), suggesting some mutual influence of the child's speech behaviors on the adult's speech rate, while stuttering appeared to elicit more rapid speech from both groups of mothers as well.

Speech rate and other temporal characteristics of dyadic interaction have been a particular focus of a number of studies of stuttering children and their parents. Schulze (1991) reported no difference in parents' speaking rate, rate of turn taking, interruptions, and requests. Kelly and Conture (1992) found no difference in speaking rate, interruptions, and time taken before responding to children's utterances. Kelly (1994) broadened the scope of her study to investigate fathers' interactions with stuttering and fluent children. No differences were found in the conversational profiles of either fathers or the children; however, relative differences between fathers' and stuttering children's speech rates were found to correlate with measures of stuttering severity. Greater difference between parental and child rate was associated with higher stuttering rates. Ryan (2000) found few measures that distinguished a cohort of 20 stuttering and 20 fluent peer children's interactions with their mothers, and no significant differences between the two groups of mothers in terms of language use and speech rate. However, for the stuttering children, frequency of stuttering was modestly correlated with their mothers' rate of speech.

Two prospective reports from the same team of researchers in the Netherlands have examined possible input precursors of stuttering. Both addressed a number of features of maternal child-addressed speech (CDS). Kloth, Janssen, Kraaimaat, and Brutten (1995a, 1995b) and Kloth, Janssen, Kraaimaat, and Brutten (1998) examined profiles of maternal speech and language addressed to 26 of 93 at-risk children of stuttering parents. In general, no patterns of child-addressed speech or language discriminated the children who did and did not develop stuttering, and the authors suggested that maternal input to young children who are perceived to be normally fluent does not contribute to later development of stuttering.

Additionally, few studies have investigated children's responses to changes in parental speech rate. Bernstein Ratner (1992) found that typically developing children did not entrain (match) changes in their mothers' speech rates across pre- and post-instruction sessions to modify interaction style, while instructions that mothers slow speech rate and simplify speech actually increased the children's patterns of normal disfluency. A similarly variable profile of normally fluent children's responses to rate modifications in maternal speech was noted by Guitar and Marchinkoski (2001). Zebrowski, Weiss, Savelkoul, and Hammer (1996) found some facilitating effects of reduced maternal speech rate on children's stuttering, as did Stephenson-Opsal and Bernstein Ratner (1988), and Guitar, Schaefer, Donahue-Kilburg, and Bond (1992). In a single case study, Jones and Ryan (2001) found that decreases in maternal speech rate to a 4-year-old boy diminished the rate of his stuttering. In general, studies find that some stuttering children's fluency is improved somewhat by a slower rate of speech from parents; notably, however, the children do not appear to reduce their own speech rate to match that of their parents. Thus, the actual mechanism by which the children profit from such adjustments is not known. We return to the question of parental input adjustments to stuttering children in Chapter 14, which surveys outcomes of treatment programs and recommendations.

Langlois, Hanrahan, and Inouye (1986) found that mothers of stutterers produced more imperative and interrogative utterances than mothers of nonstutterers. Weiss and Zebrowski (1991) found that parents of stutterers and nonstutterers did not differ in frequency of responses to children's attempts to converse as opposed to "assertive," i.e., unsolicited conversational contributions. Weiss (2002) found equivalent rates of parental recasts of children's utterances, and no tendency to recast disfluent utterances, when she compared 26 parent-child dyads, in half of which the child was a stutterer. Despite the fact that many parents have been advised not to pressure children by asking questions of them (Van Riper, 1973), neither Weiss and Zebrowski (1992) nor Wilkenfeld and Curlee (1997) found parental questioning to be associated with a higher rate of disfluency in children's responses than their other speech attempts.

Bernstein Ratner and Silverman (2000) examined stuttering and fluent children's parents' estimates of their language ability using the *Speech and Language Assessment Scale*. While both mothers and fathers of the stuttering children rated them as less advanced in a number of communicative skills than the fluent peers, their judgments were in fact better correlated with actual formal assessment results: the stutterers scored more poorly on all measures used. To test the hypothesis that parents of stuttering children exposed them to unreasonably sophisticated language models, Miles and Bernstein Ratner (2001) contrasted the difference between language profiles of stuttering children and age-, gender-, and socioeconomically matched fluent children and their individual mothers. For each dyad, the child's patterns of grammatical and vocabulary use were measured, and subtracted from his or her mother's patterns to measure relative distance or demand of maternal speech style. No differences in what was termed "relative language demand" were seen.

On the whole, the studies have not always found what many clinicians might have expected. This may be merely because the best experimental analogues of life situations are not the real thing. Or it may be that the studies argue against the indiscriminate application of some established clinical axioms. We address this problem in Chapter 14, which surveys the evidence base for fluency interventions.

Parental Standards of Fluency and Attitudes toward Stuttering To what extent parents of stutterers are specifically perfectionistic about speech fluency is a question crucial to a diagnosogenic theory, but difficult to answer. In the Iowa studies, far fewer of the stutterers' than the nonstutterers' parents agreed with the statement that "nonfluencies in speech are normal if not excessive." But the unusual concern about the fluency of their children's speech such parents expressed in response to this and other questions may just as well have been an effect of the problem as an integral part of it, as Johnson and Associates (1959, p. 85 ff.) pointed out.

Bloodstein, Jaeger, and Tureen (1952) found that parents of stutterers appeared to be somewhat unusually prone to identify tape-recorded samples of normal childhood speech as belonging to stutterers, but this was not confirmed in subsequent research by Berlin (1960). When mothers were asked to respond to individual examples of disfluency in a study by Zebrowski and Conture (1989), mothers of stutterers made more judgments of stuttering than nonstutterer's mothers in response to most disfluency types, but the difference was statistically significant only in the case of sound prolongations and broken words.

Neither Darley (1955) nor LaFollette (1956) found any difference between the two groups of parents on the *Iowa Scale of Attitude toward Stuttering*. Parents of stutterers did reveal less favorable attitudes, however, on an inventory of parental attitudes toward stuttering constructed by Crowe and Cooper (1977). They also scored lower than parents of nonstutterers on a test of factual knowledge about stuttering.

Cox, Seider, and Kidd (1984) administered the revised Erickson inventory of attitudes toward speech to nonstuttering relatives, including parents, of stutterers and nonstutterers and reported no difference between the groups. Lasalle and Conture (1991) found a significant tendency for mothers of stutterers to initiate eye contact with their children during moments of stuttering.

Parental Fluency Knepflar (1965) found that parents of stutterers had more normal disfluencies in their speech than did parents of nonstutterers. Meyers and Freeman (1985b) failed to confirm this in their study of stutterers' mothers.

SUMMARY REMARKS

We may now restate in brief the essential facts that have been learned from research on the medical, developmental, and school histories and the home environments of stutterers.

Stutterers' medical records are for the most part similar to those of nonstutterers, despite a few vague and ambiguous suggestions of more abnormal birth conditions in the case of the stutterers in both the Iowa and Newcastle studies. The possibility of more allergies, as indicated by both personal and family histories, is also still an open one. The physical examination is apt to disclose chiefly somatic symptoms of anxiety.

Stutterers as a group appear to have normal developmental histories except with regard to speech and language. A number of research findings indicate that stutterers tend to be later than nonstutterers in saying their first words, phrases, and sentences and in acquiring intelligible speech. On tests of linguistic ability, they also tend to perform more poorly at early age levels, although studies of older subjects appear to show that they soon overcome this disadvantage, at least when linguistic ability is measured by standardized tests. In contrast, there is evidence that many stutterers on therapy caseloads carry clinical diagnoses of additional speech and language impairments. Almost without exception, studies have shown that stutterers tend to have more articulation difficulties than nonstutterers. Stutterers are often regarded by their parents as being "nervous" and as exhibiting more of such behavior as fears, nightmares, enuresis, fighting, and the like, to an extent that is probably compatible with the observation that as adults they tend to be somewhat more maladjusted, anxious, or emotionally reactive as a group than are nonstutterers. Whether these symptoms represent contributors to stuttering or its possible consequences cannot yet be determined. Mild degrees of educational maladjustment also appear to be more common among stutterers, probably because of reasonable consequences of stuttering in a school setting.

While research findings make it quite clear that the intelligence of stutterers is generally equivalent to that of nonstutterers, close agreement among a number of studies suggests that when surveys are extended to include low as well as high socioeconomic segments of the population, the mean IQ of stutterers may be slightly below the general average. Moreover, stuttering appears to be unusually prevalent among those with mental retardation syndromes.

Examination of the family environments of stutterers suggests that there may be a somewhat larger proportion of only children among them than among nonstutterers, as well as a longer average separation in age from their nearest siblings, but this has not been firmly established. There is rather substantial and consistent evidence that the parents of stutterers are generally normal in adjustment, and not in any ordinary sense neurotic. But there have been conflicting findings regarding certain specific features of their personality makeup and about their behavior as parents. Earlier studies done at the University of Iowa over a period of years, and corroborated by independent research done elsewhere, show that when compared with parents of nonstutterers from the same cultural and social background, many stutterers' parents are to some extent more competitive and perfectionistic, somewhat over-concerned about their children, and more inclined to dominate them and to set unrealistically high goals for them. That may be in fact why they actively seek help for them from professionals, and come to our attention. On the other hand, comprehensive research on a group of children in Newcastle-upon-Tyne, England, offers essentially no confirmation of this view and depicts the mother instead as a person who by reason of low innate capacity tends to be poorer at creating a stable home environment than mothers of typically fluent children. More recent studies have tended to focus on traditional therapy recommendations, to ascertain whether differences in speech rate, turn-taking, or language style appear to differentiate the conversational profiles of parents of stutterers from those of fluent children. To date, no obvious differences have been found. Thus, it may always be difficult to make any sweeping statements about the nature and extent of the role that parents play in the emergence or persistence of their children's stuttering.

Chapter 10

Stuttering as a Response

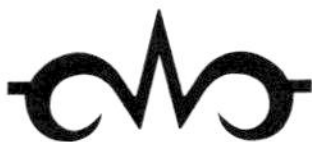

In the next two chapters we will survey a major area of research that is concerned with identifying the variables related to the precipitation of stuttering. We will shift our attention now from people who stutter to the moments of stuttering. In these chapters, we will be concerned with a single basic question, "*What is the underlying nature of stuttering as a response?*"

In Chapter 2, we discussed three general concepts about the nature of the stuttering block that have had wide influence: the *breakdown*, the *repressed need*, and the *anticipatory struggle* hypotheses. It may be helpful to keep in mind that, historically, much of the research on the moment of stuttering had its source in the anticipatory struggle hypothesis, particularly in a form of that hypothesis, advanced by Johnson and Knott in the 1930s, which asserted that stuttering was an anticipatory avoidance reaction.[1] Much that has been discovered about stuttering as a response has resulted from attempts to verify this concept. Added impetus has been given to such studies by approaches that view stuttering in the context of the psychology of learning and feedback theory.

Beginning around 1935, the intensive concern with neurophysiological data that had initially dominated research on stuttering at the University of Iowa began to give way to an interest in the objective study of psychological variables related to stuttering. A major role in this development was played by Wendell Johnson. Johnson (1933) had suggested the notion of approaching the problem of stuttering by studying the intermittent stuttering responses or "moments" individually. This led at once to the idea of measuring the amount of stuttering

[1] See Johnson and Knott (1936), Knott and Johnson (1936).

by simply counting the moments. Stuttering behavior was thus made subject to investigation by the methods of experimental psychology, an orientation that contrasted sharply with the medical model of stuttering that up to that time had dominated its investigation as a "disorder."

The basis was thus laid for an extensive research emphasis on the frequency and distribution of stuttering events, an approach that was to be for many years the distinctive contribution of American researchers to a better understanding of the nature of stuttering. In the initial research reports of a series titled, "Studies in the Psychology of Stuttering," Johnson and several of his students and coworkers in a single year, 1937, published so much fundamental work on stuttering as a response to stimuli that, for 30 years, research on the subject consisted mainly of elaboration of it.

THE DISTRIBUTION OF STUTTERING EVENTS

If we want to learn about the nature of the stuttering response, there is hardly a more fundamental question we can ask than the question of how stuttering events are distributed in the speech sequence—in essence, what words are likely to be stuttered. In view of Johnson's working assumptions, it was logical for him to have begun by raising the question of the extent to which stuttering occurred on words on which it was anticipated.

Anticipation in Relation to Occurrence of Stuttering

The phenomenon of anticipation may be looked at from a number of points of view. Clinically, it is best known as a fearful premonition of impending blockage that most stutterers begin to experience at some time in the development of their speech problem. In the laboratory, it has been studied by measurement of physiological changes occurring just prior to the block. As we will see later in this chapter, there are other ways to examine the relationship between stuttering and anticipation. To Johnson and others conducting research at the time the question first arose, the simplest objective approach seemed to be to investigate stutterers' ability to predict the occurrence of their blocks.

In general, the procedure that was followed in this type of investigation was to ask stutterers to make an appropriate signal before their attempt to say each word on which they thought they were going to stutter as they read aloud to the experimenter. From the resulting data for each participant, one may obtain two principal findings: the percentage of signaled anticipations that were followed by stuttering and the percentage of stuttered events that were anticipated. Using this method, Knott, Johnson, and Webster (1937) found that 96 percent of the signaled anticipations of their participants were followed by stuttering (see Table 10-1). Conversely, almost 94 percent of the stuttering events occurred on words on which they had been anticipated. Van Riper (1936) had reported similar findings, and Van Riper and Milisen showed that stutterers could often predict not only the occurrence, but also the length, of their blocks.

These facts are impressive. It may be argued, however, that the same facts may be interpreted as evidence *against* the anticipatory struggle hypothesis, since the relationship between stuttering and expectancy found in these studies, though high, is far from perfect. The observation that not all anticipations lead to stuttering is perhaps not difficult to explain since expectations of stuttering may often be held tentatively, conditionally, or with varying degrees of doubt. It is the apparently unanticipated block that poses a problem. If stuttering events are caused essentially by the anticipation of stuttering, it follows that every block the stutterer has must be preceded by expectancy. This is certainly not borne out by the research findings. Not only does the average stutterer have a certain percentage of ostensibly unanticipated blocks, but Van Riper (1936) found that, when such blocks occurred, the stutterer frequently reported reactions of surprise. Furthermore, as Milisen (1938) demonstrated, there are stutterers who seem to be able to predict essentially none of their blockages.

TABLE 10-1 The Relationship between Signaled Expectancy and Occurrence of Stuttering

	N	Percentage of anticipations followed by stuttering	Percentage of stuttering events anticipated
Van Riper (1936)	21	83.2	93.3
Knott, Johnson, and Webster (1937)			
Inexperienced Group	10	96.0	93.7[c]
Experienced Group[a]	12	94.0	87.3[c]
Johnson and Solomon (1937)	13	51.1[b]	62.7[b]
Milisen (1938)	26	85.0	84.6

[a]Subjects in this group had undergone considerable therapy, and several had served in another study involving prediction of stuttering.
[b]When subjects read aloud after an interval of 1–7 days following the marking of words on which they expected to stutter.
[c]These percentages were not given by Knott, Johnson, and Webster but are deducible from their data.

Anticipation as a Process Involving a Low Degree of Consciousness As a solution to this dilemma, Johnson proposed that anticipation is a process that may occur on a low level of consciousness. Evidence in support of such a concept was initially offered by Johnson and Sinn (1937). They marked stuttered words as stutterers read a lengthy passage aloud. The participants were then asked to read the passage again, using a fresh unmarked copy, this time reading aloud only those words on which they did *not* expect to stutter. Although 98 percent of the stuttering events were eliminated by this process, there remained a relatively small residue of apparently unexpected blocks. It was these blocks that formed the topic of the study. The outstanding fact that Johnson and Sinn discovered was that, to a marked extent, these blocks had occurred on words that had been stuttered in the first reading. In addition, subjects' introspections showed that, in the majority of these cases, their attention had wandered, they were reading far ahead, or they had for some other reason failed to form a judgment whether they would stutter or had forgotten to indicate their anticipation by omitting the word.

The kind of interpretation that Johnson placed on these findings was that it is possible for stutterers to anticipate blockages in a certain sense without being highly aware of it. Stuttering, he thought, might occur in response to a kind of anticipation that is fleeting and subliminal.

Johnson and Solomon (1937) performed a different type of experiment that they believed to be an analogue of the ordinary day-to-day situation in which stutterers seldom have time to form a deliberate, conscious judgment about the occurrence of stuttering in advance of their speech attempts. They had participants mark words in a reading passage on which they expected to stutter. They then read the passage aloud after an interval of 10 to 15 minutes, and then again after an interval of at least a day. In both situations, stuttering occurred on about 50 percent of the words on which expectancies had been marked, as compared with about 10 percent of the words on which they had not.

Wingate (1975) found relatively little relationship between the words on which stuttering was anticipated and those that were actually stuttered when participants read the words aloud in an altered sequence one and two weeks later. Both the Johnson and Solomon experiment and that of Wingate were concerned with an unusual sense of the term anticipation. The possibility that stuttering might be precipitated by expectancies that had occurred hours or days before, even in the same context, has rarely if ever been contemplated.

Anticipation in School-Age Children who Stutter Whatever the merits of Johnson's concept of anticipation on a low level of consciousness, it was clearly designed to account for a relatively small number of exceptions to what seemed to be the general rule that stutterers could predict the occurrence of their stuttering. It has since developed, however, that while this may be true of adults, it is not nearly so general a rule among children.

In the first place, clinical study of the course of development of stuttering in childhood seems to show that expectancy in the usual sense of the term tends to be among the last features of the problem to develop. As a result, Bloodstein (1960a) found that the question, "Can you sometimes tell that you're going to stutter on a word before you say it?" got the answer "yes" from only 45 percent of 10- to 11-year-old children, and only 38 percent of 8- to 9-year-olds. (The question was not asked of younger children.) Since stutterers themselves have provided some of the strongest support for the belief that they stutter because they expect to, the fact that so many stutterers either do not have such a belief or are unable to verbalize it cannot be ignored.

In addition, we have evidence from a study by Silverman and Williams (1972b) showing that children between the ages of 8 to 16 years vary markedly in their ability to predict the occurrence of their stuttering when reading isolated words. Although some children predicted essentially all of their blocks, others predicted few or none. About half of the children were able to predict less than 50 percent of their stuttered words. Silverman and Williams questioned whether the anticipatory struggle hypothesis can apply to all stuttering children.

If it does, the evidence for it is obviously not to be found in studies of the accuracy of prediction of stuttering. As we have seen, however, prediction is not the only possible way in which we can operationalize the phenomenon of anticipation. Bakker, Brutten, Janssen, and van der Meulen (1991) attempted to do it through a study of the eye movements of school-aged children who stutter. On a list of 144 words, the children first marked the words on which they thought they would stutter. Their eye movements were then recorded as they silently read a passage composed of those words. Finally, they read the passage aloud. The children fixated longer on words on which they subsequently stuttered than on their fluent words. Only 10 percent of the words they had previously marked were stuttered. The experimenters believed the findings showed that school-aged children anticipate stuttering events to the same extent that adult stutterers do. If so, they evidently anticipate stuttering in the sense that Johnson had in mind when he theorized that the process could occur on a low level of consciousness.

The Consistency Effect

Research on the moment of stuttering as a response had an even more fundamental beginning in the demonstration by Johnson and Knott (1937) of the consistency effect. In this investigation, Johnson and Knott noted the words on which people who stutter had difficulty as they read a brief passage 10 times in succession. They found that, for most subjects, the distribution of stuttered words was markedly consistent from one reading to the next. In short, the places at which participants blocked in repeated readings of the same material were more or less the same. The words with which they had difficulty tended to be words on which they had stuttered in previous readings. If this simple observation is considered carefully, it will be seen to have some significant implications. The truth might have been otherwise. It might have been found that all the words of the passage had about an equal chance of being stuttered on in any given reading. The consistency effect appears to show that there is something in the reading itself, some feature of the speech sequence—whether of form or content—that in some manner serves to elicit the stuttering block. As Johnson put it later, "... stuttering does not occur haphazardly or in a random or chance fashion but as a response to identifiable stimuli."

The consistency effect was confirmed by Johnson and Inness (1939) and has since been demonstrated in various other studies,[2] including two

[2] See, for example, Jamison (1955), Shulman (1955), Tate and Cullinan (1962), Cullinan (1963a), Martin and Haroldson (1967), Neelley and Timmons (1967), Williams, Silverman, and Kools (1969a), Rosso and Adams (1969), Adams and Brutten (1970), Prins and Lohr (1972), Seidel, Weinstein, and Bloodstein (1973), Hendel and Bloodstein (1973), Stefankiewicz and Bloodstein (1974), Wingate (1986).

investigations of school-age stutterers by Neelley and Timmons (1967) and Williams, Silverman, and Kools (1969a). On the whole, about 65 percent of a child's stuttering in a given reading takes place on words that were stuttered in a previous reading.[3] Zenner, Webster, and Fitzgerald (1974) showed that consistency also extends to the types of stuttering behavior that appear at the same loci.

Further work has been done in an effort to narrow down the precise meaning of the consistency effect. Johnson and Knott believed that the consistency effect showed the power of stimuli to which the stuttering had already become attached when the person came to participate in the experiment. An alternative explanation might be that the person remembers having stuttered on a given word in the previous reading and may respond by stuttering on it again. It is Johnson and Knott's interpretation that appears to be correct, at least in large part. Seidel, Weinstein, and Bloodstein (1973) interposed extraneous readings between the first and second readings of a test passage in an attempt to interfere with participants' memory of the initial stutter events; this had no effect on consistency. Stefankiewicz and Bloodstein (1974) interposed a four-week interval between two readings. This resulted in somewhat lower consistency than in successive readings of a passage on a single occasion, but the bulk of it remained. After four weeks, 49 percent of the stuttered words were words that had been stuttered originally.

Stuttering thus appears to be in large measure under the control of stimuli. When the stimulus conditions are held relatively constant, as they are in successive readings of the same passage, the distribution of stuttered words tends to be relatively constant too. This seems to be the meaning of the consistency effect. To be sure, this leaves some unanswered questions. Why is the average amount of consistency not greater than it is? Is it because of our failure to control stimuli that are subtle and fleeting? Does it reflect a churning cognitive substrate of stuttering that is beyond our control? Or is there some purely random influence on stuttering? We have barely begun to think about such questions.

The Role of Cues Representative of Past Stuttering

Once the consistency effect had been established, it was natural to look for more direct evidence of the role of cues in the precipitation of stuttering. Not only was such evidence found, but some interesting and basic properties of these cues also came to light in the process.

The Cues Are Learned The special form in which Johnson and his associates developed the anticipatory struggle concept of the moment of stuttering may be written concisely:

$$\text{Cue} \rightarrow \text{Anticipation} \rightarrow \text{Avoidance}$$

That is, a cue representative of past difficulty leads to an anticipation of stuttering, which in turn leads to the effort to avoid stuttering, an effort that is stuttering. This kind of formulation clearly implies that a segment or feature of the speech sequence acquires the power to elicit stuttering through a process of learning. Johnson, Larson, and Knott (1937) succeeded in demonstrating the potentiality of neutral cues for acquiring this power. Using a passage with a colored border, they made sure that subjects would experience a large amount of stuttering on it by having them read it to an audience. Subsequently, they found that when these subjects read to a single listener the presence of a colored border resulted in increased stuttering. In a similar manner, they showed that other cues, such as the content of a passage or diagonal lines drawn through words, could

[3]This percentage measure of consistency, originally employed by Johnson and Knott (1937), has been widely used because it is simple and intuitively comprehensible. A serious drawback of the measure is that it varies with the severity of a person's stuttering merely as a computational artifact. For example, if a speaker stutters on 100 percent of words in Reading 1, 100 percent of any words stuttered in Reading 2 will inevitably have been stuttered in Reading 1, and there will be a consistency score of 100 percent. Consequently, the percentage of consistency cannot be used in comparing different groups of stutterers, or stutterers under different conditions, unless the frequency of stuttering is constant. Tate and Cullinan (1962) and Wingate (1984a) suggested improved methods of measurement that overcome this disadvantage, among others, and that are especially useful in evaluating the consistency of individual stutterers. See also Cullinan (1988).

be made to evoke more stuttering through association with past difficulty.

Further demonstrations of this kind reported subsequently used other kinds of neutral stimuli. Goss (1956) found that once speakers had been given sufficient experience stuttering on words exposed for 12 seconds before the signal to say them was given, the 12-second interval produced more stuttering than did longer or shorter intervals. Peters and Simonson (1960) increased the frequency of stuttering on words rarely stuttered by their subjects by pairing each of these words repeatedly with a word that had often been stuttered. Fierman (1955) showed that a red border associated with reduction in stuttering by its presence during repeated readings of the same passage tended to cause a drop in the frequency of stuttering on a similar passage. Operant conditioning experiments later produced additional examples of reductions in stuttering through the influence of neutral discriminative stimuli (see Martin & Siegel, 1966a, 1966b; and Reed & Lingwall, 1980).

The Adjacency Effect Johnson and his coworkers theorized that the colored border had the power that it did because it served as a reminder of previous stuttering. Strictly speaking, the experiment proved only that stuttering could be influenced by learning. In the given experimental arrangement, the colored border might have become a conditioned stimulus for stuttering regardless of the underlying reason for which the stuttering had occurred. This fact lends special significance to another experiment in which the role played by cues was less ambiguous.

Johnson and Millsapps (1937) had each of their participants read the same passage nine times in succession. At intervals, the words that had been stuttered were blotted out by heavy pencil markings so that they could not be read, and the stutterer was instructed to continue to read the words that were visible. In view of the consistency effect, this procedure should soon have eliminated essentially all of the stuttering. For some individuals it did, but in the majority of cases, a small residue of persistent stuttered words kept cropping up in new places. Examination of the words on which these residual blocks had occurred showed something unexpected. To a significant degree, these words were adjacent to previously stuttered words that had been blotted out. In short, the blottings appeared to have served as cues capable of evoking new stuttering. This finding seemed to Johnson and Millsapps to epitomize stuttering as a response to cues representative of past speech failure. Moreover, it is not easily explained in terms of a simple conditioning scheme, since the blot neither precedes nor coincides with the original stimulus for stuttering, but covers it up.

The inference that Johnson and Millsapps drew from their study has received some support from later research. Brutten and Gray (1961) devised an adjacency condition in which the words stuttered in repeated readings of a series of nouns could be physically removed and the remaining words respaced so as to minimize the cues representing past stuttering. They compared this with a similar condition in which the word card was merely inverted so that a colored blank remained as a visible cue to the removal of the stuttered word. Brutten and Gray found that when the visible cues were removed, there was a less marked adjacency effect. The difference fell short of statistical significance, however.

Rappaport and Bloodstein (1971) put Johnson and Millsapps' inference to a different kind of test. Inferring that blots might produce stuttering for reasons other than their association with past stuttering, they compared an ordinary adjacency condition with a condition in which words were blacked out at random in a reading passage. A quite marked, unforeseen result was obtained. For half the stutterers—those who had the random blots condition first—the random cues did not evoke adjacent stuttering. In the case of the remaining speakers—those for whom the random blackout cues came second—they did. In other words, blottings scattered at random do not in themselves produce adjacency. Once the person has had the experience of having the stuttered words blotted out, however, blackout cues not only serve as stimuli for stuttering, but even have the power to do so in a new passage containing different words. It was a resounding confirmation of the conclusions to which Johnson and Millsapps had been led.

From the point of view of the anticipatory struggle hypothesis, it would be difficult to overemphasize the importance of the adjacency effect. The tendency for stuttering to occur in response to the stutterer's memory of past difficulty may be said to be the essence of the assertion that it is an anticipatory struggle reaction. Furthermore, if we were to attempt to define this type of reaction in behavioral terms without the use of such words as anticipation or evaluation, we could perhaps do so only with reference to its responsiveness to cues associated with past difficulty.

This being the case, special mention should be made of the observation that the adjacency effect is apparently to be found in children as well as adults. We have discussed the inability of many school-age children who stutter to predict the occurrence of their blocks and the questions that this has raised. In a group of 12 stutterers of elementary school age, Avari and Bloodstein (1974) were able to demonstrate the adjacency phenomenon in every case. Yet 6 of the 12 children were unable to predict the occurrence of any of their blocks in oral reading, and only one was able to do so with substantial accuracy. This suggests that the failure of many children to anticipate their stuttering in this type of task may not rule out the possibility that their stuttering events are anticipatory struggle reactions. We will return to the complex question of anticipation and its relation to stuttering later in this chapter.

A fresh approach was taken to the investigation of adjacency by Hawkins and Brutten (1964). If the obliteration of a word by means of a heavy pencil mark may serve as a cue representative of past stuttering on a word, why should not the unobliterated word do so itself, to some extent? Hawkins and Brutten had stutterers read a passage five times. For each participant, they then embedded a number of stuttered words in a new passage. In the new reading, the previously stuttered words produced adjacent stuttering not only horizontally, but also in other directions on the page. Horizontal adjacency was greater than vertical adjacency, and vertical greater than diagonal. In addition, more adjacency was produced by words that had been stuttered consistently and early in the previous readings than by words that had been stuttered late or only once.

Wong and Bloodstein (1977) tried to determine whether apparent departures from consistency in stuttering could be accounted for in part by an adjacency effect. It could not; they found little tendency for the new stuttering that occurs in repeated readings to take place on words adjacent to those previously stuttered.

Consistency in Relation to Anticipation

One more piece of evidence was needed to close the frame of interlocking observations that Johnson and his associates marshaled in support of their conception of the moment of stuttering. If stuttering events were distributed in a predictable, consistent fashion because they were responses to expectancies set off by identifiable cues, then it followed that the expectancies, too, must show a consistent distribution in repeated readings. Accordingly, Johnson and Ainsworth (1938) asked participants to indicate in two silent inspections of the same material seen from two to six weeks apart the words on which they thought they would stutter if they were reading the material aloud. They found a marked tendency for anticipations to occur on the same words. Similar findings were later obtained by Peins (1961b).

A different but related question was raised by Skalbeck (1957), who found that words on which stuttering was expected were stuttered on more consistently than words on which it was not. Going a step further, Martin and Haroldson (1967) established that the stronger the speaker's expectation of stuttering on a given word in a passage, the more consistently the word will tend to be stuttered in successive oral readings.

The Attributes of Stuttered Words

Of course, in the person who stutters' ordinary experience, colored borders or words blotted out in a reading passage do not often serve as cues for stuttering. The research we have considered so far showed clearly enough that stuttering is a response to cues, but gave little indication of the features of the speech sequence generally responsible for the consistent occurrence of stuttering in repeated oral readings, or of why these and not other cues had come to be associated with past stuttering events. This was the problem to which Johnson's colleague, Spencer F. Brown, turned his attention in a series of pioneering studies occupying a period of about 10 years.

The question of precisely where stuttering occurs has at least two distinguishable aspects that are readily investigated—its locus within the word and the locus of the stuttered word in the larger context of speech production attempts. The first question has been of lesser concern to researchers because it is so easily answered. Over 90 percent of stuttering has been found to take place on the initial sound or syllable of words.[4] It almost never occurs on the last sound of a word.[5] Stuttering is sometimes heard within the word, however—usually on accented syllables. Within polysyllabic words, accented syllables are more apt to be stuttered than unstressed ones.[6] That word accent exerts a distinctly secondary influence, however, was precisely demonstrated by Weiner (1984b). She compiled a list of two-syllable words, such as "contract," "address," or "permit," that can be accented on either syllable depending on meaning. Subjects pronounced each word twice with different meanings. Weiner found that 90 percent of the stuttering occurred on the first syllable, regardless of whether or not it was stressed. Similar findings were obtained by Hubbard (1998b), using a sentence-reading paradigm with 10 adults who stutter, although she left open the possibility that, in connected speech, stress variability that characterizes the prosodic patterns of utterances and sentences might affect stuttering loci. Using reaction time data from Dutch speakers, Burger and Wijnen (1999) also found no evidence that syllable stress posed any particular encoding difficulty for adults who stutter.

Nonetheless, these results show with particular clarity the primacy of the word in stuttering. Although people who stutter do at times have difficulty initiating syllables within words, stuttering in its developed form appears to be, above all, an inability to initiate words fluently.

It was the problem of identifying the characteristics of stuttered words that presented a serious challenge. Brown approached this task with a number of hypotheses inspired by Johnson's anticipatory avoidance model of stuttering as well as by clinical observation. Some very definite predictions about the loci of stuttering events may be deduced from this model; namely, that the difficulty will occur whenever people who stutter expect to have an interruption in their speech and are particularly anxious not to—consequently on those parts of the speech sequence that they evaluate as difficult or conspicuous. By 1945, on the basis of analysis of 10,000 words of oral reading by 32 adults who stuttered, Brown was able to announce the confirmation of each of his hypotheses: there were four principal attributes of words that seemed to determine the loci of stuttered words in oral reading and that appeared to him to be sufficient to account for essentially all of them—the initial sound of the word, its grammatical function, its position in the sentence, and its length.

The Phonetic Factor As early as 1935, Johnson and Brown had shown that for most adults who stutter, the likelihood that they would block on a given word was strongly influenced by the sound with which it began. This was, however, an individual factor to a far greater degree than a group factor; the specific sounds that gave difficulty varied markedly from person to person. For stutterers as a group, no one sound has as yet been established as being appreciably more difficult to say fluently than any other. While ranks of difficulty for various sounds have sometimes been reported, there has as yet been only limited or qualified agreement on such rankings in various studies of the

---

[4] Johnson and Brown (1935), Hahn (1942b), Taylor (1966a), Sheehan (1974), Weiner (1984b).

[5] In fact, sporadic cases of individuals with noticeable patterns of stuttering (or at least stutter-like disfluency) on the final portions of words are unusual enough to merit case study description. See Stansfield (1995), McAllister and Kingston (2005), van Borsel, Geirnaert, and van Koster (2005).

[6] Brown (1938b), Hejna (1972), Sheehan (1974), Prins, Hubbard, and Krause (1991).

phonetic factor.[7] There is, however, one major group tendency on which almost all studies agree: For stutterers as a whole, initial consonants have been clearly shown to be more difficult than initial vowels.

Brown's observation that different sounds tend to occasion trouble for different stutterers lent itself readily to interpretation on the basis of the anticipatory avoidance concept, since it would appear to follow from such a concept that it is the stutterer's attitude about the difficulty of a sound, rather than any inherent difficulty of the sound itself, that makes it likely that he or she will stutter on it. It is an interpretation that accords well with case history data suggesting that experiences of speech failure may instill in people who stutter the conviction that they are unable to say certain specific words or sounds.[8] Further evidence of the part that attitudes and expectations play in the phonetic difficulties of stutterers comes from certain other observations we both have made clinically. Words beginning with "ph" may be spoken fluently by some stutterers who are unable to say the initial "f," while "ph"-words may offer difficulty to some stutterers who are able to say "f," but not words beginning with "p." One 15-year-old boy, when asked by the first author if there were any sounds that gave him unusual trouble, replied, "The d-d-double-u sound. See, I couldn't say it just now." Another stutterer blocked fairly consistently on words beginning with "th," but generally not on initial "t" or "d," despite the fact that he spoke a New York City dialect in which all "th" sounds were pronounced "t" or "d." As a final example, we have seen stutterers who profess to have difficulty saying words such as "psychology" or "phone" because they start with their feared sound, "p."

The group tendency of people who stutter to have more trouble with initial consonants than initial vowels is not quite as easy to account for on an anticipatory struggle hypothesis. Brown (1938c) suggested that it was due in part to the greater importance of consonants for speech intelligibility, and hence meaning. Another possibility is that consonants are distinguished from vowels by a degree of stoppage or impedance of the airstream, involve a greater measure of articulatory tension, and consequently lend themselves more readily to the suggestion that they are difficult to say. Vowels are also fewer than consonants, tend not to be the first sounds in content words, and, as Taylor (1966b) has pointed out, are distributed with less "statistical uncertainty" (are easier to guess at when deleted in sentences) than consonants, and therefore carry less "information." The lesser importance of vowels for intelligibility, their lower articulatory complexity, and their smaller information value in written speech are all probably interrelated attributes; and together they probably serve to foster a folk attitude toward vowels perhaps best expressed by orthographies (e.g., Hebrew, Egyptian hieroglyphics), which either omit most vowels or represent them by means of diacritical marks.

Some findings by Uys (1970) on South African stutterers seem to suggest the importance of articulatory tension in producing the vowel-consonant difference. Unlike English, Afrikaans is distinguished by a hard attack in the articulation of initial vowels. Uys compared Afrikaans-speaking and English-speaking stutterers in the reading of lists of words beginning with vowels and consonants. As usual, the English speakers stuttered more on initial consonants than vowels, but the Afrikaans speakers did not. The Afrikaans speakers stuttered on more initial vowels than the English speakers did. In short, when vowels were more like consonants in their manner of articulation, the difference in the amounts of stuttering they produced disappeared.[9]

The assumption that consonants are stuttered more frequently than vowels because they are motorically difficult faces other challenges. Many measures of phonetic or phonological complexity do not appear to influence stuttering or differentially affect the speech of people who do and do not stutter

[7] See Johnson and Brown (1935), Brown (1938a), Hahn (1942b), Soderberg (1962a), Quarrington, Conway, and Siegel (1962), Taylor (1966a), Griggs and Still (1979), Jayaram (1983), Wells (1983).

[8] See Van Riper (1963), pp. 338–339. Connett (1955) attempted to increase the frequency of stuttering on the sound /t/ by a discussion intended to foster the impression that it was a difficult sound, with equivocal results.

[9] In Dutch, a language closely related to Afrikaans, Vaane and Janssen (1978) reported that vowels were among the most frequently stuttered sounds.

(see Bernstein Ratner, 2005a, for discussion). For example, in children who stutter, phonological complexity of words does not appear to predict stuttering (Throneburg & Yairi, 1994). The authors noted that most of the stuttered words produced by 24 children near stuttering onset contained no more late-acquired sounds, complex syllable shapes, or multiple syllables than fluently produced words, or words produced just following the stuttered words (a potential measure of planning difficulty at the phonetic or phonological level). Logan and Conture (1997) found that neither the frequency nor duration of stuttered disfluencies in the speech of school-aged boys who stutter were associated with measures of syllable complexity. Shimamori and Ito (2006) found that, for Japanese children, words beginning with phonetically more complex syllables are easier to produce than those with simpler syllables. Finally, in children who stutter and who demonstrate clinical phonological disorder, stuttering is not more likely to occur on words containing systematic speech errors (Yaruss & Conture, 1996; Wolk, Blomgren, & Smith, 2000).

Yet another problem in distinguishing a reason for the typical difficulty that many adults have been found to have with consonants, rather than vowels, is the rather dominant representation of English-speaking participants in the research literature. Bernstein Ratner and Benitez (1985) noted that their Spanish-English speaking adult stutterer had more difficulty in vowel-initiated words in Spanish than in English, potentially because vowels initiate verbs and other content words more frequently in Spanish than in English. In sum, Bernstein Ratner (2005a) notes that it is extremely difficult to sort out phonetic factors from other linguistic factors, such as lexical access and syntactic formulation, because sounds are not equally distributed across parts of speech or more and less frequently used words within the world's languages.

However, before leaving this discussion, we must note that there are a certain number of stutterers who tend to have all or most of their difficulty on words beginning with vowels. Some researchers take this as evidence that it is not so much the nature of consonants that usually makes them difficult as the kinds of evaluations that the person who stutters places on them.

The Grammatical Factor Brown discovered that most stuttering in oral reading took place on four principal parts of speech—nouns, verbs, adjectives, and adverbs—while far less difficulty was encountered on articles, prepositions, pronouns, and conjunctions. Studies by others have generally corroborated the finding that the blocks of adult stutterers occur chiefly on lexical, or content, words as opposed to function words, but have either failed to find or have failed to agree on any further ranking of difficulty of grammatical parts of speech.[10]

Brown and other proponents of the anticipatory struggle hypothesis have attributed the high frequency of stuttering on content words to the fact that these are the focal points in the stream of communication at which the meaning is most important, the speaker's emphasis is greatest, and the listener's interest is concentrated. It is here that the person who stutters is therefore most likely to anticipate difficulty and to be anxious to avoid it. It may be said that the same facts would offer little difficulty to other theories of the moment of stuttering. The grammatical factor often appears to undergo a change during the course of development of stuttering, however, since many stuttering children in the earliest phase of the disorder have a considerable amount of difficulty on function words, especially pronouns and conjunctions in English as well as other languages (Howell, Au-Yeung, & Sackin, 1999; Au-Yeung, Gomez, & Howell, 2003; Dworzynski & Howell, 2004; Natke, Sandrieser, van Ark, Pietrowsky, & Kalveram, 2004; Natke, Sandrieser, Pietrowsky, & Kalveram, 2006; see Bloodstein, 2006, for additional discussion). Whether all theories can explain this change in grammatical

[10] See Brown (1937), Hahn (1942a), Eisenson and Horowitz (1945), Quarrington, Conway, and Siegel (1962), Danzger and Halpern (1973), Griggs and Still (1979), Wingate (1979). Soderberg (1967) found the grammatical factor within the body of the phonemic clause, but not in its initial position, where many function words were stuttered. Koopmans, Slis, and Rietveld (1991) made the same observation in a study of Dutch-speaking stutterers.

focus of stuttered words over the course of development with equal readiness is a moot question. We will return to this subject in Chapter 12 when we discuss the distinct linguistic factors that appear to influence the frequency and loci of stutters in young children close to stuttering onset.

Word Position There is more stuttering on the first word and in varying degrees on other early words of the sentence than on words in other positions.[11] Explanations that have been offered, again chiefly on the anticipatory struggle hypothesis, have stressed the conspicuousness of the beginning of the sentence. This is the point at which speakers pass fairly noticeably from silence to speech, at which they renew their lease on the listener's attention, and at which they are therefore most likely to be conscious of themselves to some extent in their role as speakers. It is of interest that some individuals who stutter have relatively few blocks once they have said the first few words of a conversation or have gotten past the first few words of a reading passage.

In apparent contradiction of past findings, Tornick and Bloodstein (1976) found essentially no tendency for the first few words of long sentences to contain proportionately more stuttering than the rest of the sentence. A plausible explanation is that each of the long sentences was constructed by adding a coordinate clause to a shorter sentence. The beginnings of constituent grammatical clauses may play a role in stuttering similar to that of the initial parts of sentences. Indeed, the position effect has been found in phrases (Taylor, 1966a), in phonemic clauses[12] (Soderberg, 1967), and even in random sequences of words (Conway & Quarrington, 1963) or in counting aloud (Borden, 1983). However, Klouda and Cooper (1987) did not find any tendency for adults to stutter at the start of syntactic units when reading sentence pairs such as "When John leaves, Penelope will be upset," and "When John leaves Penelope, we'll be upset."

[11] Brown (1938b), Quarrington, Conway, and Siegel (1962), Quarrington (1965), Taylor (1966a), Griggs and Still (1979). Soderberg (1967) found this to be true in relation to phonemic clauses. Only Hannah and Gardner (1968), who examined spontaneous language, seem to have found conflicting results; they noted especially frequent stuttering in post-verbal syntactic units.

[12] Units of speech having only one primary stress and ending in a terminal juncture (Soderberg, 1967).

Word Length Brown's fourth factor was word length, although he defined this factor on the number of typed letters in the transcribed words rather than on their phonemic length, a more valid measure of word length in spoken, as opposed to written, language. Longer words have been found, other things being equal, to occasion more stuttering than shorter ones.[13] Brown and Moren (1942) attributed this to the greater prominence of longer words. Long words are also, of course, inherently more difficult to articulate, are frequently evaluated as something of a challenge by stutterers and nonstutterers alike, and may be stuttered on more often because they readily evoke the threat of failure, at least for adults, who are metalinguistically aware.

Word length in English is also inextricably linked to word frequency; longer words are typically less frequent. Word frequency is a notable influence on ease of word retrieval, and the combination of word length and word frequency is mapped to the recent concept of "sparse" phonological neighborhoods, in which longer, less frequent words may be particularly difficult to retrieve (see Newman & Bernstein Ratner, 2007, for discussion).

The facts themselves unfortunately also do not tell us whether it is the inherent complexity of longer words or the stutterer's evaluation of them as difficult that is primarily responsible for the increased likelihood of stuttering in adults; however, as we have noted, in children, multisyllabic words or those that are phonetically more complex (as typically measured by consonant clustering, which adds to word length) tend not to be stuttered any more frequently than other words (Throneburg & Yairi, 1994).

[13] Brown and Moren (1942), Soderberg (1966), Schlesinger, Melkman, and Levy (1966), Taylor (1966a), Wingate (1967b), Lanyon and Duprez (1970), Soderberg (1971), F. H. Silverman (1972), Danzger and Halpern (1973), Griggs and Still (1979). The Lanyon and Duprez study dealt with spontaneous speech.

Summary Remarks and Interpretations

There is now a considerable body of evidence confirming the relationship that Brown postulated to exist between the loci of stutterings and the four factors of initial sound, grammatical function, word position, and word length in oral reading. Furthermore, Hejna (1955), working with adults and a number of researchers working with children (whose work we will discuss further in Chapter 12) obtained essentially similar findings with regard to the spontaneous speech of stutterers. Trotter (1956) showed that not only the locus, but also the severity of the individual moment of stuttering, was related to the degree to which a word was characterized by these factors. Silverman and Williams (1967b) replicated some of Brown's basic work using alternative measures of disfluency and obtained the same results. Williams, Silverman, and Kools (1969b) found that Brown's factors characterized elementary school–aged children's stuttering. (The early stuttering of preschool-aged children seems to present a very different picture, however, as will become evident in Chapter 12.) Little work has been done on the subject in languages other than English, but Brown's factors were found to characterize stuttering in Norwegian by Preus and his coworkers (1970) and in Kannada by Jayaram (1983) and Venkatagiri (1982b).

As we will see shortly, there are still other attributes of words associated with the distribution of stutter events. Brown (1945), however, concluded that the likelihood of occurrence of stuttering was so highly related to the degree of presence of his four factors that any contribution made by others was small. In fact, Taylor (1966a) found that most of the dependence of stuttering on types of words seemed to be accounted for by only three properties—the consonant-vowel difference, word position, and word length. It must be kept in mind, however, that these factors represent generalizations about groups of stutterers. Griggs and Still (1979) demonstrated that individual cases may show departures from them and Bernstein Ratner and Benitez (1985) found that stuttered words had different characteristics in the spontaneous speech of the two languages of a bilingual stutterer.

In trying to determine the meaning of Brown's four factors, a troublesome problem that has existed from the start is that of establishing to what extent these factors are independent of each other. For example, it is probable that content words produce more stuttering than function words largely because content words tend to be longer or because many function words begin with vowels, at least in English, if not other languages. In the studies done since Brown's early work, the kinds of controls that would permit better answers to such questions have been applied with increasing ingenuity. Taylor (1966a, 1966b) made a particularly comprehensive attack on this problem as it applies to the consonant-vowel, position, and length factors and found that all three were effective independently of each other, decreasing in influence on stuttering in the order given, with the consonant-vowel effect about twice as large as that of position and about seven times as great as that of length. As Taylor pointed out, the independent influence of the grammatical factor (content words vs. function words) has not yet been rigorously demonstrated. Evidence presented by Griggs and Still (1979) suggests, however, that it is independent of both the phonetic factor and word position.

Not only stuttering but expectations of stuttering as well have been found to occur in close relationship to Brown's four factors.[14] This is consistent with an anticipatory struggle theory. As we have already noted, it is in this type of theory that the research on the loci of stuttering events originated and in terms of which the findings have been most comprehensively interpreted. That is not to say, however, that others are not to be considered. The reader who tries to explain Brown's factors in accordance with the breakdown and the repressed need hypotheses will find that these are by no means totally lacking in the ability to account for them.

---

[14] See Skalbeck (1957). Also, in an early study, Milisen (1937) found that stuttering was more frequently expected on longer words than on shorter ones, and on the first word of the sentence, with the second, third, and fourth following in order.

On the basis of the breakdown hypothesis, one might reasonably predict the occurrence of stuttering whenever speech inherently requires more complex, precise, or difficult muscular adjustments, greater linguistic complexity, and also, as we must not forget, at any point in the speech sequence at which social or emotional stress is at a peak. Brown himself (1938c) undertook, for argument's sake, the most painstaking attempt to reconcile his findings with the viewpoint that stuttering is basically a physiological disorder. Perhaps the greatest difficulty such a viewpoint encounters is presented by the phonetic factor. The larger amount of stuttering on consonants than on vowels might be expected, and the difficulty with feared sounds could be explained fairly readily. But the breakdown hypothesis might also predict that stutterers would also tend to have more difficulty as a group with certain specific consonants—those that are learned relatively late or that innately demand more complicated types of articulation. As noted, no such group tendency appears to exist,[15] even when we consider the speech of children with concomitant difficulty in articulation.

The repressed need hypothesis might lead us to expect stuttering to occur in large measure on words laden with aggressive or libidinal significance or having some relationship to the speaker's inner conflicts. Little research has been done to determine to what extent the distribution of stuttering events is influenced by specific word meanings. Degree of meaningfulness of words as a whole, as measured by means of the semantic differential, does not appear to be conspicuously related to likelihood of stuttering.[16] Some of the facts we have reviewed about the loci of stuttering events appear to be rather difficult to account for on the basis of the repressed need hypothesis.

[15] Fairbanks (1937), however, found some correlation between amount of stuttering on various speech sounds and certain measures of the difficulty of sounds. He concluded that, "... variations in physiological difficulty ... may be a partial determinant of spasm distribution over the various sounds. The individual differences among stutterers are so large, however, that no single cause may be assigned."

[16] See Peterson (1969), Peterson, Rieck, and Hoff (1969). Danzger and Halpern (1973) found no relationship between stuttering and ratings of abstractness of words.

Word Frequency

Since Brown completed his investigation of his four factors, various others have been found or hypothesized. One of these that is well documented is the frequency of occurrence of the word in the language. In general, the less frequently that a word occurs, the greater the probability of stuttering on it.[17] The influence of this factor is independent of others we have mentioned, such as word length and grammatical function, and appears to occur in children as well as adults. It does not appear to be difficult to theorize about possible reasons for this factor, since word frequency is a potent predictor of speech production difficulty in all speakers (see Gleason & Bernstein Ratner, 1998, for discussion). Perhaps it is worth noting that, if we wanted to determine the influence of reading difficulty of words on stuttering, we could hardly do it better than by studying the effect of word frequency.

Predictability of Words in Context (Information Load)

Other work on the loci of stuttering events has been concerned with the factor of information value of words, in an information-theory sense. If contextual material is presented to a listener word by word, the listener will have varying degrees of success at guessing the next word from what has gone before (see Gleason & Bernstein Ratner, 1998, for discussion of this psycholinguistic concept). By using the guesses of a fairly large number of adult language users, it is possible to obtain a reliable measure of the ease or difficulty with which each of the words in a given context may be predicted in sequence. Such a measure has interesting ramifications. A word that is easily guessed from preceding words is relatively redundant, since it adds little to what the listener already knows. A word that is difficult to guess, in contrast, communicates a large amount of new information. In a highly special but useful sense, then,

[17] Hejna (1963), Schlesinger, Forte, Fried, and Melkman (1965), Schlesinger, Melkman, and Levy (1966), Soderberg (1966), Wingate (1967b), Danzger and Halpern (1973), Ronson (1976), Palen and Peterson (1982).

the predictability of words (also referred to as their statistical uncertainty or transition probability) is a measure of the information load or value they have in a given context.

In a series of independent studies, it has been established that there is a degree of relationship between occurrence of stuttering and low predictability (i.e., high information value of words in oral reading).[18] This factor may overlap considerably with those identified before. That is, there is evidence that content words, the initial position in the sentence, and perhaps the other factors associated with the loci of stutter events are also points of relatively high information value in language.[19] This tends to raise the question of the extent to which these factors are independent of word information in their effect on stuttering. As yet, we do not know how to balance these factors appropriately. We also note that transitional probabilities lost popularity as a research topic for psycholinguists following the emergence of Chomskyan views of language (see Fodor, Bever, & Garrett, 1974, and Gleason & Bernstein Ratner, 1998, for discussion).

Quarrington (1965) showed that word position affects stuttering independently of, and more powerfully than, information value. Lanyon and Duprez (1970) found that, in both spontaneous speech and oral reading, stuttering was not related to information value when word length was held constant. Soderberg (1971), on the other hand, obtained evidence that both word length and information value influenced stuttering independently in oral reading. We note that there are inherent problems in balancing these overlapping factors: one can attempt to do this by using reading material, but only at the expense of generalization to spontaneous speech behavior. On the other hand, analysis of spontaneous speech samples cannot hope to balance these factors well.

Clearly related to information load is what Kaasin and Bjerkan (1982) were concerned with in their study of the influence of "critical words" on stuttering frequency. As an example, subjects tended to stutter on "library" and "six o'clock" when conveying a message to meet there at that time. Considerable speculation has been stirred by the relationship between information load and disfluency. This interest originally developed outside the field of speech pathology in the linguistic study of normal adult hesitation phenomena.[20] In the case of normal disfluency phenomena, the plausible inference has been drawn by linguists that hesitations occur at points of high uncertainty because the speaker is engaged in making lexical or grammatical decisions. The same reasoning may be applied to stuttering, a point of view that has been most clearly expressed by Taylor (1966b). A difficulty with the hypothesis of lexical uncertainty is that it implies a model of stuttering behavior that has not found favor among speech pathologists. It runs counter to the general clinical impression that when stutterers block on a word, they usually know very well, and often far in advance, what word they want to say and in fact tend to betray it when they stutter by repeating, prolonging, or silently mouthing the first sound of the word. Grammatical uncertainty might not seem to be a plausible explanation either, since stuttering in adults so often occurs on the last word of a sentence or other syntactic unit. Having said this, it is extremely critical to note that the time frame that psycholinguists use in experimentally evaluating the process of lexical decision is on the order of milliseconds, and is not readily observable when making such clinical observations.

Another interpretation of this hypothesis is possible. When speakers come to a point of low predictability in the speech sequence, they are indeed at a point of high uncertainty as speakers. But there is an equal amount of uncertainty for the listener. It should be considered that what stutterers are reacting to when they stutter at that point may not be any type of uncertainty of their own as much as their knowledge that the listener is unable for the moment to guess what is coming next and that they, the speakers, bear alone what Eisenson

[18] Quarrington (1965), Schlesinger, Forte, Fried, and Melkman (1965), Soderberg (1967), Lanyon and Duprez (1970), Soderberg (1971). Only Lanyon (1968) failed to find this in a study of three stutterers' spontaneous speech.

[19] The evidence is reviewed by Taylor (1966b).

[20] Lounsbury (1954), Goldman-Eisler (1958a, 1958b).

has called the burden of "communicative responsibility." There are few reactions to the speech of stutterers more calculated to result in their stuttering than the response, "What did you say?" Conversely, it is often much easier for stutterers to tell a store clerk what they want once they have totally dispelled any possible listener uncertainty by pointing to it on the shelf.

Linguistic Stress

Brown (1938b), in one of his pioneering series of studies on the loci of stuttering events, noted a tendency for stuttering to occur on accented syllables of words, as we have seen. Brown did not include word accent (lexical stress) among his four factors because it is a syllabic characteristic, and he was especially interested in the relationship of stuttering to properties of words (see Brown, 1945). Words differ, however, in the relative amount of stress they receive within the sentence (linguistic stress or focus), and a number of researchers, including Karniol (1995), Packman et al. (1996), and Wingate (1976, 1979), speculated that this exerts an important influence on the distribution of stuttering.

From a study of the interaction of grammatical function and word position in oral reading, Wingate (1979) inferred that both owe their effect to linguistic stress. Using Brown's (1937) data to examine the grammatical factor, Wingate pointed out that words that received very little stress, namely auxiliary verbs, infinitives, coordinating conjunctions, and possessive pronouns, were seldom stuttered. On the other hand, relative and personal pronouns and subordinating conjunctions, which are often stressed, were stuttered frequently, along with such other stressed words as main verbs, nouns, and adjectives. He suggested that the amount of stress that words receive may be more closely related to stuttering than is their formal designation as either content or function words. In a subsequent study, Wingate (1984b) found that occurrences of stuttering during oral reading of a passage corresponded closely to stress peaks recorded in a reading of the passage by a nonstutterer. Klouda and Cooper (1988) obtained similar findings in a study of stutterers' oral reading of sentences. Further confirmation came from an investigation of German-speaking stutterers by Bergmann (1986), in which subjects read the same sentence (e.g., "Mr. Vogt is cleaning the car"), in response to two different questions that called for differential stress in responses: "Who is cleaning the car?" and "What is Mr. Vogt doing to the car?" Recent investigations, however, have differed in their findings regarding associations between stress and stuttering: Natke, Grosser, Sandrieser, and Kalveram (2002) found that stress predicted stuttering in German-speaking adults, while other researchers have not been able to confirm a systematic influence of stress on stuttering, as we noted earlier (Burger & Wijnen, 1998; Hubbard, 1998b).

The Question of Phonatory Transitions In Chapter 5, we reviewed a considerable amount of research on the voice initiation times of stutterers that stemmed from the belief that the larynx might have a critical role to play in stuttering. The same interest led Adams and Reis (1971) to raise the question whether stuttering is frequently associated with the necessity to initiate phonation during speech. They found that in five repeated readings of a passage consisting entirely of voiced sounds, adults who stutter stuttered less than in repeated readings of an ordinary passage in which transitions from voiceless to voiced sounds were required. They also reported that more than a third of the stutters were associated with such transitions or with the beginning of a new phrase or sentence.

In actuality, the difference between the passages in frequency of stuttering was not evident on the first reading, but only appeared subsequent to it. In a later replication of their study, Adams and Reis (1974) confirmed this; in their second study, there was no difference until the fourth reading. They concluded that the need for rapid shifts from voiceless to voiced sounds served mainly to slow down the subjects' rate of adaptation to the passage.[21] Controversy developed when Young (1975a) applied a different method of analysis to the data of

[21]The adaptation effect is the tendency of stuttering to decrease in frequency with successive readings of the same material. We will consider this phenomenon in detail in the next chapter.

both studies and reported no significant effect on either frequency of stuttering or adaptation. Adams and Reis (1975) argued in defense of their findings, and Adams, Riemenschneider, Metz, and Conture (1975) presented additional evidence showing that there was more adaptation in an all-voiced passage. Later studies by Hutchinson and Brown (1978) and Runyan and Bonifant (1981) verified the fact that an all-voiced passage produces no change in frequency of stuttering in a single reading. In response, Reis and Adams (1978) contended that the effect is not strong enough to show itself except after repeated readings. McGee, Hutchinson, and Deputy (1981), however, found no significant difference in either initial frequency or adaptation of stuttering between the all-voiced and comparison passages, though they noted a slight trend toward more adaptation on the all voiced passage.

Some other work touched more directly on the influence of phonatory transitions on the loci of stutterings. Manning and Coufal (1976) found that significantly more stuttering occurred during voiced-voiced transitions in oral reading than during voiceless-voiceless, voiceless-voiced, or voiced-voiceless. In a study of oral reading of 48 Dutch stutterers aged 13 to 16 years, Vaane and Janssen (1978) found no differences in the distribution of stuttering among the four types of phonatory transitions. Currently, the evidence that voiced initiations or transitions in the speech sequence are especially likely to be loci of stuttering does not appear strong.

Cycles and Clustering Finally, we note two hypotheses about the loci of stuttering events that relate to temporal factors. Neither Pittenger (1940) nor Taylor and Taylor (1967) were able to find any evidence of a tendency for stuttering during oral reading to appear in periodic waves or cycles. The second factor is clustering. Fein (1970) observed a tendency for stuttered words to be followed immediately by more blocks. We might expect this if the block had a stimulus value for the stutterer. Taylor and Taylor (1967), however, found no evidence of any such clustering of stuttered words. Results obtained by Still and Griggs (1979) suggest that the probability of stuttering is highest on the words immediately following a block. In two of their six subjects, however, there was first an opposite tendency, as though getting through a block conferred immunity to stuttering over the next few words.

In children, clustered disfluencies are more likely to occur in the speech of children who stutter than typically developing peers. However, these clusters are often accompanied by self-repairs of speech production errors, potentially suggesting that they arise from linguistic encoding problems (LaSalle & Conture, 1995; Logan & LaSalle, 1999).

Congruity between Subjects—The Power of Individual Factors

We have just surveyed essentially everything we know at this writing about the reasons why stuttered moments occur precisely where they do in the speech sequence. What does this knowledge amount to? How well, let us say, could we predict the words on which an individual speaker would have difficulty in reading a passage from our knowledge of the factors that we have found to influence the loci of stutters? If we think about this, something notable about these factors will soon appear. With the sole exception of the individual aspect of the phonetic factor, they are all *group* factors. They tell us nothing about the reasons why one person might differ from another with respect to the words that are stuttered. To imagine that these factors would help us to predict the distribution of stuttering moments in an *individual* case, then, is to assume that this distribution is much the same from stutterer to stutterer. Is this the case?

The answer is that it is not. Hendel and Bloodstein (1973) compared the distribution of stutters in the speech of 17 male stutterers in the reading of the same passage. On average, 18 percent of the words stuttered by one person were also stuttered by another. By chance alone, this would have been 11 percent, so to some extent, group factors did influence the loci of their stutters. Yet the within-speaker consistency in reading the passage again averaged 48 percent. Thus, individual factors evidently played a much larger part in the stuttering of these speakers than did group factors.

We can only infer that the various factors we have been discussing would not help us very much to predict the occurrence of stuttering in an individual case. They represent only some broad generalizations that are useful in refining our theories about stuttering. In the final analysis, the loci of stuttering events may have their main source in each stutterer's individual history of learning experiences.

We have relatively little laboratory-based information about what such individual factors might be. Clinical experience, however, suggests that a very important role is played in stuttering by specific words and sounds that vary from case to case. We have already mentioned the individual factor of phonetic difficulty, for which essentially our only source is the early study by Johnson and Brown (1935). There has been equally little study of the individual word factor. Van Riper (1972, pp. 269, 270) contributed some clinical observations suggesting that difficulties with words may arise from memories of past failure or penalty for stuttering on them; a notable example is the difficulty that most stutterers have when saying their names. In addition, some light was shed on the potency of this factor in a study by Hamre and Wingate (1973).

Hamre and Wingate found that, of the words stuttered in a word association task, 36 percent were later stuttered again when the speakers were asked to construct sentences using these words. They interpreted this as a small amount of consistency, but we must evaluate this conclusion in relation to the conditions under which it was observed. Stimuli tend to be discriminated in relation to speech contexts. It is common in clinical experience to observe that stutterers can often avoid stuttering on some of their most difficult words simply by changing the position of the words in the same sentence. To find, then, that more than a third of the stuttered words were stuttered again in new sentences, in different tasks, on different occasions, appears to argue that the individual word, in and of itself, is a relatively powerful stimulus for stuttering. It may be that, in the aggregate, difficult words and sounds, together with all those group factors that have some influence on stuttering, largely account for the amount of stimulus control that we see reflected in the consistency effect.

THE FREQUENCY OF STUTTERING

In considering the effects of varying conditions on the frequency of moments of stuttering, we are in a sense simply extending our discussion of the basic questions just discussed. Just as stutterers do not typically block on every word in the speech sequence, they do not usually stutter in every speech situation. For many stutterers, there are consistent conditions under which they have difficulty, suggesting that not only words and sounds, but listeners, situations, and physical environments as well may serve as cues that are capable of precipitating stuttering.

Of the observations about variations in stuttering profiles, most by far are directly concerned with the conditions under which it diminishes or disappears. These conditions are quite numerous. Relatively speaking, only a small proportion of reported observations have been subjected to objective laboratory study. Consequently, we will supplement our review of laboratory findings with the results of an investigation (Bloodstein, 1950a, 1950b) that used interviews and questionnaires to study the conditions under which stuttering is reduced or absent. The observations to be reported are derived from these interviews and questionnaires unless otherwise noted.

In Bloodstein (1950a, 1950b), some 115 "conditions" were described under which fairly large proportions of people who stutter believed that their stuttering was either absent or substantially reduced. Considerable individual variation was evident; few of these conditions produced decreases in stuttering for all speakers, by their report. Much of this variation is also an artifact resulting simply from the fact that there are no definable absolute limits to what is meant by a "condition" in the context of this type of inquiry. "Speaking to your mother" is likely to represent many different conditions for different stutterers or for the same stutterer on different occasions. Even the most elaborately described conditions, therefore, remain abstractions that subsume innumerable others, and it is impossible either to count them or to make unqualified statements about their effects on stuttering.

The usefulness of a large number of observations of the conditions under which stuttering varies in frequency consists of the challenge they present to us to abstract their essential features and reduce them to a relatively small number of conditions of broad generality. Some of the conditions we will deal with will be more general than others. As a result, they will be more abstract, hypothetical, and in some cases controversial.

Communicative Pressure

An extremely large part of what we know about the way stuttering varies in frequency can be generalized by saying that it is affected by communicative pressures. These are of many kinds, and may come from the form or content of the speaker's message, the listener, the situation, or the nature of the social interaction.

Communicative Responsibility The observation that frequency of stuttering seems to be related to the extent to which a person who stutters is trying to convey information to a listener has been given particular emphasis by Eisenson. Degree of communicative responsibility is itself related to a number of different kinds of variables. One of the most important of these is the meaningfulness or "propositionality" of speech. Eisenson and Horowitz (1945) found considerably more stuttering on words in a meaningful reading selection than on the same words presented in the form of a list or in a nonsense passage. Further, stutterers may report that they can fluently speak words as words rather than sentence portions (i.e., when playing word games or when explaining what words "always" give them trouble), although such tasks are more linguistically demanding. Bardrick and Sheehan found a decrease in stuttering for numbers read aloud (see Sheehan, 1958a). Some conflicting evidence came from a study by Hegde (1970), in which 10 stutterers had as much difficulty when reading a 150-word passage composed of nonsense words as in reading a meaningful paragraph.

Swearing, singing, and counting are other examples of relatively non-propositional speech in which stuttering rarely occurs. Glover, Kalinowski, Rastatter, and Stuart (1996) observed reductions in stuttering when people who stutter were instructed to sing, even when singing was not markedly "musical" in quality. For many stutterers, there is little difficulty with the conventional verbal gestures of greeting and leave taking, commenting on the weather, or saying something "just to keep the conversation going." Stuttering may also be reduced in recitation of memorized material. However, other than reduced propositionality of speech, there are certain other variables that may serve in obvious ways to decrease communicative responsibility. Some are related to the nature of the listener. The common examples are talking to an infant or to an animal, both among the easiest of reported speaking situations for most stutterers. Finally, communicative responsibility may be affected by the nature of the circumstances. We have already noted that a person who stutters may block severely when required to repeat something that their listener has failed to "catch." Conversely, there are many conditions under which stuttering appears to be reduced, essentially because the listener already knows what the stutterer is going to say; the message is therefore redundant. Stutterers often report that they can make purchases fluently if they give the clerk their shopping list, or that they can ask for a book in the library once the person at the desk has seen the call slip, or that they can say a difficult word easily once they have spelled it aloud. It may be in part for the same reason that stutterers usually seem to be able to pronounce a word on which they are blocked if the listener supplies it. Burke (1975) noted that many stutterers could repeat sentences fluently from dictation. Stutterers can generally repeat a word without difficulty immediately after getting over a block on it.

A different type of condition producing effects that have often been attributed to reduced communicative responsibility is choral reading. The well-known fact that most stutterers can read fluently in unison with another person, whether a stutterer or a nonstutterer, was first confirmed experimentally by Johnson and Rosen (1937). Barber (1939) found that choral reading was decidedly more effective than reading together with others who were reading different material or in the presence of mere vocal or mechanical noise. Eisenson and Wells (1942) noted some tendency for stuttering to increase in a choral reading situation when people who stutter read into a microphone and were told they would be heard individually by an audience in another room. Eisenson and Wells inferred that the reason for stutterers' typical fluency in choral reading was a reduction in their responsibility for communication. On the other hand, Pattie and Knight (1944) found that in choral reading before a small audience, the additional signal was just as effective when it was conveyed to the stutterer by telephone as when the accompanying reader was present in the room. They concluded that the choral reading situation was comparable to that in which the stutterer reads in time to a metronome, the accompaniment acting as a "pacemaker." Curiously, speech rate increases have been observed in an investigation of choral reading (Freeman & Armson, 1998); as noted later in this chapter, increased speech rate has sometimes been shown to impact speech fluency adversely in stutterers. Choral reading does appear to reduce self-perceived speech effort in people who stutter, although, curiously, it appears to increase self-perceived effort in typically fluent speakers (Ingham, Warner, Byrd, & Cotton, 2006). A more recent explanation of the choral reading effect was offered by Saltuklaroglu, Kalinowski, and Guntupalli (2004). They proposed that an accompanying speech signal activates the so-called "mirror neuron" system first described in detail by neuroscientist Giacomo Rizzolatti and colleagues in the 1980s. A mirror neuron is active both when an animal (or person) performs an activity and when observing (or in this case, overhearing) the same activity. Thus, an accompanying signal could potentially "prime" less effortful and more accurate speech behavior.

Reading aloud is another condition that may alter speech fluency. On the whole, oral reading evokes less stuttering than self-formulated speech, as Young (1980) showed, and this too is easily imputed to a reduction of communicative responsibility. We note that reading does not require linguistic formulation, unlike spontaneous speech. Whatever factor is at work, however, it may be outweighed by others, since some stutterers have most or all of their difficulty in oral reading. This may be because it brings back unpleasant memories of elementary school assignments to read aloud in class, or because it does not permit the stutterer to substitute less-feared words for feared words in the reading passage.

Time Pressure A familiar form of communicative pressure apt to have a marked effect on stuttering is time pressure. It is a common clinical observation that stutterers tend to have more trouble when they feel hurried. Theoretically, time pressure could have an effect by inducing a faster speech rate, or by reducing available time to formulate speech, in addition to creating more global stress on the speaker. In a laboratory study, Johnson and Rosen (1937) found that stuttering increased when participants were instructed to speak more rapidly.[22] There was frequently little actual increase in reading rate. Vanryckeghem, Glessing, Brutten, and McAlindon (1999) had 24 adults who stutter read at three rates: their habitual rate, one that was paced to be 30 percent faster, and one that was paced to be 30 percent slower. Faster rates produced statistically more stuttering, although slowed rates did not reduce stuttering when compared to baseline. However, post-hoc analysis showed that only the more severe of their stutterers showed an adverse impact of increased rate on their fluency. Glover, Kalinowski, Rastatter, and Stuart (1996) found no impact of speech rate during speaking and singing on stuttering frequency for their study participants. As noted earlier in this chapter, Freeman and Armson (1998) found speech rate increases for people who stutter in a choral reading experiment, even though stuttering was virtually eliminated. Smith and Kleinow (2000) did find some breakdown in motor coordination when adults who stutter were asked to speak more rapidly; but some speakers demonstrated inconsistent motor

[22]Young (1974) failed to confirm this, but instructions to speak rapidly tended to increase the frequency of stuttering in a study by Kalinowski, Armson, Roland-Mieszkowski, Stuart, and Gracco (1993).

patterns even when speaking at their habitual rates. Thus, speech rate demands could increase demands on the motor system for some people who stutter.

From the perspective of speech planning time, Goss (1952) found that when the time interval between exposure of a word and the signal to say it was very short (less than two seconds), the likelihood of stuttering increased for his participants. However, Yaruss (1997) found no relationships between either speech rate or latency of response and stuttering rate for 12 young boys who stutter.

Difficulty of the Motor Plan Another type of communicative pressure results when speech is made more formidable by heavy demands on motor planning. Frick (1965) pointed out the relevance of motor planning to stuttering. Wingate (1967b) suggested that it helps to explain why stutterers tend to have more difficulty on long words than on short words or on unfamiliar words—that is, words of low frequency of occurrence in the language. The effect of reading difficulty of the material is no doubt a reflection of the same facts. Making use of graded reading material, Blood and Hood (1978) observed that stuttering in school-aged children tended to increase as the material varied in difficulty from one grade below to three grades above the readers' age levels.

Reduced demands on motor planning probably have much to do with the fact that stutterers tend to speak fluently when they use a slower rate of speech, although this finding is not universal (Vanryckeghem et al., 1999). They also generally have less difficulty in saying a series of isolated words than when speaking in phrases and sentences (Brown, 1938a), and appear to read paragraph material more fluently when they pronounce it word by word (Adams, Lewis, & Besozzi, 1973). There is rarely any difficulty at all in saying speech sounds or isolated syllables of words. Furthermore, it may be of interest from this point of view that when a difficult word is pronounced "for" stutterers—that is, when they are presumably making use of auditory assistance in their motor planning of the word, they can often say it fluently. As we have seen, they also tend to be able to say a stuttered word fluently after one or more successive productions of it on their own. Silverman and Williams (1972a) had stutterers repeat a stuttered word 180 times. Most of them quickly became fluent, though they then tended to have alternating periods of stuttering and fluency.

Stuttering also appears to be influenced by the length and complexity of sentences, particularly in children (Bernstein Ratner & Sih, 1987; Gaines, Runyan, & Meyers, 1991; Melnick & Conture, 2000; Yaruss, 1999; Zackheim & Conture, 2003), although this phenomenon appears to be reduced somewhat by adolescence (Silverman & Bernstein Ratner, 1997). Tornick and Bloodstein (1976) found that less stuttering occurred in the reading of a short sentence (e.g., "She learned to swim") when it stood alone than when it was made the initial part of a longer sentence (e.g., "She learned to swim in the clear water of the lake"). Jayaram (1984) confirmed this effect in both English and Kannada speakers and found in addition that, when the short sentence was made the end of a longer sentence rather than the beginning, it occasioned not more but less stuttering than when it stood alone. Somewhat different findings were obtained by Kleinow and Smith (2000), using a very similar paradigm. Although only fluent utterances were analyzed, speech motor coordination was markedly reduced for their stutterers when a baseline phrase was embedded so that it formed the last part of a longer utterance.

It may not be length or complexity *per se* that is the potent factor, but the anticipation of and planning for it. However, Postma and Kolk (1990) found that "tongue twisters" produced more stuttering, but instructions stressing accuracy in the repetition of sentences had no effect. Wells (1979) examined six sentences containing only one relative clause and six sentences with two relative clauses from the recorded spontaneous speech of each of a group of stutterers. A higher percentage of stuttered syllables was found on the more complex sentences. Ronson (1975), however, found no differences in stuttering in the reading of simple, active, affirmative, declarative sentences, negative sentences, and passive sentences by adult participants. In a similar study with 8- to 12-year-old children, on the other hand, Palen and Peterson (1982) reported a trend for severe stutterers to have more difficulty in the oral reading of sentences as the level of difficulty (as measured by presumed underlying transformational complexity) increased. This may be because children's linguistic systems are not yet fully mature. In studies of types of sentences in relation to stuttering, it is difficult to separate syntactic complexity from motor planning difficulty, since sentences that contain more complex language are typically, although not always, longer. The use of oral reading, however, would seem to minimize linguistic formulation complexity.

Bernstein Ratner (1997) was able to separately analyze contributions of length and complexity on children's stuttering and found complexity a better predictor of stuttering in children's elicited imitations than length. Yaruss (1999), who examined children's spontaneous speech, found length a better predictor of stuttering than complexity, but did not find either to be a strong predictor of fluency breakdown. Brundage and Bernstein Ratner (1989) contrasted the predictive power of children's spontaneous utterance lengths using three different indices: sentence length in words, in syllables (considered a more motoric measure) and mean length in morphemes (considered a linguistic complexity measure). Utterance length in morphemes was most highly correlated with stuttering.

In sum, essentially any kind of spoken language that minimizes formulation difficulty is likely to produce less stuttering. Healey, Mallard, and Adams (1976) found more fluency in the oral reading of song lyrics with which stutterers were highly familiar than in the reading of unfamiliar lyrics. As we will see later, the simplification of motor planning may also have something to do with the much-discussed adaptation and metronome effects.

Listener Reactions to Stuttering Stuttering often appears to vary with social pressures (e.g., unfavorable listener reactions) or what the stutterer perceives as social penalties for stuttering. Porter (1939) showed that the amount of difficulty speakers experienced in reading to various listeners was consistent with their previous evaluations of the listeners as "hard" or "easy" to talk to. Berwick (1955) found that this extended even to a situation in which the stutterer read to photographs of such listeners. It is evident that listeners or cues representative of them may become capable of consistently evoking stuttering. This raises the question of whether there are any definable features of listeners that tend to make them "hard" or "easy" for stutterers as a group. Comments from adults who stutter appear to indicate that one important feature is listeners' reactions to stuttering. Generally speaking, persistent stutterers have more difficulty when noting or expecting reactions of impatience, embarrassment, pity, shock, or the like by listeners (Yovetich & Dolgoy, 2001). In contrast, a close friend who no longer appears to notice the stuttering may be quite easy to talk to as may, in some cases, a stranger who is not expecting the person to block.

Stutterers' comments about the amount of difficulty experienced in speaking to their parents are often revealing. Parents characterized as easy to speak to are often described as easygoing, understanding, or the like. On the other hand, those with whom there is a great deal of stuttering tend to be described as distressed, critical, or impatient. One person who found it difficult to talk to his mother said, "When I go into a block she goes into it with me." Another said about his father, "I seem to feel that when I talk to him I must choose my words carefully." In general, it may be said that speakers typically have less difficulty when their listeners appear to accept them as individuals rather than reacting to them as stutterers.

An experimental study of the effect of listener reactions on stuttering in an audience situation was reported by Hansen (1956). By actuating feedback from the *Wisconsin Sequential Sampling Analyzer*, Hansen presented stutterers with what they believed to be listener reactions from their audience from moment to moment as they spoke or read. When unfavorable audience reactions were presented during intervals of speech difficulty, the stuttering seemed to increase. To a lesser extent, favorable reactions during fluent periods appeared to result in a decrease in stuttering.

Concern about Social Approval Communication is a social act. Communicative pressure is increased when the speaker is ill at ease, feels inferior, or expects social disapproval or rejection. Under such conditions, stuttering is liable to be intensified.

One of the outstanding examples is speaking to a person whom the stutterer perceives as important, superior, or in a position of authority. Sheehan, Hadley, and Gould (1967) showed that collegiate stutterers had more speech difficulty when speaking to faculty members dressed in suit or sport jacket and tie and addressed by the title of "Doctor" than they did in speaking to students dressed in sports shirts without jacket or tie and introduced only as "Tom Brown" or the like. They concluded that the lower the speaker's self-esteem, or the more authority-laden the listener's status, the greater the amount of stuttering.

Conversely, there is likely to be less speech difficulty when stutterers have reason to be confident about their status. They usually report that they tend to speak more fluently with people who are younger or who are in lower status to them. Ramig, Krieger, and Adams (1982) verified the observation that stutterers generally have less difficulty speaking with children than adults. Officers who stutter are often able to give orders fluently to soldiers they command, and in varying degrees this may apply to a foreman in a factory, an overseer of hired help on a farm, or even a student monitor at school. During one interview, one stutterer experienced a marked reduction of stuttering that he attributed to wearing a pair of hunting boots. His explanation was that they had virtually "the same feel" as the paratroop boots he had worn for four months while serving in an airborne unit in the army two years earlier. During those four months, he had had very little difficulty with his speech, "partially, I suppose, because other people didn't do things such as jumping out of an airplane." Soon after his return to civilian life, his stuttering became more severe, but about a month or two later he noticed that whenever he wore his hunting boots he spoke more fluently.

Speaking to members of the opposite sex represents a different type of circumstance in which concern about the listener's approval often appears to result in considerable stuttering. On the other hand, some stutterers almost never block or have any tendency to do so when on dates, and it is interesting to note in such cases that the person frequently has a history of success in social situations of this type, is confident of his or her ability to impress the opposite sex, and seems, in general, to be gifted with ease and assurance in such situations. One woman accounted for her fluency when speaking to members of the opposite sex by explaining that she felt "more free to speak" with men than with women.

There are still other conditions that illustrate the manner in which stuttering may be related to desire for approval. The difficulty of the audience situation for most stutterers is an example about which we will say more shortly. For some stutterers, speaking to a stranger appears to be an easy speech situation; they become relatively unconcerned about the listener's approval because they believe that they are unlikely to meet the person again. Stutterers also frequently explain the favorable effect of alcoholic intoxication on their speech in this way. One person commented, "You don't care if you stutter or what you do."

Audience Size Stuttering tends to increase when there is more than one listener and apparently becomes radically reduced when no listener is present. There can hardly be any better example of the effect of communicative pressure. As audience size increases, so does communicative responsibility, the threat of unfavorable listener reactions to stuttering, and concern about social approval.

Increases in stuttering in audience situations have been observed in a series of studies.[23] Porter (1939) found that frequency of stuttering increased progressively with audience sizes of one, two, four, and eight listeners, although the difference between four and eight listeners was small and not significant (see Figure 10-1). Young (1965) obtained findings to the contrary. He arranged a series of oral reading conditions in such a way that the stutterers had no

[23] Steer and Johnson (1936), Porter (1939), Hahn (1940), Dixon (1955), Shulman (1955), Van Riper and Hull (1955), Siegel and Haugen (1964), Commodore (1980).

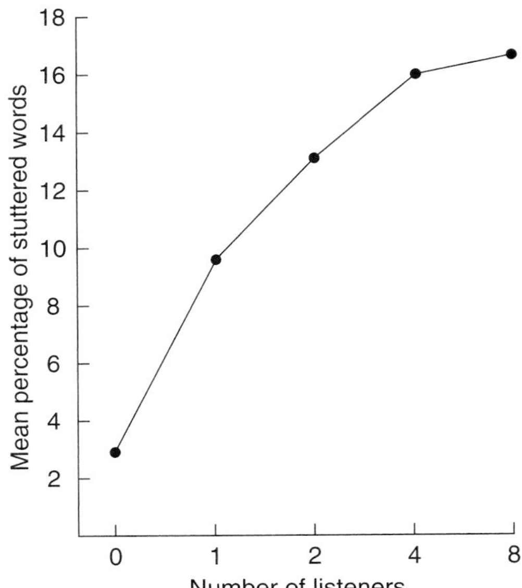

FIGURE 10-1 Mean percentage of stuttering of 13 stutterers in oral reading to varying numbers of listeners. Plotted with permission from data of Porter, H. V. K., studies in the psychology of stuttering: XIV Stuttering phenomena in relation to size and personnel of audience. *Journal of Speech Disorders, 4,* 323–33. Copyright 1939 by the American Speech-Language-Hearing Association. All rights reserved.

way of anticipating beforehand how many listeners there would be, with the startling result that variations in audience size had essentially no effect on stuttering. Armson, Foote, Witt, Kalinowski and Stuart (1997) also found no effect of audience size (2, 4, and 15 people) on adults' stuttering.

Reports by stutterers that their difficulty is very markedly reduced when they are alone have also been confirmed repeatedly.[24] The usual procedure in these studies has been to monitor stuttering by means of a concealed listener or microphone, after instructing subjects to check their own stuttered words in order to preserve the impression that they were not being observed. Bergmann (1987) observed a marked reduction in stuttering when oral reading was recorded in a sound-isolated booth without direct contact with the experimenter. Martin and Haroldson (1988) even found some reduction in stuttering when they had participants engage in monologue, apparently with no effort to convince them that they were alone. In an experiment by Hood (1975), stutterers spoke more fluently in the presence of a person whose hearing was masked and whose eyes were blindfolded than in the presence of someone who could see and hear them. Simply being heard evoked more stuttering than did just being seen. That there is any stuttering at all when stutterers are alone is perhaps due in part to the fact that they may serve to some extent as their own critical listeners. Some stutterers say that they have no blocks whatever if they are absolutely sure they are alone, but that they may stutter if they hear a footstep down the hall, or if they talk "as though" to a listener, or even if they think, "If somebody were listening to me, I would be stuttering."[25]

The Factor of Attention

Another general statement that we can make about the frequency of stuttering is that it tends to vary with the amount of attention that stutterers give to their speech, the cues that evoke stuttering, their role as speakers, or their self-concept as stutterers. When they forget that they are stutterers—for example, when acting in a play or in some cases when talking to total strangers—they may have little or no difficulty with speech. One stutterer commented that if a teacher called on him unexpectedly for a response, it was often possible for him to say three or four sentences fluently until it suddenly "dawned" on him and he would begin to stutter.

On the other hand, if the total stranger with whom the stutterer is talking fluently should turn out at some point in the conversation to be a speech pathologist, there is liable to be an abrupt recurrence of stuttering. As we have seen, there is also likely to be a sharp increase in difficulty if we fail to hear the initial message and ask the stutterer to repeat it. By

[24] Steer and Johnson (1936), Porter (1939), Hahn (1940), Razdolsky (1965), Quinn (1971), Šváb, Gross, and Langová (1972), Langová and Šváb (1973).

[25] See Bluemel (1935, p. 86), Blanton and Blanton (1936, p. 79).

doing so, we have made the person more conscious of his or her role as a speaker. Similarly, stutterers are apt to have exceptional trouble on the telephone, which reduces a person to a voice and removes nonverbal listener responses. (In recent years, many have welcomed the advent of answering machines, as well as e-mail.) Maddox (1938) found that blocks increased in oral reading when stutterers observed themselves in a mirror. Van Riper (1937c) reported more stuttering on words dictated by stutterers than on words dictated by nonstutterers.

There is an almost endless number of examples of reduction in stuttering that appear to be due to displacement of attention, or what has generally been called "distraction." It is possible to group them into several well-defined categories.

Novel Modes of Speaking Virtually any change that can be made in the way a person normally talks is apt to result in much improved or essentially fluent speech for the majority of stutterers, provided the change does not lose its novelty.[26] Such changes include singing, speaking in a sing-song or with other unusual inflectional patterns, speaking in a monotone, whispering, shouting, using an abnormally high pitch or an abnormally low pitch, adopting an unusual voice quality, speaking with exaggerated articulatory movements or with "slurred" articulation, speaking with objects in the mouth, speaking at a slow rate, speaking on inspiration of air, speaking with altered breathing, or speaking in time to rhythmical movements such as those of a metronome. Perhaps the only important exception is rapid speech, which, as we have seen, may be a source of speech pressure for many stutterers as they try to "get their words out" hastily before impatient listeners. Garber and Martin (1977) found no reduction in stuttering when speakers increased their vocal intensity. Shouting, however, has often been observed to result in more fluency.

There are many other examples of the immediate effectiveness of a change in speech pattern. Stutterers can often speak fluently when they imitate a foreign dialect, impersonate someone else, speak in a declamatory manner on the stage, or adopt an unaccustomed manner of behavior—for example, clowning, assertiveness, or the like. Cherry and Sayers (1956) found that many stutterers spoke fluently while "shadowing" or concurrently repeating another person's speech, and this was confirmed by Kondas (1971), Healey and Howe (1987), and others. Dixon (1957) obtained a reduction in stuttering in oral reading by having participants shout "Hey!" at the beginning of each sentence. In studies by Ingham, Montgomery, and Ulliana (1983), Gow and Ingham (1992), and Ingham, Kilgo, et al. (2001), stuttering was reduced by instructions, aided by visual and auditory feedback, to vary the frequency of intervals of phonation of prescribed durations. Stutterers who underwent laryngectomies and did not stutter when they learned to use esophageal speech have been mentioned by various writers, along with some counterexamples of stuttering that persisted after laryngectomy.[27]

A number of the effects we have mentioned have been investigated experimentally. Johnson and Rosen (1937) demonstrated the effects of singing, whispering, choral speaking, and changes in rate, pitch, loudness, and inflection. Other studies have been done on whispering,[28] singing,[29] high and low pitch,[30] reduction of speaking rate,[31] and the use of a monotone.[32] Speaking in time to a metronome has also been repeatedly investigated, as will be seen in Chapter 11. Perkins, Bell, Johnson, and Stocks (1979) found that reducing reading rate by pausing between words reduced stuttering, but doing so by prolonging the sounds in each syllable reduced stuttering far more. Healey, Mallard, and Adams (1976)

---

[26] Novel speech patterns may fail to work if they are used repeatedly. One stutterer, newly arrived in New York City from a small town in the Midwest and anticipating an exceptional amount of difficulty speaking, adopted the habit of speaking in a Texas "drawl" and spoke quite fluently for about a month in this way. He began to stutter again, however, as soon as the drawl became an accustomed manner of speaking.

[27] Irving and Webb (1961), Doms and Lissens (1973), Wingate (1981a), Rosenfield and Freeman (1983).

[28] Witt (1925), May and Hackwood (1968), Perkins, Rudas, Johnson, and Bell (1976), Commodore and Cooper (1978), Commodore (1980).

[29] Witt (1925), Wiechmann and Richter (1966), Healey, Mallard, and Adams (1976), Colcord and Adams (1979), Wingate (1981b).

[30] Ramig and Adams (1980, 1981).

[31] Ingham, Martin, and Kuhl (1974), Perkins, Bell, Johnson, and Stocks (1979).

[32] Adams, Sears, and Ramig (1982).

showed that fluency in singing was not due merely to familiarity with the lyrics. Several studies have attempted to pursue a suggestion by Wingate (1969, 1981b) that the choral reading effect in stuttering results from changes in the vocal pattern. Ingham and Carroll (1977) and Ingham and Packman (1979) reported that the nonstuttered speech of stutterers in solo and choral reading conditions could not always be differentiated by listeners. Adams and Ramig (1980) found decreased vowel durations in the choral reading of stutterers. By controlling for reading rates, Ingham and Packman (1979) showed that the choral reading effect on fluency could not be attributed simply to reduced rate.

The assumption that the novelty of the speech patterns we have been discussing is the chief reason for their effectiveness is based in part on the fact that practically any alteration in speech seems capable of producing fluency, at least temporarily. Although the best evidence that the effect of a mode of speech is due to its novelty is probably its failure to be of help after prolonged use, there is little reliable evidence of this kind outside of clinical experience, since it is essentially impossible to devise a satisfactory laboratory analogue of prolonged use. As is true of so many other reductions of stuttering, moreover, some of these are attributable and may indeed be due to more than one factor. Some speech patterns, such as speaking slowly, make reduced demands on motor planning, as we have already seen. Others are probably incompatible with stuttering behavior on the level of sheer execution of speech movements; examples are legato speech, speaking with gentle phonatory onsets, using soft articulatory contacts, or initiating airflow before speech attempts. Stager, Denman, and Ludlow (1997) found that improved fluency under choral reading, metronome pacing, delayed auditory feedback, and noise conditions could be correlated to changes in speech rate, consonant closure duration, amplitude and time to maximum airflow and intraoral pressure for initial plosives, and the duration and intensity of the following vowel.

In addition, Wingate (1969, 1970) offered the view that many such reductions in stuttering result specifically from altered vocalization and prosody. In a study of the speech patterns of three stutterers under a large number of fluency-inducing conditions, Andrews, Howie, Dozsa, and Guitar (1982) searched for temporal characteristics (e.g., speech rate, articulation rate, duration of phonation) common to all of them, but could find none. Wingate (1981b) studied the speech of four subjects in shadowing, singing, speaking in time to rhythm, and unison speaking. Qualitative analysis of spectrograms seemed to show some common features, chiefly reduced vocal inflection and concentration of energy in the lower harmonics.

Although other factors besides novelty may thus account for a part of the fluency produced by certain altered speech patterns, these factors can play a part in only a relatively small number of them. The best explanation is one that will help us understand why almost any and all unaccustomed ways of speaking, even imitation of the normal speech of another person, will cause an abrupt decrease in stuttering in most cases. The only explanation of this kind that has ever been offered is the novelty of the pattern.

That such novelty in itself can be the cause of fluent speech implies that some type of distraction of attention is operating. Generally, the stutterer's attention has been thought to be distracted from either speech or stuttering. It is well to consider that if novel speech mannerisms owe their fluency-enhancing effect to distraction, it can hardly be because of the very small amount of attention it takes to talk in a high pitch, in a foreign accent, or in time to rhythm, or the like. It may be instead that the interference with stuttering comes mainly from the impression stutterers receive from hearing themselves talk in a strange way and/or from awareness of the strange impression they are making on others. Support for this notion comes from a study by Kalinowski, Stuart, Wamsley, and Rastatter (1999). Under normal auditory feedback, stuttering frequency differed across a number of feedback conditions, including speaking alone, speaking alone while being video-recorded, and being recorded in the presence of two observers. When stutterers heard their fundamental frequency distorted under frequency altered feedback, listener conditions no longer affected their stuttering. To change one's voice or speech is to assume a masquerade that may serve to hide for a moment the person stutterers feel themselves to be. In short, it is perhaps not so much the difference in their speech that makes stutterers fluent as much as the perception that they are speaking differently.[33]

Associated Activity A second category of reductions in stuttering that seem to be attributable to distraction includes associated physical and/or cognitive activities of various kinds. For example, there may be little stuttering when speech is accompanied by dancing, piano playing, or swimming or when the stutterer is demonstrating how to play a musical instrument or operate a machine. Geniesse (1935) reported a laboratory investigation showing that stutterers tended to be able to speak fluently while walking on all fours. In a study by Arends, Povel, and Kolk (1988), stuttering was significantly reduced when subjects spoke while engaged in a manual tracking task that consisted of keeping a dot on a screen within a moving square. Similarly, Vasić and Wijnen (2005) found that playing the classic computer game "Pong" decreased stuttering rates in the adults they studied. However, not all dual-task conditions improve fluency. Caruso, Chodzko-Zajko, et al. (1994) found that stuttering was increased when color-word naming was compared to the well-known and cognitively demanding Stroop-test condition, in which the color of printed text must be named when it spells out a differing color word. Bosshardt (2002) found that reading while repeating words impacted fluency in persons who stutter more than it did for typically fluent adults.

The effectiveness of some of these conditions, when compared to the others, appears to stem from the fact that stutterers are able to time their word attempts with part of the action. For example, a stutterer reported that while playing the piano, he avoided stuttering by striking the keys when he was about to block. When every syllable of speech is timed with a rhythmical activity—for example, with walking or periodic movements of the arm, hand, or foot—there is particularly little probability that stuttering will occur, as Barber (1940) demonstrated experimentally. The only stutterer seen by the first author who had blocks when talking in time to a rhythmic swing of the arm was a person who had been trained to do this at a "stammering school." It is probable that the facilitating effects of this activity had worn off over time, a common feature of physical concomitants seen in some adults who stutter.

Emotional Arousal Stuttering is likely to be reduced or absent under conditions that generate motivation, excitement, or emotion so strong as to make stutterers "forget themselves." People who stutter may be able to express themselves fluently when angry or when carried away by enthusiasm. It is particularly instructive that they often tend to speak well under conditions of fear. One stutterer said that during World War II, his speech had been good enough for him to do mortar communications work, but only in the heat of combat. Another said that as a navigator on a heavy bomber, he had never stuttered when there was doubt about whether they would get back to their base. Even stage fright is occasionally mentioned by people who stutter as a condition that eliminates disfluency. A commonplace example of distraction through emotional arousal may be glimpsed in the following dialogue between a rehabilitation counselor and a young woman with a stuttering problem:

Counselor: How do you feel about drugs?

Client: (stuttering) I wouldn't have anything to do with them.

Counselor: Why not?

Client: (stuttering) Well, just because everybody else takes drugs doesn't mean I have to.

Counselor: Is that the only reason?

Client: (stuttering) They're no good. They can kill you.

Counselor: You know that, because your sister died of an overdose.

Client: (fluent for the first time in the interview) How did you know that?

[33] In Chapter 11, we will encounter further evidence of this effect in the observation that essentially any change in auditory speech feedback that causes people who stutter to hear themselves in a strange way appears to reduce stuttering.

Intense or Unusual Stimuli A variety of sensory stimuli appear to be capable of reducing stuttering. Among examples reported by stutterers are severe pain and extreme fatigue.[34] The use of drugs producing narcosis, anesthesia, sedation, vasoconstriction, and other effects has been observed clinically to remove stuttering in certain instances.[35] Hyperventilation caused a drop in stuttering in a study by Sayles (1971). Many other examples of reductions in stuttering associated with extraneous stimulation are to be found in the literature on stuttering going back many years. For instance, Gutzmann (1898, p. 433) found that some stutterers were able to speak fluently under the influence of a small but steady electric current from electrodes at the larynx and on the nape of the neck. In a few cases, he was astonished to find that mere application of the electrodes without the electrical current had almost the same effect.

Loud noise and many other kinds of alteration of the stutterer's auditory feedback are also capable of reducing stuttering. As we will see later in this chapter, however, the reasons for this are a matter of debate. Webster and Gould (1975) reported a marked reduction in the blocks of a severe stutterer following anesthetization of his larynx. Modest reductions in stuttering have been seen following laryngeal administration of botulinum toxin (now more popularly known as Botox; Brin, Stewart, Blitzer, & Diamond, 1994). Fluency gains were lost over time as the effects of the toxin wore off. On the other hand, Hutchinson and Ringel (1975) found an increase in the stuttering of six subjects as a result of anesthesia of the oral structures.

Can Someone Be Distracted from Stuttering? Throughout this discussion, we have been assuming that there is an important factor of attention in stuttering and that fluency is often achieved by distraction of this attention. This, assumption, however, has been questioned from time to time. In recent years, in particular, a tendency has arisen to regard such explanations of fluency with suspicion. Three different and mutually incompatible objections to distraction have been raised—either that it plays no part in stuttering, or that it is meaningless, or that it is inadequate to explain all of the phenomena that have been attributed to it. We will consider each of these criticisms in turn.

Doubts about the existence of distraction as a factor in stuttering were based initially on some experimentation by Beech and Fransella, who were primarily concerned with the reason for the metronome effect. After demonstrating that stutterers could speak fluently in time to a rhythmic metronome, Fransella and Beech (1965) attempted to rule out distraction as a cause of their findings by showing that fluency did not result when the subjects were instructed to listen attentively to an arrhythmic metronome beat. Recognizing that listening to an arrhythmic beat might simply not be as distracting as talking in time to rhythm, Fransella (1967) had stutterers write down a series of tape-recorded numbers while reading aloud. Again there was no effect on stuttering. Fransella concluded that the metronome effect had not been caused by distraction.

The same argument can be used equally well to reject distraction as a cause of any other effect in stuttering, of course. It therefore raises a very broad issue. If a certain degree of attention is required in order for stuttering to take place, this is a fundamental and revealing fact, though one that we have long taken for granted. If it were true that a person could not be distracted from stuttering, this would be bound to influence our perspective on it profoundly. It would make stuttering unique among behaviors that are as responsive to environmental stimuli as stuttering has been found to be.

In our opinion, the task of writing numbers while reading does not put distraction to any such critical test. There are several reasons for this. Not only must we consider the factor of the strength or magnitude of a distractor, but we must also take into account that if activities are capable of interfering with stuttering, the reverse must also be true. Unfortunately, we cannot judge from Fransella's study to what extent her participants' stuttering

[34] See Bloodstein (1950a, 1950b). In an experimental study, Curtis (1942) found a tendency, short of statistical significance, for stuttering to decrease following muscular exercise.

[35] See Bloodstein (1949). In a laboratory study by Love (1955), however, neither Nembutol (a depressant) nor Benzedrine (a stimulant) was found to have any significant effect on stuttering. See additional coverage of pharmacological treatments for stuttering in Chapter 14.

interfered with the response of writing numbers—that is, to what extent such responses were delayed while blocks were occurring.

There is, however, an even more urgent question that arises in relation to this experiment. It is quite possible that the writing of numbers was distracting enough to interfere with the act of oral reading itself. If the speaker had a tendency to stop reading momentarily when it was time to write down a number, the writing activity could not conceivably have reduced the stuttering. It is self-evident that a condition so distracting that it compels the person who stutters to take time out from speaking or reading cannot interfere with stuttering. In fact, the reason why unusual patterns of speaking give the appearance of being such powerful distractors is in all probability that they are among the few competing responses that by definition do not distract from talking.

Two additional studies have tested whether people can be distracted from stuttering. Kamhi and McOsker (1982) had stutterers step on and off a 10-inch platform while reading aloud, and Thompson (1985) had them manually track an irregular line on a rotating drum while speaking. In neither case was there any effect on stuttering. These experiments, like those of Beech and Fransella, demonstrate the peculiar difficulty of doing research regarding distraction. It is clear that the conditions employed did not interfere with stuttering; yet neither these nor an endless number of similar demonstrations could prove that there are not other conditions capable of distracting from stuttering. On the other hand, it would be easy to point to a great many conditions that do interfere with stuttering, but these are the very conditions about which controversy exists regarding whether they are examples of distraction. We are forced to conclude that this type of research is incapable of determining whether stuttering requires attention and can be reduced by diverting the stutterer's attention. Until a better approach to the problem can be devised, our only alternative may be to evaluate the concept of distraction by considering what it helps us to explain. We may now place in the balance a compelling amount of evidence in its favor.

Distraction in Psycholinguistic Models of Speech Production A recent model of stuttering places the potential role of distraction into a new light. Vasić and Wijnen (2005) suggest a role for distraction within Levelt's model of speech production and its component module, the internal monitor (see Chapter 2). The task of the internal monitor is to check the well-formedness of utterances just prior to phonetic encoding (see Gleason & Bernstein Ratner, 1998, for discussion), and some theorists have suggested that it may be dysfunctional in people who stutter. In this view, distracting conditions may prevent the internal monitor from inappropriately rejecting and reformulating speech output. As noted earlier, the authors found less stuttering when adults who stutter were required to play a computer game while speaking. This was interpreted as evidence that external attentional demands could distract the inappropriately calibrated pre-articulatory speech production monitoring system so that it would not inaccurately reject and attempt to reformulate otherwise well-formed speech output.

In brief, distraction, although an imprecise notion, helps us to account for a very wide range of observations. We may sum these up by saying that people who stutter are likely to talk more fluently when they adopt virtually any novel speech pattern or mannerism, when they are in vigorous concurrent action or problem-solving, when they are carried away by emotion or excitement, or when they are reacting to novel or powerful stimuli. It enables us to understand why some of these factors have a tendency to "wear out" when they are overused. In addition, it meshes with another set of observations that seem to be merely the inverse of the distraction effect. As we saw in Chapter 1, stuttering is capable of interfering with voluntary manual activities such as the alternate squeezing and releasing of a rubber ball. It may interfere with the perception of the passage of time. In some cases, it may reduce the perception of visual and auditory stimuli. Finally, the concept of distraction is consistent with the many indications that stuttering tends to increase in real-life circumstances that draw stutterers' attention to their speech.

We have been discussing the most sweeping objection to the concept of distraction; namely, that stutterers cannot be distracted from stuttering. A second and more valid objection to the concept is its vagueness of definition. Writers who have used the term through the years have variously held that stutterers were being distracted from their speech, their stuttering, or their anticipation of stuttering. As the work of Fransella and Beech has served to show, there is little agreement on any precise operational meaning of distraction.

The problem of describing what we mean by distraction in adequately scientific terms does not seem insurmountable, however. It reduces essentially to a description of interference between competing stimuli or competing responses. This has been a matter of concern in other areas of cognitive research as well, when dual-task designs are employed (see Lavie, Hirst, de Fockert, & Viding, 2004, for recent discussion). For example, Norman and Waugh (1968) identified both a stimulus-produced and a response-produced interference with recognition memory. Keele (1972), also concerned with the subject of memory, wrote, "When the processing of one stimulus interferes with processing another, the processing is said to take attention," and also, "When performing one task interferes with performing another, the tasks are said to require attention." This may be applied directly to stuttering. What we have called distraction appears to consist of two broad observations. One is that competing stimuli of sufficient strength or novelty may interfere with attention to the stimuli that evoke stuttering. The other is that competing responses requiring sufficient attention may interfere with the response of stuttering.

Finally, an objection to the concept of distraction that may be raised with some justification is that it has tended to be overused. Its capability to cover a multitude of circumstances makes it all too easy to invoke it as a reason for observations of fluency having no other readily apparent explanation. Alternative explanations may prove to be better in some instances. In many cases, several influences probably contribute equally to a reduction in stuttering, and distraction may serve merely as one factor. For this reason, we need to be skeptical of the uncritical use of explanations based on distraction.

Suggestion

Hypnotic suggestion was used widely in attempts to treat stuttering as early as the beginning of the nineteenth century. Its effects are often striking, though usually temporary. Moore (1946) reported a clinical investigation of hypnotic suggestion with 40 stutterers; each was worked with repeatedly for a period of at least seven weeks. Of the 40, 9 were not adequately responsive to hypnosis. Twelve spoke fluently when the suggestion was given that "hesitances would not bother," but failed to respond to posthypnotic suggestions. Eleven not only spoke to audiences without stuttering, but usually carried out posthypnotic suggestions fluently. Eight remaining subjects with "apparently little limit" to hypnotic behavior carried out posthypnotic suggestions fluently before audiences and reported that their speech continued to be "easy and relaxed" for two or three days following hypnotic sessions.

Various forms of nonhypnotic suggestion have been observed to be equally potent in removing stuttering for brief periods. Emile Coué, a Frenchman famous for his feats of suggestion, once persuaded a severe stutterer to speak before an audience by leading him to the stage and assuring him that he did not stutter. The stutterer spoke without difficulty, but within a week he appeared at a speech clinic for help, blocking more severely than before.[36] The effects of suggestion on stuttering are perhaps best known in the form of the observation that literally any form of therapy appears to be capable of producing sudden and largely temporary "cures" in certain instances. This phenomenon, which is not unlike the placebo effect discussed in Chapter 14, is not limited to stuttering.

Tension, Stress, and Generalized Anxiety

People who stutter often report that their speech improves when they are calm and relaxed. Some individuals benefit from training in voluntary

[36] See Heltman (1943, p. 78).

relaxation of their muscles. Six stutterers who engaged in the regular practice of transcendental meditation all reported to McIntyre, Silverman, and Trotter (1974) that their stuttering had been reduced as a result. This finding was confirmed by Allen and Daly (1978). Treon and Tamayo (1975) reported that two individuals reduced their stuttering moderately by self-regulation of their galvanic skin response.

Conversely, clinical observation suggests that an increase in general tension may result in more frequent blocks. For example, stutterers who tell of speaking fluently under conditions of acute fear or emotional stress sometimes report more stuttering "after it was all over." One person who had no stuttering immediately after an automobile accident said, "And then when I got home I was shot. I could hardly say one word without having a bad block." In some cases, stuttering appears to increase on almost every occasion on which the speaker is generally tense, anxious, or upset; stuttering may become virtually a daily barometer of the person's frame of mind.

Research findings that bear on the effect of stress on fluency tend to be equivocal, but this is perhaps to be expected in view of the variety of ways in which it can be defined and the difficulty of creating stress in the laboratory; however, random electric shock seems to have limited effect on stuttering.[37] Toomey and Sidman (1970) studied the frequency of stuttering during the sounding of a buzzer that warned the participants of impending shock. Of four study participants, only one showed an increase in stuttering; two stuttered less. Stressful conditions such as fatigue, pain, or hyperventilation appear to be more likely to decrease stuttering than to increase it, as we have seen. Laboratory experiences of failure seem to have little effect.[38] Confronting the person with discomforting silence does seem to produce more stuttering, according to a report by Gould and Sheehan (1967), though somewhat conflicting findings were obtained by Adams and Brutten (1970). On the basis of the well-documented premise that women tend to have higher anxiety levels at premenstruation than at ovulation, Silverman, Zimmer, and Silverman (1974) recorded the speech of four female stutterers at these two points in their menstrual cycles and found more stuttering at premenstruation in each case.

[37] Frick (1951), Bearss (1952).

[38] Lerea (1955), Trombly (1959).

The Presence or Absence of Cues

Among the conditions under which stuttering may be markedly reduced are a number that differ considerably from each other, yet seem to owe their effect on stuttering to a common underlying factor; in all of them, many of the cues to which the person habitually responds by stuttering have been removed. For example, some individuals who stutter are able to avoid stuttering effectively at times by using word substitutions. Some stutterers have difficulty at home but not at school, while in other cases the reverse may be true. One may find stutterers who have essentially all of their difficulty in oral reading, but none in spontaneous speech. Cases have been reported in which the person stuttered only on the telephone, or only when ordering a meal, or only when riding in an elevator;[39] such stutterers appear to speak normally in most situations for the same reason that most of us are nonstutterers in all of them—there are no stimulus cues for speech difficulty. Presumably, under all of these conditions, the stutterer has learned to respond discriminatively to cues associated with them as a result of specific past experiences.[40]

A stutterer may have difficulty speaking one language but not another. Sometimes it is the first-learned language in which stuttering occurs and sometimes the second. Dale (1977) described the cases of four Cuban-American adolescent boys who stuttered in Spanish but not English. All had been born in the United States, but spoke only

[39] Blanton (1931), Bender and Kleinfeld (1938, p. 243).

[40] This premise may underlie the reported success of self-modeling therapies for stuttering (see Chapter 14), in which repeated exposure to videotaped samples of a person's stutter-free speech in previously difficult settings are used to improve fluency.

Spanish at home. Dale related their stuttering to home pressures, reported by both the boys and their parents, to retain proficiency in the Spanish language. Nwokah (1988) noted that among 16 stutterers in Anambra State, Nigeria, who were equally proficient in English and Igbo, some stuttered more in one language and some in the other.[41]

Finally, some stutterers speak better in new surroundings—for example, on vacation trips, when enrolling in a new school, or on entering the armed services. One stutterer interviewed by the first author had virtually lived a nomadic life for this reason. Whenever he stayed in one place for more than a few months, his stuttering became so severe that he could hardly talk. He would then quit his job, pack his belongings, and move away to begin all over again in a new town.

Anticipation of Stuttering

It is an old observation, long antedating current anticipatory struggle theories of stuttering, that stutterers' expectations of difficulty with their speech may be a powerful force in bringing it about. This is an assumption of rather broad reach, since it can be viewed as encompassing many of the generalizations we have already made. If blocks can be evoked by the anticipation of stuttering, it is only reasonable to assume that they may come and go with fluctuations in stutterers' attention to their speech, with suggestions that instill the conviction that they will or will not stutter, with the cues to which their anticipations have become attached, and even with generalized states of tension or anxiety that are conducive to expectancy.

Ironically, it is the very prominence of this factor in stuttering that has given it its controversial aspects, since it has led to the theory that it is the essence of the difficulty. This has tended to carry with it the implication that every block that the stutterer has must be preceded by anticipation. This is a far more debatable point than the assumption that anticipation is an influential factor, and research findings have not produced conclusive evidence with regard to it. Earlier in this chapter, we saw that while many people who stutter can predict the occurrence of their stuttering, there are many exceptions to this, particularly in children and even in adults. There are, however, other ways besides speakers' predictions by which anticipation of stuttering can be studied.

The Effect of Varying the Duration of Expectancy Within certain limits, the longer the time interval elapsing between the moment of the stutterer's planned speech response and the moment that they attempt it, the greater the probability of stuttering. Stutterers who wait a long time for their turn to recite in the classroom because their name begins with "W" are apt to have a great deal of difficulty when finally called on. An observation of this sort serves both to define anticipation operationally and to suggest a systematic way to study its effect on stuttering.

Goss (1952) studied this effect experimentally by varying the time interval between the exposure of a stimulus word and a signal to the subject to say the word. For intervals from 2 to 10 seconds, he found that the amount of stuttering progressively increased with the length of the latency required to say the word. For intervals shorter than 2 seconds, there was another increase in stuttering as the interval was decreased to 1 and then 0 seconds, a finding that suggests that with the demand for an immediate or rapid response, a new source of speech pressure makes itself felt (see Figure 10-2).

In a further study, Goss (1956) varied the time interval between a warning signal and the exposure of the word, the word being spoken as soon as it was seen. Again there was more stuttering with longer intervals. It appears that not only waiting to say a specific word, but merely waiting to speak, tends to increase the probability of stuttering.

These findings appear to show not only that a relationship between stuttering and anticipation exists, but also that the relationship is dependent. Consequently, they are of considerable importance. In a somewhat similar study, however, Fransella

[41] For recent reviews of characteristics of bilingual stuttering, see van Borsel (2001) and Bernstein Ratner (2004).

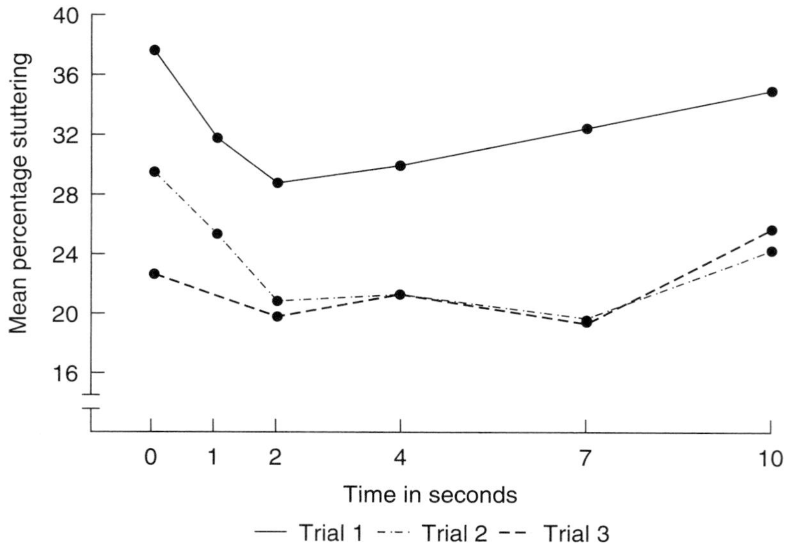

FIGURE 10-2 Mean percentage of stuttering as a function of the time interval between the exposure of stimulus words and the signal to say them, during three successive trials. Adapted from Goss, 1952.

(1971) obtained negative results. Time intervals ranging from 5 to 13 seconds between word presentation and signal to speak did not differ in their effects on stuttering, either when subjects could predict the moment of occurrence of the signal or when they could not.[42]

On the other hand, Forte and Schlesinger (1972) found the effect again. Furthermore, they found it in children. Their subjects were 20 school-aged children who stutter. Each participant took turns reading aloud with five normally fluent classmates on a series of occasions. The order in which the children read was determined by their seating arrangement, and this was systematically varied from one time to the next. The results were similar to those of Goss. The first position produced more stuttering than the second, but from the second to the sixth the stuttering increased progressively again (see Figure 10-3).

[42] Fransella's experiment was chiefly concerned with the effect of ability to predict the occurrence of the signal to speak, and it differed from Goss's in certain aspects of the method. For example, participants were allowed 10 seconds to say the word after receiving the signal.

Autonomic Arousal as a Measure of Anticipation The objectivity of measures of autonomic arousal has long been appealing to researchers who have been interested in the subject of anticipation of stuttering. In general, laboratory investigations have produced a great deal of evidence of physiological arousal just prior to the block. At an early date, Van Riper and Milisen (1939) were able to review a considerable amount of research showing that stuttering was often preceded by accelerations in pulse rate, vasoconstriction, unusual eye movements, electrodermal responses, and disturbances of breathing. Later, Tanberg (1955) reported manual motor disturbances prior to stuttering. Kurshev (1968a) and Ickes and Pierce (1973) found additional evidence of vasoconstriction. Kurshev (1969) studied galvanic skin response (GSR) measures accompanying expectation of stuttering, and Brutten (1963) traced the decline in palmar sweating as speakers' predictions of stuttering decreased in repeated silent readings of a passage. Gray and Williams (1969), however, could find no evidence of pupil dilation preceding the block. Myers (1978) studied the relationship of the sever-

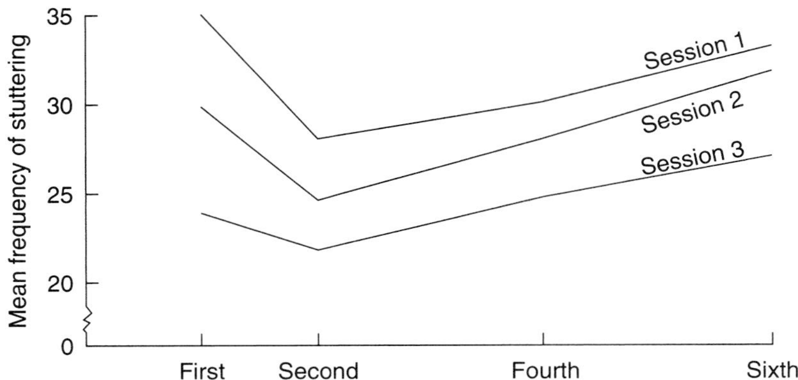

FIGURE 10-3 Mean frequency of stuttering of 20 school-aged stutterers in relation to the order in which they took their turn in oral reading with five classmates, during three reading sessions. Reproduced by permission of the publisher from " Stuttering as a function of time of expectation" by Forte and Schlesinger. *Journal of Communication Disorders*, 5, 347–58. Copyright 1972 by Elsevier Science Publishing Co., Inc.

ity of stuttering events to various measures of respiration, blood volume, skin conductance, and heart rate just prior to stuttering. Dietrich and Roaman (2001) found little correlation between stuttering adults' predictions of speech anxiety in various speaking conditions and actual skin conductance measures.

As useful as these studies have been, they have not provided any critical tests of the hypothesis that stuttering events are precipitated by anticipation. To find changes in the GSR preceding the block is interesting, and it would be even more so if we found them when the person did not consciously anticipate stuttering. But finding such changes frequently is not the same as finding them in every case. Furthermore, the absence of such signs might merely mean that anticipation may occur without a detectable degree of emotional arousal. In a study of three adults who reported that they consistently anticipated their stuttering moments, Baumgartner and Brutten (1983) found that in two cases, there was no relationship between cognitive expectancy and changes in heart rate prior to stuttering. They concluded that "for some stutterers, expectancy may reflect an objective rather than an emotional belief that speech will be difficult." The theory that stuttering blocks are caused by the conviction that the words they are attempting will be difficult, and that they must therefore use some effort, care, or special strategy for saying them, does not necessitate the assumption that stutterers are emotionally aroused, but only that they want to talk and mistakenly believe there are obstacles in the way.

Preparatory Muscular Activity Perhaps more crucial than autonomic arousal to an anticipatory concept of stuttering is some kind of inappropriate muscular preparation for speech. In an electromyographic study of a single stutterer, Bar, Singer, and Feldman (1969) found evidence of unusual laryngeal muscle activity during anticipation of stuttering. A study of 19 subjects by McLean and Cooper (1978) failed to confirm this. On the other hand, Shrum (cited by Guitar, 1975) obtained action potentials from adult stutterers' facial, neck, and chest muscles and found a rise in their amplitude preceding stuttering in almost all the muscles studied. More recently, an electromyographic study of 42 adults by Thürmer, Thumfart, and Kittel (1983) showed muscular hyperactivity at the larynx, tongue, and lip prior to stuttering. Murray, Empson, and Weaver (1987), also found evidence in action potentials at the larynx for the hypothesis that muscular preparedness for speech may play an important role in stuttering.

A series of studies has also demonstrated that adults can generally reduce their stuttering by using auditory or visual feedback to lower the electromyographic signal from their laryngeal, masseter muscle, lip, or chin areas prior to utterances.[43] The precise reasons for such reductions in stuttering are in some doubt, however, due to a number of further observations. For example, Guitar (1975) noted that the sites at which reduced preparatory muscle activity resulted in decreased stuttering were not necessarily the same sites where speech was blocked. Pachman, Oelschlaeger, Hughes, and Hughes (1978) reported on two adults for whom training of the frontalis muscle was effective in reducing stuttering and for whom such training worked whether the speaker raised or lowered muscle activity. Both Craig and Cleary (1982) and Moore (1984b) noted instances in which fluency accompanied high levels of muscle tension.

Shearer and Simmons (1965) obtained negative findings in a study of the stapedius muscle of the middle ear, which has been found to be activated concurrently with the speech musculature. Acoustic impedance measurements showed that middle ear muscle activity did not precede speech output in stutterers by a longer interval than it did in nonstutterers. Their results were confirmed by Quinn and Andrews (1976).

Other Evidence of Anticipation Peters et al. (1976) found changes in stutterers' brain potentials prior to attempts on words that they had rated as frequently stuttered. These changes appeared even when the word was not actually stuttered.

Brutten and Janssen (1979) showed that in silent reading, adults who stutter tended to have longer eye fixations on words for which they had indicated expectancy of stuttering than on words for which they had not. The participants also showed longer fixations on words on which they subsequently stuttered than on nonstuttered words when they read the passage aloud. Janssen and Brutten (1981) reported similar results for stuttering children aged 6 to 12 years, as did Bakker, Brutten, Janssen, and van der Meulen (1991).

On spectrograms of syllables spoken just prior to stuttering events, Knox (1976) found increases in fundamental frequency, decreased rate, and atypical transitions. Falck, Lawler, and Yonovitz (1985) found decreases in fundamental frequency and decreased voicing prior to blocks. The pattern of change varied, however, depending on whether the block that followed involved prolongation, repetition, or absence of phonation, suggesting that the moment of stuttering begins its characteristic pattern "considerably before it is easily identifiable." In summary, the anticipation of stuttering manifests itself in a wide variety of ways. There is little doubt that, in older subjects at least, stuttering moments tend to be closely associated with anticipatory events. Unfortunately, relatively little research has yet been done to determine whether such events occur preceding ostensibly unexpected blocks, how frequently they might be observed in young children, and whether stuttering ever appears in the absence of such events.

Anxiety about Stuttering

Since the precise role of anticipation in stuttering has not been established, it stands to reason that this is also true of that special kind of anticipation called anxiety about stuttering. In at least a loose sense, stuttering in its developed form often appears to be a kind of speech anxiety reaction. To many who have worked with stutterers clinically, this impression seems very strong. Furthermore, a difficulty that varies with communicative pressures, with attention to speech, and to a large extent with anticipation of stuttering might perhaps hardly be thought at a glance to be anything else. Bloodstein (1950b) made an elaborate attempt to show that the broadest possible generalization about the multitude of conditions under which stuttering is reduced or absent is that it declines with reduction in anxiety about stuttering. So close has such a relationship

[43] Guitar (1975), Hanna, Wilfling, and McNeil (1975), Lanyon, Barrington, and Newman (1976), Cross (1977), Lanyon (1977), Moore (1978), Craig and Cleary (1982), Moore (1984b).

appeared to be that the anticipatory struggle hypothesis (see Chapter 2) has often been expressed as the inference that stuttering is a reaction of anxiety about speech or stuttering.

It is, in fact, the very closeness of the relationship that makes counterexamples so striking. And counterexamples are to be found in ample number, even on the level of clinical observation. They are especially common in our experience with children. Although stuttering children are capable of intense speech anxiety reactions, many show little outward sign of anxiety on most occasions. The tendency of people who stutter to have more severe difficulty as a result of obvious fear of stuttering is characteristic of its most advanced forms. Moreover, even adults who stutter can be found who have some of their most severe difficulty in situations such as the speech clinic, in which their attention is strongly focused on their speech, but in which they seem to experience little if any anxiety as that term is commonly understood.

We also find counterexamples when we define anxiety in terms of objective signs of autonomic arousal. In general, such measures do tend to give abundant evidence of anxiety accompanying stuttering. We reviewed this evidence in our description of the visceral concomitants of stuttering blocks in Chapter 1 and in our discussion of the physiological studies of anticipation in the preceding section. Furthermore, certain studies have shown in a rather pointed way a tendency for GSR measures to vary concomitantly with the stutterers' speech or stuttering.[44] In other research, however, such a tendency has been missing or equivocal. For example, Gray and Brutten (1965) did not find a consistent reduction in palmar sweat measures of anxiety as the frequency of stuttering decreased with repeated readings of a passage. Neither did Ritterman and Reidenbach (1975). Nor was there any reduction in palmar sweating under white noise in a study by Adams and Moore (1972), although the noise reduced the stuttering markedly. Reed and Lingwall (1976, 1980) found no consistent tendency for GSR measures to decrease with reduction in stuttering in "punishment" experiments. Similarly, palmar sweat measures of anxiety have failed to decline concomitantly with improvement in speech during treatment.[45] In an experiment by Ickes (1975), the administration of Nembutal lowered adults' palmar sweat indices, even though it increased stuttering in some cases. Janssen and Kraaimaat (1980) found that, although the self-rated anxiety of stutterers exceeded that of typically fluent speakers during oral reading, their skin conductance and heart rates increased no differently. Similar results were obtained by Peters and Hulstijn (1984). During and just before speech tasks, stuttering and typically fluent speakers differed only in self-ratings of anxiety. Heart rate, pulse volume, and skin conductance increased to the same extent in both groups. Murray, Empson, and Weaver (1987) found that stutterers did not have elevated heart rates when they anticipated speaking. Weber and Smith (1990) recorded palmar skin conductance, peripheral blood volume, and heart rate before, during, and after reading and speaking. They found correlations between these arousal measures and stuttering that were significant but quite low. The relationship varied considerably among individuals.

We can add to this the observation that tranquilizing drugs appear to be quite variable in their influence on stuttering. Some stutterers appear to be helped by them, while some do not. Clinical reports of successful use of tranquilizers are common, but some studies have shown little evidence of effectiveness (see Chapter 14).

It is evident that anxiety is a term with many meanings. As a result, the question of how stuttering varies with anxiety about stuttering is far from simple. All that we can say is that by the definitions of anxiety that are usual in clinical and experimental work, anxiety about stuttering has a distinct but inconsistent, limited, and qualified relationship to stuttering.

[44] Berlinsky (1955), Kline (1959), Valyo (1964), Treon and Tamayo (1975).

[45] See Gray and England (1972) and Gregory (cited by Ingham and Andrews, 1971a).

SUMMARY REMARKS

In this chapter, we have dealt with the basic question of the nature of stuttering as a response. The facts that have been discovered may be summarized as follows.

The Distribution of Stuttering In general, there is a strong tendency for stuttering to occur on words on which the speaker predicts that they will occur. Stuttering events that are not predicted occur often, however, particularly in the case of children. Some older and many younger individuals who stutter are able to predict the occurrence of few of their blocks. Nevertheless, there is evidence that many of these speakers may respond to subliminal anticipations of stuttering.

In both children and adults, stuttering tends to occur as a relatively consistent response to cues in the speech context. The same cues have been found to evoke stuttering over periods of weeks, though some change appears to take place in them with the passage of time. In the laboratory, new cues may be given the power to elicit stuttering by association with conditions under which frequent stuttering occurs. There is evidence that, in both children and adults, stuttering may take place in response to cues for no other reason than that they are evocative of past stuttering.

Studies of the loci of stuttering in the speech sequence show that blocks are likely to occur on the first syllable of the word, although they may sometimes be found on accented syllables in other positions within polysyllabic words. Various attributes of words have been found to influence the distribution of stuttering in adults and children of school age. Stuttering tends to occur more often on words beginning with consonants than on words beginning with vowels (at least in English), on content words than on function words (at least in adults), on long words than on short ones, on words at the beginning of the sentence than elsewhere, on words of lower frequency of occurrence in the language, on words carrying more information load as defined by their predictability in context, and probably on words that receive more stress. It is not entirely clear to what extent these factors are overlapping and interdependent. In any case, since the distribution of stuttering events in the same reading material varies widely among different individuals, it is evident that these general features of words do not wield as strong an influence as do individual factors. Although relatively little research has been done on factors that vary from case to case, it is known that there is a marked tendency for individual people who stutter to have special difficulty with certain words or sounds, apparently because of personal histories of past failure on them, and there is some evidence that this has a fairly strong effect on the distribution of stuttering.

The fact that the distribution of stuttering is influenced by so many attributes of words may perhaps be interpreted to mean that, whatever its origin, stuttering in older children and adults is above all a difficulty in the initiation of words, rather than the execution of sounds, syllables, or other units of speech. This is corroborated by the observation that stuttering usually occurs at the beginning of a word and virtually never at the end. There is some evidence, however, that stuttering may be influenced by certain features of sentences, particularly their length or complexity, and in Chapter 12 we will see that the early stuttering of young children may consist to a large degree of difficulty with whole syntactic structures.

The Frequency of Stuttering The frequency of stuttering tends to vary markedly in response to a very large number of identifiable situational factors. All or most of these appear to be subsumed under a number of general conditions:

The frequency of stuttering tends to vary with the amount of communicative pressure imposed on the speaker by such factors as audience size, listener reactions, concern about social approval, time pressures, the degree to which the stutterer is responsible for conveying a meaningful message to a listener, and the demands that the encoding of the message makes on motor planning.

The frequency of stuttering is also affected markedly by a factor of attention, most clearly exemplified by conditions that tend to interfere with stuttering. This interference, generally known as distraction, may come from competing stimuli or competing responses. It may take the form of novel speech patterns or mannerisms of almost any kind, associated activities, emotional arousal, or strange or intense sensory stimuli. The frequency of stuttering may also be influenced by suggestion, by the presence or absence of the cues to which it has become attached, and probably also to some degree by generalized tension and anxiety. Finally, the frequency of developed stuttering often seems to vary, at least to a considerable degree, with anticipation of stuttering, and that appears to be the most general statement we are at present able to make about it.

Alternative Models of the Stuttering Response

In Chapter 2, we described three basic conceptual models that have been advanced to account for the moment of stuttering. The information outlined in this chapter represents almost all the data in our possession by which these models may be tested. We may now ask how good an explanation of the data each of them provides.

The Anticipatory Struggle Hypothesis It was largely out of efforts to substantiate a form of the anticipatory struggle hypothesis that research on stuttering as a response originated. How well has this model succeeded? On the positive side, it takes little effort of interpretation to make it fit most of the facts in an illuminating way. Stuttering appears to be a response to cues representative of past difficulty, a property that uniquely defines anticipatory struggle reactions among learned responses. The blocks appear to occur chiefly on those segments of the speech sequence that individuals who stutter tend to evaluate as difficult or important, that evoke the threat of failure, or on which stuttering is likely to be conspicuous or embarrassing. The frequency of stuttering seems to vary largely with communicative pressures and with the attention people give to their stuttering, their speech, or their role as speakers. In many individuals, stuttering seems to vary with fear or expectancy of stuttering. On the whole, the anticipatory struggle model appears to achieve a parsimonious integration of a very broad range of observations.

The model also meets with some notable difficulties, however. One of them is that stuttering can and evidently often does occur in the absence of anxiety as that term is ordinarily defined. Some might argue that essentially any awareness of the threat of something even slightly annoying or frustrating must be considered mild anxiety, regardless of what the GSR reading or the speaker says. In any case, this problem does not appear to be critical. Johnson's concept of stuttering as an anxiety-motivated avoidance reaction received wide currency, but it is not the only way to state the anticipatory struggle hypothesis. It can be expressed adequately by saying that the stuttering block may result from speakers' convictions, preconceptions, or expectations about the difficulty of the utterance they are about to attempt or from their doubts about their ability to succeed at it. Stated in terms of anxiety, the model will fit many cases. It is not without any foundation in fact. It is simply not general enough.

Perhaps a more serious difficulty is that stuttering can occur in the absence of expectancy of stuttering as defined by speakers' reports or by their ability to predict the occurrence of their blocks. It can be argued that conscious expectancy of stuttering is not necessarily implied by the theory that stuttering is due to a belief in the difficulty of speech or by the hypothesis that it is a response to cues representative of past speech failure. Nevertheless, some form of anticipation would seem to be implied. As we have seen, there are numerous ways in which anticipation may be defined operationally for the purpose of verifying its relationship to stuttering. One can, for example, vary the amount of time the person who stutters waits to say a word and see how that affects the probability of stuttering. Researchers have also investigated stutterers' brain waves, muscle potentials, visceral reactions, and eye movements just prior to stuttering and have made spectrographic analyses of the acoustic characteristics of their speech that precedes blocks. All of these studies have resulted in variable demonstrations of the anticipatory activity for which the investigators were searching. As yet, however, conclusive evidence in support of the anticipatory struggle hypothesis is lacking.

Another problem encountered by this model has to do with the role of punishment in stuttering. According to the anticipatory struggle hypothesis, stuttering should increase as a result of punishment for stuttering. There is considerable clinical impression and some experimental evidence that it does. Yet research has shown that electric shock, verbal punishers, and other typically aversive stimuli tend to reduce stuttering markedly when administered contingently, as we will see in Chapter 11. The issue is further clouded by the observation that such presumably reinforcing stimuli as cessation of loud tone and the word "right" have been found to do the same thing. It is possible that what has been called punishment is in fact stimulus-based distraction. In any case, laboratory conditions of punishment may represent poor analogues of social penalty in the world outside.

The Breakdown Hypothesis The breakdown model of stuttering implies that the block is primarily a response to stress. Perhaps all of the observations that appear to support the anticipatory struggle hypothesis can be explained without difficulty by this theory as well. It is possible to assume that anticipation of difficulty or memories of past failure in speech are factors that may powerfully affect stuttering but are not the essence of it. The essence of it may be a predisposition to motor disintegration of speech. Speech anxieties may serve, with other stressors, to trigger such disintegration.

One issue that this point of view raises concerns the relative influence on stuttering of speech-related stress and stress from other sources. In our review of the variables related to stuttering, speech-related pressures appeared to predominate by far. This may only be, however, because the person who stutters encounters speech-related stress far more often than other kinds.

The same ambiguities with regard to punishment, expectancy, and anxiety that are an embarrassment to the anticipatory struggle hypothesis create similar problems for the breakdown model. Perhaps particular difficulty is offered by the inconsistent relationship between stuttering and signs of autonomic arousal.

The Repressed Need Hypothesis Psychoanalytic theories of stuttering have been concerned with few of the phenomena that have been discussed in this chapter and do not appear to afford a satisfactory integration of many of them. There are frequent allusions in psychoanalytic writings to fluency under conditions of anger and to the ability of some stutterers to perform roles in plays fluently. In addition, there is the general implication that the difficulty varies with the ideational or emotional content of the stutterer's speech. Compared with other factors, only a small amount of research has been done on the influence of speech content on stuttering. Bernhardt (1954) reported that in response to the *Blacky Pictures Test*, certain areas of psychosexual conflict evoked more stuttering than others. In a word association study using words related to speech, security seeking, obstacle surmounting, and sex, Kline (1959) found significant differences in the amount of stuttering in verbal associations to the various word groups. On the other hand, Weisberger (1967) did not find increased stuttering in *Thematic Apperception Test* responses involving themes of sexuality, aggression, and parental authority. Most other studies of the effect of speech content have not been directly relevant to the repressed need hypothesis.[46] However, Perkins and Hagen (1965) permitted their study participants to overhear a derogatory impression of their personal adequacy. Immediately afterward, participants who were allowed to vent aggression directly by giving their frustrator an electric shock stuttered less in oral reading than those who were not. L. H. Silverman, Klinger, et al. (1972) found increased stuttering in spontaneous speech immediately after subliminal exposures of anal and oral aggressive pictures.

[46] Moore, Soderberg, and Powell (1952), Moore (1954, 1959), Bar (1969), MacKay (1969).

Chapter 11

Stuttering as a Response: Some Controversial Phenomena

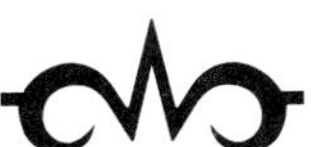

In the general review of variations in the frequency of stuttering that was provided in the previous chapter, we have purposely put off any detailed discussion of four specific conditions under which stuttering tends to diminish. Although they represent only a few of scores of such conditions, they are especially important because they have lent themselves to a great deal of research and speculation concerning their meaning. Knowing what causes these conditions to ameliorate stuttering may give us deeper insight into the possible causes of other changes in the frequency of stuttering.

THE ADAPTATION EFFECT

In 1937, Johnson and Knott issued the first published report of the observation that a reduction in stuttering usually takes place in successive oral readings of the same material.[1] Further research on the effect was done by Johnson and Innes (1939). In these and other studies that soon followed, several basic facts about adaptation became clear. It tends to be very marked during the first few readings and becomes progressively less so, generally reaching a limit beyond which repeated readings have little or no further effect. Most of the reduction that is to take place will be evident in most cases by the fifth reading. On the average, this decrease in stuttering is roughly 50 percent of the frequency of stuttering in the initial reading.

Johnson's curiosity was aroused by the adaptation effect, and it occupied his attention for a considerable time. But it was principally due to the important role that adaptation played in the

[1]According to an editorial note by Johnson, the study by Van Riper and Hull (1955) was probably the first investigation of the adaptation effect, although it remained unreported for many years.

learning-based formulations of Wischner (1950, 1952b); it was somewhat later that extraordinary interest developed in studies of this effect. As a result of decades of research we now probably know more about adaptation than about almost any other comparable aspect of stuttering.

Among the basic facts that have been learned is that the rate of adaptation decreases with an increase in the time interval between successive readings.[2] The length of the passage does not seem to be an important factor.[3] There is relatively little transfer of the adaptation effect to readings of different material.[4] Adaptation is only temporary; if the passage is read again after an interval, the frequency of stuttering will have increased again in amounts varying with the length of the interval and will be fully restored to its original level within a few hours.[5] This "spontaneous recovery" of stuttering has been of exceptional interest to those to whom it has appeared analogous to the spontaneous recovery of a conditioned response following experimental extinction trials.

The adaptation effect is to be found in the stuttering of children as well as adults.[6] Although it has been studied chiefly in oral reading, it has also been demonstrated in spontaneous speech by various means.[7] In general, during adaptation there is a reduction in essentially all of the various types of disfluency (part-word repetitions, word repetitions, phrase repetitions, etc.),[8] although some differential effects have been shown to occur in individual cases.[9]

Stutterers differ widely in the extent to which they adapt; many do not appear to show any adaptation at all, and some may show increased stuttering with repeated readings.[10] There has been a good deal of curiosity about the reasons for this individual variation. Attention has been given to the possibility that adaptation scores might be useful in measuring or predicting response to therapy, on the assumption that adaptation represents a "miniature model" of improvement. Findings so far have not provided much support for such an assumption.[11] Some attempt has been made to relate amount of adaptation to certain personality measures and behavioral characteristics.[12] The only relationship on which there is as yet consistent evidence is that less severe stuttering is associated with a more marked tendency to adapt.[13] Work has also been done on problems relating to the measurement of adaptation, and various ways of measuring it have been proposed.[14]

Theories of Adaptation

A variety of theories have been offered to account for the adaptation effect. The theory advanced by Wischner (1950) was that it represents the experimental extinction of a learned anxiety-motivated response. This point of view asserts that adaptation is an actual on-the-spot unlearning of stuttering behavior and implies that whatever reinforcement serves to maintain this behavior is diminished during successive readings of the same material.

A second theory, suggested by Johnson,[15] is that stutterers' anxieties about stuttering are reduced through deconfirmation of their expectancies. That is, their stuttering or its consequences may fail to live up to their expectations in the sense that we tend

[2] Shulman (1955).

[3] Shulman (1955) demonstrated this with passages varying from 200 to 1,000 words in length. Brutten and Dancer (1980) showed, however, that repeating each of a series of words individually results in a greater reduction of stuttering than repeating the same words the same number of times as a list.

[4] Harris (1942).

[5] Newman (1954), Jones (1955), Jamison (1955), Frick (1955), Leutenegger (1957), Peins (1961a), Gray and Brutten (1965).

[6] Neelley and Timmons (1967), Williams, Silverman, and Kools (1968).

[7] Moore (1954), Newman (1954), Schaef (1955), Bloom and Silverman (1973), Coppa and Bar (1974), Kroll and Hood (1974).

[8] Timmons (1967), Silverman and Williams (1971), Kroll and Hood (1974).

[9] Sakata and Adams (1972), Webster and Brutten (1972).

[10] Newman (1963), Bloom and Silverman (1973), Moore, Flowers, and Cunko (1981).

[11] Van Riper and Hull (1955), Quarrington (1956), Johnson, Darley, and Spriestersbach (1963, p. 268), Prins and McQuiston (1964), Lanyon (1965), Prins (1968).

[12] Falck (1956), Quarrington (1956, 1962), Agnello (1962), Gray and Karmen (1967), Sayles (1971).

[13] Van Riper and Hull (1955), Shulman (1955), Oxtoby (1955), Quarrington (1959), Siegel and Haugen (1964). Gray (1965a, 1965b) showed that it is possible to predict the course of adaptation from the participant's initial frequency of stuttering.

[14] Trotter (1955), Quarrington (1959), Tate, Cullinan, and Ahlstrand (1961), Cullinan (1963a), Silverman and Williams (1968), Bloom and Silverman (1979).

[15] See Johnson et al. (1967, p. 276) and Johnson, Darley, and Spriestersbach (1963, p. 268).

to exaggerate what we dread, and so they tend to be less fearful of stuttering and less concerned with avoiding it.

A third proposal, by Sheehan (1958a, p. 132), was that the occurrence of stuttering in itself is fear reducing. The stuttering during the first reading thus reduces fear enough to permit less stuttering on the second, and so on.

A fourth theory is that adaptation is due to reactive inhibition. In his theory of learning, Hull postulated that massed repetitions of a response produced an inhibitory potential, related to fatigue, that temporarily reduced the strength of a response in the absence of any change in learning or motivational states. This explanation of stuttering adaptation, originally weighed by Wischner (1947), was particularly developed and extended by Brutten and his coworkers.[16]

A fifth theory is that adaptation is due to rehearsal of the reading material. Various reasons why this might reduce the frequency of stuttering have been suggested. Perhaps the earliest proponent of such a theory was Eisenson (1958, p. 240 ff.), who stated that repeated readings of a passage reduce its propositional value and tend to "establish an articulatory and vocal set that approaches the automatic." Eisenson suggested that adaptation was related to the effect on stuttering of memorization of reading material.

The Effect of Varying the Reading Material

Precisely what is it that the stutterer adapts to? The most direct approach to an understanding of adaptation has been made in studies that have attempted to answer this question by varying one feature or another of the adaptation condition. One way to do this is by varying the reading material. Experiments in which stutterers have read continuously changing material have established that far less adaptation—only 10 to 20 percent, on the average—takes place under these conditions.[17]

[16] See Gray and Brutten (1965), Brutten and Shoemaker (1967, p. 67 ff.).

[17] Johnson and Innes (1939), Cohen (1953), Donohue (1955), Golub (1955), Hegde (1971c). There is even less adaptation in continuously changing spontaneous speech (Cohen, 1953; Rousey, 1958).

These findings show clearly that while some adaptation takes place to the speech situation, most of it is to the speech context. We are left, however, with the question of precisely what features of the speech context are adapted to. It is interesting from this point of view that adaptation takes place even in the repeated reading of word lists.[18] On the other hand, there is evidence that some of the adaptation to be observed in connected reading is adaptation to its prosodic features. Wingate (1966b) conducted an adaptation experiment with a series of reading passages that contained the identical sequence of words, but each of which was punctuated differently to produce a different pattern of meanings. Less adaptation occurred under this condition than in the reading of a passage that was not successively altered in this way. It would seem that the stutterer adapts to any or all features of the reading material.

The Effect of Varying the Situation

A different type of experimental attack on the problem of adaptation is one in which the speech content is held constant and some feature of the situation is systematically varied from reading to reading. Shulman (1955) took this approach in a study in which the audience of people who stutter was increased by one person with each of five successive readings of a passage to a maximum of five listeners in the last reading. The stuttering rate decreased from reading to reading despite the progressive increase in the size of the audience, but the amount and rate of adaptation were decidedly less than in an ordinary adaptation sequence. This finding was confirmed by Siegel and Haugen (1964). Wischner (1952b) interpreted Shulman's results as reflecting the interaction between specific word anxiety, which was decreased by the successive readings, and general situational anxiety, which was increased by the audience factor.

Wischner (1947) found that a sudden loud noise during the course of the readings tended to arrest the course of adaptation temporarily, and inferred

[18] Wischner (1947), Golub (1955), Peterson, Rieck, and Hoff (1969), Brutten and Dancer (1980).

that this was analogous to the phenomenon of disinhibition in classical conditioning experiments—the arrest of experimental extinction of a response by distracting stimuli. Wingate (1972) reported a similar finding, but attributed it to interference with "general psychophysiological adaptation" to the situation during the initial reading.

Daly and Cooper (1967) administered electric shock to subjects during and following stuttering blocks in the course of successive readings. They were attempting to test Wischner's non-reinforcement theory of adaptation and hypothesized that the contingent shock would prevent reinforcement and lead to an increase in the adaptation rate. It did not do so. Finally, Kroll and Hood (1976) reported that when subjects were not told beforehand that they would be required to read the passage repeatedly, adaptation was preceded by an increase of stuttering on the second reading.

The Role of Anxiety and Expectancy in Adaptation

The adaptation theories proposed by Wischner, Sheehan, and Johnson implied that adaptation is associated with a progressive decrease in anxiety. Brutten and his coworkers attempted to check this assumption directly by means of measures of palmar sweating taken during adaptation and obtained inconsistent results. Sometimes adaptation was accompanied by a decline in the palmar sweat measures and sometimes not.[19] They drew the conclusion that reduction in anxiety is not a necessary condition for adaptation.

Somewhat related to this is the question of whether there is an "expectancy adaptation effect." Wischner (1952b), who related expectancy to anxiety about stuttering, found that there was. He reported that when stutterers were asked to pick out the words on which they would expect to stutter, they tended to mark progressively fewer words in repeated silent inspections of the same reading material. While this effect was not found by Peins (1961a), Brutten (1963) found a tendency toward expectancy adaptation that approached significance.

Is the Person who Stutters Adapting to Stuttering?

Let us come back to the question of what people who stutter are adapting to. So far we have seen that they are adapting for the most part to the reading material and to some extent also to the situation. Yet if we examine the theories of adaptation enumerated earlier it will be clear that almost all of them view stutterers as adapting primarily to neither, but to their stuttering. With the exception of the point of view that the adaptation effect is due to rehearsal of the reading material, they all impute the effect for different reasons to the fact that in the course of successive readings the subject repeatedly experiences stuttering. Whether it is the fact that the stuttering fails to receive reinforcement, or that the consequences of stuttering are not as fearful as expected, or that the stuttering serves to reduce anxiety, or that the stuttering creates reactive inhibition, in all these cases it is the experience of stuttering itself that is viewed as bringing about its reduction. There is a simple way to tell whether adaptation is due to repeated stuttering, and that is to see what happens if the individual reads a passage repeatedly with little or no stuttering.

Frank and Bloodstein (1971) attempted to do this by having the people who stutter read in unison with an experimenter. After five unison readings during which there was little stuttering, the participants read the passage once more independently. Their stuttering was compared with their performance in an ordinary adaptation condition. The results were instructive. In the sixth reading of the unison condition, when the subjects read independently, the average frequency of stuttering was almost exactly equal to the average amount of stuttering in the sixth reading of the ordinary adaptation condition (see Figure 11-1). In brief, their stuttering had been reduced to the same extent by repeated reading regardless of how much stuttering they had done along the way. They had adapted to the reading, not the stuttering. These readings were

[19] Brutten (1963), Gray and Brutten (1965), Brutten and Shoemaker (1967, pp. 75, 76). See also Ritterman and Reidenbach (1975).

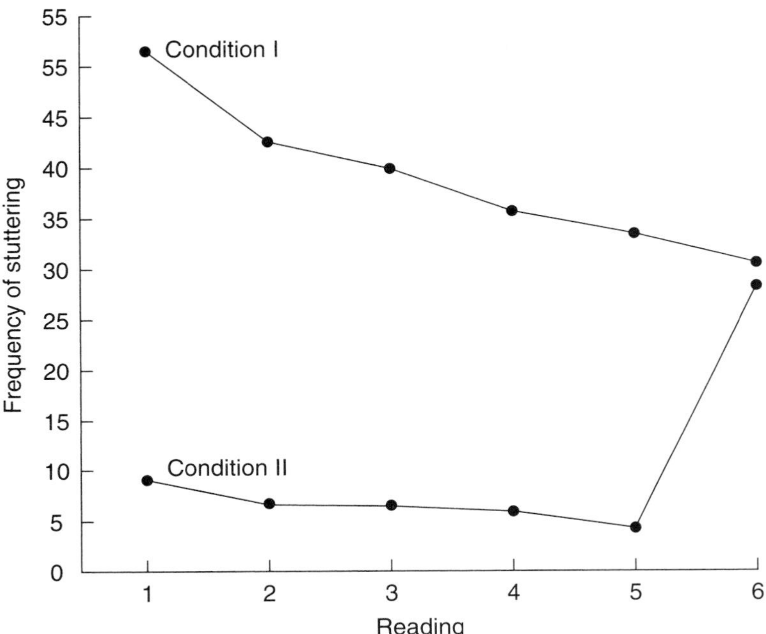

FIGURE 11-1 Mean frequency of stuttering in repeated readings of a passage under two conditions. Condition I was an ordinary adaptation series. In Condition II the subjects read in unison with an experimenter in all readings but the last. The two curves end at approximately the same point even though there has been a difference in the amount of stuttering along the way. Reproduced from Frank and Bloodstein (1971). Copyright 1971 by the American Speech-Language-Hearing Association. Reprinted by permission.

confirmed by Gold (1994) and Max, Caruso, and Vandevenne (1997).

Rehearsal Theories of Adaptation

It would appear that the rehearsal theory of adaptation is the only one that has merit. If so, this raises the question of exactly how rehearsal might lead to a reduction in stuttering. Again we have plunged into the depths of speculation since it is possible to identify some five theories about the answer to this question.

One is Eisenson's theory, already alluded to, that rehearsal minimizes the propositional value of the reading material. A related theory, proposed by Jakobovits (1966), is that the individual words tend to lose much of their meaning through "semantic satiation." The theory is based on the observation that through repetition, words tend to decrease in meaningfulness as measured by the semantic differential. Like Eisenson's hypothesis, it assumes that stuttering is influenced by the propositionality of speech.

A third theory with some connection to the first two is that in repeated reading of a passage, the words become more predictable and lower in information value. This notion was advanced by Schlesinger, Forte, Fried, and Melkman (1965). Soderberg (1969a) showed that in successive readings of the same passage, the information value of words tends to decrease according to a curve that is similar to the typical curve of adaptation.

A fourth hypothesis is that of Webster and Lubker (1968a), who speculated that, through successive rehearsals, people who stutter tend to become less dependent on auditory cues for guidance of their speech output. It is based on the premise that stuttering is due to interference with speech by defective auditory feedback. Webster and Dorman (1971) demonstrated that normally fluent speakers make fewer errors under delayed auditory feedback after they have rehearsed the reading material orally.

Finally, Bloodstein (1972) suggested that the adaptation effect is due to greater ease and conviction in the serial ordering of speech movements through rehearsal of the motor plan. Earlier in this chapter we noted instances in which fluency seemed to come from simplification of motor planning due to the person's manner of speaking or to the nature of the material. Another way to facilitate serial ordering is through rehearsal, as anyone who has ever repeated a difficult or unfamiliar word aloud in order to master its motor plan knows. This explanation is related to one that was offered by Wingate (1966b), and it was clearly anticipated by Eisenson's view that the repeated readings "establish an articulatory and vocal set that approaches the automatic." In somewhat different terms, repeated readings permit increased automaticity of the linguistic encoding processes required to generate the target utterance.

What Is the Person Who Stutters Rehearsing?

All the evidence we have reviewed hints that adaptation is basically a matter of familiarization. But with precisely what? Is it necessary, for example, for subjects to read the passage orally, or is it enough for them to read it silently or mark the words on which they think they would stutter? We can give a conclusive answer to this question. Peins (1961a) found that successive silent markings of anticipation had no influence on frequency of stuttering when the participants began to read the passage aloud, and a series of further studies has confirmed the ineffectiveness of passive silent rehearsal.[20]

The rehearsal must be oral. Must it also be vocal, or will repetition of silent speech movements do? Wischner (1947) found that after two rehearsals of a passage with silent "lip" movements, there was a reduction of stuttering that did not quite attain statistical significance. With four lipped rehearsals, Robbins (1971) found distinct evidence of such an effect. Brenner, Perkins, and Soderberg (1972) found that neither lipped nor whispered rehearsal reduced stuttering. Analysis of the data presented by Moss (1976) showed that lipped and whispered rehearsal had significant effects, but Moss found that vocal rehearsal reduced stuttering even more. In a study by Bruce and Adams (1978), whispered rehearsal had no effect. The issue is in doubt. All we can say for sure is that adaptation requires some type of active rehearsal. The more closely such rehearsal approaches the person's ordinary speech, the more unequivocal appears to be its benefit.

While the fact that active rehearsal is necessary may seem to give more support to some of the rehearsal theories of adaptation than to others, it will not, perhaps, serve to rule out any of them conclusively. Other kinds of information tend to weigh against several of these theories, however. The well-established fact that adaptation occurs in the repeated reading of word lists appears to make it unlikely that reduced contextual propositionality is a factor of major importance. In addition, the theory of increased predictability (reduced information load) is difficult to apply meaningfully in the case of a list of words.

This does not rule out reduced propositionality through semantic satiation of words, but Peterson, Rieck, and Hoff (1969) have cast some doubt on such a theory. They had adults who stutter rate selected words of a passage on the semantic differential both before and after repeated readings. In some cases, the adaptation trials produced some semantic satiation of the words; in an equal number of cases it did not, though the stuttering declined.

On the assumption that the critical factor in the rehearsal effect is improved control of phonation, Ciambrone, Adams, and Berkowitz (1983) correlated 13 participants' adaptation scores with their improvement with practice in voice initiation time (see Chapter 5). The correlation coefficient (+0.445) was too small to demonstrate that improvement in vocal initiation time is a good predictor of amount of adaptation. Similarly, Zimmermann and Hanley

[20] Besozzi and Adams (1969), Robbins (1971), Brenner, Perkins, and Soderberg (1972), Moss (1976), Murray, Empson, and Weaver (1987).

(1983) theorized that the adaptation effect would be accompanied by changes in the velocities, displacements, and durations of movement of the tongue, jaw, and lip. In a study of three participants, the hypothesis was not borne out.

Horii and Ramig (1987) found that in the course of repeated readings, both stutterers and nonstutterers increased the duration of utterances between pauses. No change occurred in the fundamental frequency of the voice. Prins and Hubbard (1990, 1992) reported that the duration of various speech segments did not change during adaptation, that adapting and nonadapting stutterers did not differ in the duration of speech segments, and that speech did not become more rhythmic during adaptation.

RESPONSE-CONTINGENT STIMULATION

In all of the attention we have given to the conditions under which stuttering varies in frequency, we have not yet considered whether it is amenable to punishment and reinforcement. Yet, as we saw in Chapter 2, the broad issue of whether stuttering is an operant response, subject to prediction and control within the framework of B. F. Skinner's operant analysis of behavior, hinges on this question. The first answer came in a report by Flanagan, Goldiamond, and Azrin (1958) that they had produced temporary fluency in three people who stutter by contingent presentations of a 105 dB tone, and had increased the frequency of stuttering by contingent cessation of the tone. Following this announcement and the publication of a theoretical paper on stuttering and normal disfluency as operant behavior by Shames and Sherrick (1965), unusual interest developed in verifying the observations of Flanagan, Goldiamond, and Azrin.

The first to do so were Martin and Siegel (1966a, 1966b). Their participants were five adult stutterers, each of whom spoke continuously in 40-minute to 1-hour sessions at intervals of a day to more than a week. With their first two participants, they made electric shock contingent upon specific stuttering behaviors such as nose wrinkling, tongue protrusion, or prolongation of the sound "s." In each case, within the first several minutes of shock, the speech behavior rapidly decreased in frequency until it had virtually disappeared. In each case the behavior continued to be essentially absent in subsequent sessions, whether or not shocks were given, as long as the electrodes remained in place on the subject's wrist. Each time the electrodes were removed the behavior rapidly increased in frequency to its original level. The only exception to this occurred after a plain nylon strap had been attached to one subject's wrist during a single 22-minute contingent shock session. In subsequent sessions there was a marked reduction of his behaviors even when the electrodes were removed, as long as the nylon strap remained in place.

With a third volunteer, shock was given during continuous spontaneous speech for any stuttering in any observable form, and virtually all stuttering was soon eliminated. In a later session during which the participant stuttered and was shocked on five occasions, a blue light was turned on during the procedure. On a subsequent occasion, the presentation of the blue light alone produced a reduction in stuttering almost to zero for a time, despite the fact that the electrodes were not in place and the participant knew that he could not possibly be shocked. Whenever the electrodes and the blue light were both removed, the stuttering returned to its usual level.

With the two remaining adults (Martin & Siegel, 1966b), a more complex contingency using verbal punishment and reinforcement was arranged. The shock was replaced by the words "not good," and the word "good" was spoken at the end of every 30-second interval of oral reading during which no stuttering had occurred. In addition, at the start of experimental sessions, the participants received instructions to read carefully and fluently, and in some of the sessions, a nylon strap was fastened to their wrists with the explanation that it was a "reminder to say each word as fluently as possible." The stuttering of both participants fell off rapidly to a very low level under these conditions.

In three later sessions, the nylon strap alone, without initial instructions or contingent verbal reward and punishment, produced a marked reduction in stuttering even when the participants read to new listeners in a different room or into a telephone. Whenever the strap, instructions, and contingent verbal stimuli were removed, the stuttering returned to its former level. When the instructions to "read fluently" were presented alone, the stuttering dropped rather sharply to about a third of its original frequency, but the reduction was not as marked as under the other experimental conditions, and the stuttering steadily rose to its base level over the next 15 minutes.

These findings of Martin and Siegel had weighty theoretical implications concerning the nature of the moment of stuttering. They served in a most compelling way to raise the question whether stuttering is to be regarded, in behavioral terms, as an operant response, subject to positive or negative reinforcement and to punishment like the instrumental lever-pressing activity of a hungry rat. Such a model appears to suggest what in everyday terms is called a "simple" habit—that is, a habit simple enough to eliminate by paying attention to it and trying hard not to do it again. To all appearances, it is in direct conflict with a considerable amount of clinical experience suggesting that people who stutter are often likely to have their most severe difficulty when fearful of stuttering, aware of the probability of severe penalties for it, and strongly motivated to avoid it. Moreover, it runs counter to the experimental data of Van Riper (1937b) and Frick (1951), which showed that, when people who stutter were told that at the end of their reading they were to receive as many electric shocks as they had blocks, their stuttering tended to increase.

There have been other experimental findings, however, that are in apparent conflict with those of Van Riper. Oxtoby (1955) reported that instructions to "try to avoid stuttering" had no effect on the frequency of stutters. Steer and Johnson (1936) found that in a series of 15 situations of varying difficulty, there was a correlation of only 0.36 between severity of stuttering and reported desire to talk without stuttering. Wingate (1959) found a decrease in stuttering when the participants were penalized after each stutter by an interruption in an electronic communication link with a listener or when each stutter was simply called to their attention by a recording counter. Furthermore, the results of Van Riper's experiment on the effect of penalty on stuttering were not confirmed either by Gross and Holland (1965) or by Williams and Martin (1974).

Additional Evidence in Support of the Operant View

A large amount of further research has been done on the question of whether stuttering may be modified by its contingent consequences, and almost invariably the answer has been that it can. Most of these studies have dealt with punishment for stuttering. This has taken the form of electric shock,[21] reprimands such as "wrong,"[22] loud noise,[23] intervals of delayed auditory feedback,[24] response-cost (money taken away),[25] time-out (an interval of several seconds during which the subject is not permitted to speak),[26] and recorded laughter.[27] It should be added that as soon as the punishment is discontinued, the stuttering generally tends to return to its original level. Hegde (1971b) found no lasting effect on stuttering in oral reading after three months of daily application of contingent noise with five participants.

Christensen and Lingwall (1983) found that contingent presentations of the word "wrong" produced its maximum effect in 20 minutes of conditioning; no further reduction in stuttering occurred after that. Christensen and Lingwall (1982) also reported that the conditioning was more effective in a laboratory than in a homelike setting, particularly when the verbal punisher was presented remotely by headset.

---

[21] Gross and Holland (1965), Daly and Cooper (1967), Daly and Frick (1970), Moore and Ritterman (1973).

[22] Quist and Martin (1967), Reed and Lingwall (1976), Mowrer (1978), Martin and Haroldson (1979), Christensen and Lingwall (1982, 1983).

[23] Murray (1969), Hegde (1971b), Reed and Lingwall (1976), Stephen and Haggard (1980).

[24] Goldiamond (1965).

[25] Gross (1969), Halvorson (1971).

[26] Haroldson, Martin, and Starr (1968), Adams and Popelka (1971), Martin and Haroldson (1971), James and Ingham (1974), James (1976), Martin and Haroldson (1979), Costello and Hurst (1981), James (1981a, 1983).

[27] Reed and Lingwall (1980).

Gross and Holland (1965) found not only that contingent electro-shock reduced stuttering, but also that it did so even when the listener was the one who received the shock. LaCroix (1973) observed that speakers can reduce their own stuttering by activating a hand counter each time they stutter. Similar results have been described by Mowrer (1978) with the self-administered verbal punisher "stop," by Hanson (1978) and James (1981b) using self-recording of stuttering, and by Martin and Haroldson (1982) and James (1983) using self-administered time-out.

Stuttering has been reduced in laboratory investigations not only by punishment, but also by reinforcing fluency. The reinforcement has generally consisted of the word "good" or a small amount of money, and the reinforced response has been a predetermined period of fluency or number of consecutive fluent words. Reinforcement of fluency has either been given alone or combined with punishment for stuttering.[28] Self-reinforcement for fluency with tokens produced reductions in stuttering in a study by Cross and Cooper (1976).

Other demonstrations of the effect of contingent stimuli on stuttering have taken a considerable variety of forms. Hutchinson and Mackay (1973) brought about increased stuttering on previously fluent words in repeated readings by shocking speakers for saying the words fluently. Hasbrouck, Graham, and Brooks (1976) reduced the stuttering of three participants by punishing them only for their normal disfluencies. In a study by Martin and Haroldson (1977), a group of participants stuttered less after watching a videotape recording of a person who stuttered severely and who experienced a marked reduction in stuttering under a contingent time-out procedure.

A unique application of punishment was made by Curlee and Perkins (1968). After being instructed to signal expectancies of stuttering prior to speech attempts, participants were intermittently shocked for doing so. Both the frequency of signaled anticipations and the frequency of stuttering decreased as a result. Daly and Frick (1970), however, obtained only a moderate reduction in expectancies and no reduction in stuttering in a similar study, while Harris, Martin, and Haroldson (1971), using time-out from speaking as a punisher of expectancy, obtained variable results with three participants. Earlier, Williams (1962) had found a marked decrease in stuttering when electric shock was made contingent on any anticipatory behavior such as tensing the jaw muscles, holding the breath, or changing the speaking rate prior to stuttering.

Dissenting Views and Counterexamples

Not all agree that the operant control of stuttering has been adequately demonstrated by the research we have just reviewed. The mildest demurrers have been on purely methodological grounds. For example, Starkweather (1971) argued that for several reasons, the usual practice of making base-rate comparisons in operant conditioning studies may be of questionable validity in research on stuttering. Adams and Popelka (1971) showed that there is some difficulty involved in making a stimulus contingent on stuttering and that attempts to do so are frequently unsuccessful. James and Ingham (1974) questioned whether stutterers' expectations of fluency might account for some of the results attributed to punishment. They found, however, that manipulating their participants' expectations did not influence the results of a time-out study.

Is Operant Stuttering Limited to the Secondary Features? A different kind of qualification was urged by Brutten and Shoemaker (1969), who argued that only the associated symptoms of stuttering are subject to modification by response-contingent stimuli and that the repetitions and prolongations are not. This is consistent with their theory that the integral symptoms of stuttering are classically conditioned, while the secondary features are acquired through instrumental (operant) conditioning (see Chapter 2). In support of this view, Janssen and Brutten (1973) reported a study of four stutterers in

[28] Russell, Clark, and van Sommers (1968), Gross (1969), Halvorson (1971), Moore and Ritterman (1973), Lanyon and Barocas (1975), Hegde and Bruttten (1977), Bastijens, Brutten, and Stés (1978), Mowrer (1978). See also Chapter 14.

which shocks that were made selectively contingent on prolongations of sound had no systematic effect on the prolongations themselves; there was an increase in the case of two participants and no change in the other two. For three of the participants, there was a decrease in the total number of moments of stuttering. Janssen and Brutten also cited an unpublished single-subject study by Webster in which part-word repetitions failed to decrease under contingent aversive stimulation. Also consistent with this point of view is the finding by Oelschlaeger and Brutten (1976) that instructions to two stutterers to try to avoid repetitions of sounds were of no avail, whereas instructions to avoid interjections such as "uh" and "um" significantly reduced these reactions. Finally, Brutten (1980) presented data on one adult who stuttered, whose prolongations increased in frequency under contingent presentation of the word "wrong."

Costello and Hurst (1981) obtained somewhat contrary results in a study of three individuals. In two cases, target behaviors such as jaw tremors and repetitions of sounds, syllables, and words were reduced by contingent time-out, along with other symptoms that were not targeted for punishment. Participant 3 was given time-out for prolongations. There was no consistent effect on the prolongations, and her hard contacts increased. The experimenters then tried to punish the prolongations with a 90-decibel burst of tone. Prolongations, repetitions, and hard contacts decreased as a result, but only moderately. Finally, the experimenters had a talk with her "to encourage harder work at fluency," following which all types of disfluency decreased further. Eventually the experimenters were able to demonstrate a distinct reduction in all disfluencies in response to the tone.

Punishment or Distraction? A more sweeping skepticism was expressed by Biggs and Sheehan (1969), who contended that the reason for the punishment effect in stuttering is not the relationship of response and aversive stimulus at all. In a modified replication of the original study by Flanagan, Goldiamond, and Azrin (1958), they placed six adults who stutterered under three conditions of 4000 Hz, 108 dB tone: presentation of the tone contingent on stuttering, cessation of the tone contingent on stuttering, and random presentation of the tone. The three conditions resulted in approximately the same amount of suppression of stuttering. Biggs and Sheehan concluded that the decrease in stuttering as a result of response-contingent stimulation is not the effect of punishment, but of distraction.

Effect of Neutral and Rewarding Stimuli There is another reason why questions have been raised about the meaning of the research findings on punishment. In many studies, the stimuli responsible for producing fluency have apparently had little aversive quality. Biggs and Sheehan's participants generally rated the loud tone as only mildly aversive. In a study by Reed and Lingwall (1976), the punishment, consisting, of 95 dB noise or the word "wrong," failed to elevate galvanic skin response (GSR) measures in 6 of 10 volunteers. In four cases, the GSR was actually lowered. In a later study, Reed and Lingwall (1980) again found that punishment, in the form of recorded female laughter, had inconsistent, variable effects on the GSR, although stuttering was consistently reduced. Adams and Popelka (1971) questioned eight participants in a study of the effect of time-out from speaking and found that six had failed to perceive the time-out as punishment, evaluating it instead as a chance to, relax. In a similar study by James and Ingham (1974), only 6 of 14 participants evaluated the time-out in terms that suggested unpleasantness. Martin and Gaviser (1971) showed that time-out was aversive enough so that normally fluent speakers who were engaged in a free-choice button-pressing activity during spontaneous speech learned to avoid the button that signaled time-out from speaking and to press the one that did not. Typically fluent speakers questioned by Yonovitz and Shepherd (1977) also tended to regard time-out as annoying, but stuttering participants did not have definite reactions, and measures of their GSR and heart rate showed little evidence that the time-out was aversive.

If the mild aversiveness of some punishing stimuli tends to raise some questions, what is the meaning of "punishers" that are on their face neutral or even rewarding? The outstanding case in point was supplied by Cooper, Cady, and Robbins (1970). They tested the effect of the words "wrong," "right," and "tree" and found that they all reduced stuttering equally. Siegel and Martin (1966) encountered a similar phenomenon in normally fluent speakers when a "neutral" buzzer reduced the frequency of disfluencies. They offered the explanation that a neutral stimulus may have an alerting or "highlighting" value in the case of responses that are socially unacceptable and that therefore "carry their own punishment."[29] Cooper, Cady, and Robbins suggested that a similar explanation might possibly account for their findings. This cannot be denied, and if it is true it is important, even more so since it seems to run counter to long-standing expectations about stuttering that have stemmed from ordinary clinical observation. We cannot overlook the fact, however, that this type of explanation has little place in the operant analysis of behavior that is concerned only with the effects of observable consequences. To resort to such an explanation is therefore to abandon the hope of prediction and control within a Skinnerian system that has been the ultimate goal of efforts to demonstrate the operant nature of stuttering.

Within the operant framework, a punisher is defined only as a contingent stimulus that reduces the rate of responding. To remain within this frame we must forego any "explanation" of the Cooper, Cady, and Robbins findings and simply define them as punishment. It is irrelevant that the words "right" and "tree" do not strike us as punishing or may not be evaluated negatively by the participants. At first glance, this may seem to be a simple way to dispose of a troublesome problem, but the impression proves to be illusory. The difficulty is not merely the artificiality of this use of the term punishment, but the conclusions to which it leads. It is paradoxical within the operant frame to find that a stimulus that decreases the rate of occurrence of one response increases the rate of another. Judged by its consequences, the word "right" is as effective a generalized reinforcer as can be found. To observe it acting as a punisher is anomalous and contradictory.

Daly and Kimbarow (1978) replicated the Cooper, Cady, and Robbins experiment with school-age children who stutter and obtained the same results. Several additional attempts have been made to test the effect of contingent presentation of stimuli that are presumably neutral or reinforcing.[30] The reinforcers have usually been money or a signal in lieu of money. The results have been somewhat inconsistent and confusing, but there is a distinct tendency for the stuttering of most people to decrease just as it does when presumably aversive stimuli are used. Lanyon and Barocas (1975) found that an audible signal contingent on stuttering reduced stuttering about equally whether it meant monetary gain or loss, but that random presentation of the signal had no effect.

No satisfactory explanation has yet been advanced for the fact that virtually any contingent stimulus seems capable of reducing the stuttering of most study participants. Hanson (1978) attempted to test the hypothesis, already mentioned, that by drawing the speaker's attention to the stuttering moments, the stimulus somehow makes it possible for the person to speak more fluently. Hanson reasoned that if this were the case, stutterers' heightened awareness of their stuttering would be reflected in a tendency to identify more stuttering in their own speech. In an experiment, two participants were instructed to first depress a switch to note each stuttering event that they detected in their own speech. In a subsequent session, Hanson administered a neutral stimulus in the form of a brief flash of a small light. The participants' attentiveness to stuttering was then measured once again by having them detect stuttering in their speech. In the case of one participant, the light flash reduced the stuttering, but had no effect on her subsequent count of her own stutters. In the other case, the light flash had no effect on the stuttering, but the participant's count of her stutters increased. As Hanson concluded,

[29] See also Siegel (1970).

[30] Patty and Quarrington (1974), Lanyon and Barocas (1975), Oelschlaeger and Brutten (1975), Starkweather and Lucker (1978), Corcoran (1980), James (1981a).

each person failed in a different way to confirm the hypothesis that contingent stimuli reduce stuttering by calling people's attention to their stuttering.

In a study by James, Ricciardelli, Rogers, and Hunter (1989), a group of stutterers who were not highly responsive to time-out from speaking became more so after completing a program of training in syllable prolongation. It was concluded that the contingent stimulus became more effective because it encouraged the subjects to use their "fluency skills" during the time-out period.

In Chapter 14, we will review a clinical trial of a time-out treatment for stuttering (Hewat, Onslow, Packman, & O'Brian, 2006). Relatively little work has been done to determine how time-out reduces stuttering, or what trade-offs might occur in other aspects of speech production, such as speech rate or linguistic variables, following contingent feedback. Onslow, Bernstein Ratner, and Packman (2001) studied two boys whose stuttering was decreased under response-contingent time-out; one reduced linguistic complexity but did not alter speech duration characteristics, while the inverse was true of the other child. The authors concluded that time-out might induce changes in verbal output that would need to be studied in greater detail. To date, the major work has only demonstrated fluency outcomes.

In the years since the last edition of the *Handbook*, the major clinical implementation of response-contingent feedback has been the Lidcombe program for the treatment of early childhood stuttering. We discuss the outcomes of this program, and meta-analyses of its possible mechanisms of action further in Chapter 14.

Summary Remarks The results of a number of studies have caused some researchers and clinicians to be skeptical about the interpretation placed on the effects of contingent stimuli in so much past research on stuttering and to question whether the operant model of behavior is an adequate representation of the stuttering response. Such doubts have been strengthened by other apparent discrepancies between predictions from the model and observation. It would be reasonable to predict, for example, that punishment for operant behavior would be more effective if delivered immediately contingent on the response than if it were delayed. Williams and Martin (1974) compared the effect of electric shock immediately after each stutter with a condition in which the participants received the appropriate number of shocks following every sentence. Stuttering was reduced by the same amount under both conditions.

We would also expect a large amount of punishment to have a greater effect than a small one. Yet, in a study of the effect of time-out from speaking, James (1976) found that enforced interruptions of speech of 1, 5, 10, and 30 seconds reduced stuttering to about the same extent. James suggested that the punishment in this procedure might be the initial interruption rather than the time-out from speaking.

Finally, it has been difficult for researchers to account for anomalous and idiosyncratic individual responses to the operant conditioning paradigm. One example was a study of punishment and negative reinforcement of stuttering with five participants by Martin, St. Louis, Haroldson, and Hasbrouck (1975). Punishment consisted of electric shock. Negative reinforcement, under which stuttering should have increased, took the form of brief periods of cessation, contingent on stuttering, of a steady electric shock. Under negative reinforcement, there was an increase in stuttering in two participants, a decrease in one, and no change in two. In the punishment condition, two participants stuttered less, two stuttered more, and one was not affected. The authors concluded that, "Results of the present experiment yield only very equivocal support to the notion that stuttering is an operant response class." Equally contradictory or inconsistent results of response-contingent stimulation were reported by Hegde (1971a), Cross and Cooper (1976), and others.

Summary Remarks: Response Contingencies

Almost all research findings point to the conclusion that response-contingent stimuli have a broad potential to reduce the frequency of stuttering. The reason for this reduction, however, is far from clear. What was at first widely thought to be a punishment effect that contradicted long-standing clinical assumptions about the effect of aversive reactions to stuttering now seems more and more to represent another kind of process, as yet poorly understood, in which the aversiveness of the contingent stimulus is irrelevant and that has little in common with the social penalty that often appears to increase the severity of stuttering. Three alternative hypotheses have been advanced to account for the effect of contingent stimuli. One is that it represents a form of operant conditioning. A second is that contingent stimuli help the speaker to avoid stuttering by calling attention to it. A third is that some type of distraction is at work.[31] As yet there is little evidence to support any of these explanations. Stuttering is an ephemeral, elusive phenomenon that is responsive to subtle psychological states. The application of contingent stimuli, whether aversive or not, generally appears to create a psychological state in which stuttering tends to diminish. The nature of that state remains to be clarified.

The outstanding triumph of the operant model of stuttering was the unexpected demonstration that stuttering appeared to be subject to punishment within B. F. Skinner's operant conditioning paradigm. The model would now seem to have produced research findings that are anomalous within this paradigm, and not everyone is agreed that what is taking place in so-called operant conditioning experiments is learning or conditioning.

There is a further problem with which the operant model must deal. Operants represent an extremely broad category of behavior. The statement that stuttering is operant behavior is therefore relatively empty in itself. It acquires significant content only to the extent that we can specify at least in general terms the contingencies by which the behavior is governed. At this writing, as in the last edition of the *Handbook*, we do not seem to be closer to being able to do so than we were in 1958 when it was first reported that stuttering had been brought under "operant control." That is, we lack elementary knowledge of the reinforcements by which stuttering is maintained. We could not take any steps to extinguish it by withholding reinforcement. We do not know what satiations would serve to decrease it or what deprivations would tend to make it more frequent.

THE WHITE NOISE EFFECT

For many years, it had occasionally been noted that people who stutter are likely to have less speech difficulty in the presence of loud noise—for example, near ocean surf, a waterfall, or a passing train. Kern (1932) demonstrated this effect experimentally by means of a Barany drum. Then in 1955, Shane in the United States and Cherry, Sayers, and Marland in England reported that binaural masking with white noise at high intensity brought about the virtual elimination of stuttering in most laboratory participants. In both cases, the inference was drawn that it was the inability to hear one's own speech that produced the effect, rather than mere distraction. Since then, the white noise effect has been verified repeatedly.[32] The reductions in stuttering achieved tend to vary from person to person and often fall considerably short of complete fluency. Conture and Brayton (1975) observed the chief effect of the noise to be on part-word repetitions, but in a study by Hutchinson and Norris (1977), most disfluency types were found to be reduced.

The great majority of studies have been concerned with oral reading. In spontaneous speech, both Hutchinson and Norris (1977) and Mallard and Webb (1980) found no significant reduction in stuttering for participants as a group. That the white noise effect can be demonstrated in the spontaneous

[31] The distraction hypothesis should not be dismissed lightly. Participants receiving an unusual or inappropriate stimulus immediately after every stuttering event are soon conditioned to expect the stimulus at each instant they expect to stutter. The distraction, if distraction it is, may thus come at a critical moment.

[32] Maraist and Hutton (1957), Sutton and Chase (1961), Shrum (1962), May and Hackwood (1968), Burke (1969), Murray (1969), Webster and Dorman (1970), Adams and Moore (1972), Adams and Hutchinson (1974), Conture (1974), Garber and Martin (1974), Conture and Brayton (1975), Dewar, Dewar, and Anthony (1976), Dewar, Dewar, and Barnes (1976), Yairi (1976), Altrows and Bryden (1977), Garber and Martin (1977), Hutchinson and Norris (1977), Brayton and Conture (1978), Lechner (1979), Martin and Haroldson (1979), Ingham, Southwood, and Horsburgh (1981), Zsilavecz (1981), Martin, Siegel, Johnson, and Haroldson (1984), Martin, Johnson, Siegel, and Haroldson (1985).

speech of people who stutter is evident, however, from a series of studies.[33]

Theories of the White Noise Effect

Several points of view have developed about the reason for reductions in stuttering under masking noise. The conclusion to which Cherry and Sayers came from their study in 1956 was that stuttering is a perceptual rather than a motor abnormality. At about that time, interest had begun to develop in Lee's discovery that delayed auditory feedback could produce "artificial stutter" in many normally fluent speakers, and an analogy with clinical stuttering had already been drawn (see Chapter 2). To some researchers, the white noise effect seemed an illuminating confirmation of the hypothesis that the basic cause of stuttering was a disturbance of auditory feedback, since it was easy to imagine that the noise served to mask the interfering feedback. Maraist and Hutton (1957) put this in servo-theory terms when they said that in stuttering, a person "misevaluates his own speech output at some point in the control system and finds error where, in reality, no error exists." When their auditory feedback is interrupted, stutterers cease their efforts to correct their nonexistent error and so temporarily stop stuttering. It is this general point of view, expressed in various ways by Yates (1963), Webster and Lubker (1968a), and others, that has perhaps been chiefly responsible for the continued interest in the white noise effect.

A second interpretation was advanced by Shane (1955). She suggested that when stutterers were unable to hear their own speech, they were "relatively free from the anxiety-producing cues involved" in hearing themselves stutter. Others would have said hearing themselves "speak." In either case, the explanation is based on the anticipatory struggle concept of stuttering, particularly as expressed by Johnson.

A third possibility, suggested by Wingate (1970), is that fluency under white noise results from an increase in the intensity of the person's voice or from other vocal changes of the Lombard effect. A fourth theory is that the noise acts as a distraction. This simple viewpoint has not often been advocated, but it has been recognized from the beginning as a possibility.

Must People Fail to Hear Their Own Speech?

In trying to narrow down the possible reasons for the white noise effect, we would obviously find it helpful to know if the critical factor is the person's inability to hear their own speech. Shane (1955) believed it was and offered as evidence the finding that white noise that had a marked effect on stuttering at 95 dB had essentially no effect at 25 dB. Cherry and Sayers (1956) found that high-frequency masking noise was considerably less effective than low-frequency noise (below 500 Hz). They concluded that the reduction in stuttering was due to the stutterers' failure to hear the low-frequency components of their speech.

On the other hand, the research findings as a whole have tended to weigh against the assumption that people must fail to hear their own speech. In the first place, both Shane (1955) and Adams and Moore (1972) found that the great majority of their study participants reported hearing their own speech above the noise. In addition, ample evidence exists that white noise will reduce stuttering in forms allowing individuals considerable ability to hear their speech. Maraist and Hutton (1957) studied the effect at masking levels of 30, 50, 70, and 90 dB above normal threshold and observed a progressive decrease in the amount of stuttering, with a particularly marked decline beginning at 50 dB, where the participants' speech must have been clearly audible to them. Murray (1969) found that random bursts of noise produced a decided reduction of stuttering, though not as much as continuous noise. Both May and Hackwood (1968) and Conture (1974) found that high-frequency masking (above 500 Hz) resulted in as much fluency as low-frequency masking. This finding conflicts with Cherry and Sayers' results referred to previously, but even Cherry and Sayers observed distinctly reduced

[33] Garber and Martin (1974, 1977), Dewar, Dewar, and Barnes (1976), Martin and Haroldson (1979), Ingham, Southwood, and Horsburgh (1981), Martin, Siegel, Johnson, and Haroldson (1984), Martin, Johnson, Siegel, and Haroldson (1985).

stuttering under high-frequency noise. Moreover, Barr and Carmel (1969) reported a decrease in stuttering with only 50 dB of high-frequency narrow-band masking noise delivered to only one ear. Yairi (1976) also found that stuttering decreased under monaural noise, though not to the same extent as under binaural masking.

These conditions did not all reduce stuttering equally, and it might be argued that there are various possible degrees of interference with the ability to hear one's own speech. For this reason, exceptional interest was stirred by a study by Sutton and Chase (1961), in which reduced stuttering was apparently achieved by white noise without any masking of speech at all. Using a voice-actuated relay to turn the noise either on or off while the participants read aloud, Sutton and Chase tested the effect of three experimental conditions: continuous noise, noise present only during the phonation of sounds, and noise present only during the silent periods. They found that all three conditions were equally effective.

This prompted a rejoinder by Yates (1963) that we normally hear the feedback from our speech with a slight delay; moments of feedback do not coincide exactly with moments of phonation. For this reason, Yates believed that at least part of this feedback was masked in both of Sutton and Chase's discontinuous noise conditions. Later, a somewhat similar objection was raised by Webster and Lubker (1968b). They pointed out that it takes time for a voice-actuated relay to respond to phonation since the intensity of the voice must reach a required level. Consequently, they reasoned, in the condition in which the noise was turned off by phonation, the speakers' auditory feedback must have been masked during the critical fraction of a second when phonation was being initiated. In reply, Chase and Sutton (1968) agreed that such a delay existed and that it was added to by mechanical lag in the relay itself. With reason, however, they pointed out that the same delay that was present when voice turned the masking off must also have been present in the condition in which voice turned it on. Using the argument that the initial part of the phonation is critical for stuttering, it thus becomes difficult to explain why stuttering was reduced when noise was present only during phonation, the initial portions of these phonations not having been masked.

Subsequently, Webster and Dorman (1970) performed the same experiment using a list of single words in place of connected reading material and obtained the same results: Stuttering was reduced equally whether the noise was started by onset of phonation, stopped by phonation, or continuous. Altrows and Bryden (1977) repeated this experiment using sentences in place of words. Controlling the noise manually, they found that noise presented only before initiation of a sentence and terminated following the first audible speech sound had no effect on stuttering in the sentence as a whole. This is perhaps no more than would be expected considering that there was no noise during almost the entire reading of the sentence, but they also found no effect on stuttering on the first word, despite the masking of its initial sound. When they presented the noise continuously or concurrently with the reading of each sentence, stuttering was reduced.

What results of these three studies suggest is that the noise works grossly and not by virtue of any selective effect on the initial portion of a word, that the noise must be present for a substantial part of the time during which the person who stutters speaks, but that it need not be concurrent with intervals of phonation. If this is so, our best judgment at present would probably have to be that the white noise effect does not depend on masking of speech. This means that neither Cherry and Sayers' theory that the noise masks a perceptual defect nor Shane's inference that it obliterates anxiety-producing cues would seem to have sufficient support. With respect to anxiety reduction, it may be pertinent that Adams and Moore (1972) found that the white noise had little effect on stutterers' levels of autonomic arousal as measured by palmar sweating.

The Influence of Vocal Changes

If the improved fluency of people who stutter while under white noise has little to do with difficulty in hearing their own speech, it is perhaps unlikely that it is due to the Lombard effect. Nevertheless, the increase in vocal intensity that usually occurs with exposure to loud noise had frequently been considered as a possible cause of the reduction in stuttering. There is ample evidence that, at least as a group, people who stutter do increase their vocal loudness under masking (see Chapter 6, footnote 12). The question is whether this is the factor responsible for the gain in fluency. One way to test such an assumption is to instruct or train individuals to maintain a normal level of vocal intensity while exposed to the noise. This was done in three separate studies with the same result: The stuttering decreased in noise despite the absence of increased vocal intensity.[34] A second strategy is to study the effect of raising vocal intensity without masking noise. Again the results conflict with the vocal intensity hypothesis. Shrum (1962) found significantly greater reduction of stuttering in people who stutter under masking than when they read at the same high intensity level without masking. Garber and Martin (1977) found no decrease in stuttering with increased vocal intensity and no masking. Further difficulties for the hypothesis are presented by reports of individual cases in which the person's vocal intensity in noise failed to vary concomitantly with stuttering frequency. For example, Yairi (1976) noted that in two of his six experimental participants, decreases in stuttering in noise were not always accompanied by increases in vocal level, and in a study by Martin, Siegel, Johnson, and Haroldson (1984), the amount of reduction in stuttering was unrelated to the change in intensity of the participants' voices.[35] There seems, then, to be little evidence to support the hypothesis that increased vocal loudness alone can account for the white noise effect. Wingate (1970) pointed out that we must also consider the effects of noise on the stutterer's vocal pitch and duration, but relevant research findings as yet have been sparse and ambiguous. Brayton and Conture (1978) found (as did Lechner, 1979) that the fundamental frequency of stutterers' voices did tend to rise in noise, but the participants with greater increases in fundamental frequency tended to show smaller decreases in stuttering. For seven participants, decreases in stuttering showed a modest correlation with increases in vowel duration ($r = 0.41$), but in the remaining two cases, there was apparently little relationship between the two measures. Increased vowel duration may possibly be part of the reason that people who stutter tend to speak more fluently in noise, but, as is true of increased vocal intensity, it is evidently not the whole reason.

Finally, Hayden, Jordahl, and Adams (1982) explored the possibility that stutterers' fluency in masking noise is due to a favorable effect of noise on voice initiation time (see Chapter 5). Contrary to their hypothesis, however, participants' vocal initiation time proved to be slower rather than faster under noise.

We are left with one remaining explanation—that the white noise is distracting. This is a prosaic hypothesis, but it has at least one strong source of support. Evidence suggests that almost any novel form of auditory feedback is capable of reducing stuttering.

EFFECTS OF OTHER FORMS OF ALTERED AUDITORY FEEDBACK

Harris (1955) found that merely amplifying the speaker's voice reduced the frequency of stuttering. Ham and Steer (1967) observed less stuttering in some participants with amplification, delay, or frequency filtering of their auditory feedback. The effect of distorting the stutterer's auditory feedback by frequency filtering was confirmed by Howell, El-Yaniv, and Powell (1987) and by Kalinowski, Armson, Roland-Mieszkowski, Stuart, and Gracco (1993). Unison reading reduces stuttering even when the second person reads different material.[36] Adamczyk and his colleagues found that

[34] Cherry and Sayers (1956), Dewar, Dewar, and Anthony (1976), Garber and Martin (1977).

[35] See also Conture (1974), Mallard and Webb (1980). Moore and Adams (1985), however, found that instructions and practice did not completely reduce participants' vocal intensities to pre-noise levels, although the difference was not apparent to the ear.

[36] Barber (1939), Cherry and Sayers (1956), May and Hackwood (1968). The effect is greater when the material is the same, however.

reverberation had a marked effect on stuttering.[37] Stephen and Haggard (1980) obtained reductions in stuttering with delayed auditory feedback, with a four-speaker babble of voices played backwards, delayed, or synchronous, contingent on speech or continuous; with a speech-contingent low-frequency tone that was either synchronous or delayed; and with a continuous low-frequency tone. Stuttering has also been reduced by frequency filtered delayed auditory feedback (Adamczyk & Kuniszyk-Jóźkowiak, 1987), by phase shifted feedback of the vocal tone (Webster, 1991), and by a click at the onset of each syllable activated by the intensity of the sound (Howell & El-Yaniv, 1987). Not all of these conditions reduced stuttering to the same degree, but the observations suggest that just as it is difficult to find a novel method of speaking that does not alleviate stuttering, it may be difficult to find an unusual kind of auditory speech feedback or auditory perceptual field that does not do the same thing.[38]

Martin, Siegel, Johnson, and Haroldson (1984) found that amplification of stutterers' feedback of their own voices resulted in greater fluency only when following a condition in which their stuttering had been reduced by masking noise. Curious about whether it was the noise or the fluency that had caused this effect, they repeated the study with the addition of a rhythmic speech condition. Again the amplified side-tone reduced the speakers' stuttering when preceded by the noise condition, but not when preceded by rhythmic speech (Martin, Johnson, Siegel, & Haroldson, 1985).

Howell (1990) investigated the effect of altered feedback of several kinds on the intensity of the voice. He found that both stutterers and normally fluent speakers increased their voice levels under delayed feedback and white noise and reduced them slightly under frequency shifted and amplified speech feedback.

[37] Adamczyk, Sadowska, and Kuniszyk-Jóźkowiak (1975), Adamczyk, Kuniszyk-Jóźkowiak, and Smolka (1979), Adamczyk and Kuniszyk-Jóźkowiak (1987).

[38] The first author was acquainted with a stutterer who was in the habit of drawing his record player up to the telephone when he had a call to make.

Delayed Auditory Feedback (DAF)

Although masking noise was historically the first form of altered auditory feedback to be investigated in relation to effects on fluency in stuttering, it has not been extensively studied in recent years (Lincoln, Packman, & Onslow, 2006). In contrast, one of the most thoroughly investigated forms of altered auditory feedback, because of the applications it has found in the treatment of stuttering, has been delayed auditory feedback (DAF).[39] Its effect on the person who stutters is often just the reverse of its effect on the typically fluent speaker, despite some inconsistency. In such speakers, it tends to increase disfluency, although earlier reports that it induces behavior comparable to stuttering have been called into question when the disfluency patterns are examined closely (Stuart, Kalinowski, Rastatter, & Lynch, 2002). A frequent report is that some people who stutter, especially in milder cases, tend to experience increased difficulty, much as do normally fluent speakers. Most people who stutter appear to improve under DAF, however, at least under limited laboratory conditions, particularly those that involve oral reading. Whether or not this phenomenon can be successfully exploited to create durable therapeutic improvements in fluency in spontaneous speech outside the research laboratory or clinic is still under investigation, as we will discuss further in Chapter 14.

There is reason to believe that more than just novel auditory feedback is involved in this improvement. In the effort to overcome the disruptive effect of the DAF, most speakers tend to slow their rate of speech, run their words together, concentrate on proprioceptive and tactile monitoring, or

[39] Nessel (1958), Soderberg (1960), Chase, Sutton, and Rapin (1961), Lotzman (1961), Neelley (1961), Goldiamond (1965), Ham and Steer (1967), Webster and Lubker (1968a), Curlee and Perkins (1969), Soderberg (1969a), Langová, Morávek, Novák, and Petřík (1970), Webster, Schumacher, and Lubker (1970), Gibney (1973), Hutchinson and Burk (1973), Macioszek (1973), Burke (1975), Treon and Tamayo (1975), Hayden, Scott, and Addicott (1977), Hutchinson and Norris (1977), Novák (1978), Timmons and Boudreau (1978a, 1978b), Lechner (1979), Martin and Haroldson (1979), Stephen and Haggard (1980), Zsilavecz (1981), Howell, El-Yaniv, and Powell (1987), Kalinowski, Armson, Roland-Mieszkowski, Stuart, and Gracco (1993).

over-articulate.[40] Stutterers who do these things in order to "beat" the DAF effect are incidentally doing things that are likely to decrease their stuttering as well and are often targeted in the "fluency shaping" therapies discussed in Chapter 14. Stager, Denman, and Ludlow (1997) found, for example, that improved fluency for adults under DAF was also characterized by reductions in peak air flow and peak pressure from baseline; similar patterns correlating with improved fluency were also found for choral reading and metronome-paced speech. This may be the reason why stutterers who speak fluently under DAF appear to be miraculously avoiding both their stuttering and the disfluencies that are a usual consequence of DAF.

However, some researchers have found that stuttering can be reduced under DAF without changes in speech rate, or even at increased speech rates (MacLeod, Kalinowski, Stuart, & Armson, 1995). This implies that something other than altered speech production behaviors under DAF are responsible for fluency improvement.

Frequency-Altered Feedback

In recent years, there have also been a number of studies of the fluency-enhancing effects of frequency-altered feedback (FAF), which, thanks to newer digital technology, can adjust the fundamental and resonant frequencies in the speech signal without altering speech rate. Options can include a feedback signal much higher or much lower in frequency than the speaker's normal pattern.

Early studies suggesting that FAF can reduce stuttering rate in adults came from Kalinowski, Armson, Roland-Mieszkowski, Stuart, and Gracco (1993) and Ingham, Moglia, Frank, Costello-Ingham, and Cordes (1997), among others. Because some studies placed participants under FAF for only a few moments to measure outcomes, Armson and Stuart (1998) examined response to FAF by 12 stuttering adults over the course of an hour of short periods of exposure to FAF alternated with normal side-tone. There was large variability in results under FAF—during reading, three participants showed clear response to FAF that disappeared with removal of the altered feedback, six participants showed an initial response that diminished over repeated exposure, and three participants showed little effect of the treatment. Fluency during conversational monologue, a more typical speaking task for adults, was not improved, for the most part, under FAF. Natke (2000) did not find FAF to have fluency-enhancing effects for 12 adults who stutter, and concluded that its potential for therapeutic use is limited. Howell, Sackin, and Williams (1999) noted that older children (average age of 9 years) did not respond as well to FAF as did adults; their stuttering decreased from a mean of approximately 12 percent stuttered syllables to roughly 9 percent, while the stuttering rate for the adults decreased from an average of about 13 percent to 4.6 percent.

Stuart, Kalinowski, Armson, Stenstrom, and Jones (1996) examined the extent to which the speaker's fundamental frequency must be shifted to obtain maximal fluency. They suggested that only a one-quarter octave shift appeared to generate fluency enhancement. In contrast, some subjects in a study by Hargrave, Kalinowski, Stuart, Armson, and Jones (1994) required one-half to 1 full octave shift to experience benefit.

A few studies have compared the relative fluency-enhancing effects of DAF and FAF in the same participants. Zimmerman and Kalinowski (1997) found relatively similar reductions in stuttering frequency during counter-balanced use of either in scripted telephone conversations for a group of nine adults. Stuart, Kalinowski, and Rastatter (1997) found that both DAF and FAF reduced stuttering at roughly equivalent rates of approximately 60–75 percent; binaural presentation was more advantageous than monaural presentation.

Combined DAF and FAF

Some recent investigations of altered auditory feedback have investigated combining DAF and FAF; this mix is the basis for the SpeechEasy©, an in-the-ear feedback device marketed as an assistive device

[40] See discussions by Soderberg (1969b), Van Riper (1970), and Wingate (1970).

for the out-of-clinic treatment of stuttering. When combined together, these two feedback signals can best be compared to the feedback heard during choral reading, also known to exert a fluency-enhancing effect. As noted in Chapter 14, there is laboratory and clinical evidence that the combined signal can reduce stuttering substantially in some participants (Armson, Kiefte, Mason, & De Croos, 2006; Stuart, Kalinowski, Saltuklaroglu, & Guntupalli, 2006; see also discussions by Lincoln, Packman, & Onslow, 2006; Ramig, Ellis, & Pollard, 2007); this finding has prompted some companies to produce such devices for therapeutic use (Lincoln, Packman, & Onslow, 2006).

How Does Altered Auditory Feedback Achieve Its Effect?

It is possible that both DAF and FAF may also derive a large share of their power over stuttering simply because they create a novel change in the stutterer's auditory-perceptual field, since Langová, Morávek, Novák, and Petřík (1970) found that DAF that had been made almost unintelligible by frequency filtering had as beneficial an effect on the speech of stutterers as did unfiltered DAF. Rami, Kalinowski, Rastatter, Holbert, and Allen (2005) found this generalization to be only partially true for their participants: conversational speech low-pass filtered at 500 Hz (voicing source plus first formant) and 1000 Hz (voicing source plus first two formants) facilitated fluency for 12 adult stutterers, but speech filtered at 100 Hz (fundamental frequency only, with no segmental information) did not. However, Rami and Diederich (2005) also found fluency-facilitating effects for reversed conversational speech played back at slow rate, a condition that can not be considered analogous to any typical aspects of speech feedback while speaking. Similarly, Kuniszyk-Jóźkowiak, Smolka, and Adamczyk (1996) found that auditory feedback was not necessary to improve fluency: in their sample of 120 stuttering children and adults, some degree of fluency enhancement could be obtained with delayed visual feedback of the speaker's face or vibrotactile feedback of the speech signal.

In view of all these findings, it is perhaps not too soon to conclude that virtually any change in stutterers' accustomed way of hearing themselves speak is likely to alleviate their speech difficulty. This calls to mind a similar observation we made in Chapter 10—namely, that any change in the stutterer's accustomed way of speaking is likely to result in immediate fluency. Is the parallelism merely a matter of chance? In Chapter 10, we ventured to suggest that it is not the negligible effort it takes to adopt an artificial speech pattern that diverts the speaker's attention from stuttering, but the bizarre way in which he hears himself talking. It may not be far-fetched to suggest that in reviewing the effects of artificial speech patterns on stuttering, we are dealing with one and the same observation.

It can be argued that it is something in the signal besides mere novelty that achieves increases in fluency, in view of the differing effects of specific delayed feedback times on stuttering rates. Lincoln, Packman, and Onslow (2006) note that optimum fluency enhancement occurs between 50–75 msec. delay, and not less. It is of course possible that longer delays are simply more perceptible and more novel than shorter delays.

Returning to the white noise effect and the supposition that it acts as a novel form of feedback, there is one final question that is crucial for essentially all explanations based on distraction but rarely easy to answer. Does the effect wear off with loss of novelty? The evidence we have is too meager to permit a confident answer. We know that of the volunteers tested by Cherry, Sayers, and Marland (1955) the only one who failed to improve under white noise worked in surroundings with a high ambient noise level. We also have a report by Guttman (1960) that in Leningrad portable hearing aid–like masking devices for stutterers were abandoned after a few years "because stutterers did not experience lasting improvement and found it cumbersome." On the other hand, Trotter and Lesch (1967) reported the successful use of such a device by a college teacher for two and a half years. He normally used it during lectures, committee meetings, and telephone conversations, turning it on whenever he stuttered or thought he was about to stutter. Garber and Martin (1974) had three participants talk spontaneously during a series of 6 to 11 50-minute sessions in which white noise was on continuously for alternate 5-minute periods. In two of the three cases, there was no substantial "long-term" effect on stuttering, although their stuttering had been reduced by 82, 15, and 38 percent, respectively, during the first five minutes in which noise had been presented. Many of the participants studied by Armson and Stuart (1998) showed initial response (in reading) to altered auditory feedback that was not maintained over repeated exposure to the signal. By contrast, a stutterer tested by Dewar, Dewar, and Barnmes (1976) showed no habituation to the noise in 22 biweekly sessions. The difficulty with all such observations is that we know too little about the effect of novel conditions on stuttering to say whether an adequate test of this effect requires days, weeks, or many months.

The Auditory Feedback Theory of Stuttering

In stuttering theory, the white noise effect has been important chiefly in relation to speculations about defective auditory feedback mechanisms as the underlying cause of stuttering (see Chapter 2). A theory has several possible relationships to the facts. It may be in conflict with them, it may be irrelevant to them, it may manage to account for them, and it may illuminate them with meaning. The auditory feedback model is the kind of theory that brightly illuminates a few facts, but stands in weak or ambiguous relationship to most of them. It has given a simple meaning both to the white noise effect and to what would otherwise have been merely a chance resemblance between stuttering and the speech breakdown of normally fluent speakers under delayed auditory feedback. It has also been made to account for several other facts about stuttering, but appears irrelevant to most of them. Since it is questionable whether the white noise effect depends on masking of speech, the explanation provided for it by the theory seems to be of doubtful validity. It remains to be seen whether the resemblance of DAF speech disruptions to stuttering fares better with careful investigation.

Hutchinson and Ringel (1975) reported that complete deprivation of oral sensation in six adults who stutter caused an increase in the frequency and severity of stuttering. Although the significance of this finding is obscure, some may be inclined to speculate that the loss of oral sensation increased the participants' dependence on their auditory feedback.[41] If the finding is confirmed, the theory of defective auditory feedback may therefore have scored another enlightening explanation. On the debit side, no satisfactory answer has yet been made to the objection of Morávek and Langová (1967) that stuttering tends to occur at the moment of initiation of speech units before auditory feedback has begun to arrive.

THE METRONOME EFFECT

Most stutterers can talk with exceptional fluency when they time their speech to a rhythmic beat such as the ticking of a metronome. This finding played a part in both early and more recent attempts to treat stuttering. Laboratory studies have repeatedly confirmed the metronome effect.[42] Both syllables and words have been timed with the metronome with striking results. Auditory, visual, or tactile rhythmic stimuli have all been found equally effective. The effect has been demonstrated in both oral reading and spontaneous speech. Trotter and Silverman (1974) reported that a portable metronome device continued to reduce stuttering after 16 months of continuous use by one of the authors (Silverman), but the effect was greatest during the first 3 months. Later, Silverman (1976b) related that over a three-year period the benefit he received from the device steadily decreased, and in the final six months, it had very little effect on the frequency or severity of his

[41] The interpretation suggested by Hutchinson and Ringel was that the loss of sensory feedback may have impaired the participants' ability to minimize stuttering by appropriate oral movements.

[42] Barber (1940), Fransella and Beech (1965), Azrin, Jones, and Flye (1968), Brady (1969), Jones and Azrin (1969), Greenberg (1970), Silverman and Umberger (1974), Trotter and Silverman (1974), Silverman (1976b), Hanna and Morris (1977), Hutchinson and Navarre (1977), Hutchinson and Norris (1977), Brayton and Conture (1978), Martin and Haroldson (1979), Wingate (1981b), Hayden, Adams, and Jordahl (1982), Martin, Johnson, Siegel, and Haroldson (1985).

stuttering. Barber (1940) and others have regarded the metronome effect as an example of distraction. Fransella and Beech (1965) questioned whether this is an adequate explanation, however, and so have others since. In discussions of distraction as a possible cause, there has sometimes been some confusion between the distraction, if any, that might come from the sound of the rhythmic beat and the distraction that might be involved in the use of the rhythmical pattern of speech. Experimental work attempting to rule out distraction has been inconclusive, as we saw in our discussion of distraction in Chapter 10. Perhaps the only undisputed fact that has been learned from explorations of the basis for the metronome effect is that it is not due primarily to reduced rate of speech. Brady (1969) set the metronome at a rate corresponding to that of the participants' unaided oral reading. Fransella and Beech (1965) used their volunteers' rates of nonstuttered reading as predicted from their silent reading rates. Hanna and Morris (1977) used their reading rates in free speech. Both Barber (1940) and Hanna and Morris (1977) tested the effect of a metronome rate that made study participants speak even faster than usual. In all cases, the metronome remained highly effective, though slower rates tended to result in still less stuttering.

There are two other identifiable effects of the metronome condition besides the effect it may have on rate. One, of course, is the unusual regularity or rhythm it imparts to speech. The other is the effect it has of breaking speech up into very small units for isolated articulation, particularly when speakers time their speech to the metronome syllable by syllable. It is a good guess that something might be learned by separating the effects of these two factors.

The Factor of Syllabification

A separation of syllabification from rhythmicity was accomplished by two studies, one of which was done by Brady (1969). He had adults speak one syllable per beat in time to both a rhythmic metronome and a metronome that produced beats in accordance with no regular pattern. In both cases, there was little stuttering. Significantly less stuttering occurred in the rhythmic condition, but the difference was slight.

It might have appeared from Brady's study that rhythm had little to do with the metronome effect. He suggested that the beat had a "cue" function, signaling to the participant when the next sound was to be said. Fransella (1971), however, found that such a signal has little effect on stuttering, even when it is predictable. Brady's findings are not difficult to account for on the basis of the observation that under both of his metronome conditions, speech was reduced to a string of isolated syllables. Syllables tend to be extremely easy for most people who stutter to say in isolation. In part, it appears to illustrate a general factor that we discussed earlier in this chapter, the tendency for stuttering to diminish as the motor plan of speech becomes easier.

The Factor of Rhythmicity

As we have seen, Brady studied the effect of syllabification removed from rhythmicity. Azrin, Jones, and Flye (1968) did the opposite; they studied the effect of rhythmicity independently of syllabification. Like Brady, they had subjects speak in time to a rhythmic and arrhythmic metronome—in actuality a vibrotactile pulse. Unlike Brady, however, they instructed subjects to speak one whole word to each beat, except that words that were too long were to be syllabically divided between beats.[43] This was an important difference in procedure. Isolated words tend to be stuttered far more often than isolated syllables, probably because many of them are polysyllabic and require more complex serial ordering and because they have more meaning. The results were instructive. The rhythmic condition reduced stuttering sharply. In the arrhythmic condition, however, with neither syllabification nor rhythmicity to help them, the subjects stuttered as much as they did without any metronome.

It is evident that rhythmicity has a very strong effect of its own on stuttering, apart from the powerful

[43]The participants were reported to have followed these instructions with no apparent difficulty. When a word was long, either one or two syllables were usually spoken during a beat.

effect of syllabification. Why this is so may be open to debate. When virtually every unusual pattern of articulation, voice, stress, inflection, or phrasing that can be invented for that purpose seems to reduce stuttering markedly, however, it would be gratuitous to assume that speaking rhythmically is an exception. On the other hand, Brady (1969) argued that the metronome effect is greater in magnitude than that of most other speech patterns. This gains support from the study of Johnson and Rosen (1937) in which a metronome condition produced more fluency than high or low pitch, high or low intensity, slow rate, or whispering. It was on a par with singing, speaking in time to an arm-swing, and speaking in a sing-song, all of which have a rhythmic element.

Considered solely as an unusual speech pattern, however, rhythmic speech is obviously a compelling one. Perhaps the reason for this can be glimpsed in the finding of Azrin, Jones, and Flye (1968) that a rhythmic beat produces a synchronization effect; vocal and motor responses of normal subjects tend to become timed with it. In contrast, speaking in time to an arrhythmic beat, though it is difficult and confusing, as Brady remarked, is hardly a speech pattern at all, in the usual sense. Since the beat is unpredictable, subjects are forced to wait for it and then say their word or syllable. In the rhythmic condition, on the other hand, they do not literally time each word or syllable to the beat. They extract from the beat the information they need to program their speech so that its rhythm coincides with that of the metronome. It is this programmed aspect that gives it the character of a speech pattern. As unusual patterns go, it can hardly be denied that rhythmic speech is a bizarre one.

The evidence we have considered suggests, then, that at least two factors underlie the metronome effect. One is that people who stutter tend to become fluent when they find themselves speaking in almost any way strange to them. In this respect the metronome effect is allied to the fluency that people who stutter experience when they assume a dialect or imitate another person's speech. The other factor, especially strong when the speaker times each syllable to the beat, is a drastically reduced demand on motor planning.

Throughout this discussion we have tacitly discounted the effect of any distraction that might come merely from hearing a rhythmic metronome. Although such an effect seems improbable, studies by Greenberg (1970) and Brayton and Conture (1978) force us to think about it since they found that a rhythmic metronome reduced stuttering even when the participants were not instructed to pace their speech with it. We must recall that Azrin, Jones, and Flye (1968) found a rhythmic beat to have a synchronization effect on vocal responses. Greenberg's comments, furthermore, suggest that the participants often spontaneously "fell into rhythm" with the metronome. Presumably, this was the cause of their fluency.

SUMMARY REMARKS: FEEDBACK EFFECTS

Many types of feedback have been found to alter the frequency of stuttering in laboratory experiments, and, as Chapter 14 will show, have been employed as therapeutic agents in treating the disorder. While it is fairly clear that consequation of stuttering within an operant framework, altered auditory feedback while speaking, or the challenge to speak in time to an exogenous signal all appear to reduce stuttering for some speakers, and for various lengths of time, there is much that we yet need to learn about all three of these controversial sets of findings. First, it is not entirely clear how these fluency-enhancing outcomes, when they are observed, are brought about. As we discuss, most theories that have been advanced to explain the phenomena do not stand up under close scrutiny. It is clear that individual responses are varied enough to question how much they tell us about the underlying cause of stuttering or factors that maintain it. Finally, because durable fluency benefits have not yet been documented in long-term, out-of-laboratory studies, it is not yet clear how well these phenomena can guide improvements in therapeutic intervention, although, as Chapter 14 will show, all have been tested to some extent with varying results.

Chapter 12

Early Stuttering and Normal Disfluency

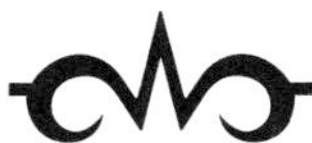

Stuttering usually develops in the early years of childhood, as we have seen. It tends to undergo many changes over the course of time. To try to glimpse something of its etiology in the mass of information we have accumulated on adults and school-aged children is a little like viewing it through a dense screen. In this chapter, we will be concerned with the relatively small but increasing amount of knowledge that we have about the moment of stuttering in its earliest forms.

Most of the work that has been done on early stuttering has been inspired by theories about its relationship to the disfluency that is so commonly observed in the speech of young children. We will therefore need to be concerned with this as well. It is possible to take essentially three points of view about normal disfluency in relation to early stuttering: (1) that it has nothing to do with stuttering, (2) that stuttering begins as an effort to avoid it, and (3) that stuttering develops as certain forms of normal disfluency become more frequent and severe. We might narrow the search for the cause of stuttering considerably if we could choose among these points of view.

THE AVOIDANCE HYPOTHESIS

Wendell Johnson was not the first to take notice of the fact that most young children are exceptionally disfluent at the same age at which a certain number of them begin to stutter. However, it was the central role that this fact played in his diagnosogenic theory that was primarily responsible for the important place that normal disfluency assumed in thinking and research on stuttering. His theory stated that some parents or other adults are unusually anxious or perfectionistic about the child's speech fluency. Such adults tend to react to the child's essentially normal disfluencies as a speech impairment. The child may then develop anticipatory avoidance reactions through anxiety about the speech hesitancy. Before its diagnosis as stuttering, this hesitancy may, to a greater or lesser degree, be affected by factors of environment, personality, or heredity, but in most cases, according to this theory, it does not differ markedly in amount or quality from that of other children who do not come to be regarded by their parents as stutterers.

Johnson's theory challenged an older viewpoint about the origin of anticipatory struggle behavior, one that assumed that it came about as a reaction of fear and avoidance to a stage of *abnormal* repetitions or prolongations in a child's speech. In short, one of the most basic issues that his theory raised was whether a so-called primary stage of stuttering existed. Johnson said it did not; the disfluencies that others had described as primary stuttering Johnson regarded as normal. This theoretical issue had a clinical counterpart. How did one tell the difference between a normally disfluent child and an incipient stutterer? Prior to Johnson, it was widely assumed that if the parents said the child was a stutterer, their word could be taken for it. Johnson's theory made it plain that the question was not so simple. It was true that many youngsters brought for treatment as stutterers could have raised few doubts in anyone's mind that their fluency was atypical. Furthermore, when speech interruptions did appear to leave room for some uncertainty, the parent was apt to state flatly that the child was not stuttering that day. Nevertheless, there were instances in which many speech clinicians believed they had genuine reason to be perplexed, and it was soon evident that little agreement existed on any reliable objective criteria for making a distinction between a stutterer and a nonstutterer in early childhood.

Other questions, more easily answered by investigation, were raised by the diagnosogenic theory. The theory implied that a relatively large amount of disfluency was to be found in the speech of normally developing children. This was amply confirmed in a series of studies.[1] The early research of Adams (1932) and Fisher (1932) also showed that speech repetitions in children tended to decrease with age. Other students of early childhood development described what they called "stuttering" as a common occurrence in preschool children.[2] They seemed to be referring to identifiable episodes of speech difficulty, but its nature was not well described.

The diagnosogenic theory also implied that adult listeners were apt to differ appreciably in their view of speech behavior that warranted the label of stuttering. Tuthill (1940, 1946) found evidence that this was true not only of ordinary listeners, but also of so-called experts. Various efforts to determine whether parents of stutterers had higher standards of fluency than parents of nonstutterers produced results that were inconsistent or difficult to interpret.[3] While some studies described in Chapter 9 show parents of stuttering children to have relatively high standards of behavior for their children, others have failed to find any such trend. When all of these pieces of evidence are carefully weighed, it is apparent that they fall short of furnishing conclusive proof of Johnson's theory. Furthermore, not one of them is, strictly speaking, necessary to the proposition that stuttering is caused by a misdiagnosis of normal disfluency. There is perhaps only one underlying assumption crucially important to the theory; namely, *that at the moment of initial diagnosis the speech of children who come to be regarded as stutterers does not differ in essential respects from that of children who do not come to be so regarded.* This is the essence of the diagnosogenic concept, upon which it stands or falls.

Unfortunately, it is extremely difficult to submit such an assumption to an objective scientific test, since the investigator is almost never present in the role of a detached observer at the moment of original diagnosis. We cannot do it in a speech clinic since, as Johnson emphasized, children's speech a month, a week, or even a day following the diagnosis may differ from their speech prior to the diagnosis as a re-

[1] Davis (1939, 1940), Branscom, Hughes, and Oxtoby (1955), Egland (1955), Mann (1955), Johnson and Associates (1959, chap. 8), Winitz (1961). See also Starkweather (1987).

[2] Ilg, Learned, Lockwood, and Ames (1949), Métraux (1950).

[3] Bloodstein, Jaeger, and Tureen (1952), Berlin (1960), Johnson and Associates (1959, p. 85 ff).

TABLE 12-1 Percentages of Comparison and Experimental Group Parents Who Reported That the Child Was Performing Each of the Indicated Speech Reactions When They First Thought the Child was Nonfluent or Stuttering, Respectively

	Repetition			Other nonfluency			
	Syllable	Word	Phrase	Sound prolongations	Silent intervals, pauses	Interjections	"Complete blocks"
Control							
Fathers (N = 69)	4	59	23	3	36	30	0
Mothers (N = 80)	10	41	24	4	41	21	0
Experimental							
Fathers (N = 143)	57	48	8	15	7	8	3
Mothers (N = 146)	59	50	8	12	3	9	3

Source: Wendell Johnson and Associates, *The Onset of Stuttering*, University of Minnesota Press, Minneapolis. Copyright © 1959 by the University of Minnesota. By permission.

sult of the negative evaluations placed upon it. The major method found practicable to date, that used by Johnson and his coworkers, has been based upon parents' descriptions, supplemented by imitations, of the earliest stuttering of their children obtained some time after the onset of the problem.[4] The disadvantage of such a procedure is partly in its reliance on parents' memories, which can seriously distort past events. A further weakness of such a procedure results from the fact that language, which in large part intervenes between the observer and the observed, is a great leveler of distinctions. Nevertheless, the issue has been of such importance to many fluency researchers and clinicians that the findings have been of outstanding interest despite these limitations.[5]

[4]An innovative exception to studies that have been limited to scrutiny of children after referral for stuttering was a series of articles by the team of Kloth, Janssen, Kraaimaat, and Brutten (e.g., Kloth, Janssen, Kraaimaat, & Brutten, 1995a, 1995b, 1998; Kloth, Kraaimaat, Janssen, & Brutten, 1999) that identified children at genetic risk for stuttering and began following them before stuttering was diagnosed. However, the published study results did not address pre-onset fluency characteristics, and children were not studied immediately after parents became concerned that they were beginning to stutter.

[5]Johnson himself was well aware of these limitations; his defense of the method was, in essence: if you don't study it this way, how do you study it? Since Johnson, there has been little attempt to study the "onset" of stuttering through interviews with parents. See Yairi (1983) and Yairi and Ambrose (1992b, 2005), however.

In Chapter 9, we cited findings from a series of investigations referred to as the Iowa studies, in which parents of stutterers and nonstutterers were interviewed intensively by Johnson and his coworkers. If our interest were solely in the validity of the diagnosogenic theory, essentially all of these findings could probably be ignored except for one particular portion of the results obtained in Study III (Johnson & Associates, 1959, chap. 6). In this portion of the study, mothers and fathers of stutterers, who were interviewed, on the average, about 18 months after the reported onset of stuttering, were asked to "*imitate and describe what the child was doing in his speech when he first stuttered.*" A comparison group of mothers and fathers of nonstutterers were asked to report similarly on the first nonfluencies that they recalled having observed in their children's speech.

The results are summarized in Table 12-1. It takes hardly more than a glance at the Table to see that there were distinct differences in the descriptions offered by the two groups of parents. The earliest normal disfluencies were characterized by phrase repetitions, pauses, and interjections far more often than were the earliest remembered stuttering events. The earliest stuttering behaviors, on the other hand, were more often described as syllable repetitions and sound prolongations. Word repetitions were identified as stuttering with great frequency, but with about equal frequency as normal disfluencies. In addition to the differences shown in Table 12-1, the parents' responses indicated that the earliest stuttering events were more frequently accompanied by unusual force, effort, or muscular tension in "getting words out" than were the earliest normal nonfluencies. This was reported by 36 percent of the mothers and 34 percent of the fathers of the stutterers, as compared with 17 percent of the mothers and 13 percent of the fathers in the comparison group (Johnson & Associates, 1959, Table 47, p. 145).

In short, the central premise of the diagnosogenic theory would not appear to have been borne out by the group data. Did this mean that the theory had been proved wrong? Johnson argued staunchly that it did not. He reasoned that there was not a single type of nonfluency that separated the two groups of children without very considerable overlap between them. The very same things that most parents had described as initial stuttering had been classified by some others as normal disfluencies, and the same things that most parents had described as normal disfluencies had been identified by some as stuttering; consequently, stuttering was, at least in part, a perceptual problem.

The same overlapping distribution extended to reports of "unusual effort or tension." Not only did most parents of stutterers report that the earliest stuttering that they remembered was devoid of any signs of tension, but, curiously, a few of the *nonstutterers* were reported to have shown signs of tension, awareness of speaking differently or incorrectly, surprise, irritation, or displeasure in connection with their earliest nonfluencies, despite the fact that any child who had ever even briefly been regarded by anyone as a stutterer had been systematically excluded from the typically fluent comparison group (Johnson & Associates, 1959, Appendix, pp. 79, 80). Clearly, the overlapping distributions required as much explanation as did the differences. Johnson's point was, in essence, that if the parents' evaluation of a child as a stutterer was influenced solely by the child's excessive or unusual disfluencies, there should have been little or no overlap between the two groups with respect to the phenomena they had respectively labeled stuttering and normal disfluency.

Accordingly, Johnson did not abandon his theory. He did revise it, however. In place of the simple statement that stuttering was caused chiefly by its own diagnosis, he substituted an "interaction hypothesis." This said that stuttering was most appropriately defined, not as a feature of a child's speech, but as a perceptual and evaluative problem that arises for a listener as the result of an interaction involving three major variables—the listener's sensitivity to the speaker's nonfluency, the degree of nonfluency of the speaker, and the speaker's sensitivity to his or her own nonfluency and to the listener's evaluative reactions to the nonfluency (Johnson & Associates, 1959, chap. 10).

THE CONTINUITY HYPOTHESIS

Johnson might have drawn a different conclusion from the overlapping data that he observed. If parents of stutterers and nonstutterers tended to a notable extent to describe the same disfluencies in their children's speech, this might have been because stuttering and certain kinds of normal disfluency in young children are not categorically different things. Johnson did not draw this conclusion. His basic philosophy about stuttering was that it was something to be sharply differentiated from the normal. This dichotomous view had been inherent from the start in his theory that stuttering was the child's effort to avoid normal disfluency. When the overlap he found between stutterers' and nonstutterers' behaviors seemed to show that no feature of speech would serve to differentiate them categorically, he defined stuttering as a problem that arose for a listener. It was the only way to maintain a clear-cut distinction between them.

Consequently, it remained for others to propose the continuity hypothesis on the basis of the work Johnson had done to make such a theory virtually inevitable. The suggestion has been made in more than one form. It was discussed by Bloodstein (1961a, 1970, 1975) as the view that mild tensions and fragmentations are an ordinary feature of the speech of young children as a result of commonplace communicative pressures and difficulties. When the tensions and fragmentations become magnified by communicative pressures or failures that are severe and chronic, they tend to be identified as episodes of stuttering, according to this viewpoint.

Shames and Sherrick (1965) also advanced a continuity hypothesis in the context of their analysis of stuttering and normal disfluency as operant behavior (see Chapter 2). They suggested that what comes to be called stuttering may be normal disfluency that has increased in frequency due to inadvertent reinforcement by individuals in the child's environment.

LISTENER IDENTIFICATION OF STUTTERING

The moment it was recognized that there was such a thing as normal disfluency in the speech of young children, the words *stutterer* and *stuttering* acquired a degree of ambiguity that they have never lost. The fact that this ambiguity played a special part in Johnson's theory, furthermore, insured that it would become an important subject for research.

The usual procedure in studies conducted to test the theory has been to present recorded samples of speech to listeners for identification. Both the identification of disfluencies as occurrences of stuttering and the identification of speakers as stutterers have been investigated. The speakers have been adults as often as children, but in either case, the ultimate focus of the research has been the diagnosis of stuttering in young children.

Listener Agreement

The initial study of listener identification, done by Tuthill (1940, 1946) under Johnson's direction, was concerned almost solely with determining how well listeners tend to agree on the occurrence of stuttering blocks. For this purpose, Tuthill performed three experiments. In the first one, he made a phonograph recording of the speech of adult stutterers and normally fluent speakers. He played this recording to three groups of listeners: speech clinicians, normally fluent speakers with no training in speech pathology, and stutterers. As the participants listened, they marked the stuttered words on a transcript of the recording. The results showed marked disagreement among listeners in all three groups concerning places at which stuttering had occurred. A considerable number of "stutterings" were identified in the speech of nonstutterers. The clinicians showed no more agreement than the untrained normally fluent speakers.

In the second experiment, Tuthill played a recording of a stutterer's speech to 11 experts on stuttering, to 7 janitors, and to 6 mothers of preschool-aged children. Each of the experts had a Ph.D. in speech pathology, seven were directors of university speech clinics, and four were Fellows of what was then called the American Speech Correction Association (now the American Speech-Language-Hearing Association). Despite this, the experts ranged from 34 to 89 in the number of blocks heard and did not agree better among themselves on the occurrence of stuttering than did the untrained listeners.

Tuthill's third experiment was essentially a replication of the first—with sound film replacing a phonograph recording. The addition of visual cues did not increase observer agreement materially. Of 219 words marked as stuttered, half were marked by less than 25 percent of the listeners, only 39 were agreed on by 75 percent of participants, and 45 were identified in "normal" speech.

Further evidence of listener disagreement on the occurrence of stuttering has been obtained in successive studies.[6] In an investigation by MacDonald and Martin (1973), a group of college students observed videotaped samples of the speech of adult stutterers and identified both the "speech disfluency" and the "stuttering." No more than 13 percent of all the events judged as stuttering were agreed on by the majority of observers. Curlee (1981) reported that giving observers a definition of stuttering had no effect on extent of agreement; Martin and Haroldson

[6] Emerick (1960), MacDonald and Martin (1973), Young (1975b), Coyle and Mallard (1979), Curlee (1981), Martin and Haroldson (1981), Martin, Haroldson, and Woessner (1988).

(1981) found that it actually resulted in significantly lower agreement.

It should be noted that the evidence of observer disagreement relates mainly to the identification of individual moments of stuttering. This finding should not be surprising, in fact, given the notoriously poor reliability of transcription found for either suprasegmental, hesitation, or narrow phonetic transcription tasks in a number of studies (see, for example, Patterson, Neupauer, Burant, Koehn, & Reed, 1996, for low levels of agreement on pauses and intonational characteristics, Ferber, 1991, for speech errors, and Stockman, Woods, & Tishman, 1981, for phonetic detail). In this regard, the task of judging individual words as stuttered or not may be as difficult a perceptual task as that required in noting and locating "clicks" interspersed inside of utterances, a notoriously difficult task to perform accurately, as discussed in most psycholinguistics texts (see Berko Gleason & Bernstein Ratner, 1998, for discussion). Even when given repeated opportunities to replay small segments of digitized speech to code disfluencies for clinical or research purposes, many clinicians and researchers note that achieving good intra- as well as inter-rater reliability is difficult, and cannot simply be ascribed to different "standards" for what constitutes normal vs. disfluent speech production. In this sense, we must be careful not to over-interpret some of the past literature that shows poor listener agreement for moments and types of disfluent behaviors.

However, not everyone agrees that listeners have difficulty in reaching consensus regarding fluency judgments (see Yairi & Ambrose, 2005, p. 88, for detailed discussion). For example, Curlee (1981) obtained high agreement among observers on frequency *counts* of stuttering despite low observer agreement on individual occurrences of stuttering. Hubbard (1998a) found similarly high agreement for judgments of both disfluency types and stuttering in children's speech. In evaluating the research literature published between the 1980s and 1990s, Yairi and Ambrose (2005) report reasonably high reliability estimates for fluency coding judgments that range from 0.82 to 0.93. In contrast, Ingham and Cordes (1992) reported marked differences in frequency counts of stuttering by different judges.

Some studies have asked listeners to judge small intervals of speech, rather than longer samples or individual instances. Wingate (1977) found relatively high agreement and accuracy among judges asked to identify *samples* of the speech of adolescent and adult individuals as belonging to stutterers or nonstutterers. Armson, Jenson, Gallant, Kalinowski, and Fee (1997) found reasonably good agreement for judgments of stuttered utterances. Judgments of stuttering were highly predicted by perceptions of audible struggle, rather than by presence of absence of particular fluency types. Cordes and Ingham (1994) found increased reliability of judgments about stuttering when listeners were exposed to short intervals and asked to discriminate them as stuttered or not. For both experienced and naive listeners, longer intervals were more likely to be judged as stuttered, but the two groups did not vary markedly in their decisions. Highest agreement was found for intervals in the range of 3–5 seconds in length.

Variables Related to the Identification of Stuttering

In some work, the disagreement among listeners has generally been taken for granted. Rather, interest has centered around the question of what factors tend to influence the identification of stuttering.

Speech Variables As might be expected, the identification of speakers as stutterers from recorded samples of their speech increases with the frequency, extent, or rated severity of their disfluency.[7] The type of disfluency is also a factor. In general, sound or syllable repetitions and sound prolongations tend to incline listeners to identify stuttering more than do revisions and interjections, which are more likely to be evaluated as normal disfluencies.[8] With respect to syllable repetition, however, Sander (1963) found that it made a considerable difference whether the

---

[7] Boehmler (1958), Berlin (1960), Sander (1963), Hoops and Wilkinson (1973), Huffman and Perkins (1974).

[8] Boehmler (1958), Williams and Kent (1958), Huffman and Perkins (1974).

speaker used single-unit repetitions such as *th-this* or double-unit repetitions such as *th-th-this*. Sound prolongations, in research by Lingwall and Bergstrand (1979), were judged to be stuttering events if they exceeded 912 milliseconds in duration.

In some of the studies we have cited, whole word repetitions occupied a somewhat anomalous position with respect to listener judgments, since they were readily evaluated as either stuttering or normal disfluency. The frequency and extent, of such repetitions have proved to be critical factors. Curran and Hood (1977b) found that double-unit word repetitions (e.g., *like like like this*) tended to be identified as stuttering events, whereas single-unit word repetitions did not. Multiple iterations of repeated segments do in fact characterize the speech of a large number of the stuttering children seen close to onset, as we shall see. In a study by Hegde and Hartman (1979b), however, even single -unit word repetitions were judged to be stuttering events when they were frequent enough; a majority of listeners judged speech samples as stuttered when 15 percent of the words were repeated. Hegde and Hartman (1979a) and DeJoy and Jordan (1988) found that even interjections of "uh" evoked a judgment of stuttering by large numbers of listeners. As noted, Armson, Jenson, et al. (1997) found that degree of audible struggle, rather than type of disfluency *per se*, was an extremely high predictor that a listener would judge a disfluency as stuttered. By manipulating temporal characteristics of children's disfluencies, Amir and Yairi (2002) found that shorter vowel durations and shorter inter-iteration intervals between repeated segments were more likely to contribute to judgments of stuttering.

Listener Variables: The Set to Observe Stuttering From the point of view of Johnson's avoidance or interaction hypothesis, the effect of listener variables on the identification of stuttering is of particular interest. Several listener variables have been studied. One of these is the set that may be given to listeners by instructing them to listen for stuttering. In a study by Williams and Kent (1958), college students listened to a recording of an adult speaker imitating various types of disfluency. On one occasion, they were instructed to mark all "stuttered" interruptions on a transcript of the recording. On another presentation of the same recording, they were told to mark all "normal" interruptions. The results showed that, to a considerable degree, they tended to hear what they were instructed to listen for. Many of the interruptions marked as stuttered under one set of instructions were marked as normal interruptions under the other.

The tendency of observers to identify the same interruptions as both stuttering and normal disfluency on different occasions was referred to as "confusion" by Williams and Kent (1958) and as "ambiguity" by MacDonald and Martin (1973). In the study conducted by MacDonald and Martin, college students observed videotaped samples of the speech of adult stutterers and evaluated them once for the occurrence of "speech disfluency" as differentiated from stuttering, and again for the occurrence of "stuttering." They found that of all the events identified as stuttered words, 29 percent were also judged to be disfluencies by one or more of the observers. A similar investigation by Curlee (1981), even with some improvements in procedure, produced considerably higher measures of ambiguity.

In a different type of study by Berlin (1960), several groups of mothers evaluated recorded samples of children's speech. Berlin found that mothers of children who stuttered or had other speech impairments were more likely to evaluate a child as a stutterer if the word *stuttering* was used in the instructions than if it was not.

In contrast, Curran and Hood (1977a) found results that conflicted with those of previous studies. College students listened to samples of the speech of three young children who had been trained to imitate various disfluency types. Attempts to influence the listeners' judgments by telling them that the children were stutterers or nonstutterers had little effect on the evaluation of the speech as stuttered or normal. In a study by Bar (1967), listeners who were instructed to attend to the manner of a stutterer's speech and listeners who were instructed to attend to the content did not differ significantly in their estimates of the percentage of stuttering.

Other Listener Variables It has generally been found that speech clinicians, students in speech-language pathology programs, or others who have some professional knowledge about stuttering tend to make more identifications of stuttering or stutterers than do laypersons.[9] For example, Brundage, Bothe, Lengeling, and Evans (2006) found that highly experienced clinicians identified more than twice as much stuttering as did less experienced clinicians or student clinicians, although each group was internally consistent in their judgments. Tuthill (1940) and Lickley et al. (2005) also found a higher propensity for stutterers to identify stuttering events. Similar findings with regard to parents of stutterers were obtained by Bloodstein, Jaeger, and Tureen (1952), but not by Berlin (1960) or by Curran and Hood (1977b).

Sander (1968) had mothers of typically fluent children listen to a recording of a child with mild and ambiguous disfluencies and then questioned them about some of their attitudes and reactions. He found two assumptions that were significantly related to a judgment that the child was stuttering—that the child not only looked upon speaking as something difficult to do, but also showed signs of emotional disturbance. Sander discovered, in addition, that mothers who did not believe that the child was stuttering were just as likely to say that they would try to correct the child's speech as were mothers who did feel that the child was stuttering. In short, the failure to apply the label "stuttering" did not necessarily mean the absence of concern.

Gately (1967) found that the recorded speech of a stutterer more often evoked a judgment of stuttering from listeners who had high scores on the *Taylor Anxiety Scale* than from those with low scores, but this tendency did not reach statistical significance. Responses to questions about the speaker and his manner of speaking suggested that the anxious listeners were more sensitive to and critical of the disfluencies.

Giolas and Williams (1958) investigated the reactions of kindergarten and second grade children to adult disfluencies. They reasoned that if children tend to label the disfluencies of others as "different," they may react similarly to disfluencies in their own speech. The children listened to tape-recorded stories told by fluent and disfluent speakers and were then asked which stories they liked best and which person they would prefer as a teacher. The disfluencies markedly affected the children's choice of a teacher, and their comments showed that they were aware of the disfluencies and reacted to them. Several of the second graders were already using the term "stuttering." Culatta and Sloan (1977) obtained similar findings in a study of children from first to fourth grades, and Norbut (1976) reported that children from kindergarten to sixth grade readily differentiated fluency from disfluency. Langer (1969) even found expressions of negative attitudes in preschool children when he questioned them about their reactions to filmed examples of stuttering. Ezrati-Vinacour, Platzky, and Yairi (2001) used puppets to model a variety of fluency behaviors for Hebrew-speaking children ages 3 through 7 years of age. Many 3-year-olds could discriminate fluent from stuttered speech, and by age 4, most children gave such speech rather negative evaluation, even when they could not label it using the Hebrew word for stuttering.

THE FEATURES OF EARLY STUTTERING

The findings that we have just reviewed show that listeners may experience a certain amount of confusion about what to call stuttering and normal disfluency, even in the speech of adults. This suggests that even adults, and so presumably young children as well, are not divided into two totally distinct categories with respect to the amount or kind of disfluency they exhibit in their speech. Such an assumption was basic to Johnson's hypothesis that stuttering is largely a disorder in the evaluations placed upon a child's fluency. It is also basic to the outlook that what are called stuttering and normal disfluency in young children are largely different degrees of the same thing. We will now take stock

[9] Tuthill (1940), Boehmler (1958), Emerick (1960), Ward (1967), Hoops and Wilkinson (1973). Conflicting findings were obtained by Schiavetti (1975) and Curran and Hood (1977b).

of the information we have about the early disfluencies of children from this point of view.

The Iowa Study

Normative data on the types of disfluency observable in the speech of young stutterers and nonstutterers are not abundant. Until recently, the largest proportion of the available data came from the study by Johnson and Associates (1959, chap. 8). That study consisted in part of an analysis of recorded samples of the speech of 68 boys and 21 girls "alleged" to have been stuttering for periods ranging from a month to over three years and a like number of nonstuttering children matched for age, sex, and socioeconomic status of the family. The children's speech samples, about 500 words in length on the average, were analyzed for the occurrence of the eight kinds of disfluency listed in Table 12-2 and also described in Chapter 1.

Two cautions should be observed in accepting these data as a valid description of early disfluency. One is that they omitted both silent intervals and such symptoms of effort or tension as hard attacks on sound, gasping, or audible glottal straining, shown earlier in this chapter to affect stuttering judgments. All of these can be heard in examples of early stuttering and, potentially, in normal childhood disfluency. The other caution is that the children, though 5 years old on average, ranged from about 2.5 to slightly more than 8. As we will see, there is evidence that well before the age of 8, changes occurring in early stuttering may affect the relative frequency of certain disfluency types.

TABLE 12-2 Mean Number of Disfluencies per 100 Words of 68 Male Stuttering and 68 Male Nonstuttering Children

	Stutterers	Nonstutterers	P*
Interjections	3.62	3.13	NS
Sound and syllable repetitions	5.44	0.61	0.01
Word repetitions	4.28	1.07	0.01
Phrase repetitions	1.14	0.61	0.01
Revisions	1.30	1.43	NS
Incomplete phrases	0.34	0.23	NS
Broken words	0.12	0.04	0.05
Prolonged sounds	1.67	0.16	0.01
All categories	17.91	7.28	0.01

*Level of significance of the difference between stutterers and nonstutterers.
Source: Wendell Johnson and Associates, *The Onset of Stuttering*, University of Minnesota Press, Minneapolis. Copyright © 1959 by the University of Minnesota. By permission.

Differences between Stutterers and Nonstutterers With these qualifications in mind, we may review the results of the Iowa study. A significant portion is summarized in Table 12-2. The table shows the mean number of disfluencies of each type per 100 words for the male stutterers and nonstutterers.[10] The stutterers exceeded the nonstutterers in the frequency of most types of disfluency. There was no significant difference, however, in the frequency of interjections (such as "uh"), revisions, and incomplete phrases. The data provide an empirical basis for excluding these types from a definition of stuttering. Significant differences between the two groups appeared in the case of sound and syllable repetitions, word repetitions, phrase repetitions, broken words, and prolonged sounds. If we take into consideration the fact that certain disfluency types were far more frequent than others in general, the groups differed mainly in the number of sound, syllable, and word repetitions. Not only did the stutterers tend to have more of these repetitions, as shown in Table 12-2, but they also significantly exceeded the nonstutterers in the mean number of units per repetition. This was also true of interjections and, in the case of females, phrase repetition. The average stuttering child tended to have one- to three-unit repetitions, while the average nonstuttering child tended to have repetitions of one or two iterations (Johnson & Associates, 1959, pp. 212–14).

So much for the differences. Johnson considered them to be the result of an "undeliberated

[10] The data for the females were essentially the same, except that the groups were smaller and that two differences significant in the case of the boys (phrase repetitions and broken words) were not significant for the girls.

experiment" in which two groups of children whose speech was "presumably more or less similar" to begin with were subject to different evaluative reactions to their speech by parents for varying periods of time.

Do Stutterers Have More of the Same Disfluencies than Nonstutterers Do? In addition to statements about differences, two general statements can be made regarding similarities between the two groups of children. One is that, as Table 12-2 shows, no broadly defined types of disfluency exhibited by the stutterers were absent from the speech of the nonstutterers, not even those most clearly differentiating the two groups. As far as it goes, this observation makes it possible to entertain a continuity hypothesis about the relationship between stuttering and normal disfluency. Stutterers appear to do the same things nonstutterers do, only—in the case of some of these things—more so. It does not lend particular support to Johnson's interaction or avoidance hypothesis, since it is possible to assume that whether children come to be perceived as stutterers is essentially a matter of how much of certain kinds of disfluency they exhibit in their speech, or aspects of their quality, and has little to do with any eccentricity of the perceiver.

The Overlapping of the Distributions There is, however, a second statement that can be made about the relationship between the two groups of children that supports the interaction theory, and Johnson gave it great emphasis. It was the observation that even where the stutterers showed more of a given type of disfluency than the nonstutterers, there was a marked overlap of the two distributions. In the case of sound or syllable repetitions, for example, about 20 percent of the male nonstutterers had more of them in their speech than did 20 percent of the male stutterers. In the case of word repetitions, 20 percent of the male nonstutterers exhibited more than did 20 percent of the male stutterers. With respect to total number of disfluencies of all kinds, 20 percent of the male nonstutterers exceeded 30 percent of the male stutterers. The fact that certain children bore the label "stutterer" though they were more fluent than certain children who were called "normal speakers" seemed to Johnson to be evidence of perceptual and evaluative factors at work. He argued that there were no "natural lines of demarcation" between "normal" and "abnormal" fluency. Consequently, there was no way to define stuttering as a feature of a child's speech that would serve to differentiate it operationally from normal disfluency. Stuttering therefore could only be defined, he said, as an evaluative reaction of a listener (Johnson & Associates, 1959, pp. 205, 218–20). As we have seen, for Johnson the distinction between stuttering and normal disfluency was by definition a sharp and categorical one.

The Illinois Study

The second major study of children at the onset of stuttering and peers who were considered normally disfluent is the cross-sectional and longitudinal study conducted by Ehud Yairi and colleagues at the University of Illinois beginning in the early 1980s. Yairi and Ambrose (2005) provide a detailed summary of this program of research that followed 163 children referred for stuttering.[11] Of these, 146 were referred within the first year following onset of stuttering symptoms and 17 were referred more than one year following onset. These children were compared to a comparison group of gender- and age-similar children considered to be normally fluent. Fluency characteristics of the children in these groups are shown in Table 12-3. Yairi and colleagues isolated what they termed stutterlike disfluencies (SLDs), and contrasted them with other forms of disfluency. In contrast to Johnson, they found relatively little overlap between the stuttering children and those considered by their parents and the researchers to be normally fluent.

As the authors noted, the total frequency of part-word repetitions, monosyllabic word repetitions, and disrhythmic phonations in the speech of stuttering children was approximately eight times that seen in normally fluent children (11.3 percent

[11] It is beyond the scope of this chapter to do justice to the many analyses reported from this longitudinal project. The reader is referred to Yairi and Ambrose (2005) for full discussion.

TABLE 12.3a Post-onset Interval, Mean, and Proportion of Stuttering-Like Disfluencies (SLD) for Experimental and Comparison Groups in Previous Studies

Study and Group	Post-onset interval (months)	*N*	Mean SLD	Proportion of SLD to total disfluency
Yairi and Lewis (1984)	≤ 2			
Experimental		10	16.43	0.77
Comparison		10	3.02	0.49
Hubbard and Yairi (1988)	≤ 6			
Experimental		15	16.88	0.75
Comparison		15	2.59	0.43
Zebrowski (1991)	≤ 12			
Experimental		10	9.63	0.78
Comparison		10	1.83	0.37
Yairi and Ambrose (1992a)	≤ 12			
Experimental		27	10.87	0.73
Yairi, Ambrose, and Niermann (1993)	≤ 3			
Experimental		16	11.99	0.69
Ambrose and Yairi (1999)	≤ 6			
Experimental		90	10.37	0.66
Comparison		54	1.33	0.24

Source: Yairi and Ambrose (2005).

TABLE 12-3b Mean Frequency and Standard Deviation of Specific Disfluencies per 100 Syllables for Stuttering and Comparison Groups

Disfluency Type	Stuttering children	Comparison children
Stuttering-Like Disfluencies		
Part-word repetitions	5.64 (4.28)	0.55 (0.43)
Single-syllable word repetitions	3.24 (2.01)	0.79 (0.74)
Disrhythmic phonations	2.42 (2.62)	0.08 (0.12)
Total	11.30 (6.64)	1.41 (0.96)
Other disfluencies	5.79 (2.75)	4.48 (2.41)

Source: Yairi and Ambrose (2005).
Note: Standard deviations in parentheses.

spoken syllables vs. 1.41, with no overlap when mean and standard deviations are considered). The frequency of other types of disfluency was also statistically elevated for the stuttering children, but was much closer in terms of absolute proportion, and did show overlap.

The Illinois group also highlighted additional findings that seem to categorically distinguish typically fluent children from those referred for stuttering. One is the proportion of stutter-like disfluencies to other forms of disfluency. For stuttering children, this value was approximately 66 percent, while for typically fluent children, the proportion was approximately 28 percent. A second was the number of iterations in repeated segments. For stuttering children, the mean was 1.56, with a range of between one and over five iterations during sound, syllable, or word repetitions. For normally fluent children, the mean was only slightly over 1 (1.13), with an average range of one to less than two repeated segments. When Yairi et al. applied their weighted disfluency formula, which loads blocks and prolongations as well as the number of iterations in repeated segments, the stuttering group achieved a score of over 20, while the normally fluent group had a mean score of 1.72. In summarizing their data on frequency, typology and duration of disfluencies in young children diagnosed as stutterers, Yairi and Ambrose (2005) state flatly that, "from the time when stuttering is said to begin in preschool children, their disfluent speech is markedly different from that of normally fluent children" (p. 138). This lead them to reject Johnson's theory, saying that, "the data leave little doubt that, in most cases, parents who believe that their child has begun stuttering do not exercise erroneous judgment but are reacting to real changes in the child's speech."

Further Work on the Features of Early Stuttering

Most other work has left little doubt that young stutterers tend to have more disfluencies in their speech than young nonstutterers. The questions that have arisen have been concerned mainly with the form of the disfluencies. Yairi (1972) and F. H. Silverman (1974) gathered data on elementary school–aged children that appear to be in general agreement with Johnson's with respect to the disfluency types that tend to differentiate groups of stutterers and nonstutterers. We can form a preliminary conception of early stuttering from the data gathered by Johnson and Associates (1959) on a group of children ranging up to 8 years of age. At least with respect to the frequency of word repetitions, the information may be misleading. Although Johnson's data showed word repetitions to be very prominent in the speech of stutterers and indicated that they are more than four times as frequent as in the speech of nonstutterers, the data showed them to be less common than sound and syllable repetitions. Clinical experience suggests that, in the very earliest phase of stuttering, between ages 2 and 5 years, the reverse may be true in many, if not most, cases. In an analysis of the disfluencies of five preschool stutterers by Bloodstein and Grossman (1981), word repetition proved to be the most frequent aspect of the disfluency in three cases, part-word repetition in only one. Word repetition was the only feature forming a conspicuous element of the pattern for all five subjects. Part-word repetition was a prominent element in two cases. This is in agreement with observations made by Westby (1979), but conflicts with those of Culp (1984) and Meyers (1986), who reported part-word repetition to be the most common type of disfluency in preschool stutterers.

Part-word repetitions were also the most frequent type in the speech of 10 2- and 3-year-old stutterers studied by Yairi and Lewis (1984), but these unusual cases, collected over a 10-year period, involved children brought for examination only two months or less after the reported "onset" of stuttering. In our experience, few parents seek help quite so soon if the child's difficulty is largely confined to whole word repetitions.

The longitudinal work that Yairi and colleagues report in Yairi and Ambrose (2005) is subject to the same concern. However, with the growth of the Internet and web-related resources for parents who have concern about their children's fluency development, this profile is likely to continue, even as studies attempt to determine the nature of stuttering at its onset by actively recruiting families very soon after behaviors of concern are noted. That is, since organizations such as the Stuttering Foundation of America and National Stuttering Association, among others, emphasize the importance of part-word repetitions, blocks, prolongations, and dis-rhythmic phonation in characterizing a child at risk for stuttering, we might logically expect to see larger distributions of these items in the speech of children observed by professionals soon after symptom onset.

Thus, not everyone has accepted the assertion that early stuttering cannot be categorically distinguished from normal disfluency on the basis of features of a child's speech. To Wingate (1962a), McDearmon (1968), and Kools and Berryman (1971), the evidence that certain types of interruption are more typical of children called stutterers, while others are equally characteristic of stutterers and nonstutterers seems to justify the outlook that there is a difference in kind between stuttering and normal disfluency as forms of speech behavior. In support of this, Floyd and Perkins (1974) found no evidence suggesting overlap or even continuity between the disfluencies of 4 preschool stutterers and 20 preschool nonstutterers. The lowest percentage of disfluent syllables in the speech of a stutterer was 7.28, whereas the highest among the nonstutterers was 2.58. Although recognizing that their sample was too small for generalization, they pointed out, "The fact that within each group the scores are closely spaced, whereas between the two groups a large gap in the scores exists, suggests that the preschool stutterers and nonstutterers of this study were discretely different."

Other Research on Normal Disfluency in Young Children

As we have seen, there is a body of research that has suggested that the kinds of disfluency most typical of stuttering are also found abundantly in the speech of nonstuttering children, although their frequencies and more specific characteristics may vary somewhat. E.-M. Silverman (1972a) found that so-called stuttering-type disfluencies occurred frequently in the speech of 10 4-year-old normally fluent children. She observed marked variation from child to child and from one speech situation to another in the most frequently occurring types of disfluency and found that almost all of the children exhibited "stuttering-type" interruptions—chiefly part-word repetitions and prolongations—as their most frequently occurring disfluency types on at least one of three days on which their speech was sampled.

Westby (1979) examined the disfluencies of three groups of kindergarten and first grade children: 10 stutterers; 10 children who were not regarded as stutterers, but who were judged by their teachers to be highly disfluent; and 10 typically disfluent children. She found that both the stutterers and the highly disfluent normal speakers had more disfluencies of all types than the typically disfluent normal speakers, but were quite similar to each other in both amount and type of disfluency. Word repetitions and interjections were the most frequent types of disfluency for both stutterers and highly disfluent normal speakers, and interjections were the most common type for the typically fluent speakers. The stutterers and highly disfluent normal speakers differed most from the typically fluent speakers in frequency of word and part-word repetitions. A suggestion that emerges from Westby's study is that one might find children in whom stuttering lies latent during their early years, although they are by any ordinary definition normally fluent speakers. However, the quality of these moments of disfluency is unknown.

Similarly, Yairi (1982), in an early study following the development of fluency in 33 2-year-old children for the space of a year, observed disfluencies that "may be regarded by parents or other observers as stuttering." Large increases and decreases in disfluency occurred in the speech of many of the children, although part-word repetitions decreased progressively with age. Yairi (1981) noted the possible existence of two subpopulations of children, a large number of fluent children and a much smaller number of highly disfluent ones.

In a study of 50 normally fluent 2- to 6-year-olds, Ito (1986) found that disfluency increased with age until it reached a peak at age 4 years, then decreased in the 5- and 6-year-old children. At the early age levels, those using more complex sentences exhibited the largest amounts of disfluency. Of one particularly disfluent child who was studied over time, Ito reported, "The highest observed frequency of dysfluency corresponded with the period when she began to use longer and more complicated sentences. Furthermore, her dysfluency began to improve at approximately the same time that she began to use those sentences constantly." Wijnen (1990) reports a case study that shares many similarities to this observation.

Additional studies of the disfluencies of typically fluent preschool children have been reported. Like those already mentioned, they have shown that young nonstutterers exhibit all of the types of disfluency found in the speech of children who stutter.[12] Bjerkan (1980) identified virtually no part-word repetitions, sound prolongations, or blockings in the speech of 108 normally fluent nursery school children, although the speech samples were, on the average, over 300 words in length. At the same time, he found that two children who were regarded as

[12] Haynes and Hood (1977), Colburn and Mysak (1982a), Wexler (1982), Wexler and Mysak (1982), Yairi (1982), Culp (1984).

stutterers exhibited no more "word repetitions" (by which Bjerkan meant repetitions of words, phrases, or sentences) than did the nonstutterers. Bjerkan concluded that early stuttering is qualitatively distinguishable from normal disfluency as fragmentation of words.

Weighting Frequency Measures to Describe Patterns of Early Disfluency

Measures that combine frequency counts for different types of disfluencies as well as weights for their characteristics (e.g., numbers of iterations per repetition episode) may be able to identify nonoverlapping groups of typically disfluent and stuttering children. Ambrose and Yairi (1999) developed such a diagnostic taxonomy based on their longitudinal research. Their fluency measure takes the weighted sum of part- and one-syllable word repetitions and disrhythmic phonation per 100 syllables. In addition, the mean number of iterations in repetitive disfluencies and disrhythmic phonations are weighted more highly and are factored into the computation. A discriminant analysis using these values was correctly able to assign 90 stuttering and 54 nonstuttering children to the appropriate diagnostic category. However, as Natke, Sandrieser, Pietrowsky, and Kalveram (2006) note, Yairi et al.'s original selection criteria maximized behavioral separation between the groups by specifically requiring nonstuttering children to show no more than three stutter-like disfluencies per 100 syllables and children who stutter to have no fewer than three stutter-like disfluencies. The same was true for work conducted by Conture and colleagues (Pellowski & Conture, 2002), who also found little overlap in behaviors between preschool children referred for stuttering and typically fluent peers.

Natke et al. (2006) set no such exclusionary criteria for study of 24 pairs of German preschool children who did and who did not stutter, who fell between a wide range of times post-onset of symptoms. Both groups exhibited all types of stutter-like disfluencies. However, all types of stutter-like behaviors, as well as the total of such behaviors, were significantly more frequent in the speech of children classified as stutterers. The two groups did not differ in frequency of normal disfluency, except for repetitions of multisyllabic words, which were more likely to be seen in children who stutter.

The cut-off of 3 percent stutter-like disfluencies has been employed by a number of researchers, who find it useful in discriminating between stuttering and nonstuttering children, even if rare stutter-like disfluencies can be observed in children not considered to be at risk for stuttering. Natke et al. (2006) found that 94 percent of their study children could be correctly classified in this way. Using the weighted score proposed by Yairi and Ambrose (1999) did not improve accuracy of classification and produced more false negative classifications (considering a child who stuttered to be normally fluent). The authors concluded that even at a very early stage post-referral, children who stutter differ in their fluency characteristics from children who are perceived to be normally fluent. Although each type of disfluency was found in each group, stutter-like disfluencies were much more frequent in the speech of stuttering children and rarely, if ever, observed in the speech of children thought to be typically fluent.[13] "Stuttering is distinctly different from normal speech (even at an early age) and can be clearly diagnosed in the majority of cases. The opinion that stuttering constitutes a common phase in normal language development is not supported by the data reported here" (Natke et al., 2006).

Qualitative Analyses of the Moments of Disfluency

It is evident that the question of how to draw a line between cases of early stuttering and normal disfluency has continued to challenge workers who are investigating both the avoidance and continuity hypotheses. One obvious answer is to find qualitative differences in the actual disfluent events seen in speech perceived to be stuttered rather than normally disfluent. Stromsta (1965, 1986) suggested that such

[13] Essentially similar findings were reported by Juste and de Andrade (2006) for Portuguese-speaking children.

a distinction might be made by spectrographic study of children's disfluencies. Of 38 children who were examined because their parents were concerned about their disfluencies, the speech of 27 yielded spectrograms characterized by experienced judges as having "a lack of formant transitions and abrupt phonatory stoppages in association with prolongation and clonic-type disfluencies." Ten years later, Stromsta determined the status of these children by questionnaire. Of the 27 children with abnormal spectrograms, 24 were still stuttering, while of the remaining 11 cases with normal-appearing spectrograms, 10 were not stuttering. Yaruss and Conture (1993) noted the same spectrographic features that Stromsta had observed, but the abnormalities failed to distinguish a group of children thought to be at high risk from a group thought to be at low risk for continuing to stutter.

Other researchers have continued to look for evidence of specific features of early disfluency that differentiate the normal from the abnormal in a categorical way, but with limited success. Caruso, Conture, and Colton (1988) compared the respiratory, laryngeal, and labial activity of 3-year-old stutterers during stuttering with that of nonstutterers' fluent speech. They observed essential similarity of functioning between the two and concluded that the speech coordination of the stutterers and nonstutterers differed in degree, rather than kind. Healey and Bernstein (1991) reported no differences between the repetitions of preschool stutterers and typically fluent peers in variability of vocal fundamental frequency. Zebrowski (1991) found that young stutterers and normally fluent speakers did not differ in the length of their sound prolongations or the number of repeated units of sound or word repetitions. Yairi and Hall (1993) found no difference in durational features of children's word repetitions, except for a possible tendency for children who stutter to have faster repetitions. A follow-up of this work by Throneburg and Yairi (1994) did identify statistically shorter inter-iteration intervals in the repetitions of children who stutter than in the repetitions of children considered to be typically fluent.

Hubbard and Yairi (1988) found that disfluencies occurred in clusters in both stutterers' and nonstutterers' speech, although this tendency was greater in the case of the stutterers. LaSalle and Conture (1995) obtained similar results in their analysis of speech samples from 30 pairs of preschool children. They noted that stuttering children often produced clustered stutters. While their normally fluent children occasionally produced stutter-like disfluencies, they were never observed to produce such clusters.

Finally, Einarsdöttir and Ingham (2005) argue against using any of these kinds of taxonomies to evaluate whether there is continuity between the speech characteristics of children who are perceived to be typically fluent and those who are judged to stutter. In a comparison of diagnostic labels used across a wide number of studies conducted by Johnson and Associates and others over the past 50 years, they note wide disagreement in terminology and findings. They conclude that most existing terminology has failed to capture the essential features that differentiate normal from pathological fluency, even though listeners can reach agreement on this construct if given intervals of speech to judge.

THE DISTRIBUTION OF EARLY DISFLUENCIES

The question we have been discussing is whether stuttering and stutter-like normal disfluencies are merely different degrees of the same thing, or whether they are two quite different kinds of speech behavior, with entirely different sources, that by accident resemble each other. Can there be "stuttering" and "nonstuttering" repetitions? This serves to raise the question whether the disfluencies of stuttering and normally fluent young children tend to vary under the same conditions and in general respond to the same stimuli. The question can be raised separately for different types of disfluency. There are large gaps in our knowledge of this broad subject. Such information as we have is chiefly about the distribution of the disfluencies in the speech sequence.

Consistency and Congruity

Stutterers The evidence about the consistency effect, though meager, suggests that it is present in the disfluencies of young children who stutter. Bloodstein (1960a) tested 14 stutterers between the ages of 3 and 6 years by having them repeat a list of simple sentences from dictation twice in succession, and found percentages of consistency ranging from 50 to 100 with a mean of 71 percent. Neelley and Timmons (1967) found a mean consistency of about 40 percent in 30 3- to 8-year-old stutterers, using a similar method. None of the individual consistency scores of their children was statistically significant, but the test was very brief. It appears likely, as Neelley and Timmons stated, that the consistency effect as it is found in young stutterers is an early form of the adult phenomenon. The findings therefore suggest that stuttering is a response to stimuli even in its incipient stages.

Is it heavily influenced by individual factors, as is fully developed stuttering? To answer this question, the first author reanalyzed the data of the Bloodstein (1960a) study of the consistency effect in young children who stutter to compute the amount of congruity among the children. By eliminating some children and some sentences, it was possible to isolate a series of five consecutive sentences that had been said in identical form by seven children. The average congruity was 42 percent. That is, on the average, each child had stuttered on 42 percent of the words that were stuttered by any of the other six children. This was significantly higher than chance. The average consistency of these children, however, was significantly higher still, amounting to 75 percent in their two utterances of these sentences. Just as in the case of older stutterers (see Chapter 10), the responsiveness to cues that was evident in their consistency scores appeared to reflect their unique learning experiences as individuals to a greater extent than it reflected the influence of factors operating for the children as a group.

Nonstutterers The consistency effect has also been found repeatedly in the disfluencies of typically fluent children. It was reported in elementary school–aged children studied by Williams, Silverman, and Kools (1969a), in 5- to 8-year-olds by Neelley and Timmons (1967), in 4- to 6-year-olds by Bloodstein, Alper, and Zisk (1965), and in 3- to 4-year-olds by Wynia (1964). Neelley and Timmons observed that it tended to be lower in magnitude than the consistency of stutterers of comparable age. None of the children had consistency scores that passed individual tests of statistical significance, but it is difficult to tell to what extent this was due merely to inadequate sampling of their performance.

The Loci of Disfluencies in the Speech Sequence

There appears to be a broad similarity between the factors affecting the loci of disfluencies of stutterers and nonstutterers at various age levels, as well as a few differences. In normally fluent adults and older schoolchildren, the factors seem to be essentially the same as those discussed in Chapter 10 in connection with stuttering. In this age range, normal disfluencies are more likely to occur on content words, longer words, words beginning with consonants, and words of lower predictability in context.[14] One exception is position of the word in the sentence, which seems to be an important factor only in the youngest nonstutterers.[15] Another unexpected observation made by Lanyon (1968) was that in the spontaneous speech of adult nonstutterers, disfluency was not related to the predictability of words in context, as it was in oral reading.

The outstanding difference in the loci of disfluency, however, is not between stutterers and nonstutterers. It is between children of preschool age and older children, whether stutterers or not.

The Loci of Disfluencies in Preschool Children Are Anomalous It was in stutterers that the anomalous pattern of distribution of early disfluencies first showed itself. In a clinical study of developmental forms of stuttering by Bloodstein

[14] Lounsbury (1954), Mann (1955). Goldman-Eisler (1958a, 1958b, 1961), Maclay and Osgood (1959), Blankenship (1964), Blankenship and Kay (1964), Silverman and Williams (1968), Chaney (1969), Williams, Silverman, and Kools (1969b), F. H. Silverman (1972).

[15] Silverman and Williams (1968), Chaney (1969), Williams, Silverman, and Kools (1969b).

(1960b), several distinctive aspects of the earliest phase of the disorder appeared to emerge. Among these was a tendency for almost all of the stuttering events to take place at the beginning of the sentence for most children. A second feature was a tendency for most stuttering to occur on function words, especially pronouns, conjunctions, and prepositions. This finding, that early stuttering and normal disfluency tends to cluster on function words, regardless of position within the sentence, has been replicated by a number of other researchers since that time: Bernstein (1981) for English, Dworzynski, Howell, and Natke (2003),[16] and Natke, Sandrieser, Pietrowsky, and Kalveram (2006) for German, Au-Yeung, Gomez, and Howell (2003) for Spanish.

Still another was a tendency toward frequent repetition of whole words. This all added up to typical sequences such as "*And-and-and-and Ira's cousin came too*," or "*Her-her-her-her name is Leslie. I-I-I-I told you already*." These were by no means wholly new observations. Bluemel (1932), in his original description of what he termed "primary" stuttering, said ". . . it commonly assumes the form of repetition of the first word of the sentence. . . . Often we hear repetition of initial consonants or initial syllables of words, and especially of introductory words to sentences."

Furthermore, the statement that referred to prepositions in the same breath as pronouns and conjunctions eventually needed to be qualified. Several years later, Bloodstein and Gantwerk (1967) did a quantitative study of the grammatical factor in the disfluencies of 13 stutterers from about 3 to 6.5 years of age. Two main findings appeared. In the first place, the grammatical factor as it exists in developed stuttering was absent. Stuttering tended to occur on all parts of speech, for the most part in proportion to how frequently the various parts of speech were represented in the child's verbal output. Second, there was a distinct tendency for pronouns and conjunctions (but not prepositions) to be stuttered on more often than would have been expected by chance.

[16]Although the age range in this study was from 7–11 years of age.

This was an unusual departure from previous findings on older stutterers, and it seemed even more remarkable when a study of elementary school–aged children by Williams, Silverman, and Kools (1969b) showed that, with just a few years of development, the grammatical factor seemed to change abruptly to conform to the adult pattern. What did it mean? The interpretation that Bloodstein and Gantwerk (1967) offered of their findings of patterns observed in preschool stutterers was based on the premise that when stutterers repeat a sound or syllable, they are repeating the initial fragment of a word because they feel helpless to say the word in its entirety. They speculated that young children often tend to fragment sentences rather than words. This would explain the unusually frequent repetition of the first words of sentences. Since the first words of sentences are often pronouns or conjunctions, this seemed to them to account for the high frequency of repetition of these parts of speech. Inspection of the transcripts confirmed that stuttered words at the beginnings of sentences were indeed often pronouns and conjunctions. Bloodstein and Gantwerk suggested that the grammatical functions of words acquire their influence on stuttering only as the child begins to find individual words forbidding and begins to fragment words rather than sentences. It was an explanation that seemed to catch a number of elusive facts in one net, but it ultimately proved to be in need of refinement. Bloodstein and Gantwerk did not suspect that in obtaining their findings, they had touched the edge of something that probably involves much more than just the grammatical factor alone.

A logical next step would be to find out whether these curious features of early stuttering were present in the disfluencies of preschool nonstutterers as well. In time, it became clear that they were. In the first place, E.-M. Silverman (1972b) reported that word repetition was exceedingly common in a group of 4-year-old typically fluent children. Then Helmreich and Bloodstein (1973) and E.-M. Silverman (1974) independently investigated the grammatical factor in the disfluencies of 4-year-old normally fluent children, and both found an unusually large amount of disfluency in only two categories—pronouns and conjunctions.[17]

Word Repetitions Occur at the Beginnings of Syntactic Units E.-M. Silverman (1974) reported two other notable findings. One was that there was a significant tendency for the normal disfluencies of 4-year-olds to occur on the first words of sentences. This was as expected. In addition, however, she reported that her children's disfluent pronouns and conjunctions very frequently occurred within the sentence as well as at the beginning. This observation, if it were to prove true of stutterers as well, would of course give little support to Bloodstein and Gantwerk's attempt to explain the high frequency of stuttering on pronouns and conjunctions as a consequence of the fact that these parts of speech are often located at the beginnings of sentences.

Why would a child repeat a pronoun or conjunction in the middle of a sentence? To illustrate the point, we can examine some samples of the recorded speech of preschool stutterers made by the first author. In these samples, virtually all of the word repetitions, and even the majority of the part-word repetitions, occur at the beginnings of syntactic units—that is, at the beginnings of sentences, clauses, verb phrases, noun phrases, or prepositional phrases. We will now examine one of the samples.[18] In the following transcript, an arrow following a sound means a prolongation of the sound. The horizontal line indicates a silent interval.

> *Once upon a time there w . . . th-there-there-there was a _______ a sailor, and he . . . and his name was Ira, and-and then a-a big whale and . . . came along, and-and-and no one could catch that whale e-except-except Ira, and it was M → by Dick. N-no sai → lors could catch him. And so once upon a time all the sailors came out to see Ira catch that whale, and (swallow, gasp) and-and-and-and Ira's cousin came too. So they . . . I-Ira (unintelligible fragment) with the harpoons, and Ira got a harpoon, a-and-and they . . . But Moby Dick has-has-has harpoons in-in himself, Moby Dick.*

This sample abounds in word repetitions. Note that each one occurs at the beginning of a clause, such as "*and no one could catch that whale*," a verb phrase such as "*has harpoons in himself*," a noun phrase such as "*a big whale*," or a prepositional phrase such as "*in himself*." In no case is a word repeated at the end of a sentence or at the end of a constituent syntactic unit within a sentence. That is, there are no utterances such as "*Once upon a time-time all the sailors . . .*," or "*No sailors could catch him-him*," or "*Moby Dick-Dick has harpoons in himself*." As examples of stuttering, these are as eccentric as "*look-k-k*" or "*Bob-b-b*."

In the other samples, the same rules were observed. Four were fairly good illustrations of the tendency of word and part-word repetitions to occur very frequently on the first words of sentences There were many examples such as "*He-he-he-he . . . h → is fathers' _______ name _______ is Stevie too*," "*'Cause-'cause-'cause-'cause I'll get sick*," and "*Weh-weh-weh well I think you forgot wuh-one other thing*."

The remaining case was in marked contrast to the others. There were no word repetitions. The stutterings consisted chiefly of sound repetitions, prolongations, and hard attacks on sound. An example was "*I → have t → wo s → s-sisters*." The stuttering was not confined to the first words of syntactic units, but was distributed as typically found in developed stuttering. If the child's repetitions were fragmentations of anything, they were clearly fragmentations of words. It was an example of stuttering in a more advanced form. In our experience, such early cases of more advanced stuttering are not rare, but they are not typical of children brought for treatment as stutterers in the earliest years.

In brief, these observations suggested that there are certain regularities that govern the distribution of early stuttering in its typical form. To verify them, Bloodstein and Grossman (1981) subsequently ex-

[17] There were also some respects in which the findings differed from those that had been obtained on stutterers. In the Bloodstein and Gantwerk study, the increase in disfluency on pronouns and conjunctions was at the expense of nouns and interjections. In the Helmreich and Bloodstein study, it was largely at the expense of nouns, verbs, and prepositions.

[18] For a more detailed report of this study, see Bloodstein (1974).

amined longer samples of the speech of five additional preschool stutterers. Of the 135 words that these children were heard to repeat, all except one were the first word of a syntactic unit.[19] To be sure, the other features of their disfluency, such as part-word repetitions and prolongations, also showed a strong tendency to occur at the beginnings of syntactic units, but 18 percent of such features appeared at other loci. In the case of word repetitions, we seem to be dealing, not with a tendency, but essentially with a rule. Word repetitions appear to occur at the beginnings of syntactic structures as often as sound or syllable repetitions occur at the beginnings of words.

In confirmation of this hypothesis, Bernstein (1981) conducted a statistical analysis of the spontaneous speech of eight young children who stuttered. She confirmed that stuttering occurred at syntactic constituent boundaries, rather than on words inside of sentential constituents, at a much higher level than would be predicted by chance.

Further Inferences and Questions What does this regularity mean? In the first place, it would seem that the features of early stuttering that appear anomalous—its frequent occurrence on function words, its strong affinity for the beginnings of sentences, and the numerous repetitions of whole words—can all be accounted for by supposing that stuttering has its origin in an early stage of fragmentation of syntactic units. The essence of this assumption is that children repeat the initial word of the unit because to attempt the unit as a whole is too difficult. Repetition allows time for the child to plan and then execute the remainder of the constituent.

Sometimes children may repeat whole phrases for the same apparent reason; phrase repetitions occur regularly at the beginnings of syntactic units too. It also seems probable that many if not most of the sound and syllable repetitions of young children have the same meaning. The great majority of them occur at the beginnings of syntactic units, often in conjunction with word repetitions (as in "*a-and-and-a-a-a-and*"). Wall, Starkweather, and Cairns (1981) found them in nine young stutterers mainly at the beginnings of clauses, especially "and" clauses. Bernstein (1981) found them chiefly at the beginnings of sentences in nonstutterers and at the beginnings of sentences and verb phrases in stutterers. Bloodstein and Grossman (1981) found them in five stutterers primarily at the beginnings of sentences or clauses and also at the beginnings of verb phrases, noun phrases within sentences, prepositional phrases, and infinitive constructions beginning with "to." There was essential consistency among all three studies. Similar findings were reported by Howell and Au-Yeung (1995).

The difference in the case of part-word repetitions is that they can also be viewed as fragmentations of words. When a part-word repetition occurs on the last word of a syntactic unit (as in "*I painted a h-house*"), it must, in fact, be viewed as such if it is a fragmentation at all. Sound and syllable repetitions in places other than the beginnings of syntactic units are far more frequent, however, in the stuttering of older children and adults. In general, disfluencies in the later constituents of grammatical units are rare at the onset of stuttering. In an analysis based on the cohort studied by Bernstein Ratner and colleagues (e.g., Bernstein Ratner & Silverman, 2000), Bernstein Ratner and Wijnen (2007) report that only a single whole-word repetition was found in utterance-final position for their study children, and other constituent-final disfluencies were extremely rare as well.

While the hypothesis that early stuttering represents the fragmentation of syntactic units may give us an inkling of what the child is doing, we are left with the question of the ultimate reasons for the behavior. Since syntactic units are likely to be natural units of motor planning, one possibility is that the child's fragmentations may reflect difficulty in the ability to execute the motor aspects of speech production. The results of a study by DeJoy and Gregory (1973) on normally fluent 4-year-old children seem to support this view. They found that the amount of disfluency in the initial segments of the children's sentences increased with the length of the sentences, but had

[19] One child repeated the word "school" at the end of a noun phrase: "My school school my my my my my school's gonna have a big cake . . ."

no relationship to their syntactic complexity. On the other hand, the basic problem might be more closely related to grammatical uncertainty, since this would seem to accord well with the fact that many stutterers experience some early difficulty with language acquisition (see Chapter 8) and that many studies to be discussed later in this chapter suggest that linguistic factors influence the frequency of stuttering in the speech of young children (see Hall, Wagovich, & Bernstein Ratner, 2007, for more detailed synopsis of such research). In this case, the difficulty would be with linguistic encoding of the utterance targets rather than their motor execution. It is still difficult to choose between these options, which may not be mutually exclusive. As Anne Smith and her colleagues have shown (Chapters 4 and 8), difficulty in linguistic encoding may cascade into stability of motor gestures.

There is another pressing question. What is the reason for the early transition that stutterers seem to make from fragmentation of syntactic units to fragmentation of words? Again we are without an answer, but not totally without some basis for speculation. Few persons are aware of syntactic units as such, but essentially all speakers of a language develop an awareness of individual words. Speech consciousness means, above all, word consciousness. As Kamhi, Lee, and Nelson (1985) have shown, however, preschool children tend to have an incompletely developed awareness of words, and are not very metalinguistically mature. Perhaps as this awareness of language and its characteristics grows, whatever generalized sense of difficulty in speaking they have acquired therefore begins more and more to develop into a sense of the formidability of words. This feeling may be exaggerated in the case of stutterers, but it may also have much to do with the part-word repetitions of children who are regarded as normally fluent speakers.

Do Word-Bound Factors Influence the Loci of Early Disfluencies? In Chapter 10, we saw that the stuttering of older children and adults tends to be influenced by certain attributes of words. For example, they are more likely to stutter on content words, words beginning with consonants, and longer words. If early stuttering consists for the most part of fragmentation of syntactic units rather than words, this would appear to imply an easily verifiable prediction. The loci of early stutterings should not be strongly influenced by word-bound factors, except to the extent that such factors may happen to characterize the first words of syntactic units. It would also be of interest to learn to what extent this is true of the early disfluency of normally fluent speakers, since we would like to know whether normal disfluency is related to stuttering.

The evidence so far supports this prediction in the speech of both preschool-age stutterers and nonstutterers. For example, an analysis by Bloodstein and Grossman (1981) of five children's repetitions, prolongations, and hard attacks on sound showed little influence of word-bound factors. As in the study by Bloodstein and Gantwerk (1967), there was no grammatical factor as such; pronouns and conjunctions, rather than content words, were stuttered on to an unusual degree, evidently because they were so often the first words of syntactic units. Only one child showed any significant preponderance of stuttering on consonants over vowels. None of the children stuttered more on polysyllabic than monosyllabic words; there was, in fact, a distinct tendency in the opposite direction, apparently because so many of these children's sentences and clauses began with such words as "he," "and," "but," and "so." As expected, stuttering occurred with great frequency on the first words of sentences. The failure of initial consonants to elicit more stuttering than initial vowels was also reported by Wall, Starkweather, and Harris (1981) in their study of nine preschool stutterers.

As noted in Chapter 8, there has been a general failure to link *stuttering* frequency to phonetic variables (Bernstein Ratner, 2005). Throneburg, Yairi, and Paden (1994) could not associate stuttering with traditional measures of phonological complexity in young children. Logan and Conture (1997) found that neither stuttering frequency nor duration were significantly associated with syllable structure measures in children's spontaneous utterances. Bernstein Ratner (2001) found disproportionately high frequency of stuttering on early acquired, rather than late-acquired, sounds in the speech of preschool-aged children who stutter, presumably because the words containing these sounds were almost universally function words that initiate questions (e.g., *who, what, where, how*), known to be linguistically challenging for young children.

In the case of *normal* disfluency, independent investigations by E.-M. Silverman (1974) and Helmreich and Bloodstein (1973) showed, as we have already seen, that the grammatical factor is absent. Sichel (1973) investigated the phonetic (consonant versus vowel) factor in a group of typically fluent preschool children. This too was absent. The children tended to have a somewhat unexpected amount of disfluency on words beginning with vowels, in large part because of the frequency with which they repeated the word "and" at the beginnings of sentences and clauses. Finally, E.-M. Silverman (1975) studied both the phonetic factor and the influence of word length in normally fluent 4-year-olds in a preschool classroom situation and in a structured interview situation. No phonetic factor was observed in either situation. Word length had no influence on disfluency in the classroom situation. In the interview situation, there was slightly more than expected disfluency on monosyllabic words, which may have reflected other properties of the words, other than their syllable structure.

The influence of word frequency on stuttering in children close to onset was examined in an unpublished report summarized in Yairi and Ambrose (2005, p. 248). B. Johnson et al. (2001) found no overall word frequency effect for young children, unlike that seen in older stutterers. However, a complex relationship was found once only stuttered words were considered. If a low-frequency word was stuttered once, it was likely to be stuttered again, while no such relationship was found for high-frequency words. The authors proposed that a single incident of difficult phonological encoding was influential in conditioning the likelihood of future stuttering on rarely used words.

So far in our research, neither early stuttering nor the disfluencies of normally fluent young children seem to be notably influenced by the word-bound factors that operate in the case of older speakers. It seems very clear to us that both early disfluency and early stuttering reflect difficulty in the encoding of syntactic units. How these patterns contribute to patterns of older speakers' normal disfluencies and stuttering will require further investigation in order to be better understood.

Other Factors A number of attempts have been made to test additional hypotheses about the loci of early disfluencies. In a study of nine preschool-age stutterers, Wall, Starkweather, and Harris (1981) were concerned with the influence of voicing transitions. Their main finding was that stuttering most often occurred following a pause, regardless of the type of voicing transition.

In a study of four typically fluent children aged 2 to 3 years, Colburn and Mysak (1982b) found little support for the hypothesis that normal disfluencies would be associated with semantic structures just emerging in the children's grammar (e.g., action, intention, negation, etc.). Disfluency occurred more often on well-learned and practiced structures. Both E.-M. Silverman (1973a) and Colburn (1985) found a significant tendency for early normal disfluencies to cluster on the same or consecutive words.

VARIATIONS IN FREQUENCY

A great deal can be learned about early stuttering and its relationship to normal disfluency through research on the conditions under which the disfluencies of stuttering and nonstuttering children vary in frequency. The promise of this approach is underscored by the very considerable amount of data showing that among adults and older children, normal disfluencies tend to vary under some of the same conditions as does stuttering. For example, there is a large amount of evidence that normally fluent speakers exhibit something highly similar if not identical to the adaptation effect in stutterers.[20] Normal disfluencies of adults are also influenced by

[20] Starbuck and Steer (1953, 1954) Brutten (1963), Gray (1965a), Gray and Karmen (1967), Williams, Silverman, and Kools (1968), Soderberg (1969a), F. H. Silverman (1970b, 1970c, 1970d), Silverman and Williams (1971), Silverman and Bloom (1973), Kroll and Hood (1976), Miller and Miller (1977), Moore, Cunko, and Flowers (1979).

response-contingent stimuli in essentially the same way as is stuttering.[21] F. H. Silverman (1971) showed that the normal disfluencies of adults diminish when speech is timed to a rhythmic stimulus, and both Silverman and Goodban (1972) and Sherrard (1975) found that normal disfluency in oral reading was reduced under masking noise. The relationship of normal speech interruptions to anxiety has been extensively studied, chiefly in adults, by Mahl (1956, 1961) and his coworkers, and others.

Despite the many similarities found in these and other studies between the variables affecting the frequency of stuttering and normal disfluency in adults, research has also disclosed occasional differences. It is impossible to know whether such differences are basic or merely reflect divergent processes of development. We believe that it is only in the study of the relationship between stuttering and normal disfluency in their earliest phases that some possibility exists for obtaining answers to questions about the origin of stuttering.

Nonstutterers

Conversational Context Davis (1940) observed the situations in which each of 62 typically fluent 2- to 5-year-old children exhibited speech repetitions of all types during an hour of free play in a preschool situation. She found that repetitions tended to occur with outstanding frequency under certain conditions—for example, when the child was excited over his or her own activity, wanted to direct the activity of another child, was attempting to attract the attention of another child or of the teacher, was forced by the teacher to change an activity, or wanted an object in the possession of another child. In a study of children's interactions with their own and other children's mothers, Meyers and Freeman (1985b) observed that normally fluent 4- to 5-year-olds tended to be more disfluent when interrupting a mother.

Other studies have attempted to vary the frequency of normal childhood disfluency experimentally by varying the listeners or situations.[22] In this way, more disfluency has been found in a structured interview than in a preschool classroom situation, in socialized than in egocentric speech, and in solitary play than in conversation with an adult. Newman and Smit (1989) found increases in the disfluency of normally fluent 4-year-olds when the experimenter decreased her response time from three seconds to one second in conversational interaction with the children. Bernstein Ratner (1992) found that slowing mothers' speech rate reduced the rate of their children's disfluency, while both slowing rate and attempting to simplify language input increased both the rate of children's interrupting behaviors as well as their disfluencies.

Language Complexity Among the more interesting findings have been those dealing with the influence of language complexity on normal disfluency.[23] Haynes and Hood (1978) studied the effect of adult modeling of simple and complex language on the fluency of typically fluent 5-year-old children. The instructions to each child were, in part: "*I'm going to look at these pictures and say something about each one. Listen very carefully to my sentences so you will know what kinds they are. Later, we will take turns making sentences and I want you to try to make your sentences like mine.*" After listening to the experimenter model a series of sentences, the children were asked to make up their own sentences for each of a new series of pictures. In the simple condition, the experimenter used sentences that contained no major transformations[24] and few pronouns or auxiliary verbs. In the complex condition, sentences were of comparable length and

[21] Siegel and Martin (1965a, 1965b, 1966, 1967, 1968), Brookshire and Martin (1967), Brookshire (1969), Brookshire and Eveslage (1969), Siegel, Lenske, and Broen (1969), Siegel and Hanson (1972), Hutchinson and Mackay (1973), Kazdin (1973), Hasbrouck and Martin (1974).

[22] Egland (1955), E.-M. Silverman (1971, 1972a, 1973b), Martin, Haroldson, and Kuhl (1972a, 1972b), Martin and Haroldson (1975), Wexler (1982).

[23] A tabled summary of many of the studies conducted in this area of inquiry may be found in Hall, Wagovich, and Bernstein Ratner (2007).

[24] In this study and some others conducted in this general time period, principles of transformational-generative (TG) grammar were used to define complexity of sentence structures. Although changes have occurred in linguistic theory over the years, there is still evidence that the basic ordering of complexity used in these studies corresponds to gradations in linguistic encoding difficulty (see Berko Gleason & Bernstein Ratner, 1998).

involved pronouns, negatives, and more difficult transformational rules. Analysis showed that the two conditions did, in fact, produce a difference in the syntactic complexity of the children's language, their mean length of response, and their disfluency. The disfluencies that increased in frequency in the complex condition were chiefly word repetitions, revisions, incomplete phrases, and "disrhythmic phonations" (prolongations, hard attacks, or broken words).

In a study by Pearl and Bernthal (1980), normally fluent 3- and 4-year-old children repeated the experimenter's production of sentences representing several basic grammatical types. The passive sentences, typically among the last to be acquired by children, occasioned more disfluency than the others. Simple, affirmative, active sentences were the most fluently produced. The 5-year-olds studied by Gordon, Luper, and Peterson (1986) did not demonstrate this effect when simply repeating sentences after an experimenter, but did so in a sentence modeling procedure similar to that used by Haynes and Hood. The passive construction also elicited more stuttering in a study by Gordon and Luper (1989), although Gordon (1991) failed to confirm this. Bernstein Ratner and Sih (1987), using a sentence imitation procedure, and McLaughlin and Cullinan (1989), using a sentence modeling procedure, found that the disfluencies of preschool-age nonstutterers increased with sentence complexity. Modeling of sentences produces more stuttering than simple sentence imitation, as Gordon, Luper, and Peterson (1986), Gordon and Luper (1989), and Gordon (1991) all showed.

In analyzing spontaneous speech samples from preschool-age children, Yaruss, Newman, and Flora (1999) found more disfluency in utterances that were longer (contained more clausal constituents) and more syntactically complex. Logan and LaSalle (1999) found that utterances with both single and clustered disfluencies were longer in terms of syllables, clauses, and clausal constituents than were fluently produced utterances in typically fluent young children's speech. Zackheim and Conture (2003) found that normal disfluency rates in preschool-aged children increased when children produced conversational utterances that exceeded their typical mean length of utterance (MLU).

With children able to read (third to sixth grade), Cecconi, Hood, and Tucker (1977) found that the amount of disfluency in oral reading varied with the reading difficulty of the material. The disfluencies most affected were word and part-word repetitions, "disrhythmic phonations," and "tense pauses." In a single-subject investigation of the oral reading of a 5-year-old boy, Hegde (1982) analyzed the antecedents of disfluencies of various types. By far, the most frequent antecedent was poor lexical control (unacceptable pronunciations of unfamiliar words), which resulted in disfluencies of all types.

Stutterers

Context and Feedback Conditions There are now a number of reports describing conditions under which the frequency of stuttering varies in young children. A tendency of 5- to 8-year-old stutterers to show adaptation was reported by Neelley and Timmons (1967). In two preschool stutterers, Martin, Kuhl, and Haroldson (1972) found a decrease in stuttering as a result of contingent time-out procedures (this response is described in greater detail in Chapter 11). Razdolsky (1965) reported the interesting observation that of a group of 32 stutterers between 2 and 6 years of age, the majority stuttered as much or almost as much when they were alone as when they were speaking to a listener. By contrast, most of a group of school-age stutterers spoke appreciably more easily when they were alone. The only preschool stutterers who did so to a marked degree were said to be three bright 6-year-olds who were embarrassed by their stuttering. In contrast, Meyers (1989, 1990) studied the disfluencies of 12 2- to 6-year-old stutterers in dyadic interactions with mother, father, and a familiar playmate. Frequency of stuttering did not vary with conversational partner, nor was there any evidence that stuttering was affected by the positive or negative intent of the partner's verbal interactions or by whether the partner's interactions consisted of comments, questions, interruptions, or imperatives.

Linguistic Complexity In a study of nine stuttering children aged 4 to 7 years, Stocker and Usprich (1976) employed a series of questions with increasing levels of communicative demand[25]—for example, about a toy car: (1) Is it hard or soft? (2) What is it? (3) Where would you keep one? (4) Tell me everything you know about it. (5) Make up your own story about it. The frequency of stuttering increased with levels of demand, with a particularly marked increase occurring between levels 3 and 5. There was much less stuttering in a similar condition requesting responses identical to those given previously (e.g., "*This is what you told me about the car last time ... Now tell it to me again*").

A replication of the Stocker and Usprich study by Martin, Parlour, and Haroldson (1990) did not unequivocally confirm the inference that early stuttering varies with level of linguistic demand, but the question of a link to language difficulty was pursued in other forms. Bernstein Ratner and Sih (1987) had 3- to 6-year-old children imitate utterances varying in 10 stages of syntactic complexity from simple active affirmative declarative sentences to those involving varying forms of embedded clauses. In stutterers and nonstutterers alike, the amount of disfluency was generally correlated with documented order of development of the sentence types in children's spontaneous speech. Gaines, Runyan, and Meyers (1991) found that young children's stuttered sentences in spontaneous speech tended to be longer and more complex than their fluent sentences. Weiss and Zebrowski (1992) also observed more stuttering on longer and more complex utterances produced by children 4 to 10 years of age. Zackheim and Conture (2003) found more stuttering in preschooler's conversational utterances with their mothers that exceeded their typical mean length of utterance. Logan (2003) found that longer utterances were likely to be accompanied by higher rates of stuttering, but that utterances embedded in multiple utterance turns did not produce more stuttering than length-matched single utterance turns.

Logan and Conture (1997) collected conversational samples from young stuttering children conversing with their mothers; their stuttered utterances contained more clausal constituents than their length-matched fluent utterances. In general, most recent research has found that stuttering increases with linguistic complexity variables, such as Developmental Sentence Score (Gaines, Runyan, & Meyers, 1991; Ryan, 2000) or Mean Length of Utterance (Brundage & Bernstein Ratner, 1988).

Disfluency clusters (multiple stuttering events in sequence within an utterance) were found to be associated with increases in utterance length as measured in syllables, clauses, and clausal constituents by Logan and LaSalle (1999). Gordon (1991) reported that preschool children stuttered more on a sentence modeling than a sentence imitation task but failed to find that syntactic complexity of sentences had any effect. Kadi-Hanifi and Howell (1992) found that 2- to 6-year-old stutterers and nonstutterers were more disfluent on simple sentences in spontaneous speech than on complex ones. Older children were more disfluent on complex sentences.

Any impact of syntactic complexity on both stuttering and normal disfluency appears to disappear by the later years of childhood. Silverman and Bernstein Ratner (1997) found that normal disfluencies, but not stutters, increased with manipulation of sentence complexity in an elicited imitation task for adolescents who stutter.

Trautman, Healey, and Norris (2001) did find that conversational tasks affected fluency rates in children who stutter (as well as typically fluent children and children with language impairment): stuttering was increased under conditions where children had to provide decontextualized scripts (without picture or object prompts) or re-tell a story, compared to contextualized language production demands.

LANGUAGE ABILITIES OF YOUNG CHILDREN WHO STUTTER

As noted in Chapter 8, an enlarging body of literature suggests that individuals who stutter show subtle depression of language abilities when contrasted with appropriately matched groups of typically fluent speakers. In this section, we wish to highlight only a few findings that specifically pertain

[25]The Stocker Probe technique. See Stocker and Gerstman (1983).

to analyses of children observed close to stuttering onset.[26]

A few studies have shown no observable differences between the language abilities of children close to onset and their fluent peers (Watkins, Yairi, & Ambrose, 1999; Bonelli, Dixon, Bernstein Ratner, & Onslow, 2000). Others have shown subtle, subclinical depression of language abilities in this population (Ryan, 1992; Silverman & Bernstein Ratner, 2000, 2002; Anderson & Conture, 2000, 2004). One report from the Illinois project suggested that stronger language abilities, as measured by the *Preschool Language Scale*, at first diagnosis were a significant predictor of recovery (Yairi, Ambrose, Paden, & Throneburg, 1996), while another report suggested that patterns of increasingly complex spontaneous language use by the same group of children was associated with failure to recover from stuttering (Watkins, 2005).

OTHER ATTRIBUTES OF THE SPEECH OF NORMALLY DISFLUENT CHILDREN

If stuttering and normal disfluency in early childhood are related kinds of behavior, we might reasonably expect the more disfluent of a representative sample of normal speakers to have some of the same personal attributes that distinguish stuttering children as a group.

One basic personal attribute is age. Since there is a decline in the frequency with which cases of onset of stuttering are reported from year to year during childhood (see Chapter 3) it may be of some significance that with few exceptions, studies have found that the disfluency of typically fluent children also tends to decrease with age. For a brief period at about 2 years of age, children may show considerable variation in amount of disfluency with age, as both Colburn and Mysak (1982a) and Yairi (1982) observed in longitudinal studies. Evidently some children become more disfluent as language emerges. However, across the early childhood period as a whole, the decrease has been clearly apparent in most investigations.[27] DeJoy and Gregory (1985) found the decrease to be in word, part-word, and phrase repetitions; incomplete phrases; and "disrhythmic phonations" (prolongations, broken words, or hard attacks).

Another attribute is the child's gender. In view of the sex ratio in the incidence of stuttering, it would be interesting to know whether there is a difference in the amount of disfluency in the speech of normally fluent boys and girls. There is evidence that the sex ratio in stuttering tends to decrease as we go back into childhood from age level to age level, as we saw in Chapter 3. Glasner and Rosenthal (1957) found that among 153 children who were reported by their parents to have stuttered at some time before entering the first grade, the sex ratio was only 1.4 to 1 when corrected for a sex difference in the total sample surveyed.[28] Månsson (2000) found a ratio of 1.6 to 1, while Kloth, Janssen, Kraaimaat, and Brutten (1995) found a ratio of 1.65 to 1. There are some data that address the extent to which boys and girls differ in degree of normal disfluency. Fisher (1932) and Davis (1939) found somewhat more repetition, chiefly of syllables, among boys than girls. Essentially no sex differences were found, however, in later studies of young children by Johnson and Associates (1959, p. 208), Kools and Berryman (1971), Haynes and Hood (1977), Ratusnik, Kiriluk, and Ratusnik (1979), and Carlo and Watson (2003), who studied Spanish-speaking preschoolers.

Still a third characteristic about which we have some information is language and speech development. Young children who stutter often tend to be somewhat slow in the development of linguistic and articulation skills, as we saw in Chapter 8. With respect to normal disfluency, there have been somewhat inconsistent findings. In 62 2- to 5-year-old

[26] See also Table 9-1 in Hall, Wagovich, and Bernstein Ratner (2007).

[27] Adams (1932), Fisher (1932), Davis (1939), Branscom, Hughes, and Oxtoby (1955), Yairi and Clifton (1972), Haynes and Hood (1977), Wexler (1982), DeJoy and Gregory (1985).

[28] Andrews and Harris (1964, p. 31) found, however, that sex ratios based on incidence figures such as these tend to be lower than ratios based on the prevalence of stuttering at a given time, possibly because episodes of stuttering tend to be briefer in girls than in boys. They reported that for small numbers of children who were stuttering in a given year during the first five years of the Newcastle survey the sex ratio averaged 2.6 to 1.

children, Davis (1940) found essentially no relationship between amount of speech repetition and such measures of language maturity as mean length of response, amount of verbal output, vocabulary, number of correct speech sounds, intelligibility, and percentage of functionally complete responses. Likewise, Berryman and Kools (1975) found that among 92 first graders, disfluency was unrelated to reading ability, intelligence, or judges' ratings of language level, while among children aged 4, 6, and 8 years examined by Haynes and Hood (1977), there was no relationship between disfluency and syntactic proficiency as measured by Lee's Developmental Sentence Score. Enger, Hood, and Shulman (1988) reported no significant difference in language measures between highly fluent and highly disfluent young children in a school program with a preponderance of gifted children with advanced language development.

On the other hand, Borack (1969) found that elementary school–aged children with articulation problems were significantly more disfluent than a comparable group with normal articulation. Muma (1971) carried out an analysis of the language performance of carefully selected highly fluent and disfluent typically developing 4-year-olds. The two groups did not differ in their use of various sentence types, but the highly fluent group tended to use more sentences characterized by what linguists then termed double-base transformations. Similarly, DeJoy and Gregory (1976) selected from a group of 60 samples of the speech of 3-year-old and 5-year-old children the 10 with the highest number and the 10 with the lowest number of disfluencies of various types and compared the two groups of samples with respect to Developmental Sentence Scores. The disfluent children scored lower in syntactic maturity than the fluent ones in the case of word repetitions, pauses, incomplete phrases, and, for the 5-year-olds, in the case of part-word repetitions. Stocker and Usprich (1976) found more disfluencies in preschool children who had articulation problems and delayed language development than in children who did not. Similar findings were obtained by Ragsdale and Sisterhen (1984) for 5- and 6-year-olds with articulation difficulties and by Lybolt (1986) for eight children with expressive language deficits. Work done both by Hall, Yamashita, and Aram (1993) and Boscolo, Bernstein Ratner, and Rescorla (2002) suggest that children with disordered or delayed language abilities tend to produce more disfluent speech (see Hall, Wagovich, & Bernstein Ratner, 2007, for summary discussion). In particular, Boscolo, Bernstein Ratner, and Rescorla found that the stutter-like disfluency rate was sufficiently elevated in children with a history of expressive language delay that such children could, in principle, be misdiagnosed as children who stutter. However, disfluencies were produced without any evident signs of struggle or awareness. Merits-Patterson and Reed (1981) reported the interesting finding that young children receiving language therapy produced more disfluencies, in the form of word and part-word repetitions, than children with normal language development, whereas comparably language-delayed children not getting treatment did not.

The findings of these studies suggest that a relationship does exist between normal childhood disfluency and speech and language skill, but that it can be demonstrated only in children with wide disparities either in fluency or in speech and language skill. This was given a special kind of emphasis in a study by Westby (1979), in which stutterers, highly disfluent normal speakers, and typically disfluent normal speakers in kindergarten and first grade were compared on several measures of grammar, vocabulary, and semantic aspects of language. The highly disfluent typical children scored significantly lower than the typically fluent children on most of the measures. There was no difference between the highly disfluent typical speakers and the children who stuttered.

Finally, the familial tendency in the incidence of stuttering suggests the possibility that more disfluent children in general tend to have more disfluent parents. Yairi and Jennings (1974) correlated the number of disfluencies of various types to be found in the speech of a group of typically fluent preschool boys with the amount in the speech of their mothers and fathers, but could find essentially no evidence of a relationship.

SUMMARY REMARKS

The main purpose of this chapter has been to consider what relationship, if any, there is between stuttering and normal disfluency in young children. The basic empirical question is whether any "natural lines of demarcation" exist between the disfluency of those who are called stutterers and those who are called normal speakers. If, as Johnson asserted, there were not, we could draw either of two conclusions. These would depend on how we define what we mean by "abnormal" in relation to fluent speech. If, like Johnson, we viewed the abnormal as something that is by definition qualitatively distinct from the normal, we would have to conclude that stuttering had to be defined at least in part on the basis of the evaluative judgments of listeners, but might be located in subtle production characteristics yet to be identified. If, on the other hand, we were willing to accept a relative, quantitative, or dimensional concept of abnormality, we could if we wished define stuttering in young children as a relatively severe degree of normal disfluency or of those specific types of normal disfluency from which it could not be readily demarcated.

The first alternative is embodied in Johnson's avoidance or interaction hypothesis. The second is what we have called the continuity hypothesis. In effect, the avoidance theory says that if one child's speech repetitions are normal, there is little justification for calling another child's speech repetitions anything else just because there are more of them. By contrast, the continuity hypothesis says that if one child's speech repetitions are stuttering, there is little reason to call another child's repetitions anything else merely because there is a relatively normal amount of them. While these two statements appear to represent only differences in definition of stuttering, there is a vast distinction between them in their ultimate implications for theory and therapy. In the first instance we must look for the source of the child's problem largely in the perceptual distortions of a listener by reason of which the child comes to regard disfluencies as a matter for concern and to struggle to avoid them. In the second case, we must look for the causes of the problem largely in the nature of the stutters that are latent in almost all children's speech and in the variety of possible factors that might tend to increase them.

Some readers might reject both of these approaches to the etiology of stuttering because they do not accept the assumption that stutterers' and nonstutterers' disfluencies cannot be sharply differentiated empirically in early childhood. Increasing efforts have been made to find out whether any natural lines of demarcation between the two exist, either in the nature of the disfluencies themselves or in the stimulus variables that determine their distribution and frequency. Considerable evidence has accumulated that the essential features of what is generally called stuttering in young children are similar in kind to some of the features of disfluency that appear in the speech of many children who are not called stutterers. There also appears to be a striking similarity in the manner in which these features are distributed in stutterers' and nonstutterers' speech. Nevertheless, no broad consensus exists on the question of whether early stuttering and certain types of normal disfluency are united by a single continuum. The question has many aspects still open to further investigation.

It may not have been lost on the reader that in pursuing the main purpose of this chapter, we have been led repeatedly by different paths to another subject, the relationship between stuttering and language development in young children. The pieces of evidence suggesting that early stuttering may be fragmentations of syntactic structures, that the more disfluent normally fluent children are poorer in language skill, that normal disfluency varies in frequency with changes in language complexity, that stutterers are more often delayed in language development than nonstutterers—all these observations are obviously capable of being related to each other, particularly in light of emerging data that show subtle language weakness in adults who stutter as susceptibility of speech motor control to linguistic stressors. As to whether and how they are connected, however, all that anyone can as yet offer are inferences and speculations.

Chapter 13

Inferences and Conclusions

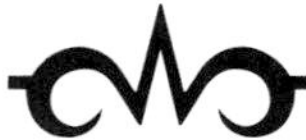

The purpose of this chapter is to draw some inferences about the meaning of the research findings we have reviewed in the preceding chapters. If we summarize the general conclusions of these chapters, much of the significant information we have gained in our survey of research may be contained in the following statements.

SUMMARY

Stuttering consists of a variety of types of involuntary speech interruptions. It affects speech rate, respiration, and phonation and leaves its imprint on such physiological activities as heart rate, blood distribution, and brain waves. Much of the stutterer's functional problem, however, consists of maladaptive attitudes and coping mechanisms that develop with the passage of time.

Stuttering generally begins in the preschool years, more commonly in boys than girls. A large proportion of those who begin to stutter recover spontaneously early in childhood. Stuttering is found the world over in essentially every distinguishable type of population. The disorder tends to run in families. Familial studies and research on twins show that the transmission is genetic, although environment also appears to play a part. At this writing (2007), research has not yet disclosed conclusive evidence of the type of genetic transmission or the chromosome on which the gene or genes that predispose to stuttering are located.

No major personality differences between stutterers and nonstutterers have been discovered despite prolonged and exhaustive research efforts. Stutterers are not markedly distinguished by any specific character traits. They more often than nonstutterers exhibit mild degrees of maladjustment that are readily attributable to the effect of stuttering.

Numerous studies have been done on the stutterer's motor skills, sensory abilities, physiological functions, and integrative cortical processes. This research has been carried out mainly on adults. It has often tended to result in findings that are conflicting, or that are open to the interpretation that they are an effect rather than a cause of stuttering. Although these studies have not produced clear evidence of a physical deficit underlying stuttering, hints of possible deficits, particularly at the level of central neurological control of speech and language production, have continued to motivate research on the neurophysiological characteristics of people who stutter.

Stutterers are often, although not always, reported to be delayed in speech and language development. In early childhood, they exhibit subtle deficiencies in language skills more often than other children. They are distinctly more prone to have profiles of delayed or disordered articulation.

In its developed form, stuttering is distributed in the speech sequence largely in response to features of words that tend to make them difficult, conspicuous, or evocative of past speech failure. Stuttering varies in frequency from situation to situation, chiefly in response to such factors as communicative pressure and awareness of oneself as a speaker or stutterer. In the absence of such factors, it may be absent altogether.

Certain types of disfluency—especially part-word repetition, repetition of whole words, and prolongation of sounds—tend to occur more often in the speech of children regarded as stutterers than in the speech of children who are not. Evidence suggests that the speech repetitions of young children are related to difficulty with whole syntactic units (aspects of grammatical processing) rather than to difficulty with words.

INFERENCES

What conclusions about the origin and nature of stuttering has all of this research led us to? For a significant portion of the twentieth century, a prevailing notion was that stuttering was a psychoneurotic disorder. This gave rise to a wealth of studies of the stutterer's personality, many of which appeared to be strenuous efforts to prove the theory correct. Sober reviews of this research finally led to the theory's downfall.

This era was followed by another distinct theoretical approach to stuttering, during which it was almost generally accepted that the disorder was brought about by parental diagnoses of children's normal disfluency as stuttering. The result was a massive research effort known as the Iowa Studies. The studies were essentially an attempt to prove the diagnosogenic theory correct. The principal investigators, like so many others, had little doubt that the theory was valid. Eventually it was discredited, in part by the revelation that stuttering was a heritable disorder. If stuttering can be inherited, parents who believe their child is stuttering are responding to something more than a product of their imagination.

To many, it has seemed to follow that if stuttering is not an "emotional" disorder, then it must necessarily be a "neurological" one. If it is, the neurological disorder must be of a kind that selectively affects the function of speech, since the typical stutterer appears normal on routine neurological examination. Accordingly, the view has developed that stuttering is a specific disorder of speech motor control. This inference has been pursued in a multitude of studies of stutterers' nonspeech oral-motor abilities, studies of stutterers' ostensibly fluent speech, and brain-imaging studies of stutterers during both speech comprehension and production. As we write this edition of the Handbook (2007), the findings have been promising, although somewhat conflicting or ambiguous and have not produced notable agreement about the nature of the posited neurolinguistic or neuro-motor basis of stuttering.

In the meantime, a complementary kind of research effort has developed on the basis of the supposition that stuttering begins in some sense as a disorder of language encoding. Ever since Bluemel (1932) suggested that stuttering in its incipient phase differs categorically from the fully developed form of the disorder, various distinctive aspects of early stuttering have come to light: early stuttering tends to come and go during language development in the form of episodes; it occurs invariably on the first word of a syntactic structure; as a result, the stuttered word is very often a function word, in contrast to developed stuttering, which generally occurs on content words; unlike developed stuttering, it does not seem to be markedly influenced by word-related factors such as word length or grammatical part of speech; it very frequently takes the form of repetitions of whole words in which the word itself is produced fluently. These observations lend themselves readily to the inference that early stuttering is essentially a difficulty in the execution of syntactic structures, in contrast to developed stuttering, which is so conspicuously a difficulty with individual words (Bloodstein, 2006). Moreover, it has not escaped the attention of researchers that preschool children rarely stutter on one-word utterances; that the onset of stuttering is rarely if ever reported prior to the acquisition of multiword phrases; that stuttering most often begins during the years in which children are learning the elements of syntax; that relatively large numbers of children recover from stuttering at just about the age when the acquisition of syntax is essentially complete; and that boys outnumber girls in the earliest stage of stuttering.

Complementing these facts is the mounting evidence from studies of the language abilities of children and adults who stutter. The majority of this evidence supports the view that, on the average, stutterers tend to develop language somewhat later and perform at subtly depressed levels on many types of language assessments when compared to typically fluent children. As in the case of research on speech motor control, the evidence is often conflicting. All that we can say for sure is that the current stage of our knowledge offers us a choice between two broad viewpoints, one neuromotor and the other linguistic. While often viewed as opposing models of the disorder, they may be complementary. Recent studies show that people who stutter may have speech motor systems that are particularly vulnerable to destabilization under conditions of relative linguistic stress. It is likely that much can be gained by seeing potential interactions among primary systems that have been implicated in stuttering, be they motoric, linguistic, cognitive, or emotional. Additionally, it should not be forgotten that there appears to be an underlying genetic basis for stuttering. What is genetically transmitted, in terms of predispositions in any of the abilities that subserve fluent speech production, is not yet clear. This may become clearer when the research that has begun to identify the gene or genes for stuttering has fulfilled its promise. With identified genes, we may better understand their impact on the child who begins to stutter, the child who spontaneously recovers, and the child who does not.

A separate issue, but one that bears directly on the etiology of stuttering, is whether there is a relationship between early stuttering and normal childhood disfluency. That they differ can hardly be disputed. The theory that parents cause stuttering by diagnosing perfectly normal disfluencies as stuttering has been discredited. The question that remains is whether the difference between early stuttering and normal disfluency is one of kind or degree. Although by no means all researchers agree, there are a number of reasons for considering the possibility that early stuttering is essentially an extreme degree of certain types of disfluency to be found in the speech of most young children. In the first place, they both occur invariably on the first word of a syntactic structure, usually a conjunction or pronoun, and in both, the dominant fluency type is whole word repetition.[1] In the second place, parents of preschool children often report episodes of stuttering of such brief duration that the incidence of the disorder in the early years is a matter of considerable vagueness and appears to depend in part on what we are willing to call stuttering. We are perhaps justified in wondering how much more often young children experience intervals of difficulty

[1]This is true when the comparison is made with stutterers who are commonly brought to the speech clinic. A curious paradox becomes evident when the comparison is made with children who are carefully selected for recent onset of stuttering. Most parents tend to wait for months before seeking help, as clinical experience and research findings indicate. It is chiefly when the speech difficulty is extreme that they bring the child for examination soon after onset. Such children are consequently not representative of stuttering children as a group.

so inconsequential that they may escape even the parents' notice or are shortly forgotten. It may be a reasonable inference that we are dealing here with something essentially equatable with the "stuttering" that Metraux (1950) and others have studied as a characteristic phenomenon in the speech of preschool children.

Third, we may recall the overlap that Johnson and his associates found to exist between the early disfluencies of stutterers and those of nonstutterers as described by parents. A considerable portion of the nonstutterers were reported to have had more prolongations and sound and syllable repetitions in their speech than did many of the stutterers. It is an interesting feature of this overlapping distribution that not only some of the stutterers, but some of the nonstutterers as well, were said to have shown signs of effort, tension, awareness, bewilderment, irritation, or the like in connection with their earliest disfluencies, despite the fact that all children who had ever been regarded as stutterers had been excluded from the comparison group. A plausible interpretation might seem to be that many ordinary young children frequently "stutter" somewhat and that a sharp distinction between the "normal" and the "abnormal" is simply not to be made. Nevertheless, this view, which has been referred to as the continuity hypothesis, is by no means accepted by all researchers. To some, the difference between normal and abnormal childhood disfluency is sufficient to suggest that they are distinct phenomena with different etiologies.

Finally we must consider the question of how incipient stuttering changes into a disorder of older children and adults in those instances in which the child fails to recover spontaneously in the early years. The difference between early and later stuttering is stark. Early stuttering is episodic, occurs on function words, occurs invariably on the first word of a syntactic structure, abounds in repetitions of whole words, and does not appear to be influenced by attributes of words. By contrast, developed stuttering is persistent, occurs on content words, may occur on the last word of a syntactic structure, far less often takes the form of whole word repetition, and is markedly influenced by attributes of words. In brief, stuttering changes from a difficulty with syntactic units to a difficulty with words.

Awareness also appears to play a role. Bluemel (1932) suggested that what he termed "primary" stuttering turns into "secondary" stuttering as the child becomes aware of his or her disfluency as a thing to be avoided. If this is so, the persistent form of stuttering is due to no more or less than a belief in the difficulty of speech. For most of us from an early age, speech means, above all, words. And so the beliefs that instigate the potential for stuttering soon center about individual words.

That beliefs may be the cause of violent emotions is all too well known. We have also all heard about "self-fulfilling prophecies." It should occasion neither surprise nor skepticism that they may cause moments of stuttering. Underlying the stutterer's array of beliefs about the difficulty of words is the dogma that he or she is a defective speaker who is helpless to speak in any other way. As a result, stutterers experience particular speech difficulty in circumstances that amplify their awareness of their role as speakers, and they tend to speak more fluently under conditions in which they forget that they stutter.

One way to express this inference is to say that stuttering is anticipatory struggle behavior. If a more specific description of the moment of stuttering is desired, it may perhaps be found in the statement that underlying the surface features of stuttering are the two elements of tension and fragmentation in speech. Tension is most readily observed in the prolongation of continuant consonants and also in hard attacks on stop consonants, essentially a lengthened stop phase followed by an over-aspirated plosive phase. Fragmentation of words is evident in the repetition of initial sounds or syllables and appears to result from the stutterer's conviction that the word is too difficult to attempt in its entirety. Such a view of repetitions is supported by the observation of Sheehan (1974) that some repetitions involve successively larger samples of the word, as in "th-thir-thirty-five." Repetitions are not so much repeated utterances as repeated stoppages.

Whatever appeal this or any other concept may have, it should not allow it to dull the sharpness of our perception that the stuttering moment remains an obscure phenomenon and that there are as yet no conclusive answers to such basic questions as whether it is "voluntary" or "involuntary" in nature, autonomically or centrally controlled, respondent or operant, learned in itself or an unlearned resultant of learned behaviors. The same may be said about the etiology of stuttering. Although we have ventured some inferences about it, we must conclude that there are few grounds for zeal in support of any single theory. It is hoped, however, that this book has helped to clarify some of the questions that are central to a solution of the problem.

Chapter 14

Treatment

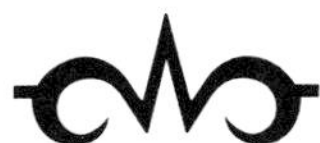

Views regarding the best approaches to the treatment of stuttering, like views of its etiology, are a matter of considerable controversy. The methods that have been attempted with some degree of success are extremely varied, and the recorded history of their use goes back in some cases to classical antiquity. In this chapter, we will briefly survey some of the principal remedial approaches, with emphasis on current practices.

PRINCIPLES OF EVIDENCE-BASED PRACTICE

Before reviewing the available research on the treatment of stuttering, it is worthwhile to consider criteria for the evaluation of this body of literature. Since the last edition of the *Handbook,* there has been a strong movement to ensure that health interventions are based on appropriately gathered and interpreted evidence. The movement, sometimes called Evidence-Based Practice, Medicine, or Treatment (EBP/EBM/EBT) or Empirically Validated Treatments (EVTs), is often referenced back to the work of David Sackett and colleagues within the medical profession (Sackett, Rosenberg, Gray, Haynes, & Richardson, 1996; Straus & Sackett, 1998). While no health care practitioners deliberately utilize interventions that they know to be ineffective, unfortunately many do employ treatments that are outdated, for which evidence does not meet more current standards for well-designed research, or that has not been shown in appropriately designed and implemented trials involving reasonable numbers of individuals to work for a large and/or representative sample of people.

In addition, repeated studies have shown that speech-language pathologists often feel their training to treat stuttering has been less than optimal

(Cooper & Cooper, 1996; Crichton-Smith, Wright, & Stackhouse, 2003; Klassen & Kroll, 2005),[1] at the same time, many if not most do not actively pursue postgraduate information or experiences to remedy these weaknesses (Klassen & Kroll, 2005; Nail-Chiwetalu & Bernstein Ratner, 2007). Such patterns can be found in other health care professions as well, and are the motivation for the EBP movement.

Some criteria for the determination of evidence-based practice involve transdisciplinary practices on the part of all health care professionals. Readable introductions to the concept as it applies to speech-language pathology and/or stuttering treatments specifically may be found in special issues of the following journals devoted to discussion of EBP: *Journal of Communication Disorders* (*37,* 5, 2004), *Journal of Fluency Disorders* (*28,* 3, 2003), and *Contemporary Issues in Communication Sciences and Disorders* (*33,* Spring 2006).

As noted by Sackett and colleagues, and as embedded in revisions to the ASHA Standards for the Certificate of Clinical Competence in speech-language pathology (ASHA, 2004), evidence-based practice first of all requires thorough identification and appraisal of the research literature on potential interventions for the disorder at hand (Nail-Chiwetalu & Bernstein Ratner, 2006), a process known as information literacy. Any information obtained must be further evaluated for relevance to the characteristics of the case at hand (the client's age, complicating features, and personal preferences of the client and/or family). Finally, no matter how well-documented, the effect of the treatment on the individual client must be evaluated; if the intervention is not producing the desired outcomes, alternatives must be considered. It is likely that no single treatment will be best for all patients.

Other EBP principles that transcend treatment of individual specific disorders involve the appropriate design of studies that can evaluate treatment outcomes. Robey (2004) reviews guidelines for preferred treatment outcome research in health-related professions. Medicine has tended to position the randomized clinical trial (RCT) above other categories of intervention effectiveness appraisal. However, as Bernstein Ratner (2005b) and Bothe, Davidow, Bramlett, and Ingham (2006), among others, note, RCTs are better designed for some sorts of medical interventions than they are for treatments in speech-language pathology, education, or psychology. That is because RCTs require double-blinded, randomized assignment to treatment groups; in nonmedical treatments, it is difficult to develop or implement "placebo" interventions, for example. Moreover, it is difficult to "wash out" treatments or use crossover designs, as may be done with drug regimens. Thus, a much wider variety of treatment designs and reports are discussed in this chapter.

HOW TO DETERMINE THE EFFECTIVENESS OF STUTTERING TREATMENTS

Still other principles are more relevant to the evaluation of treatments for stuttering, specifically. We have suggested a list of *12 tests that a method of treating stuttering must meet before it can be considered successful.*

1. *The method must be shown to be effective with an ample and representative group of individuals who stutter.* The single-subject design has a place in scientific research, particularly when appropriate designs are used (Millard, 1998). We believe that it has been widely misused, however, in the area of research on stuttering therapy, where most single cases written up for publication are apparently chosen for the precise reason that they were successes. This practice produces a distorted picture. In the end, we learn little from it beyond what we already know—that somewhere, at some time, almost any therapy can achieve a remarkable result for some stutterers.

A more subtle question may be how to define effectiveness, or what criteria will be applied to show some meaningful level of improvement or inversely, evidence that an intervention was not, in fact, very effective. What constitutes a meaningful outcome in stuttering therapy? Is total absence of stuttering a realistic goal? Onslow (in press) discusses a number of approaches to this problem that have been offered over the years. A review by Andrews et al. (1980) used effect size (specifically the difference between pre- and post-treatment means of the behavior

[1] In the United States, Great Britain, and Canada, respectively.

of interest—in this case, stuttering frequency—divided by the pre-treatment standard deviation), and a treatment sample of at least three individuals. Onslow (in press) suggests a similar approach, using percentage change in outcome measures as an index of effect size: changes of less than 70 percent reduction from pre-therapy values could be considered a small effect, reductions of between 70–90 percent representative of a medium effect, and reductions exceeding 90 percent considered a large treatment effect. In contrast, Bothe, Davidow, Bramlett, Franic, and Ingham (2006) and Bothe, Davidow, Bramlett, and Ingham (2006) suggested that post-treatment stuttering rate needed to fall below 5 percent as basic evidence of effectiveness. There is probably no single best answer to this question.

2. *Results must be demonstrated by objective measures of speech and nonspeech behavior, such as frequency of stuttering or rate of speech and by judges' ratings of severity.* Such measurements should be made before, during, and after treatment by observers other than the experimenters themselves or without knowledge that might influence their judgment (blinding), and due account must be taken of the observers' reliability. By *themselves,* subjective impressions of experimenters, stutterers, or family or friends of stutterers are inadequate because they may be colored by hopes, expectations, denial, or other psychological factors. They can, of course, accompany objective report measures of outcome. The influences that affect subjective judgments may be subtle and difficult to predict. Lanyon, Lanyon, and Goldsworthy (1979), for example, found that clinicians' judgments of stutterers' success in mastering a biofeedback treatment procedure was significantly related to those stutterers' eagerness to present themselves in a favorable light as indicated by their K scores on the *Minnesota Multiphasic Personality Inventory;* however, the stutterers' K scores had little relationship to their progress as measured objectively.

Current Evidence-Based Practice goals do position patient/client self-report as a crucial component of outcomes assessment. For this reason, it is increasingly important to develop and validate patient self-report measures. Huinck and Rietveld (2007) found that a very simple self-assessment scale, on which the stutterer measured progress by marking status on a scale from 1–10, was very highly correlated with objective measures of speech and stuttering rate, severity, and struggle.

3. *Reports of therapeutic success must be based on repeated evaluations and adequate samples of speech.* The great variability of stuttering from time to time and under different conditions is liable to result in assessments that are unrepresentative, in both pre- as well as post-treatment measures. Measures taken in the clinic immediately following treatment do not suffice in this regard. F. H. Silverman (1975) tested 51 elementary school stutterers, 39 secondary school stutterers, and 25 adult stutterers in a clinical situation. Only a third in each group said their stuttering had been typical of their usual stuttering. The same is true of intake measures of stuttering rate. Many clinical trials of stuttering interventions now routinely utilize repeated baseline measures prior to treatment to meet this challenge, rather than a single pre-intervention fluency sample.

4. *Improvement must be shown to carry over to speaking situations outside the clinical setting.* One of the best known and most frequently ignored facts about stuttering is that, in the special environment of the speech clinic, the speech of most stutterers is likely to become steadily more normal for reasons that have little to do with the effectiveness of the treatment. Such changes have been a frequent source of gratification to unsuspecting speech clinicians, and enthusiastic before-and-after tape recordings in these cases have sometimes created impressions of improvement that seemed little short of magical, although the stutterer had made few or modest gains outside the clinic.

5. *The stability of the results must be demonstrated by long-term follow-up investigations.* Many methods for making stuttering disappear have been known for many years; the great and persistent problem of stuttering therapy is how to keep the stutterer from relapsing. As we shall see, many gains evident at the end of therapy are lost to some degree at long term follow-up, when such follow-up is done.

A difficult question to answer is how long an interval we should allow to elapse between the end of treatment and the follow-up study. This is equivalent to asking how long a stutterer must talk normally or with improved speech before we can assume that the change is permanent. We do not know the answer to this question, but clinical experience prompts us to assert that a few months is not enough. Experienced clinicians can remember too many stutterers who relapsed after talking well for that long. For the same reason, a year seems inadequate. Perhaps 18 months to 2 years is the shortest interval after which most experienced clinicians would not feel unduly optimistic in hoping that the improvement was lasting.

The follow-up evaluation is likely to be biased if it is done in the same clinical environment in which the treatment was administered. Boberg and Sawyer (1977) demonstrated this experimentally when they retested stutterers by taking them to another part of their college campus and instructing them to engage in conversation with a confederate of the experimenters posing as a student. The clients stuttered more there than when speaking with a stranger in the familiar clinical surroundings. When the surroundings as well as the persons conducting the follow-up study were associated with the stutterer's recovery, the results were even more likely to be misleading. One stutterer described to the first author a follow-up evaluation that he had received at a speech clinic that claimed a high rate of success with the form of therapy that it employed. He had relapsed considerably after treatment, but once back in the familiar clinical setting and finding that the person conducting the assessment was his former clinician, he spoke and read with little tendency to stutter.

Not only should the evaluation be conducted outside the clinic, but, with the individuals' prior permission as now required by most Human Subjects Research protocols worldwide, it is probably best done without the individuals' knowledge that their speech is being evaluated. The reason for this is that clients who are motivated to create a favorable impression of their therapeutic outcomes may be able to muster better performance than usual for the purpose of an overt test. This was observed by Andrews and Ingham (1972a). At the end of intensive treatment by a token economy system combined with "prolonged" speech, 24 adult stutterers' average percentage of stuttered syllables in a spontaneous speaking task had dropped from 16.41 to 0.11. In a similar test nine months later, the mean percentage of stuttered syllables was still only 0.5. Eighteen months after treatment, however, recordings of the speech of 17 of the participants were obtained in their homes by a student who pretended to be interested in their responses to a personality test in order to fulfill a psychology course requirement. The average percentage of stuttered syllables had increased to 7.8.

In a later study, Ingham (1975) compared overt and covert assessments made after the same interval of time following treatment and again found that the stutterers generally tended to speak more fluently when they knew that their progress was being evaluated. Howie, Woods, and Andrews (1981) even found a small but significant difference between overt and covert measurements immediately after treatment. On the other hand, Howie, Tanner, and Andrews (1981) found essentially no difference between overt and covert follow-up evaluations. Neither did Andrews and Craig (1982) for stutterers as a group, though they pointed out that differences appeared in individual cases. As yet, we do not know just how vital covert assessments are, but it is difficult to ignore the possibility that at least some individuals may be apt to give misleading impressions of their fluency gains in long-term overt examinations.

Precisely how stutterers manage this we do not know, but when treatment is based on a change of speech pattern such as slow or rhythmic speech, at least part of the explanation is not difficult to discern. The chances are that stutterers seldom use these patterns for so long that their effectiveness literally "wears out." Andrews and Ingham, Perkins, and others who have described the results of such therapies with objectivity and candor suggest that when regression occurs, it generally does so much earlier if the stutterer is resistant to the embarrassment and bother of an unnatural way of speaking. If that is the case, it is probably a simple matter for stutterers to "turn on" their fluency again in the presence of their examiners. Curlee and Perkins (1973) evaluated their clients' progress in conversational rate control therapy by sending them out to record their own speech in outside situations. "On several chance meetings," Curlee and Perkins wrote, "clients were observed to be stuttering more than their tape recordings represent . . . Consequently, the measures of generalization reported in this study probably are best interpreted as being indicative of a client's ability to speak fluently when he chooses to maintain relatively stutter-free speech."

Boberg and Kully (1994) attempted to provide such covert assessment of follow-up by making surprise telephone calls to their therapy program alumni. Participants in the therapy program were tape recorded during phone calls prior to the intensive program and then telephoned at random during the following year. Results showed that fluency had in fact improved markedly following therapy, although gains were reduced over the longer term follow-up period.

6. *Suitable control groups or control conditions must be used to show that reductions in stuttering are the result of treatment.* There are other variables besides adaptation to the clinician or clinical situation that may create a false impression of successful therapy. One is spontaneous recovery. Although this is especially common in children, degrees of spontaneous improvement can be found in adults. A troublesome feature of the fluctuations in severity that occur over periods of time, as Hanna and Owen (1977) pointed out, is that stutterers (or their parents) have a natural tendency to seek help when speech difficulty is extreme. As a result, the stuttering is likely to become less severe in time merely by virtue of "regression to the mean."

Except in the case of preschool children, the effect is not likely to be large, however, as studies of stutterers who have been placed on waiting lists for treatment show.[2] Andrews estimated the average regression to be about 15 percent on the basis of data available in the literature.

Another factor that must be taken into account is the temporary fluency that so often results from the stutterer's belief in the effectiveness of the therapy. In certain cases, as when testing the effects of drugs or biofeedback training, placebo treatments have been used to control for this effect. The necessity for this was strikingly demonstrated by Prins, Mandelkorn, and Cerf (1980) in their study of treatment by haloperidol when they found that a placebo had a measurable effect.

In more typical behavioral treatments, it is not feasible to administer a dummy treatment as a control. In such cases, another method of therapy has sometimes been used as a basis for comparison, although "head-to-head" comparisons of treatments are rare (Bothe, Davidow, Bramlett, & Ingham, 2006; Herder, Howard, Nye, & Vanryckeghem, 2006). An alternative to a control group or a contrasting therapy is a waiting list condition such as that employed by Andrews and Ingham (1972a). In this case, the improvement, if any, that takes place in speech during a period of months prior to therapy serves as a basis of comparison for the change that occurs in the same individuals' stuttering during treatment. Waitlists have been used in a number of the trials of the Lidcombe program for treatment of stuttering in very young children, as described later in this chapter.

7. *The person's speech must sound natural and spontaneous to listeners.* This is an especially important part of the evaluation of all therapies that teach people who stutter to change their manner of speaking. Residual elements of slowness, monotony, or stereotypy in people's speech may seem more peculiar to listeners than the stuttering itself. Stutterers are justified in rejecting such strangeness. Increasingly, more researchers have been concerned with such questions as whether and how listeners can distinguish therapeutically derived fluency from normal speech and how to measure and enhance the naturalness of the post-treatment speech.[3] As

[2]Andrews, Guitar, and Howie (1980), Ingham (1980), Andrews and Harvey (1981).

[3]Silverman and Trotter (1973), Perkins, Rudas, Johnson, Michael, and Curlee (1974), Frayne, Coates, and Marriner (1977), Ingham and Packman (1978), Runyan and Adams (1978, 1979), Mallard and Meyer (1979), Metz, Onufrak, and Ogburn (1979), Prosek and Runyan (1982, 1983), Runyan, Hames, and Prosek (1982), Metz, Samar, and Sacco (1983), Iacono (1984), Martin, Haroldson, and Triden (1984), Ingham, Gow, and Costello (1985), Ingham, Martin, Haroldson, Onslow, and Leney (1985), Ingham and Onslow (1985), Mallard and Westbrook (1985), Robb, Lybolt, and Price (1985), Shenker and Finn (1985), Onslow and Ingham (1987), Ingham, Ingham, Onslow, and Finn (1989), Metz, Schiavetti, and Sacco (1990), Runyan, Bell, and Prosek (1990), Franken, Boves, Peters, and Webster (1991, 1992), Martin and Haroldson (1992), Onslow, Adams, and Ingham (1992), Onslow, Hayes, Hutchins, and Newman (1992), Onslow, van Doorn, and Newman (1992), Kalinowski, Noble, Armson, and Stuart (1994), Schiavetti, Martin, Haroldson, and Metz (1994).

Bothe, Davidow, Bramlett, and Ingham (2006) note, relatively few studies have assessed naturalness of speech following stuttering treatment, but this outcome is undoubtedly critical to evaluation of the effectiveness of therapy. For example, Tasko, McClean, and Runyan (2007) found that participants in an intensive fluency-shaping program who showed the largest reductions in stuttering severity were rated as most unnatural-sounding at program completion. The consequences of this finding for long-term maintenance of therapy gains are not fully known, but, as noted, probably contribute to either disuse of the instructed speech pattern or relapse, at least for some individuals.

8. *The clients must be free from the necessity to monitor their speech.* Like unnaturalness, reduced automaticity of speech is a problem that plagues the most commonly used behavior therapies and is even more intractable. Yet fluency can hardly be considered normal as long as continual attention on the part of the speaker is required to maintain it.

9. *Treatment must remove not only stuttering, but also the fears, the anticipations, and the person's self-concept as a stutterer.* To judge the outcome of therapy solely on the basis of frequency counts of stuttering, ignoring the stutterer's perceptions and attitudes is as extreme and unacceptable a procedure as relying solely on stutterers' accounts of their subjective impressions. This is particularly true when treatment has consisted of a change in the stutterer's accustomed manner of speaking. Sheehan (1984) put it incisively:

> *A stutterer may feel miserable at the strain and vigilance required to keep an artificial pattern going. But the resulting monotone might dramatically lower the frequency count. Conversely, a stutterer might relax his suppressive vigilance enough to feel much freer and more open, even though the frequency count might be reported as higher by an objective observer. Which one feels better about himself? Who is ahead in a genuine therapeutic sense?*

Howie and Andrews (1984), in their account of the Prince Henry "prolonged speech" program, wrote, "In general, while some clients are never heard to stutter, most still regard themselves as stutterers who are now able to speak fluently . . ." This has become a familiar comment in assessments of treatment programs.

In a number of studies, the *Erickson S-scale* of communication attitudes or Woolf's *Perceptions of Stuttering Inventory* have been used in evaluating the outcome of therapy.[4] The more recently developed *Overall Assessment of the Speaker's Experience of Stuttering* (*OASES;* Yaruss & Quesal, 2006) is a more extensive and norm-referenced tool that may be used in this regard. Silverman (1980a) developed an inventory for the specific purpose of measuring improvement in such dimensions as avoidance of words and situations, modification of attitudes and feelings about stuttering, modifications in the personal-social area, as well as changes in speaking behavior. Such instruments must be administered prior to therapy as well as at the end of therapy to adequately gauge the impact of therapy on cognitive and affective components of stuttering. Some recent trials of stuttering treatments have conducted such pre- and post-therapy assessments and we will note them as we discuss them later in this chapter.

Andrews and Cutler (1974) observed that removal of symptoms by behavior therapy brought only a partial improvement in clients' attitudes toward speaking. These attitudes approximated those of normally fluent speakers only after they had completed a program of supervised speaking experience outside the speech clinic.

10. *The success of a program of therapy should not be inflated by ignoring dropouts.* The problem presented by stutterers who drop out of treatment was pointed out by Martin (1981) many years ago. Estimates of the amount of improvement during therapy are often based exclusively on those who complete the clinical program. For example, in the Shames and Florance *Stutter-free Speech Program* (1980), it appears that nearly 40 percent of stutterers did not complete the full course of therapy. Similarly, in a report of the Camperdown prolonged speech-shaping program to be described in greater detail later in this chapter (O'Brian, Onslow, Cream, & Packman, 2003), only about half of the original cohort recruited for the

[4]Andrews and Cutler (1974), Guitar (1976), Guitar and Bass (1978), Helps and Dalton (1979), Mallard and Kelley (1982).

therapy program completed it fully. While most participants did not complete for reasons that would be considered unavoidable in a research study (such as moving, or family circumstances), a few could not achieve program targets or did not like the "feel" of the speech style being taught.

On its face, ignoring dropouts may seem only reasonable, but people may drop out because they are not benefiting or do not like the final product of the therapy process, and when a considerable number of such dropouts are omitted in the final tabulation of results, a distorted picture of the effectiveness of the treatment is likely to be presented. The same applies to long-term follow-up studies; when they are limited to those participants who respond to the invitation to appear for reassessment, the findings may be severely biased.

11. *The method must be shown to be effective in the hands of essentially any qualified clinician, including those without unusual status, prestige, or force of personality.* Some, but not many, studies have accomplished this by using a number of clinicians to administer the treatment. A recent report of a highly programmed prolonged speech-based therapy administered by student clinicians is one example of an assessment trial meant to test this criterion for effective interventions (Block, Onslow, Packman, Gray, & Dacakis, 2005). Results of the trial showed that outcomes were equivalent (and positive) across a large number of student clinicians.

12. *The method must continue to be successful when it is no longer new and the initial wave of enthusiasm over it has died away.* There is reason to believe that such enthusiasm alone is capable of bringing about a large number of short-term recoveries from stuttering.

We will attempt to evaluate the therapies discussed in this chapter by reference to some of these principles. However demanding this list may appear to be, it is by no means exhaustive, as a number of researchers and clinicians have suggested some reasonable additions to it. For example, as noted earlier, Bothe, Davidow, Bramlett, and Ingham (2006) have suggested some criterial level of resulting fluency should be considered in deciding whether or not a stuttering intervention is effective. They review a number of possible "normalcy criteria," which range from less than 5 percent stuttered syllables to less than 1 percent. In addition, they and Yaruss (2001) suggest that cognitive and affective handicaps associated with stuttering, particularly in adults and older children, should be objectively and measurably improved as a function of the intervention. As noted, this criterion requires that measures beyond behavioral measures of stuttering severity be appraised as part of the pre-therapy assessment process. In addition to measures discussed in Chapter 1 that are specific to stuttering, other appraisals, such as general quality of life indices, common in medical practice, may have a valuable place in assessment of stuttering as well as evaluation of its best treatment (Bramlett, Bothe, & Franic, 2006).

We now turn to the treatments that have been developed, more specifically. We start with a historical overview, and then group more currently utilized approaches by their conceptual underpinnings or treatment focus. As we shall see, a number of currently utilized approaches have their bases in methods first developed many years ago, and differ from them primarily in refinements in method, delivery framework (for example, more and less intensive fluency instatement component), and in how robustly they have been evaluated in terms of their effectiveness.

METHODS IN EARLY USE

Modifying the Speech Pattern

In Chapter 10, we saw that people who stutter are likely to speak fluently as soon as they adopt almost any novel manner of speaking. From ancient times to the present, this has been persistently discovered and rediscovered as a remedy for stuttering in a variety of ingenious forms. Demosthenes' famous pebbles, if the old story is true, were an expedient of this type. Two thousand years later, they appeared in more refined form as an ivory "support" for the tongue. In the past 200 years, this general approach to therapy has been represented chiefly by methods that teach the stutterer to talk in time to rhythmic movements of the arm, hand, or finger or to adopt other unusual speech patterns. People who stutter have been advised to speak slowly, in a sing-song, or in a monotone, to slur consonants and prolong vowels, to shorten vowels and stress the consonants, to hold the tongue this way or that way, or to pay attention in one manner or another to their rate, phrasing, or breathing.

Almost nothing appears to remove stuttering as quickly and completely as do devices of this kind. Unfortunately, in many cases, the benefit proves to be merely temporary. Furthermore, when people relapse after having been "cured" in this way, there is often a tendency for the mannerism that they have developed to become part of their stuttering pattern and to increase the unnatural quality of their speech. For these reasons, clinicians held a strong suspicion of such methods for many years, particularly in the United States, where this kind of therapy was largely confined to commercial "stammering schools" until the 1960s, when certain advances occurred in therapeutically programming speech modifications that were considered to create better and more durable results.

The invention of new ways of altering speech production patterns to treat stuttering has persisted over time, but changed from some of its original specifications. Froeschels's chewing method was a classic example from the last century. Stutterers learned to speak fluently by performing chewing movements together with speech. They then gradually attenuated the chewing activity and finally merely imagined themselves to be chewing (Froeschels, 1943). Ventriloquism, another technique suggested by Froeschels (1950), made use of the art of speaking with a minimum of lip movement. Cherry and Sayers (1956) introduced a therapy they called "shadowing," based on their observation that stutterers tend to speak fluently when producing a running copy of another person's speech. Such methods do not have a reasonable evidence-basis to justify their therapeutic use with any confidence at this time.

Eventually the advent of what are now often called "fluency shaping" therapies brought additional, often programmed modifications of the speech pattern into frequent use again, as we will see. At this time, methods that alter the way in which people who stutter are asked to speak in order to achieve fluency are among the most popular and most well-documented intervention approaches in use. Because of this, specific programs and their particular emphasis in changing speech production behaviors will be described in detail in the sections that follow.

Suggestion

Another powerful method of eliminating stuttering temporarily is suggestion. This has been used consciously and deliberately with stutterers ever since the phenomenon of hypnotism became widely known in the early nineteenth century. It was probably employed long before that, however, unwittingly and in non-hypnotic forms. The older literature on stuttering contains references to a large variety of therapeutic techniques that apparently owed whatever effectiveness they had to the person's belief that they would help. Among these were "hunger cures" and other forms of punishment, regulation of diet, periods of enforced silence, bloodletting, tongue surgery, articulation drills, and breathing exercises.

In more recent times, there have been many attempts to treat stuttering by posthypnotic suggestions of fluency, hypnotic suggestions repeated regularly over long periods, and autosuggestion. Those who can be hypnotized tend to gain marked immediate relief from their difficulty, but the majority relapse fairly soon. No studies of hypnosis using appropriate clinical design have produced credible data suggesting its appropriate use as a validated treatment for stuttering. Consistent with the lack of documented outcomes in peer-reviewed studies, when Hayhow, Cray, and Enderby (2002) surveyed members of the British Stammering Association (BSA), more than 50 percent of respondents had tried courses of hypnotherapy, but few indicated that it had been helpful to them and many more reported that it was of no value. Yaruss et al. (2002) found much the same opinion in surveying members of the American National Stuttering Association.

At least part of the reason for the temporary nature of recovery from stuttering reported in some studies appears to be that this general type of therapy makes little fundamental change in the fear of stuttering and speaking that adults who stutter are likely to have. They may tell themselves with conviction that they will not stutter and talk fluently while the conviction remains strong; however, as long as they still regard stuttering as an intolerable stigma, the most trifling counter-suggestions of imminent failure in the form of certain sounds, words, situations, or listeners to which they had learned to react with expectancy may be enough to undermine their synthetic "confidence" and precipitate relapse. Furthermore, when recovery has been based for the most part on hope and faith, relapse may be accompanied by severe demoralization.

The fact that some individuals who stutter may be helped temporarily by practically any type of therapy in which they believe strongly has some important implications. It means that they may be especially likely to obtain short-term benefit from a therapist who is deeply convinced of the effectiveness of the methods used, who happens to be charismatic, or who has a prestigious role (e.g., physician, psychiatrist, or the like).[5] A corollary hypothesis for which there is considerable evidence in the history of stuttering treatments is that almost every new movement in therapy is likely to enjoy a kind of honeymoon during which successes occur in part as a result of the hope and enthusiasm of clinicians. Therapeutic allegiance can be a very potent influence on therapy outcomes (Wampold, 2001). To the extent that this is true, evaluating the results of any new departure in therapy is obviously no simple matter.

Relaxation

An old method still in fairly wide use in the day-to-day practice of speech pathologists is relaxation. This would seem to have a certain basic appropriateness in the case of a disorder consisting essentially of struggle behavior (Gilman & Yaruss, 2000). It seems almost impossible to be relaxed and to stutter at the same time. As a result of long experience, however, some dissatisfaction with this approach has arisen among clinicians. A few individuals who stutter seem to learn the trick of relaxing their muscles so effectively that they have little further difficulty with their speech. But such persons appear to be rare. Usually, stutterers tend to speak better in a treatment environment while practicing relaxation. Outside that environment, however, they may find it impossible to relax precisely in those situations where it is most important for them to do so. Anxiety and tension are difficult to separate. Consequently, most clinicians employ relaxation only in certain special forms or in conjunction with other types of therapy. As we will see later in this chapter, relaxation has been used more recently as a feature of a conditioning therapy known as systematic desensitization, and it has also been employed to target specific speech muscles through electromyographic (EMG) feedback. It does not appear that generalized relaxation alone has been widely applied as a stuttering treatment in recent years.

Psychotherapy

Early in the twentieth century, what was then a radically new method of treating stutterers was tried for the first time. Freud wrote comparatively little about stuttering, but what he did write left little doubt that he considered it a neurotic symptom rooted in unconscious conflicts. By 1920, various followers of Freud, among them Brill and Coriat, had treated a considerable number of people who stutter by employing psychoanalytic therapy, and this then gained recognition rapidly as a reasonable way to treat the disorder. From the beginning, the psychoanalysts directed their efforts against what they regarded as the cause of stuttering through the resolution of inner personality conflicts. The older methods of distraction, suggestion, and relaxation were for the most part rejected as superficial attempts to deal with symptoms alone, and some psychoanalysts warned that the elimination of stuttering by such techniques

[5]This phenomenon is not unique to stuttering, as Wampold and others show in their work on therapist effects on outcomes, discussed later in this chapter under the topic of "common factors in therapy outcomes" (Baskin, Tierney, Minami, & Wampold, 2003; Wampold, Minami, Tierney, Baskin, & Bhati, 2005).

represented a premature and dangerous removal of the stutterer's neurotic defenses.

If hope ever existed that psychoanalysis would immediately provide an essential solution to the problem of stuttering, this hope was soon dispelled by Brill (1923). Brill, who clearly understood that the difficulty in stuttering treatment was not so much the failure of stutterers to respond to treatment as their great tendency to relapse, was one of the few clinicians of his day employing any type of stuttering therapy to make careful follow-up studies. He reported that, of 69 adult stutterers whom he had treated regularly "for a few months to a year or even longer," the great majority at first appeared to have regained essentially normal speech, but that after 11 years, only 5 of the 69 patients whom he had discharged as recovered were "really well." He commented, "Most of the others seem to be satisfied that they have been improved, although they have their ups and downs."

Other clinicians—for example, Travis (1957) and Glauber (1958)—were more optimistic about the results of psychoanalysis, and it might reasonably be argued that clinical techniques of psychoanalysis are now much advanced over those available to Brill, but further follow-up studies of any importance have not been reported. Many psychoanalysts appear to have come to the conclusion from their experience with stutterers that the majority of them are unusually "resistant to therapy"—or at least, their symptoms are.

Classical Freudian psychoanalysis is not, of course, the only existing form of psychotherapy. Stutterers have been treated by various neo-Freudian forms of psychoanalysis, by group psychotherapy, by nondirective therapy, psychodrama, gestalt therapy, rational-emotive therapy, and most other varieties of psychotherapy. There is as yet little evidence that any of these has proved outstandingly successful or has more of the usual potential for reducing stuttering temporarily that is inherent in virtually any remedial measure. Furthermore, the absence of conclusive research evidence that stuttering is an attempt to satisfy unconscious needs or that it is wholly or necessarily a symptom of personality conflict (see Chapters 2 and 7) does not encourage confidence that future efforts to treat it through psychotherapy will be more successful. We do not have any systematic reports of the effectiveness of psychotherapy in treating stuttering at this time, although it appears to be of clear benefit in other conditions (Wampold, 2001).

THE HISTORICAL ROOTS AND DEVELOPMENT OF THE "IOWA" THERAPIES

In the 1930s, another challenge arose to the older methods of treating stuttering. Although this was primarily the work of three persons, Bryng Bryngelson, Wendell Johnson, and Charles Van Riper, it may be best understood in the context of certain broader historical events to which it was related. In the early decades of the twentieth century, speech and language pathology did not exist as its own profession. Although a number of phoneticians, psychiatrists, and other professional workers were making significant early contributions to this area of knowledge, whatever speech therapy that existed was largely in the hands of classroom teachers with more good intentions than training or commercial speech "specialists," who frequently had neither. During the 1920s, the first active stirrings that were to develop into the scientific study and treatment of speech, language, and hearing problems as a nonmedical field of professional specialization made themselves felt.

One of the more significant of these beginnings took place at the University of Iowa as a clearly deliberated step undertaken by the noted psychologist Carl Emil Seashore, who was then dean of the Graduate College. Johnson (1955b) told the absorbing story of the manner in which Seashore's special kind of imagination contributed to the establishment of a new academic and professional program of study at the University of Iowa. Recognizing that the initial need was for a research program to provide a better scientific understanding of speech and hearing disorders and that no single academic department then existing could offer all of the basic knowledge and skills for such a program, Seashore proceeded to break down departmental barriers. He selected a promising student to direct the development of the program and, with the cooperation of the departments of psychology, speech, physics, psychiatry, neurology, otolaryngology, and other university departments, he prepared him for a career as a new kind of specialist.

That student, Lee Edward Travis, was, in Johnson's words, probably "the first individual in the world to be trained by clearly conscious design at the doctoral level for the definite and specific professional objective of working experimentally and clinically with speech and hearing disorders." In 1927, Travis became the first director of the University of Iowa Speech Clinic. Under his supervision, a group of researchers and clinicians was soon engaged in work on a variety of problems of speech and voice. Chief among Travis's own personal interests was stuttering, and the decade that he remained at the University of Iowa was a period of unparalleled ferment in research, theoretical speculation, and clinical experimentation in this area. In all of this intense activity, the remarkable scope of the training that Travis had received by Seashore's careful design was clearly visible, but the new concepts of therapy that emanated from this activity, and that were so profoundly to influence the treatment of stuttering in the United States, have come to be associated with the names of three of Travis's early students who were directly responsible for the development and elaboration of these concepts.

In brief, the new therapeutic approach for which Bryngelson, Johnson, and Van Riper opened the way was aimed at a reduction in the fear and avoidance of stuttering, while at the same time attempting to reduce the stuttering itself directly through gradual modification based on study and understanding of the behavior of which stuttering consisted. This approach represented a sharp departure from the philosophy on which the older methods were based. Bryngelson, Johnson, and Van Riper were severely critical of those methods. They argued that they merely gave the person who stutters a temporary crutch on which to lean and that quick recovery almost inevitably portended sudden relapse. Above all, such methods served in the long run to intensify rather than decrease fear because in effect they said to the stutterer, "Don't stutter. Swing your arms or talk in some odd and unnatural way, but whatever you do, don't stutter." And the implication was that hardly anything was more unusual or grotesque or more to be feared and avoided than stuttering. By contrast, the new approach was to say to the stutterer, "Go ahead and stutter. But learn to do so without fear and embarrassment and with a minimum of abnormality."

In precisely what manner and for what reasons this particular point of view arose in the atmosphere of the University of Iowa Speech Clinic of the 1930s is a difficult question to answer simply. Unquestionably, an influence of the utmost significance was Travis's interest in "mental hygiene" and the psychology of adjustment. Another factor of probable importance was that two of the three chief promulgators of this point of view began their professional careers as severe stutterers. They had had personal experiences of short-lived success and intense discouragement with older methods of therapy and, moreover, had intimate knowledge of the manner in which fear and stuttering were related. At any rate, this was the general clinical outlook that they more or less jointly formulated. It was an outlook that lent itself with great vitality to modification and development in highly individual ways, and anything further that is to be said about it must concern itself with the distinctive contributions of the three men who shared it.

Bryngelson: Voluntary Stuttering and the Objective Attitude

The phrase "objective attitude" in connection with stuttering therapy appears to have been first used, at least with the precise systematic implications that it came to have for most speech pathologists, by Bryngelson. Oddly enough, this basic goal of stuttering therapy initially took on significance in conjunction with the attempts to treat stutterers by means of laterality training that were made at the University of Iowa during the 1930s. Shortly after the Iowa clinical and research program was established, Travis, together with Samuel T. Orton, head of the department of psychiatry at the University of Iowa, formulated a concept of stuttering as a symptom of conflict between the two cerebral hemispheres (see Chapter 2). It is a curious feature of an essentially neurophysiological breakdown theory that it permits considerable emphasis in therapy on the attitudes of the person who stutters and adjustments to them. One reason for this is that, if individuals who stutter can avoid some of the strong emotional reactions that ordinarily accompany stuttering, they may thereby eliminate a major source of the external pressures presumed to precipitate breakdown of their vulnerable neuromuscular system.

Bryngelson, as Travis's student, followed his lead in attempting to develop the "native dominance" of stutterers as a major concern of therapy, but he also put very great emphasis on the cultivation of attitudes of acceptance and objectivity in relation to their speech difficulty. To Bryngelson, an objective attitude on the part of people who stutter meant the ability to discuss their stuttering freely and casually with others. It meant the willingness to enter difficult speech situations and the refusal to make use of word substitutions or other tricks for avoiding stuttering. In general, the goal was to bring the problem out into the open and to be willing to stutter. This lent itself to the use of group therapy in which people who stutter were encouraged to ventilate their feelings about their speech problem before an audience of other people who stuttered and in which they could be helped to gain objectivity by the examples set by others. It also led to a great emphasis on "situational" work in which clients were taken outside the speech clinic and challenged to demonstrate their ability to maintain an objective attitude in feared situations. The elements of Bryngelson's remedial program that were concerned with laterality have passed into disuse, but the teaching of an objective attitude through situational work is today still used by many speech pathologists as a major aspect of stuttering therapy with people in the most advanced phase of the disorder.

A particularly distinctive contribution that Bryngelson made to this type of therapy was a technique he termed "voluntary stuttering." Practically as soon as it became evident to the Iowa group that the fear of speaking could often be very markedly reduced, it was apparently recognized that this approach when used alone had its limitations. Not only was it useless to try to eliminate all fear of stuttering in most cases, but, very frequently, a considerable amount of stuttering remained after the fear had been substantially reduced. From the very beginning, therefore, the work on attitudes toward speech was combined with efforts to modify the stuttering behavior directly. This was the primary purpose of voluntary stuttering as it was first suggested by Bryngelson. In 1932, Knight Dunlap authored a book entitled *Habits: Their Making and Unmaking,* which proposed a technique termed "negative practice" for the elimination of an undesirable habit. Dunlap's principle was that, by practicing the error deliberately, it could be removed from the realm of the habitual and automatic and dealt with appropriately in a conscious, purposeful way. Bryngelson took this device and applied it to stuttering with a somewhat modified rationale. He suggested that clients learn to stutter voluntarily as a means of fighting for conscious control of their "spasms." Thus, for Bryngelson, the principal objective of voluntary stuttering was the exercise of control.

Clients were instructed to practice the technique before a mirror until they had thoroughly mastered it. They were then to voluntarily stutter in speech situations outside the clinic. If attempts to stutter voluntarily on a difficult word resulted in an involuntary reaction, clients were to repeat the attempt until the block was completely under their control. In principle, Bryngelson advocated that stutterers learn to imitate the basic components of their own characteristic stuttering behavior, but he found that it was usually easier for stutterers to stutter on purpose when they produced a simple, effortless repetition of initial sounds. Bryngelson was not oblivious to other benefits that voluntary stuttering provided, in addition to the element of control. He saw it as a means of learning to stutter without the avoidances, starters, and other tricks and devices with which stutterers frequently complicated their difficulty. He also recognized in it the psychological benefit of deliberately facing what one was ordinarily inclined to avoid or hide.

Voluntary stuttering has been employed widely in stuttering therapy, particularly by clinicians who are able to develop a high level of morale in the client. It is not, as may be imagined, an easy talent for the typical stutterer to learn or for parents to understand when the need for this arises. For a number of years, a tendency toward less use of voluntary stuttering in its original form was discernable, perhaps as part of a trend on the part of some speech pathologists toward greater concern about the clinician-client relationship,[6] but voluntary stuttering may be experiencing a resurgence, as seen in reports of stutterers' clinical experiences in surveys (Yaruss et al., 2002) and on Listservs such as Stut-L (see discussion of Internet-based consumer-group organizations for stutterers, their families, and speech-language pathologists later in this chapter). Voluntary stuttering exerted considerable influence on Johnson and Van Riper as they developed their therapeutic approaches, and in direct and indirect ways, this technique has played an important part in the history of stuttering therapy.

Johnson: Perceptual and Evaluative Reorientation

A product of substantially the same influences that motivated Bryngelson to advocate voluntary stuttering and the objective attitude, Wendell Johnson formulated a therapeutic program based on similar goals, but with certain differences that were eventually to lead to his own distinctive form of treatment. Johnson's outlook on therapy was markedly affected by his growing conviction that there was little physical or organic basis for stuttering and by his development in the late 1930s of a "diagnosogenic" theory of its origin (see Chapter 2). Like Bryngelson, he believed that it was necessary to reduce the fear of stuttering as much as possible. Additionally, he believed that a chief objective in therapy was for people who stutter to learn to handle speech situations adequately as stutterers without apologizing for their disfluencies or allowing themselves to be handicapped by their speech difficulty. For Johnson, however, fear was at the heart of the problem. He believed that stuttering was an avoidance reaction motivated by anxious anticipation of speech interruption and that the way to start talking normally was to stop trying to avoid stuttering.

This premise also lay behind the particular kind of use that Johnson made of Bryngelson's voluntary stuttering. For Johnson, the value of voluntary stuttering had little to do with the aim of gaining control over the stuttering reactions. The very notion of control was one to which he was unsympathetic. He felt that people who stutter tended to be overly cautious and perfectionistic in the manner in which they went about speaking to begin with and that what they needed was to be not *less,* but *more* spontaneous about it. Voluntary stuttering, as Johnson applied it, was an exercise in throwing caution to the winds. In being disfluent on purpose, people who stutter weakened their tendency to avoid disfluency and consequently their tendency to stutter. From this point of view, it was desirable to perform the voluntary pattern simply and easily, without the hurry and tension that characterized typical avoidance behavior. Gradually, Johnson believed, it would be possible for stutterers who used these techniques to slow down, delay, and simplify their stuttering reactions until they became essentially like normal disfluencies.

In this connection, he pointed out that most normal speech contained large numbers of disfluencies of some sort. The difference between stutterers and people perceived to be normally fluent speakers was that people who stutter reacted emotionally to their disfluencies. By the same token, learning to speak normally was ultimately in large measure a matter of stutterers' evaluations; it was something that would result when they could produce disfluencies without reacting to them as speech difficulties that required some sort of active response.

Perhaps the most potent factor that contributed to the development of Johnson's thinking about stuttering was the general semantics writings of Alfred Korzybski (1941) and he is generally identified with an essentially semantic approach to therapy. As Johnson saw it, the things that prevented stutterers

[6] See, for example, Cooper and Cooper (1969), Cooper (1966, 1968, 1971), and Manning and Cooper (1969) for work on this relationship.

from talking normally were simply the things they did to keep themselves from stuttering; if they were to proceed on the assumption that there was nothing to prevent them from talking adequately, they would speak without any trouble. Consequently, stuttering was caused by a peculiar set of perceptions and evaluations that people who stutter entertained about their speech. As such, it was a kind of behavior influenced by the language they used in talking and thinking about their speech and was subtly and pervasively conditioned by primitive, animistic, and naive conceptions inherent in that language.

For example, Johnson pointed out, people who stutter often tended to talk about their speech difficulty very much as though it was caused by demons inside of them that played hob with their oral apparatus; they were likely to say, not "I press my lips together too hard when I talk sometimes," but "My lips come together too hard," or "My tongue pushes against my teeth," or "My throat shuts tight." If stuttering were chiefly a matter of erroneous assumptions or inferences, then its chief antidote was the checking of these inferences by means of scientific observations, or what, as a general semanticist, he called "extensionalization," and in time this became an important feature of Johnson's therapy. Clients carefully observed their stuttering behavior before a mirror and by means of tape recording to determine just what they did to prevent themselves from speaking. They systematically observed what happened when they spoke in time to rhythms or when they were alone in order to verify the fact that there was nothing wrong "inside" to keep them from talking normally. They observed the disfluencies of normal speakers in order to discover that normally fluent speech was not perfectly fluent speech. They made scientific observations of the reactions of their listeners to find out that, by and large, listeners were more tolerant of their stuttering than they had assumed.

This type of treatment involved creating important changes in the stutterer's perceptual and evaluative reactions. Ultimately, perceptual and evaluative reorientation based upon general semantics became Johnson's chief method of attack on the problem. In this, he was influenced considerably by the work of Dean E. Williams (1957), who extended and developed this approach to therapy. Johnson finally discarded much of his earlier therapy, including the technique of voluntary stuttering. His basic clinical procedure became one of training stutterers to be conscious of the inappropriateness of the language they tended to use in talking about their problem. In group or individual discussions, individuals who came for treatment were taught to examine carefully what they meant when they referred to themselves as "stutterers," as though assuming that there was something about them that marked them as basically different from other people, or when they referred to what they did when they talked as their "stuttering" or "it" as though their problem was not what they did when they talked, but a thing inside of them that they needed to manage, stop, or control. Current research and treatment that examine the impact of locus of control (LOC) on therapy outcomes in stuttering and other disorders is consistent with this particular focus of Johnson's work. We shall return to this issue in particular when we discuss predictors of therapy relapse later in the chapter.

Finally, they were trained to set aside, at least temporarily, such words as "stuttering" in order to talk descriptively about their problem, with the expectation that, as they became aware that there was nothing to prevent them from going on except the things they themselves did when they talked, they would gradually become better able to talk without doing these things. On the basis of this sort of semantic reorientation, then, Johnson proceeded to place major emphasis on a great deal of actual speaking by stutterers—an increase both in speaking time and in the number of situations in which speech was attempted—with attention to "going ahead and talking" on the assumption that there were no basic physical or emotional reasons for not doing so.

Van Riper: Cancellations, Pull-outs, and Preparatory Sets

When Charles Van Riper left the University of Iowa in 1936 to establish a speech clinic at what is now Western Michigan University, it was with the determination to devote himself to finding more effective methods of treating stuttering. To accomplish his purpose, he resolved that he would select a small group of severe stutterers each year, vary his therapy, keep careful records, and employ a five-year follow-up study to evaluate the results. His account of this activity is a remarkable record of therapeutic experimentation over a period of more than 20 years (see Van Riper, 1958). During this period, he apparently tried almost every known and many unknown methods of treating stutterers and evolved a therapeutic program going considerably beyond that which had developed in the early years at Iowa. This program, however, may be regarded fundamentally as an extension of the Iowa concept of therapy, since it stresses the reduction of anxiety about stuttering and the deliberate modification of the stuttering behavior based on analysis and understanding.

Although Van Riper was continually concerned with the treatment of stutterers' fears and developed a variety of original techniques for desensitizing people who stutter to their difficulties and reducing their avoidances, perhaps his major contributions concerned the problem of modifying the behavior itself. If there is a single term used by Van Riper that epitomized his approach to this problem, it is the term "fluent stuttering." From the beginning, he regarded the stuttering moment as, in large part, learned behavior. It appeared to him that whether the disorder had a neurological, neurotic, or any other type of origin, it soon tended to become self-perpetuating, most of the abnormality consisting of anticipatory reactions for avoiding stuttering and reactions of frustration in response to the experience of stuttering. This suggested the possibility that one could learn to stutter with a minimum of abnormality. It was necessary to substitute for the habitual stuttering reactions a smooth, simple pattern of interruptions without struggle, and free from the devices for avoidance, postponement, starting, and release that frequently complicated them. The goal, in short, was not to speak without stuttering, but to stutter "fluently."

As a substitute method of fluent stuttering, Van Riper first tried the simple repetitive pattern that Bryngelson had termed "voluntary stuttering," but soon found it unsatisfactory for this purpose, and retained it only in the form of "faking" or "pseudo-stuttering" on non-feared words as a mental hygiene device. The pattern that seemed to fulfill his requirements as a method of stuttering more normally was a smooth, prolonged speech pattern. He found that effective employment of this pattern created an open, straightforward kind of stuttering, free from much of its usual complexity, and gave an ongoing, essentially "fluent" quality to stutterers' speech. The more skilled that stutterers became at performing the pattern, the more brief and effortless their stuttering moments became and the more normal their speech sounded.

This was true if stutterers did it effectively. Some appeared to manage it quite well. All too often, however, particularly under communicative stress, the smooth prolongations tended to give way to the tremors and spasmodic tensions of uncontrolled stuttering, despite all that the speakers could do to prevent this. Some method of teaching clients how to "smooth out" their stutters was evidently needed. As he worked on this problem, Van Riper noted that stutterers' abnormal attacks on feared words were due to the manner in which they behaved just before they said the word. During the period of anticipation prior to the word-attempt, there often appeared to be fragmentary silent rehearsals of the difficulty that was about to occur. Stutterers seemed to place themselves in a particular kind of tense preparatory set when it was necessary for them to say what they thought was a difficult word. Apparently, it was this set that gave rise to the stutter and that seemed to determine even the length and very form of it.

As Van Riper studied the preparatory set, he discovered that it had several more or less distinct features. One was a tendency on the part of people who stutter to tense the muscles of the speech mechanism as they readied themselves to say the word. A second was a peculiar inclination to say the first sound of a feared word with a fixed position of the articulators, rather than as a normal movement leading smoothly into the next sound. This was a set that appeared to reflect the stutterer's characteristic tendency to think of the initial sound in isolation from the rest of the word as a principal obstacle to be hurdled. A third was a habit of "pre-forming" the first sound, or placing the articulators in position for the sound well in advance of the attempt to say it.

It is evident that, in the brief period of anticipation just prior to the attempt on the feared word, behavior took place that was of crucial importance in the precipitation of the stutter. It occurred to Van Riper that this period afforded the best opportunity to modify the stuttering. If so, it was necessary to teach people who stutter to react to their feelings of expectancy as a signal to assume certain new preparatory sets in place of the old ones. The new preparatory sets were, first, to begin the word with the articulators in a state of rest; second, to say the first sound as a movement leading into the next sound; and, third, to initiate voice or airflow immediately on the attempt to say the word. These sets, if carried through with essential completeness, would result in normal speech. Van Riper's immediate goal was not normal speech, however. Altered preparatory sets were chiefly a means of helping stutterers to achieve their objective of learning to stutter "fluently."

The new preparatory sets served this purpose with marked success in some cases, but there were still some serious difficulties. The chief problem was that it was difficult for most stutterers to monitor their speech as painstakingly as this technique required them to and still communicate adequately. Van Riper found a partial solution to this problem in a device that he termed "pull-outs." When stutterers were unable to change their preparatory sets effectively in their attempt on a given word and had begun to stutter on it in their usual way, they were trained to finish the word with a smooth, controlled, gliding prolongation. Since a large part of the abnormality of stuttering often consists of the frantic struggle to terminate the stutter, this tended to have the immediate effect of increasing fluency. Even more important, as clients learned to "pull out" of their stutters with greater ease, their altered behavior gradually came to be initiated progressively earlier in the course of the stuttering until it began to reflect itself in changes in their preparatory sets.

Pull-outs seemed to work unusually well, far better than anything he had yet tried, but still Van Riper was not satisfied. Too often, stutterers found that they had completed their disfluencies in the old manner before they had a chance to do anything about them. It was in the attempt to cope with this difficulty that Van Riper finally came to use a technique he referred to as "cancellation." When clients failed to use an easy prolongation or to pull out of stutters successfully, they paused, studied their feelings and behavior, and immediately tried the word again. The object was not to say the word fluently on the second attempt, but to make some change for the better in their way of stuttering. Once clients had gained the ability to cancel their failures, it was a relatively short step to more satisfactory pull-outs.

Together, preparatory set, pull-out, and cancellation proved to constitute a useful set of practical techniques for modifying stuttering. In teaching them to stutterers, Van Riper frequently began with the concept of cancellation and proceeded systematically to the notion of pull-outs and then preparatory sets. When all three had been mastered, clients employed them in reverse order on a given word, first attempting to manipulate their anticipatory set and using each in turn only as the others failed. As Van Riper viewed these procedures, they were not mere mechanical devices, but in their deeper purpose, a kind of psychotherapy. Cancellation, for example, may be seen as a basic form of therapeutic self-confrontation; as stutterers make use of their disfluencies as opportunities to battle for control of their fears, maladaptive attitudes, and abnormal initiation and release of sounds, they may be compared with neurotic persons who gradually succeed in the course of the psychotherapeutic process in taking responsibility for their maladjustive behavior.

Among the important products of Van Riper's work were the findings of his five-year follow-up studies of small groups of stutterers whom he selected each year for eight months of intensive treatment (see Van Riper, 1958). They showed that about half the stutterers that he treated had very fluent or essentially normal speech, were largely free from fear and avoidance, and were socially adequate five years after treatment. Many more were apparently much improved. The results, in short, were encouraging, although they indicated that much further progress remained to be made in the development of a satisfactory therapy for people who stutter.

This approach to therapy, often now described as "stuttering modification" (Guitar, 2006), is a popular therapy in many places, although large-scale data verifying its effectiveness are still relatively sparse more than a half century after initial reports of its use. Thematically related programs, such as the Successful Stuttering Management Program (SSMP), a short-term (three-week) intensive program that combines a major focus on desensitization with the therapy components listed previously, have been in popular use in the United States and elsewhere. An analysis of the immediate and long-term (six months post-treatment) outcomes of this therapy was reported by Blomgren, Roy, Callister, and Merrill (2005) for a group of 19 adult stutterers. Both stuttering frequency and severity were assessed, along with a number of cognitive and affective variables. In their study, the program did not produce statistically significant changes in fluency, but did produce some long-term changes in avoidance and expectancy scores on the *PSI* and two affective subscales of the *Multicomponent Anxiety Inventory IV (MCAI-IV)*.[7]

An additional, limited report of the effectiveness of SSMP therapy was provided by Eichstadt, Watt, and Girson (1998). Five of eight stutterers who attended a version of the program in Johannesburg, South Africa, were followed up two years later. Data are provided for individuals, who varied considerably not only in their follow-up fluency characteristics, but in their interim therapy experiences.

Few studies have examined listener reactions to the techniques employed in this type of stuttering modification therapy. In a listening experiment in which a single speaker modeled stuttered speech and cancellations and pull-outs, Manning, Burlison, and Thaxton (1999) reported that listeners found both cancellations and pull-outs less natural and less preferred than unmodified stuttered speech. However, they appeared to prefer cancellations to pull-outs in terms of naturalness.

Sheehan: Avoidance Reduction Therapy

Joseph Sheehan, a psychologist at UCLA from 1949–1983, borrowed concepts from both conflict theory and role theory to develop the principles of avoidance reduction therapy for stuttering (Sheehan, 1953, 1970, 1975). *The Conflict Hypothesis* illustrated how the person who stutters experiences competing drives to both approach and avoid speaking due to anticipation of two opposing outcomes, either successful communication or shame related to perceived negative listener reaction. Stuttering is partially an identity problem, "a disorder of the social presentation of the self" (Sheehan, 1970). *Role conflict,* according to Sheehan, helped to explain the fact observed by most people who stutter that they could be perfectly fluent when speaking alone in a room. The experience of speaking fluently, at least some of the time, led to expectations (hopes) of continued fluency, heightening anxiety and leading to increased stuttering.

Within such a framework, treatment for stuttering involves both reducing efforts to avoid *showing* stuttering, as well as efforts to conceal one's *identity* as a person who stutters. Through avoidance reduction therapy, fluency is achieved as a byproduct of self-acceptance and letting go of efforts to control speech.

Helltoft Nilsén and Ramberg (1999) employed an intensive therapy based on these principles with 13 adolescents. Stuttering rate and other measures of stuttering severity decreased significantly. However, locus of control, which was thought to be an active component of the therapy approach, did not change between pre- and post-intervention measures.

CURRENT BEHAVIORAL THERAPIES

An approach to stuttering therapy that underwent rapid development after the 1960s was the use of so-called behavior modification techniques, which followed changes in thinking about the treatment of behavioral disorders generally. Accepted methods of

[7]Additional commentary and response on this report appear in the December 2006 issue of the *Journal of Speech, Language and Hearing Research.*

psychotherapy, based to a large extent upon psychoanalysis, had been challenged by a growing number of therapists. These clinicians were skeptical of the effectiveness of these methods, the factual basis of their theoretical assumptions, and their medically oriented model of maladaptive behavior, which assumes that stuttering is a symptom of an underlying "neurosis." Instead, behavior therapists attempted to view maladjustment conceptually as a matter of learned responses to demonstrable stimuli and to manipulate these responses by applying basic principles discovered by careful laboratory investigation of learning and behavior.

The learning-oriented discussions of stuttering offered by Wischner and Sheehan had done much to prepare a favorable reception for this outlook in the field of speech pathology, and stuttering therapy quickly began experimenting with behavior modification. The outstanding effect of this development was to encourage a spirit of innovation in the treatment of stuttering for which not even the emergence of Iowa therapy in the 1930s provides an adequate parallel.

As interest in behavior modification grew, so did the number of different kinds of therapies to which the term has been applied, and thus, it is difficult to give a simple definition of behavior therapy as used for stuttering. We will outline here essentially all of the principal procedures for treating stuttering that are generally referred to as behavioral therapies. They include both classical and operant types of conditioning procedures as well as techniques that are not based primarily on conditioning at all.

Systematic Desensitization

Among the most common maladaptive reactions are those that involve irrational fears of identifiable things such as authority figures, high places, sexual inadequacy, spiders, or speech. Since fear is a classically conditioned response, an important place exists in behavior modification for classical conditioning techniques. Such a procedure, designed to extinguish fear responses, was designed by Wolpe (1958) and is referred to as reciprocal inhibition, or systematic desensitization. Wolpe noted that certain responses tended to inhibit anxiety—for example, relaxation, eating, motor activity, or assertive behavior. He found that if such responses could be made to occur in the presence of the stimulus that evoked the anxiety, its tendency to do so would be weakened. For example, a child might lose a fear of dogs if fed repeatedly in the vicinity of one.

Of course, the reverse might happen too. The child might lose all appetite for food in the presence of the dog. It was important to make sure that the fear did not overcome the response designed to inhibit it. Wolpe therefore introduced the concept of a hierarchy of fear-evoking stimuli varying progressively in strength. On the first occasion, the dog might be tied up far enough from the child so that the eating response inhibits the fear. On successive occasions, it might then be moved closer by degrees.

This would not be practical with thunderstorms, an impatient boss, or many other objects of irrational fear that are not so easily controlled, however. For this reason, Wolpe trained patients to fantasize their fears and applied his hierarchical concept of deconditioning to imagined rather than actual feared objects. This procedure has been widely used in the treatment of a large variety of phobias.

Wolpe's methods were first applied in stuttering therapy by Wolpe himself, Walton and Mather (1963), and Brutten and Shoemaker (1967), and have since been employed by others.[8] They were developed for use specifically with stutterers by Brutten and Shoemaker (1967, chap. 5) and are highly consistent with their viewpoint that the integral features of stuttering represent disruptions of speech by visceral fear reactions that have been classically conditioned to speech sounds, listeners, situations, or other neutral stimuli (see Chapter 2).

Brutten and Shoemaker made use of relaxation training for this purpose. With the stutterer in a sufficiently relaxed condition to inhibit anxiety, fantasy is employed to present a hierarchy of feared speech

[8] Rosenthal (1968), Tyre, Maisto, and Companik (1973), Burgraff (1974), Lee, McGough, and Peins (1976), Moleski and Tosi (1976), Azrin, Nunn, and Frantz (1979), Alarcia, Pinard, Serrano, and Tetreault (1982), Zibelman (1982), Atkinson (1983), Mehta (1985).

situations repeatedly until they no longer serve as stimuli that elicit fear.

For the elimination of the associated symptoms of stuttering, which they regarded as instrumentally conditioned responses, they advocated the application of reactive inhibition through massed practice of such reactions. They referred to their therapy, in consequence, as a "two-process" one. On the basis of three years' experience with this approach, they reported that, while not "universally" effective, it resulted in marked improvement for most of the stutterers with whom they had worked.

In general, most reports of the use of systematic desensitization as the sole agent in stuttering therapy are relatively old at this point in time, and results of these studies are decidedly mixed with regard to its effectiveness. When used in current treatment, desensitization is usually included as part of a "hybrid" or integrative therapy approach, as discussed in a later section of this chapter.

Operant Conditioning

A different type of conditioning therapy for stuttering is based on the methods developed by B. F. Skinner and his followers. These have lent themselves to use in clinical work with stuttering in a variety of ways.

Punishment of Stuttering As we saw in Chapter 11, there have been a large number of laboratory demonstrations of temporary reductions in stuttering caused by contingent application of such stimuli as shock, noise, verbal disapproval, response-cost, and time-out from speaking, among others. In earliest treatment studies, only time-out was put to repeated use in therapy.[9] Martin, Kuhl, and Haroldson (1972) reported its successful use with two preschool children. Each child had weekly conversations with Suzybelle, a puppet whose voice was provided by a speech clinician through an electronic connection from an adjoining room. During periods of time-out, Suzybelle's illuminated glass case was darkened and she was silent for 10 seconds. For one child, time-out was made contingent on every stuttering event. In the other case, in which stuttering was very frequent, time-out was at first administered only for stutters that were at least two seconds in length until these disappeared. Both children improved markedly, and a one-year follow-up showed only a low rate of stuttering in each case.

In a clinical application of verbal punishment, Reed and Godden (1977) reduced the stuttering of two preschool children by using the words "slow down" as a contingent stimulus during 20 twice-weekly sessions. Tape recordings showed a decrease in stuttering at home.

James (1981a) notes that the concept of punishment can be amorphous; in some studies it has been an aversive stimulus; in others, simple signaling of stuttering or time-out from speaking has been used. He suggested that terminology used in describing the therapy approach within an operant framework might be less important than understanding how the intervention reduces stuttering behaviors. We will return to this question later, in particular as researchers attempt to better understand the very well documented effectiveness of Lidcombe therapy in treating stuttering in young children.

Reinforcement of Fluency In other clinical applications of operant conditioning procedures, the stuttering has been ignored, and reinforcement has been given for fluent utterances or stutter-free intervals of time. With a 9-year-old boy, Rickard and Mundy (1965) began by increasing his verbal output by verbal rewards or points earned for progressively longer utterances. They then reinforced his fluent verbalizations. The result was decreased stuttering, but a six-month follow-up showed that not all the improvement had lasted.

Leach (1967) tried something similar with a 12-year-old who stuttered severely. In the first six sessions, the child earned two cents a minute for each minute of talking. Thereafter, during half of each session, he earned an extra cent for each 15-second period of fluent speech. After 42 sessions,

[9] Haroldson, Martin, and Starr (1968), Martin and Haroldson (1969), Egolf, Shames, and Seltzer (1971), Martin, Kuhl, and Haroldson (1972), Costello (1975).

the stuttering was reduced to less than two stutters per minute, and outside the clinic, the speech was reported to be normal. A two-month follow-up, however, showed a partial return of stuttering.

Shaw and Shrum (1972) administered reinforcement for fluency with three school-aged children who stutter between the ages of 9 and 11 years. The immediate reinforcement, given for each 5 seconds of fluent speech in the case of one stutterer and for each 10 seconds of fluency in the other two cases, was a mark on a sheet of paper. A sufficient number of marks brought a reward in the shape of a toy or a piece of candy that the children had selected beforehand. In addition, the children were informed at the start about the contingency. In the course of four 20-minute sessions on consecutive days, there was a marked improvement in speech that carried over spontaneously into everyday situations and, on follow-up, had apparently persisted for two months in one case and four months in another. The children had previously had other types of stuttering therapy for periods ranging from two months to three years without noticeable improvement.

Using essentially the same procedure with three children aged 6, 9, and 11 years, Manning, Trutna, and Shaw (1976) found that tangible rewards were not necessary. Verbal rewards chosen by the children (e.g., "good speech," or "You sounded real nice") proved as effective as the tangible ones.[10] Similarly, the Lidcombe program for treatment of stuttering in very young children (Onslow, Andrews, & Lincoln, 1994; Onslow, Menzies, & Packman, 2001; see additional information under "Combined Punishment and Reward") provides a mix of positive reinforcement of fluent speech with much less frequent requests that the child re-attempt the stuttered utterance.

Time-Out from Speaking As noted in Chapter 11, time-out from speaking, contingent upon moments of stuttering, has been shown to reduce stuttering in laboratory settings, particularly when it is self-administered. Hewat, Onslow, Packman, and O'Brian (2006) review the small number of case studies in which time-out induced fluency gains in the clinic setting generalized sufficiently well to motivate them to conduct a clinical trial of the procedure. Thirty adults and adolescents were seen in a group setting, and instructed in monitoring and consequating moments of stuttering. Clients were required to reduce stuttering by 50 percent in response to clinician-administered time-out in order to be considered good candidates for participation. In the self-administered time-out program, initial stage instatement and generalization were carried out both in- and out-of-clinic. Second phase monitoring occurred in six monthly post-treatment visits, in which the client and clinician reviewed actual speech samples and the clinician counseled the client in how to maintain speech fluency.

In Hewat et al.'s clinical trial, 23 participants (77 percent) successfully completed the first phase of the program. The average reduction in percent stuttered syllables was 53 percent, with good naturalness ratings that compared favorably to typically fluent speakers and were markedly better than ratings obtained from prior team studies of prolonged speech. However, there was a wide range of response, with some participants benefiting very little, while others benefited more extensively. For nearly half of the participants, fluency did not improve to a clinically meaningful degree, according to the study authors. Secondary analyses revealed that more severe stutterers tended to make the most improvement, a finding contrary to outcome results in most therapy trials we discuss in this chapter. A number of the clients who responded most favorably to the intervention had received prior therapy involving fluency-shaping strategies; this finding is consistent with others (e.g., James et al., 1989), which suggest that time-out "may increase the effects of other treatment procedures" (p. 40), potentially by giving clients a chance to re-implement prior therapy skills. Changes in language use were not analyzed; there has been one report that use of time-out with children may, at least in the case of one child who participated in such a treatment, lead to reductions in spoken language complexity to accomplish the fluency gains (Onslow, Bernstein

[10] A critical review of attempts to treat stuttering by reinforcement of fluency was contributed by Hegde (1978).

Ratner, & Packman, 2001). Finally, most clients in the Hewat et al. study reported little use of the procedure on follow-up, finding it difficult to use in everyday settings.

Combined Punishment and Reward In the mid-1990s, Mark Onslow, Ann Packman, Michelle Lincoln, and their colleagues at the University of Sydney developed an operantly based program for the treatment of early childhood stuttering called the Lidcombe Programme[11] (Harrison & Onslow, 1999; Onslow & Packman, 1999; Onslow, Menzies, & Packman, 2001; among multiple other peer-reviewed publications reporting on the program's outcomes). Lidcombe is parent-conducted and combines contingent praise for fluent speech attempts, combined with less frequent feedback that either acknowledges the stuttering or requests re-attempts of the stuttered utterance. Because this approach is for exclusive use with young children who stutter, rather than all age groups, we will discuss it in greater detail later in this chapter when discussing treatment of early stuttering.

Token Economy At the Prince Henry Hospital in Sydney, Australia, Ingham and Andrews and their coworkers treated stutterers in an experimental token economy program in which methods were varied systematically in order to test various clinical hypotheses.[12] Generally, a small group of adult stutterers spent most of their waking hours together for three weeks. Periodically throughout the day, counts were made of the percentage of stuttered syllables in their conversation, and tokens were either earned or lost in proportion to decreases or increases in their stuttering from session to session. Tokens were the only means by which they could buy food or other items such as cigarettes and magazines. Ingham and Andrews frequently combined this procedure with syllable-timed or "prolonged" speech patterns.

The three-week program generally resulted in fluent speech by the end of treatment. In one study (Andrews & Ingham, 1972a), a group of adults who stuttered on a mean of about 18 percent of their syllables before treatment had almost no stuttering at the end of treatment and a mean of 7.8 percent on follow-up 18 months later.

Modifying Thematic Content In the applications of operant conditioning procedures that we have touched on so far, the target behavior has been either stuttering or fluency. In their attempts to achieve immediate fluency, such applications are, of course, opposed in basic philosophy to Iowa therapy. Shames, Egolf, and Rhodes (1969), however, described an operant conditioning program designed to modify stuttering symptoms in the gradual, stepwise manner of Iowa therapy. They also attempted to deal with the stutterer's assumptions and attitudes by conditioning the verbal behavior by which these are represented. The stutterer was systematically given approval such as "good" or "you're right" for positive verbal responses and disapproval such as "no" or "I don't agree" for negative verbal responses. Examples of positive responses were those that reflected the stutterers' insights into the nature of their speech difficulty ("I blink my eyes when I stutter"), expressed favorable feelings, or reported constructive actions or intentions ("I think I'll call him on the phone tonight"). Negative verbal responses included expressions of negative emotion ("Sometimes I hate everybody in the world"), or statements about stuttering that were not descriptive or reflected helplessness ("I can't get the word out").

Shames, Egolf, and Rhodes (1969) and Rhodes, Shames, and Egolf (1971) reported that positive verbal expressions tended to increase and negative ones tended to decrease as a result of this procedure. In addition, they found that a concomitant decrease in stuttering tended to take place even though the stuttering received no direct attention.

Even more frankly concerned with the stutterer's subjective experiences was the "cognitive conditioning therapy" described by Berecz (1973, 1976). He had stutterers vividly imagine a cognitive cue that usually triggered their stuttering (e.g., "They're

---

[11] We will use the American convention of "Program" in referring to the treatment in other places in this chapter.

[12] Ingham, Andrews, and Winkler (1972), Andrews and Ingham (1972a, 1972b), Ingham and Andrews (1973a)

all expecting me to speak" or "My throat is tense"). They then immediately self-administered a painful electric shock and substituted a more desirable cognition. Such an approach strayed relatively far from Skinnerian behaviorism, of course, but Berecz asserted that "if emphasis . . . on overt behavioral analyses results in ignoring cognitive parameters, we are left with a 'black box' approach, which is necessary in the animal laboratory but hardly sufficient for human clients."

Changing the Speech Pattern

Still other behavior therapies seek fluency enhancement through a change in the stutterer's manner of speaking, without the use of concurrent assistive feedback. Schwartz (1976) popularized a technique that relied on airflow management, in which the stutterer permits some breath to flow out passively before initiating each utterance. Azrin and Nunn (1974) offered a regulated breathing therapy. Peins, McGough, and Lee (1972, 1984) introduced the therapeutic use of legato speech, in which sounds, syllables, and words were smoothly linked by continuous phonation and flow of air. Webster (1974, 1979a) developed a program that emphasized gentle onsets of phonation; it was later refined to become Precision Fluency Shaping, described in greater detail elsewhere in this chapter. Weiner (1984c) described a treatment method based essentially on training in good vocal usage, including adequate breath support and optimal voice quality.

Prolonged Speech The prolongation of speech segments, first observed to be effective in controlling stuttering in adults, has, over recent years, become the most typical speech production style taught in stuttering treatment programs in many settings (see Onslow, Costa, Andrews, Harrison, & Packman, 1996, and Packman, Onslow, & Menzies, 2000). Prolonged speech (sometimes abbreviated PS) is often embedded into highly programmed, short but intensive (e.g., two week) programs. In these programs, clients are intensively instructed, often in a highly programmed, criterion-dependent manner, to prolong segments in spoken utterances, especially voiced components such as vowels, glides (in English, w/y), liquids (r, l), and syllabic consonants (m, n).

Because such intensive speech re-training programs may be difficult to fit into the typical working adult's schedule and occupy substantial commitment of clinician time, there have been a number of efforts to alter the basic delivery format of PS therapies. Harrison, Onslow, Andrews, Packman, and Webber (1998) condensed conventional programming into a single 12-hour day, with virtually identical immediate post-treatment values to longer programs.

O'Brian, Onslow, Cream, and Packman (2003) were also concerned that clinicians often find it difficult to operationalize, describe, or evaluate the accuracy of PS targets when administering therapy. To this end, they developed an alternative format for instating fluency via PS that they dubbed the Camperdown Program.[13,14] Rather than detailed instruction in specific speech targets, participants in the program imitate a videotaped model of the desired speech pattern until clinicians agree that the speech pattern resembles that of the model. Then participants may adjust their speech pattern in any way that they wish to eliminate stuttering during a requisite three-minute monologue. This is then followed by an intensive group practice day, in which participants also learn to monitor their speech fluency and naturalness. Fluency instatement is then followed by weekly problem-solving sessions and patients move to a Performance-Contingent Maintenance Phase after three weekly sessions in which within- and beyond-clinic fluency and naturalness measures reach a set criterion. Following a model advanced by Ingham (1980), this gradually "weans" clinical contact by moving clinical consultation meetings to 2-, 4-, 8-, 12-, and 24-week intervals. For 16 individuals who completed the program, fluency outcomes were still positive a year later; stuttering rate decreased from a mean range of about 7–9

[13] Camperdown, like Lidcombe, the name of the Australian Stuttering Research Centre's (ASRC) well-known early stuttering intervention program, is the name of a Sydney neighborhood near the Research Center.
[14] Basic program components for the ASRC programs are made available to the general public at http://www.fhs.usyd.edu.au/asrc//.

percent stuttered syllables across a variety of speaking contexts, to less than 1 percent SS, with reasonably good speech rate and naturalness ratings. However, almost half of the original participants in the study did not complete the program and can be considered "drop outs." Moreover, many also reported that they stuttered more in everyday life than was reflected in the outcome speech measurements that were obtained and some felt more comfortable stuttering than using the modeled speech pattern. Similar reactions to PS speech patterns were also noted by Cream, Onslow, Packman, and Llewellyn (2003). The primary result of the Camperdown trial appears to have been that PS can be taught using fewer hours of clinic instruction than some older programs targeting the same speech behaviors, and yield essentially similar results.

While PS can facilitate fluency, it does not remove affective and cognitive concerns that most individuals who stutter have about their speaking and fluency, nor will it remove anxiety or self-concept as a person who stutters. Because PS requires continuous practice and vigilance, fluency failures may be construed by the client as personal failures in skill, motivation, or commitment, according to post-therapy narrative accounts of 10 adults who participated in a PS program (Cream, Onslow, Packman, & Llewellyn, 2003).

Relatively few studies have tracked the outcomes of children who have been treated using variants of prolonged speech programs. Hancock et al. (1998) suggest that treatment gains were comparable in older children and adolescents who received either an intensive speech shaping program or one that was partially conducted in the home combined with a parent counseling component. At an average of four years following completion of therapy, percent stuttered syllables was diminished to about a level of 2.5 percent, from the children's pre-therapy mean of roughly 11 percent.

Ingham, Kilgo, Ingham, Moglia, Belknap, and Sanchez (2001) described a computer-assisted program that selectively shaped reduction of short phonation intervals, rather than stretching speech segments, which has been a more conventional target. For five adults, normally fluent and natural-sounding speech was achieved and maintained through one-year follow-up assessment.

PROGRAMMED APPLICATIONS

The behavior therapies that have tended to have the most appeal for many speech clinicians are those in which clients progress in treatment by small, well-defined, easily attained steps in accordance with a highly structured program. We will describe some of the best-known examples here.

The Monterey Program

Devised by Ryan (1974, 1979, 2001a),[15] the program originally used at the Behavioral Sciences Institute at Monterey employs two alternative schedules for establishing fluency, GILCU (gradual increase in the length and complexity of utterances) and DAF. In the GILCU program, which is based on operant principles, a stutterer is instructed to begin by reading fluently one word at a time. Each fluent word is reinforced by the word "good" or a token. If the word is stuttered, the clinician says, "Stop. Say it fluently." If necessary, the client may be shown how to say the word fluently in a slow, prolonged manner. After reading 10 consecutive fluent words, the client proceeds to read two words at a time to a criterion of 10 consecutive fluent pairs of words, then three, four, five, and six words at a time in the same way; next, one sentence at a time to a criterion of five consecutive fluent sentences; then, successively two, three, and four sentences at a time. Following achievement of this criterion, the client is instructed to read continuously. Reinforcement is given first after 30 seconds of fluent reading, then at progressively longer intervals. After reading continuously for five minutes without stuttering, the client is considered to have established fluency in reading. The same steps are now repeated as the stutterer engages in monologues and later in conversation. In both cases, the ultimate goal is 0.5 stuttered words or fewer per minute for five minutes.

[15]The 2001 book is a revision of the 1974 text, with additional data and discussion.

Concurrently with this program for establishing fluency in the clinic, the client is conducted through a program designed to transfer fluency to other situations and settings. This involves activities in the home, at school, at work, with strangers, on the telephone, and so forth, and is structured in considerable detail. Finally, there is a maintenance program in which the client returns for reevaluation at progressively increasing intervals and may be recycled through those segments of the program for which performance does not satisfy specified criteria.

The DAF program is an alternative designed chiefly for older children and adults with relatively severe stuttering. It differs from the GILCU program in the method of establishing fluency. With the help of delayed auditory feedback, the client is trained to read and speak in a slow monotone in which all sounds are prolonged and articulation is slurred or deemphasized. Data to support the effectiveness of the Monterey Program are provided in Ryan (2001a),[16] but attracted critical commentary by Onslow (2004) and Manning (2004).

The Hollins Precision Fluency Shaping Program

Webster (1974, 1979a) designed an intensive three-week, all-day program in which fluency is achieved by training the stutterer to use gentle onsets of phonation. For this purpose, the client is first taught to use an exceedingly slow rate of speech. This is done in work directed in turn at so-called stretched-syllable, smooth-transition, slow-change, and full-breath targets, in which the client learns to hold each syllable for two seconds, to eliminate breaks between and within syllables, and to avoid running out of breath when speaking in the resulting slow-motion manner.

After three days devoted to developing these skills, the gentle onset target is introduced. The stutterer learns to initiate all voiced sounds very softly, increasing the intensity of the voice gradually from a barely audible to a normal level. All sounds are practiced individually and in syllables with the aid of a computerized voice monitoring instrument that indicates correct or incorrect phonatory onsets. The speech sounds are worked on in a group setting. Stutterers are taught to articulate the voiced consonants by starting the gentle onset on the consonant itself, and the voiceless fricatives and stop-plosives by starting the gentle onset on the vowel that follows.

By the end of the second week, the stutterer has progressed to two-syllable words. In the third week, the prolongation of syllables is gradually reduced and rate of speech is increased, more complex speech is introduced, the voice monitoring instrument is dispensed with, and transfer is made to speeches, conversation, the telephone, and speech situations in shopping centers and elsewhere outside the treatment center.

Peters, Boves, and van Dielen (1986) described an instrument for detecting the abruptness of vocal onsets that offered some advantages over Webster's voice monitoring device. They also demonstrated that trained observers could make fairly reliable judgments about the abruptness of voice onsets, at least for isolated vowels.

Very little published data have emerged from the Hollins program over the years, although it is a very well-known and active clinic for stuttering treatment. Since the last edition of the *Handbook,* only one report appeared, of three adults, whose speech motor abilities were assessed following participation in a version of the therapy program administered by one of its trainees (Story, Alfonso, & Harris, 1996). However, numerous adaptations of the Hollins approach exist and have produced outcome reports.

For example, the Kassel program based in Germany is based on its principles; there is a German-language report of results from over 700 patients (von Gudenberg, 2006), and reference to its effectiveness appears in the research report by Neumann et al. (2005) regarding the effects of fluency shaping therapy on functional brain-imaging profiles.[17] In this latter study, nine adult stutterers'

[16] See discussion regarding evaluation of therapy outcomes by Manning (2004), Onslow (2004), and Ryan (2004).

[17] Neumann et al. also reference another German-language report of the effectiveness of Kassel therapy by Euler and von Gudenberg (2000), which does not carry an English-language abstract.

percent stuttered syllable rates were reduced from a mean of almost 10 percent before intensive therapy to less than 1 percent following therapy, with concurrent increases in speech naturalness and speech rate. Neumann et al. (2003) report favorable outcomes following this intervention for a smaller group of five adults who stutter.

Similarly, therapies used by De Nil and Kroll and colleagues at the Clarke Institute of Psychiatry in Toronto are modeled after the Hollins program (for a summary of their work, see Kroll & Scott-Sulsky, 2007). De Nil and Kroll (1995) followed up 13 of 21 adults who had participated in their precision fluency shaping therapy two years after completion of the intensive program. Prior to treatment, the average conversational rate of stuttered words was 17.5 percent, while at completion of therapy, it was 2.7 percent. At two-year follow-up, stutter rate had increased significantly, to 7.7 percent, but was still significantly improved from pre-treatment values.

Franken, Boves, Peters, and Webster (1995) report results from a Dutch stuttering treatment program that utilized the Hollins program. Thirty-two adult male stutterers were assessed prior to therapy, at its conclusion, and six months later. Mean pretreatment percent stuttered syllables was 20.5; at end of treatment it was 4.5 percent, with an upswing to 11.5 percent at six-month follow-up. Speech rate did not change appreciably at the various measurement points, and speech naturalness was judged to be only slightly less than that of typically fluent comparison speakers.

Similarly, the Walter Reed Stuttering Treatment Program (see Tasko, McClean, & Runyan, 2007) shares many features with the intensive fluency shaping programs surveyed here. For a cohort of 35 adults, *Stuttering Severity Instrument (SSI-3)* scores fell from a mean of 26 to 9.3; however, some of the participants showing the greatest reductions in stuttering severity were also the least natural sounding at conclusion of therapy.

Finally, a number of the techniques employed in the Hollins program have been incorporated into what we term "hybrid" or "integrated" therapy programs, discussed later in this chapter. In the reports that come out of such programs, it is difficult to ascertain what portion of improvement is specifically attributable to these particular techniques, but they appear to combine with other techniques to produce good outcomes for many stutterers.

Stutter-Free Speech

Shames and Florance (1980) combined techniques borrowed from operant conditioning, counseling, and psychotherapy in an innovative attempt to solve some of the problems encountered by behavior therapies for stuttering. The format for their program, which they called "Stutter-Free Speech," is a client-centered, nondirective interview session that is used in part to encourage the stutterer to explore and clarify feelings of anxiety, inadequacy, indecision, and resistance with regard to speech and therapy. In the course of these sessions, the stutterer is trained with the aid of DAF to speak fluently at a slow rate with continuous phonation and airflow. From the beginning, the stutterer is taught to avoid the robot-like quality of this pattern by prolonging only on stressed words and aiming at normal inflection. In concept, this program is a combination of approaches to treatment that we call "hybrid" later in this chapter; however, it is so highly structured that we include it here as a programmed therapy.

Once stutterers learn to monitor their speech to the degree that they can produce slow, fluent utterances without the aid of DAF, they are taught to self-reinforce this response by allowing themselves frequent brief intervals of spontaneous, unmonitored speech. Fluency is now transferred to the stutterer's daily life by means of written contracts that specify the times, places, and situations in which speech will be monitored, the target behaviors, and their reinforcements. The contract is negotiated by the stutterer and the clinician and is signed by them as well as by others, such as parents, when appropriate. The number of contracts is gradually increased until speech is being monitored throughout the day. When the stutterer's unmonitored speech begins to take on the slow, fluent quality of the monitored pattern, training in unmonitored speech begins. The brief intervals of reinforcement with unmonitored speech are now made longer and more frequent step by step until the stutterer is speaking spontaneously most of the time and monitoring infrequently. Therapy then enters a maintenance phase in which clinical contacts occur at progressively less frequent intervals.

Data for this program were reported in its original published manual; 35 of 37 participants were judged to be stutter-free at follow-up made up to five years after therapy ended. However, almost 40 percent of participants did not complete the program and were lost to follow-up.

Smooth Speech

There has been a recent report of an intensive, highly programmed and manualized program based on prolonged speech principles termed Smooth Speech by its study authors. Block, Onslow, Packman, Gray, and Dacakis (2005) provided both short-term and extended follow-up data for 68 of 78 participants of such a program studied between three and five years after treatment in an Australian university-based program where treatment was provided by student clinicians. Most treatment studies have utilized more highly trained clinicians, and thus the report is an interesting test of the notion that a good therapeutic intervention should be effective when administered by virtually any properly trained individuals. The program reduced percent stuttered syllables from a mean of 5.4 percent to 1.8 percent immediately post-therapy and to 1.6 percent at between 3.5 and 5 years post-therapy. Speech naturalness was minimally but statistically significantly reduced. Patient self-report scores were comparable to those reported by O'Brian et al. for the Camperdown program. Craig (2007) describes a hybrid approach that integrates Smooth Speech and cognitive behavioral therapy.

Summary Remarks: Programmed Applications

We note before leaving this section that other programmed therapies include Lidcombe and Extended Length of Utterance (ELU). These will be discussed more fully in the section on therapies specifically designed for young children.

As in many fields, desire to ensure treatment fidelity and uniformity (in other words, to ensure that treatments are administered as trialed) has led to an increase in manualized therapies that rather extensively detail steps, stages, and "branching procedures" used to implement therapy components and problem-solve difficulties that may be encountered. Because such approaches tend to better lend themselves to large-scale, multi-center trials of therapy outcomes (Tanenbaum, 2005; Bernstein Ratner, 2006), there is concern that they may come to dominate the array of approaches used in treating many of the disorders treated in clinical psychology and other allied health and educational settings, such as speech-language pathology. We shall address this issue further when we discuss determinants of treatment outcomes later in this chapter.

Self-Modeling

A recent approach to stuttering treatment has been the implementation of self-modeling paradigms, which have been documented as effective interventions for a wide number of complex and difficult-to-treat psychological conditions and behavioral problems (see Dowrick & Raeburn, 1977; Dowrick, 1999, for history of the technique's development and review of its common applications). In self-modeling interventions, the client is repeatedly exposed to his or her error-free, target behavior, usually accomplished by editing video to select segments portraying desired performance. Given the adaptation effect, such self-modeling videos are not terribly difficult to construct for individuals who stutter; a target behavior can be practiced until fluent to create the stimulus materials. Thus, in 1996, Bray and Kehle first attempted to extend the technique to fluency treatment in work with three teenage boys. These adolescents had received prior therapy, but had high stuttering rates for three weeks pre-intervention as obtained in multiple baseline measurements. They then viewed three sets of five-minute videos of themselves speaking fluently six times over a five-week period. At termination of the intervention, stuttering rates had decreased from 36 percent to 5 percent, 40 percent to 9 percent, and 18 percent to 4 percent stuttered syllables, respectively, with good naturalness ratings. Two years later, one boy retained post-treatment improvement, one showed no stuttering at all, and the third had relapsed substantially, from 9 percent to 24 percent stuttered syllables. Further follow-up at four years post-treatment in 2001 showed that fluency was still improved from pre-treatment measurement for all participants with stuttering rate at between 1 and 5 percent stuttered syllables.

In 1998, the same authors conducted an intervention with four children, ages 8–13. These children were much milder stutterers, with rates ranging from roughly 6 to 9 percent stuttered syllables. While all of the children made substantive improvements in fluency post-intervention, two of the children had experienced a significant degree of relapse at two-year follow-up. However, all follow-up stuttering rates were under 4 percent stuttered syllables.

Webber, Packman, and Onslow (2004) conducted a trial of self-modeling using two men and one adolescent boy. None had had recent stuttering therapy. Three five-minute videos were constructed for each. During a single day, participants spoke with an interlocutor, interspersed with opportunities to view the self-modeling videos. Additionally, in one condition, participants were explicitly asked to speak in the same way as shown in their modeling tapes. Results of this short, intensive application of self-modeling provided partial support for results of the Bray and Kehle studies, which had programmed exposure over longer periods of time; two of the three reduced stuttering following exposure to their self-modeled tapes, although one participant only benefited when explicitly instructed to speak in the manner shown in the video. Additionally, although decreases in stuttering rate were observable,[18] stuttering rates did not for the most part decline to rates that might be considered to fall within ranges for typically fluent speech (e.g., less than 2 percent stuttered words).

"HYBRID" OR "INTEGRATED" INTERVENTIONS

A number of therapy programs combine various features of the intervention approaches discussed earlier in this chapter. Some authors have called such blended therapy programs "integrative" (Guitar, 2006). A number of such programs have reported good gains in both fluency and cognitive/affective measures, and are summarized below.

Hasbrouck (1992) reported an intensive stuttering treatment program for members of the military, based in part on the Hollins program, but with additional features. He reported on 117 adult stutterers who were treated in a program that included airflow management, progressive relaxation, EMG biofeedback, and desensitization. Hasbrouck reported that all patients met the criterion of less than 1 percent stuttered words on discharge, with 42 tracked patients maintaining normally fluent speech for various extended periods of time.

Many other intensive programs primarily combine aspects of fluency shaping and cognitive behavioral therapy. Among the better known and documented is one conducted at the Institute for Stuttering Treatment and Research (ISTAR) program at the University of Alberta, Canada, called Comprehensive Stuttering Therapy (CST) (Boberg & Kully, 1985; Langevin, Huinck, Kully, Peters, Lomheim, & Tellers, 2006; Kully, Langevin, & Lomheim, 2007). The CST program combines "speech restructuring" that resembles aspects of the Hollins program targets with stuttering modification in a "Van Riperian" framework and cognitive-behavioral therapy to address the emotional and attitudinal aspects of stuttering. Langevin et al. (2006) report on 25 adults treated with the program in the Netherlands and 16 clients treated in Canada (some of whom had been reported on in earlier publications). Both groups started with about equal levels of stuttering severity (about 12 percent stuttered syllables). At the end of three-week intensive

[18] We do not report mean numbers here, as the paper provided only graphed data points for the multiple observation periods.

workshops, the Canadian group produced fewer than 1 percent stuttered syllables, while the Dutch group had slightly higher values; both groups had good naturalness scores. Attitudes, as measured by three separate assessment tools, were also improved significantly. Two years later, mean speech fluency had regressed noticeably, but stuttering was still at roughly half the pre-treatment value. A similar profile was seen for the attitude measures.

Catherine Montgomery has reported on favorable short-term outcomes in patients seen in a program that combines Hollins-type training with cognitive-behavioral objectives (Montgomery, 2006). In Germany, Baumeister, Caspar, and Herziger (2003) utilized a hybrid fluency shaping and stuttering modification program embedded in a summer camp program with 37 children and adolescents ages 9–19. Mean stuttering rate before therapy was 22 percent, with a wide range (some children were very mild, while 8 children had mean stuttering frequencies approaching 40 percent). Average stuttering rate declined to approximately 9.5 percent with improvement on speech rate and self-report measures as well. However, follow-up measurements were taken only two months after termination of therapy.

TREATMENT IN EARLY CHILDHOOD

The remedial measures that have been discussed so far were developed chiefly for use with the adolescent, adult, or school-aged child whose stuttering is in its relatively developed form. Historically, far less work has been done on the treatment of the earliest phase of the disorder, although this trend is changing. Until the 1930s, almost all the therapy that was available for young children in the age range of 2 to 6 years consisted of the traditional parental injunctions to speak slowly, take a deep breath, think before speaking, or the like—a form of help now widely regarded as just as likely to intensify the problem as to alleviate it.[19] With the growth of speech pathology as a profession, a basic orientation with regard to the treatment of stuttering in early childhood was gradually established. This orientation emphasized alteration of the child's environment through parent counseling. It grew out of two main influences. One was the concept of primary and secondary stuttering advanced by Bluemel in 1932 and given wide currency by Van Riper (1939). Bluemel's theory held that "primary" stuttering would disappear of its own accord if the child was not helped or admonished for it. The other major influence was the diagnosogenic theoryof Wendell Johnson. To some extent, the parent counseling orientation also reflected the point of view that stuttering is an emotional disorder of childhood.

In recent years, an increasing number of clinicians have begun to favor a more direct method of treatment of early stuttering than was afforded by the parent counseling programs of Johnson and Van Riper. The result has been the application of modified forms of behavior therapy to increasingly younger children who stutter. In addition, parent counseling advisements have also undergone some degree of research validation absent throughout the many years that they became conventional recommendations to the families of young children who stutter.

Parent Counseling

With the approach that has been in common use for many years, parents are persuaded to refrain from criticizing, correcting, or helping the child or from reacting negatively to the speech difficulties in any way and are advised to see that the speech interruptions are not brought to the child's attention by others. This appears still to be a primary form of advisement offered by pediatricians, to whom parents are most likely to turn first if concerned about their child's speech (Bernstein Ratner & Tetnowski, 2006).

In such an approach, every opportunity is taken to improve the parent-child relationship, as well as to problem-solve the contexts in which disfluency is most evident. For some clinicians, for

[19] Although a relatively recent study commissioned by the Stuttering Foundation of America still found that parents were likely to advise their children in this way, should they observe them stuttering.

whom this is essentially the only important aspect of treatment, this means play therapy for the child and psychotherapy for the parents administered by qualified specialists. Most others, who consider this merely an adjunct to therapy, advocate psychotherapy only in certain instances. In most cases, their interest is primarily in making direct attempts to change some of the parents' child-training practices that might aggravate the child's fluency problem. This concern is based on the belief that an adverse parental environment may increase disruption of fluency and foster anxieties about speech or fluency.

Attempts are also made to eliminate any factors or conditions that appear to increase disfluency. Careful observation indicates that children often have unusual difficulty when fatigued, excited, or speaking under pressure of some kind. Some immediate improvement in fluency may be achieved in some cases when the child is not compelled to speak to unresponsive listeners, to compete with others for the chance to talk, or to speak when upset, tense, or excited for other reasons. For example, a case study by Winslow and Guitar (1994) showed that, by extending turn-taking intervals and reducing interruptions during meal times, the child's stuttering rates could be markedly reduced.

In some cases, it is thought that parents unwittingly set unrealistic goals for the child by their own excessively rapid rate of speech or by the use of too much vocabulary that is over the child's head, and that they may need to be guided to speak more slowly and simply to the child. This is a major tenet of so-called "Demands and Capacities"–based therapies. Cooper and Cooper (1996), in surveying American speech-language pathologists, found that 92 percent agreed that "parent counseling is the critical factor in helping the preschool stutterer." At the same time, very few believed that parental behaviors were influential in causing stuttering (see Bernstein Ratner, 2004, for additional discussion on this apparent contradiction in speech-language pathologists' beliefs and practices).

In view of the frequency with which parents of young stutterers have been advised to decrease the rate of their own speech,[20] some, but relatively little, effort has been made to test the efficacy of this recommendation. Stephenson-Opsal and Bernstein Ratner (1988) and Guitar, Schaefer, Donahue-Kilburg, and Bond (1992) found limited support for this manipulation; however, the first study looked at only two children, while the second followed only one child. Guitar and Marchinkoski (2001) and Zebrowski, Weiss, Savelkoul, and Hammer (1996) studied slightly larger samples, but also noted that some children appeared to profit more than others from such input speech modifications. Additionally, when parents' rates are much faster than that of their own children, or characterized by interruptions or simul-talk (parallel or cross-talk among participants), fluency breakdown may be statistically more frequent (Kelly & Conture, 1992; Ryan, 2000). Thus, Bernstein Ratner (2004) concluded that, "counseling in the area of parental speech rate may be motivated by research and may yield therapeutically valuable results" (p. 48). However, it is clear that much more work needs to be done to validate this practice, especially because, in virtually all cases, slowing of parental rates does not appear to cause slowing of the child's speech rate. Thus, the mechanism by which children's fluency improves is not yet understood.

Bernstein Ratner (1992) could find no evidence that typically fluent children either spoke more slowly or were more fluent when their mothers reduced their speech rates. Moreover, no advantage was seen when mothers simplified language input; their children neither simplified their own language nor were more fluent. In fact, normal disfluency rate rose in this condition, along with children's interrupting behaviors. No other study has, to our knowledge, specifically investigated the results of instructions only to reduce language complexity when speaking to stuttering children. Moreover, the complexity of input language is a very potent predictor of children's later language profiles—greater sophistication in parental

[20] Bernstein Ratner (2004) finds advisement that parents should slow and simplify speech patterns to the young stuttering child to be virtually universal in major texts used in training speech-language pathologists.

input language is positively associated with children's language proficiency. For this reason, Bernstein Ratner (2004) took strong issue with the evidence-base for this particular advisement to parents.

As previously noted, there have also been limited investigations of the effectiveness of changing turn-taking patterns (e.g., Guitar & Winslow, 1996). Lengthening of adult turn-taking latency has been shown to reduce children's disfluency (Newman & Smit, 1989) and appears to be a natural consequence following instructions to slow parental speech rate (Bernstein Ratner, 1992). When parents wait longer to respond to their child's utterance, children appear to mirror this behavior, which can be fluency enhancing. Again, however, the numbers of children observed in these studies are very small.

"Indirect" interventions of this kind may not be effective by themselves in eliminating the problem, but any change in the child's environment that serves to lessen the intensity of the stuttering probably helps in some measure to prevent the development of negative attitudes toward speech and consequently contributes to the likelihood that the child will in time "outgrow" the disorder. It is probable that stuttering serves as its own stimulus in the development of behavioral, cognitive, and affective responses to the disorder, and any reductions in stuttering frequency are probably valuable. However, it is unclear whether such interventions can be considered curative rather than palliative.

Moreover, it is quite important that advisements to parents to alter the child's communicative environment not convey the impression that parental behaviors were the origin of the child's difficulties—we have little research evidence to suggest this. The second author has suggested a useful analogy in comparing advisement to parents of children who stutter to those of children with asthma—in the latter condition, the dustiness of a house is not known to cause the child's asthmatic reaction; however, alterations to décor (taking down the drapes), lifestyle (considering the impact of pets), and changing housekeeping may treat the child's condition to some extent. We believe that the same is true of stuttering. Parents do not cause the child's problem, but are capable of responding in ways that alleviate its symptoms somewhat.

Finally, a general theme of indirect interventions is to strengthen the child's anticipation of normal speech and self-assurance as a speaker. The chief method used is to give the child every opportunity to experience fluency and to gain a sense of enjoyment, adequacy, and success in speech situations. During periods of relatively fluent speech, the child is encouraged to speak as much as possible. During episodes of unusual difficulty, the parents may be trained to provide successful speaking experiences through the use of choral speaking, singing, recitation of nursery rhymes, rhythmic speaking, or puppetry. Similar techniques are frequently used by speech pathologists when they work directly with the young stutterer in conjunction with counseling of the parents.

In addition to these widely used measures, a number of other procedures have been developed within the orientation to early stuttering as essentially a problem of the parental environment. One method of dealing with environmental pressures that tend to increase the child's disfluency is the desensitization therapy described by Van Riper (1972, pp. 299, 300). This attempts to build up the child's tolerance for "fluency disruptors" by controlled exposure to speech pressures and frustrations administered by the speech pathologist during the clinical session.

Another example is the application of "filial therapy" to stuttering in children offered by Andronico and Blake (1971). This is a procedure for helping the parent to develop empathy with the child through training in the technique of play therapy. Egolf, Shames, Johnson, and Kasprisin-Burrelli (1972) also described an experimental program in which the parent was directly involved in the therapy process. They first observed the interaction between parent and child in a waiting room situation and identified parental behavior, such as silence, verbal aggression, or interruption, which seemed calculated to maintain stuttering in the child. In a series of therapy sessions, a clinician then interacted with the child in a contrasting manner. Later the parent was introduced to this situation and, with the clinician serving as a model, learned new ways of reacting to the child. Such case studies are instructive in helping clinicians and parents to "problem-solve" the contexts in which children's fluency waxes and wanes, but do not offer convincing evidence of treatment efficacy when used as the sole approach to fluency treatment.

Within the same environmental orientation is Yovetich's "message therapy" (1984), who trained parents of preschool children who stutter to monitor the child's utterances as message units. The goal was to redirect the child's attention from the how of speaking to what he or she says. Langlois and Long (1988) offered a program in which parents were taught to facilitate the child's language by such techniques as reflecting and expanding the child's utterances, self-talk, parallel talk, and slowing down their own speech. However, the meta-analysis conducted by Bothe, Davidow, Bramlett, and Ingham (2006) did not find language therapy by itself to be effective in producing normally fluent speech.

The Demands and Capacities Model was employed by Starkweather, Gottwald, and Halfond (1990), who used parent counseling alone in their treatment of 16 children seen at the Temple University Stuttering Prevention Clinic. These children maintained normal fluency at up to two years post-therapy (see also Starkweather & Gottwald, 1990; Gottwald, 2007).

Direct Behavior Therapy for Early Stuttering

Family-Based "Integrated" Therapies Most behavior modification approaches for preschool stutterers teach a slow, smooth, relaxed pattern of speech by modeling.[21] The usual practice is to progress systematically from one- or two-word utterances to longer and more complex sentences. This type of approach has generally been combined with parent counseling in which parents are assisted with what might best be described as "problem-solving" the child's fluency pattern, with a mix of indirect advisement as appropriate to the child and family dynamics and some direct fluency training components.

Starkweather, Gottwald, and Halfond (1990) and Starkweather and Gottwald (1990) combined indirect therapy counseling techniques with direct treatment for 32 children and 14 children, respectively. In the first cohort, 29 children completed the program with normal fluency, maintained for up to two years post-therapy; in the second cohort, all did (one child whose family declined to complete therapy still stuttered on follow-up). Gottwald (2007) reports results from another 27 families with children aged 2;10 to 6;2 who completed the program. Fluency improved from roughly 9 percent stuttered syllables pre-treatment to an average of 1.5 percent stuttered syllables post-intervention.

Conture and Melnick (1999) reported on application of a program combining indirect advisement and direct treatment of the child to a large group of 200 families. Seventy percent achieved a criterion of 3 percent or less stuttered syllables within 12–36 weeks; another 10 percent achieved criterion with longer periods of the same therapy approach.

An illustration of such programs' typical components might be illustrated by the approach taken by Yaruss, Coleman, and Hammer (2006) (see Figure 14-1). In their published trial with 17 children, ages 31 to 62 months, parental components were extensively described: they consisted of clinician-assisted problem-solving of the child's fluency stressors, parent education about the nature of stuttering, and instructions on how to chart or monitor the child's fluency, as well as advisement on indirect therapy techniques. Emphasis was placed on modeling slow, "easy" speech, reducing communicative stressors, and rephrasing and recasting the child's speech to support language development. Mean pre-treatment stuttering rates for the children, who had been stuttering for a mean of 10 months (with a wide range), were an average of 15 percent stuttered syllables, while mean post-treatment was 3 percent. Therapy was conducted over a mean of 12 sessions. Eleven children achieved normal fluency after receiving only the parent counseling component and were judged as normally fluent from 1 to 2.5 years post-intervention. The

[21] Guitar (1982), Wall (1982), Culp (1984), Gregory and Hill (1984), Shine (1984), Starkweather (1984).

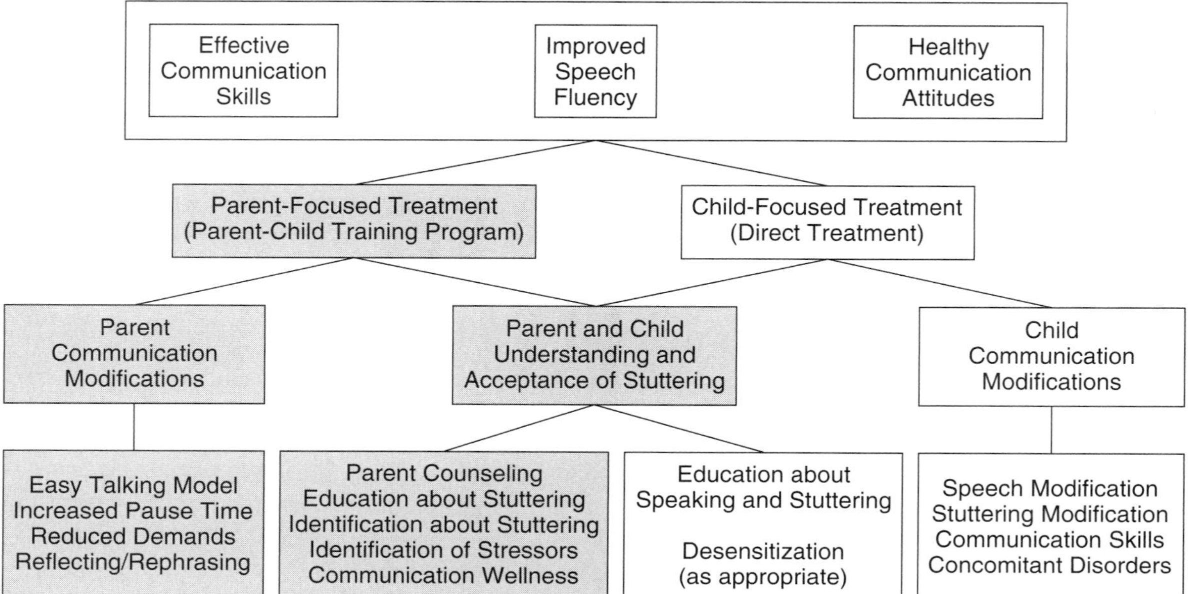

FIGURE 14-1 A family-focused treatment approach for preschool children who stutter. The shaded areas represent the parent-focused components of treatment that are described and evaluated in this article. Yaruss, Coleman and Hammer (2006).

six remaining children required the child-directed component of therapy, but were all reported to demonstrate much-improved fluency during the same follow-up period.

In a rare comparison of two alternate therapy approaches for early stuttering, Franken, Kielstra-Van der Schalk, and Boelens (2005) randomized 12 and 11 children respectively to a program consisting of parental indirect environmental modifications based on the Demands and Capacities Model (DCM) of stuttering (see Chapter 2) and the Lidcombe program, an operant-based program discussed next. All children had been stuttering for at least six months, to minimize spontaneous recovery effects, and were an average of slightly more than 4 years of age. The DCM program counseled parents to provide periods of protected talk time daily for the child, reduce parental speech rate, modeling slow and easy speech, increased turn-taking latencies, reducing complexity of speech addressed to the child, and reducing other emotional and environmental stressors. By the end of therapy, children in the DCM arm had reduced stuttering rate from about 8 percent stuttered syllables to approximately 3 percent stuttered syllables. These values were virtually identical to those seen in the children treated with the Lidcombe program.

Operant-Based Programs Operant conditioning is combined with graduated changes in the child's length of utterance in some programs we report here. Costello (1983) and Ingham (1999) developed a clinical program (Extended Length of Utterance; ELU) in which children receive social rewards or tokens for fluent utterances and are told to "stop" whenever they stutter. This therapy was evaluated (Riley & Ingham, 2000) in a head-to-head comparison of results obtained with ELU and speech-motor training (SMT, described in a following section). Six children, ages 3;8 to 8;4, participated; stuttering frequency was reduced from a mean of 4.25 percent SS to 1.89. As in some other operant programs, largest improvements were seen for the most severe children, a finding not normally observed in studies of other types of treatments. Statistically, the program yielded better results than speech-motor training (64 percent vs. 37 percent decrease in stuttering rate); additionally, some acoustic changes in speech production were observed in the speech-motor training group that were not observed in the ELU group.

Johnson (1984) trained parents to eliminate all attending responses to stuttering and to increase attention to fluent utterances. Stocker and Gerstman (1983) described a program in which they reinforced reductions in stuttering with bits of candy or pennies. (We note that it would no longer be considered safe or appropriate to reward children with food products.) We have already mentioned use of the doll Suzybelle in a time-out procedure with two preschool stutterers by Martin, Kuhl, and Haroldson (1972).

The Lidcombe Program

As noted earlier in this chapter under discussion of operant treatments for stuttering, extensive work has been done to develop and test an operantly framed treatment for early stuttering at the University of Sydney. This work, conducted by Mark Onslow, Ann Packman, Michelle Lincoln, and colleagues, has shown good outcomes from a treatment regimen administered by parents, in which children's fluent and stuttered utterances are consequated on a general schedule of one correction/request for recast for each stuttered utterance to every five positive responses/praise for fluent speech (Onslow, Costa, & Rue, 1990; Onslow, Andrews, & Lincoln, 1994; more detailed information on the program components in Onslow, Packman, & Harrison, 2003). The program involves an extensive parent counseling and training program, and a high emphasis on documentation of the child's level of fluency, both during short daily treatment sessions, and, as the child's fluency improves, in a variety of the child's day-to-day settings. The mean number of clinic visits required to reduce stuttering rates to near zero has been reported as 11–12, spread out over gradually increasing intervals (Jones, Onslow, Harrison, & Packman, 2000). To date, there have been numerous reports of positive fluency outcomes, including trials in which a wait-list control has been observed (Jones, Onslow, Packman, Williams, Ormond, Schwarz, et al., 2005), and analysis of factors that predict more or less favorable response to the treatment (Jones, Onslow, Harrison, & Packman, 2000; Kingston, Huber, Onslow, Jones, & Packman, 2003; Jones et al., 2005). Treatment effects appear to be long-lasting, at least up to from two to seven years post-therapy in a series of 43 treated children followed for that long (Lincoln & Onslow, 1997). It is, by and far, the most extensively documented early stuttering intervention in the literature to date.

Because the publication record for this program is relatively large, we will use a relatively recent report of a randomized clinical trial to illustrate typical therapy outcomes and limitations. In the Jones et al. (2005) trial, children ages 4–6 years who had begun stuttering more than six months previously (to partially control for spontaneous recovery) were randomized to waitlist ($N = 20$) or treatment ($N = 25$).[22] Mean stuttering rate was similar for both groups pre-treatment (6.4 percent SS – 6.8 percent SS, with similar severity distributions). At the end of treatment, at a nine-month post-baseline follow-up, the treated group had a mean stuttering rate of 1.5 percent, while the untreated waitlist group had also improved, as might be predicted during a time when spontaneous recovery is likely, but had a mean stuttering rate of 3.9 percent, a statistically significant difference in outcome.[23,24] The treated group had an almost equal number of children falling below 1 percent stuttered syllables and above (14 vs. 13), while in the untreated group, only 3 children met this criterion and 17 exceeded it. Some factors thought to predict differences in outcome were explored (e.g., gender, age, pre-treatment severity in percent stuttered syllables, family history of early recovery from stuttering). Of these, the only one to predict outcome was family history, with children coming from families having a history of persistent

[22] More children were originally enrolled, but a few cases were lost in both arms of the trial—we report here only final data from children whose follow-up were included.

[23] Many of the treatment reports include individual plots that show rather precipitous declines in stuttering severity following quite quickly on the heels of program implementation, making it less likely that differences in spontaneous recovery per se can account for therapy outcomes.

[24] An earlier study (Harris, Onslow, Packman, Harrison, & Menzies, 2002) found quite similar profiles in a much smaller cohort of children randomized to treatment and waitlist.

stuttering statistically much less likely to reach criterion.

Despite the number of positive reports, a certain degree of controversy surrounds this program. As Bernstein Ratner (2005) notes, operant procedures are not entirely consistent with current etiological models of stuttering. Moreover, adults who profit from operant interventions often appear to have a history of prior therapy experience that enables them to respond to consequation with altered speech production strategies; these would be unavailable to a young child being treated for the first time.

Thus, a number of authors have endeavored to interpret the Lidcombe program using alternative conceptual frameworks. These include Bonelli, Dixon, Bernstein Ratner, and Onslow (2000), Bernstein Ratner (2005), Bernstein Ratner and Guitar (2006), and Zebrowski (2007), among others. There has been speculation that the program could achieve its positive outcomes through a number of means not overtly captured by the therapy design. For example, some children appear to produce conversational speech following therapy that reflect a presumably temporary slowing of expressive language growth rates, observed to be well above typical expectations prior to the intervention in some Lidcombe-treated cohorts (Bonelli, Dixon, Bernstein Ratner, & Onslow, 2000). Put more simply, some children enrolled in the program appear to be producing utterances too long and complex for age expectations before therapy; by therapy end, they seem to have responded to the contingencies with shorter and simpler (yet still age-appropriate) utterances that conceivably permitted a higher degree of fluency (see Chapter 9). Both Bernstein Ratner and Guitar (2006) and Zebrowski (2007) note that parent involvement and parent-child cooperation during treatment are possible active factors in the children's progress; parental involvement and extensive parent counseling have been shown to be influential factors in predicting positive treatment response in other developmental conditions.

Consistent with the potential that the Lidcombe program is not best viewed as a purely operant program are data on the effectiveness of Lidcombe therapy that suggest that children must be of a certain level of cognitive awareness to profit maximally from it. Thus, it is not currently recommended as most appropriate for children under the age of 3 years (Jones, Onslow, Harrison, & Packman, 2000; Kingston, Huber, Onslow, Jones, and Packman, 2003).

The apparently widespread acceptance of Lidcombe therapy in Australia and New Zealand has not been matched by widespread endorsement of the program in the United States as this edition of the *Handbook* goes to press. Bernstein Ratner (2005) reviews some potential reasons for this. Unlike Australia and New Zealand, American clinical training programs for speech-language pathologists are much more numerous, and have many differing historical biases toward "best" treatment approaches, the variety of which is evident in reading this chapter alone. Furthermore, operant-based approaches in speech-language pathology and education went through a period of disfavor in the United States and other countries starting a number of years ago (Crichton-Smith, Wright, & Stackhouse, 2003; Kuhr, 1994). Finally, there is still a certain degree of distrust, perhaps the legacy of Johnson's diagnosogenic theory, in direct behavioral intervention with very young children, particularly any that calls specific attention to the child's stuttering moments, the basic tenet of the Lidcombe approach. Research to examine whether children demonstrate affective changes following treatment has emerged (Woods, Shearsby, Onslow, & Burnham, 2002), and preliminary data seem to indicate favorable affective outcomes. Increased numbers of confirmatory reports as well as additional exploratory investigations of the mechanisms by which children in the therapy achieve fluency will undoubtedly make strong inroads in increasing the popularity of the program in other countries in the years to come.

Other Approaches to Early Stuttering Intervention

Other methods that have been attempted in the direct treatment of early stuttering are rhythmic speech (Coppola & Yairi, 1982; Trajkovski et al., 2006) and electromyographic biofeedback (St. Louis, Clausell,

Thompson, & Rife, 1982). Riley and Riley (1984) included training in oral motor coordination, sentence formulation, and auditory processing in their program when the need for these appeared to be indicated by diagnostic tests. This approach was developed into a speech motor training program (SMT) (Riley & Riley, 1999). SMT was trialed in a report by Riley and Ingham (2001) that contrasted it with the Extended Length of Utterance (ELU) program mentioned earlier in the chapter. For six children, ages 4;6 to 7;0 years of age, mean syllables stuttered were reduced from 7.8 percent to 4.6 percent. The program was statistically effective in reducing stuttering, but did not fare as well as ELU; average decrease in percent stuttered syllables was 37 percent, compared to 64 percent for ELU.

Reports of success in therapy with young stutterers based on virtually all approaches are common, and there appears to be a widely held belief among clinicians that the disorder is usually easily treated in early childhood. Because of the transitory nature of so many cases of early stuttering and its generally agreed-upon 75–80 percent spontaneous recovery rate, however, it is very difficult to assess the validity of such reports. In an early study of this problem by Panelli, McFarlane, and Shipley (1978), 15 children who had been examined because of stuttering during their preschool years but not treated were reevaluated at age 7 to 14 years. Of the 15, 12 were judged to have recovered. More recently, substantial amounts of spontaneous recovery have been observed in clinical trials of the Lidcombe program (Jones et al., 2005). However, it should be kept in mind that older children who stutter are not as likely to achieve recovery without treatment (Ramig, 1993), and that it is evident that children who are treated may experience relapse (Hancock & Craig, 2002).

ASSISTIVE DEVICES

In the intervention approaches that follow, fluency has been induced by the use of assistive devices that either perturb or mask auditory feedback, or encourage the speaker to keep time to an external signal. We first discuss the techniques in historical perspective, then return specifically to the question of the effectiveness of assistive devices in the treatment of stuttering.

Delayed Auditory Feedback (DAF)

In Chapter 11, we saw that many stutterers can speak fluently under delayed auditory feedback (DAF), in large part because the delay forces them to speak more slowly. This expedient has been used widely in stuttering therapy, often with encouragement that the stutterer fall into the slow, prolonged pattern to which the DAF is conducive.[25] Thus, it has often been used to introduce prolonged speech targets. However, its roots were in fact in operant conditioning, where DAF was used as a form of punishment or negative reinforcement. The first to do so was Goldiamond (1965).

Goldiamond had been engaged in a program of laboratory research on stuttering as operant behavior in which he was using aversive stimuli such as loud tones as punishment and negative reinforcement. In the course of this work, he decided to test the effect of a brief period of delayed auditory feedback as an aversive stimulus. First he tried it as a punisher, turning it on each time the participant stuttered. The stuttering sharply diminished. The next step was to demonstrate its effectiveness as a negative reinforcer. The speaker was now placed under continuous DAF, and the DAF was turned off for 10 seconds on the occurrence of every stutter. By all the rules of operant conditioning, the stuttering should have increased in frequency. Instead, something unexpected happened—speech was produced fluently in a slow, prolonged manner. The DAF was rarely turned off because the person rarely stuttered.

Goldiamond saw an opportunity to devise a method for treating stutterers clinically. Using the facilities of the conditioning laboratory, he developed a program in which a slow, prolonged pattern of fluent speech was first produced by the administration

[25] Nessel (1958), Adamczyk (1959, 1965), Lotzmann (1961), Goldiamond (1965), Zemeri (1966), Soderberg (1968, 1969b), Webster and Lubker (1968a), Curlee and Perkins (1969, 1973), Webster (1970), Ingham and Andrews (1971b), Perkins (1973b), Perkins, Rudas, Johnson, Michael, and Curlee (1974), Ryan and Van Kirk (1974).

of DAF in the manner just described. Then the DAF was gradually attenuated until the stutterer was speaking in the same pattern without its help. Finally, a normal rate of speech was gradually restored by machine control of successive displays of reading material. Goldiamond reported marked success with this method, including carry-over to outside situations in many cases.[26]

Goldiamond's reports of success received wide attention and considerably influenced others who were attracted by the operant model of behavior modification. Curlee and Perkins (1969) and Perkins (1973b) described a program of therapy in which slow, fluent speech was first established by DAF with a delay of 250 milliseconds, and the DAF was gradually faded out by reducing the interval of delay in 50-millisecond steps. Ingham and Andrews (1971b) used DAF in conjunction with their token economy program to aid in the establishment of fluency. They referred to the slow speech pattern that resulted from the prolongation of syllables as "prolonged speech." A study by Howie and Woods (1982) seemed to show that the syllable prolongation worked just as well without the tokens as with them. Ryan and Van Kirk (1974) made DAF the basis for programmed therapy in which systematic attention was given to transfer of the slow, fluent pattern of speech to a variety of situations outside the clinic and to the maintenance of normal speech once it was attained. They reported successful transfer to outside situations in a series of 50 cases. Therapists employing DAF often expressed the belief that the use of a slow pattern of speech with prolongation of sounds or syllables in imitation of speech under DAF might be just as effective in producing fluency as DAF itself, and this was demonstrated by Ryan (1971) and by Watts (1971).

As noted earlier, in many clinical settings, the practice of a slow rate of speech through prolongation of syllables, with or without DAF, is now a common form of behavior therapy. We discuss the prolonged speech therapies that do not employ DAF in a separate section of this chapter. However, there has long been interest in portable devices that might provide the person who stutters with types of auditory feedback that have been shown to facilitate fluency in experimental settings, as we discuss later.

Frequency Altered Feedback (FAF)

We include discussion of the use of frequency altered feedback here because it is now sometimes offered as an alternative to DAF in devices vended for the purpose of reducing stuttering. However, the method by which FAF is presumed to induce fluency is described quite differently, usually in terms of the choral speaking effect. FAF creates feedback that emulates choral speech (see Chapter 11), and is also thought by some to stimulate mirror neuron systems that might, hypothetically, prime or ease an individual's own speech production (thus providing a reason for the choral reading effect; Kalinowski & Saltuklaroglu, 2003a; 2003b; see Chapter 2 for discussion of the mirror neuron system and its possible role in stuttering). Data to support the effectiveness of FAF in treating stuttering while the speaker wears the device is currently scanty, although in an emerging status, if recent conference presentations eventually result in peer-reviewed publication (see more later when we discuss portable devices). FAF is receiving current attention in the popular media, despite the fact that its empirical support and clearly understood mechanism of action are still lacking (see Finn, Bothe, & Bramlett, 2005). Thus, its use is "controversial" in the sense that we discussed in Chapter 11.

Masking Noise

As we saw in Chapter 11, loud masking noise is another condition that is likely to bring about immediate fluency for many stutterers. A number of attempts have been made to exploit this effect by designing portable masking devices for use in stuttering therapy.[27] The person who stutters wears the

[26] See Goldiamond (1965) and his personal communication cited by Soderberg (1968).

[27] Guttman (1960), Parker and Christopherson (1963), Derazne (1966), Trotter and Lesch (1967), Perkins and Curlee (1969), Donovan (1971), Trotter and Silverman (1973), Dewar, Dewar, and Barnes (1976), Küppers and Wünschmann (1985).

masking unit as one would wear a binaural hearing aid and turns it on when blocking or anticipating a stutter. Trotter and Silverman (1973) reported clinical results showing that some stutterers may get some benefit from this technique over trial periods of weeks. One stutterer reported on by Trotter and Lesch (1967) was still being helped more than two years later. Some disadvantages were discussed by Perkins and Curlee (1969) as a result of their experience with three cases; they included the conspicuousness of the double earplugs, the slight hearing loss they produced while they were being worn, and the fact that the device was of little help on the telephone. Some of these disadvantages were minimized by a voice-activated unit known as the Edinburgh Masker.[28] Although it is not generally regarded as an adequate method of treatment in itself, clinical experience suggests that it may be a practical source of help in some cases. Block, Ingham, and Bench (1996) trialed the Edinburgh Masker with 18 adults, both in and beyond clinic use. Stuttering was decreased by a mean of approximately 50 percent for the group as a whole, but was not eliminated for any participants save one. Listeners rated the masked speech as less natural than speech produced without masking noise. The authors concluded that the Masker could provide benefits for some individuals who stutter, but does not eliminate stuttering in most cases or produce speech that sounds like typically fluent speech.

Portable Feedback Devices

Muellerleile (1981) and Craven and Ryan (1984) described the early use of portable delayed auditory feedback devices. With increases in digital technology, such devices have become more feasible and increasingly concealable, adding to their attractiveness to patients. Several are now marketed, including a patented in-the-ear device called the SpeechEasy®, which has received substantial media attention in recent years. It must be emphasized that the major advance offered by the device is its size, and therefore its concealability, rather than offering a new treatment approach, *per se.* At the time that this edition of the *Handbook* goes to press, there have been few published reports on short- and long-term benefits of use of the device, although unpublished conference papers are beginning to emerge in number. The SpeechEasy is premised directly on the choral reading effect, and offers both DAF and frequency-altered feedback (FAF). To date, most clinical (as opposed to laboratory) reports of user efficacy have been by the device's developers at East Carolina University (see Stuart, Kalinowski, Rastatter, Saltuklaroglu, & Dayalu, 2004; Stuart, Kalinowski, Saltuklaroglu, & Guntupalli, 2006) and have used only nine participants. A short-term laboratory study (Armson, Kiefte, Mason, & De Croos, 2006) of 13 adults showed very mixed benefit across people and speaking tasks and could not evaluate potential adaptation by users, which would progressively limit its effectiveness. Major conceptual concerns with the use of altered auditory feedback (AAF) as a treatment technique were voiced by Lincoln, Packman, and Onslow (2006), and included the following caveats for potential users and therapists: Although some people benefit from AAF in the laboratory, not all do; results of long-term use and adaptation are basically unknown but could be substantial; and there are no data on use by children. Even the developers stress that devices are best used as adjuncts to therapy, not as alternatives. Systematic critiques by Bothe, Davidow, Bramlett, Ingham (2006) and McAuliffe and Bernstein Ratner (2007) do not currently substantiate the evidence base for the widespread use of such devices, although more information is being accumulated that may change this evaluation by the time of the next edition of the *Handbook*.

Before leaving this topic, it is clear that some individuals have found some degree of benefit from limited usage of altered auditory feedback devices. Bakker (2006) explores some practical concerns in evaluating such assistive devices. In particular, he notes that it is wise for anyone considering their use to see whether or not they respond to AAF with improved fluency, since not all speakers do. As he notes, there are free or low-cost programs on the

[28] See Dewar, Dewar, and Barnes (1976), Ingham, Southwood, and Horsburgh (1981).

Internet that allow individuals to trial their speech under AAF before going to the additional considerable expense of having ear molds constructed to use concealable devices and purchasing the devices.

Biofeedback

An approach that can be classified under the category of assistive devices is the use of various forms of biofeedback. Guitar (1975) presented a laboratory model of EMG biofeedback therapy using a device in which electrical potentials from surface electrodes over a muscle were converted into a steady low-frequency tone. When a threshold voltage, which could be selected by the therapist or experimenter, was exceeded, the frequency of the tone increased in proportion to the voltage and therefore to the tension in the muscle. With each of three participants, Guitar conducted successive experiments with the electrodes at the larynx, chin, upper lip, and, for purposes of control, the frontalis muscle. In each case, the stutterer first remained at rest and tried to keep the tone at the lowest frequency. Successively lower threshold voltage levels were set until the person had attained the lowest level possible. Participants then read a list of sentences containing their most difficult sounds in initial position, with instructions to keep the muscle potentials below threshold while awaiting the signal to say each sentence. Trials in which the participants received auditory feedback were alternated with trials in which they did not.

The procedure resulted in reductions of stuttering in all three cases. Training at the lip and larynx proved especially effective. Training at the frontalis muscle produced no effect. With an additional participant, Guitar undertook a clinical program of biofeedback therapy consisting of five 40-minute sessions. In the first two sessions, the stutterer was trained to reduce the muscle potentials at the site selected, the chin. The remaining three sessions were devoted to conversational speech during which the speaker practiced reducing the voltage levels whenever he anticipated stuttering. In the first of the three speech sessions, he received auditory feedback; in the last two he did not. The participant was successful in maintaining below-threshold voltage levels, and fluent speech, without feedback. He was then instructed to reduce levels during phone calls at work. After tape recordings of such calls demonstrated fluent speech for 10 days, treatment was discontinued. Nine months later, analysis of tape-recorded conversation and telephone calls showed that the participant was still speaking without stuttering.

A number of other researchers and clinicians have experimented with EMG biofeedback in what were for the most part laboratory studies for the purpose of developing treatment methodologies.[29] As we noted in Chapter 10, experiments have also been concerned with whether it is actually the muscle relaxation or some other factor that is responsible for the effect on stuttering.[30] Electromyographic feedback seems uniquely calculated to help stutterers eliminate the excessive tension that appears to be the immediate underlying cause of so much of their speech difficulty. For this reason, it may hold considerable promise both as a method in itself and as an adjunct to other therapies.

Dembrowski and Watson (1991a) described the use of combined plethysmographic, pneumotachographic, and electroglottographic biofeedback for the purpose of helping stutterers to maintain normal breathing, airflow, and phonation during speech. Gow and Ingham (1992) conducted two single-subject interventions (one adult, one adolescent) using biofeedback to identify phonated intervals that they targeted for modification. Fluency was improved for both participants.

Craig et al. (1996) conducted what is probably the largest controlled study of the use of biofeedback to date.[31] Twenty-five children, ages 9–14

[29]Aten and Blanchard (1974), Hanna, Wilfling, and McNeil (1975), Lanyon, Barrington, and Newman (1976), Lanyon (1977), Moore (1978), Gordon, Gordon, Gordon, Shapiro, Mentis, and Suchet (1981), Craig and Cleary (1982), St. Louis, Clausell, Thompson, and Rife (1982).

[30]Cross (1977), Moore (1978), Pachman, Oelschlaeger, Hughes, and Hughes (1978).

[31]This study also reported comparable data from two other forms of intervention (an intensive program to teach "smooth speech" as well as a home-based program with the same therapeutic goal) as well as a control group who did not receive treatment. Findings from these interventions are addressed elsewhere in this chapter. All treatment groups achieved high levels of fluency that were maintained over time; the no-treatment group did not experience any significant improvement in fluency during the period of the study.

years, were randomized into an intensive EMG program modeled after Craig and Cleary (1982). They were treated in small groups, for more than six hours per day for a week. The goal of the program was to reduce muscle tension in the articulators during the production of increasingly longer stretches of speech. After three days of training, the children were "weaned" from the feedback. Fluency was improved by 90–95 percent immediately post-treatment, and was 80 percent improved when measured three months post-treatment. At one year post-intervention, fluency was still 70 percent better than at study intake; speech quality was rated as the most natural of the treatment groups in the study. Roughly 75 percent of the children demonstrated fewer than 2 percent stuttered syllables on one-year follow-up. Measures of state anxiety were also improved. In a replication of Craig et al.'s EMG intervention, Block, Onslow, Roberts, and White (2004) found that conversational fluency was improved by more than 36 percent after 12 children and adolescents were trained to use EMG feedback in an intensive intervention program that lasted for six hours per day for five days. However, conversational speech rate was much slower than would be typical, and fluency benefits were more modest than those reported by Craig et al. The authors concluded that biofeedback might be a useful adjunct to other forms of therapy, but would be unlikely to succeed in inducing and maintaining both natural and stutter-free speech by itself.

Rhythmic or Metronome-Timed Speech

Like slow speech, rhythmic speech is a remedial method going back many years that owes its recurrent popularity both to the evolution of behavioral treatments and to advances in electronic engineering. Most applications have employed a miniaturized electronic metronome device that the stutterer wears like a hearing aid.[32] Brady indicated that of 26 stutterers that he treated, 21 were able to speak with markedly increased fluency even without the device after several months of therapy, and of 20 cases followed up for periods ranging from 16 months to 4.5 years, only 3 experienced partial relapses. Stager, Denman, and Ludlow (1997) found a possible reason for the fluency-enhancing properties of metronome-timed speech: both stutterers and typically fluent speakers decreased vowel intensity and peak pressure and increased subglottal pressure rise time under metronome-paced speech. Such changes might logically relate to the production of more fluent speech.

Rhythmic speech can be learned and practiced without the use of a pacing device and will tend to eliminate stuttering as effectively. This was amply demonstrated by Andrews and his coworkers in their use of syllable-timed speech, a form of speech that is produced one syllable at a time with even stress and timing.[33]

Since pacing words or syllables with a metronome tend to produce an unusual mode of speech, at least in English, which is not a syllable-timed language, Silverman and Trotter (1973) made an evaluation of listener reactions to several stutterers who used such a device. Although the observers consistently rated the stutterers as more fluent with the aids than without them, they did not necessarily have more favorable reactions. This depended on the severity of the stuttering. Mallard and Meyer (1979) found that naive listeners generally preferred the metronome-timed speech of a moderate and severe stutterer to their stuttered speech. Brady (1971) tried to impart a degree of naturalness to metronome-timed speech by teaching patients to time whole phrases to the beat rather than just words or syllables.

Trotter and Silverman (1974) reported a series of probes to determine if the effectiveness of a miniature metronome would wear out with continued use. In one test, three adults who stuttered maintained their fluency in oral reading on each of 18 days. In a second study, one schoolchild continued to benefit from the device through 14 sessions of

[32] Meyer and Mair (1963), Brady (1968, 1969, 1971), Horan (1968), Wohl (1968, 1970), Brady and Brady (1972), Trotter and Silverman (1974), Öst, Götestam, and Melin (1976), Silverman (1976b), Mallard (1977).

[33] Andrews and Harris (1964, chap. 8), Ingham and Andrews (1971b), Andrews and Ingham (1972a, 1972b), Helps and Dalton (1979).

reading and speaking, while another child benefited through 26 sessions. In a third, an adult who stuttered used a miniature metronome all day for a period of 36 days with no diminution of the effect. Finally, Silverman, who was a moderately severe stutterer, wore the device 12 to 16 hours a day for 16 months. While its effectiveness did not cease, it was not as great at the end of this period as it had been during the first three months. Subsequently, Silverman (1976b) reported that he had continued to use the same miniature metronome for three years. Its effectiveness diminished gradually until, in the final six-month period, it was of little benefit. "I found myself," Silverman wrote, "attending less and less to the metronome beat while I spoke and becoming less and less certain that using the device would have a significant impact on the severity of my stuttering."

Most work with syllable-timed speech has been conducted with adults. However, Trajkovski, Andrews, O'Brian, Onslow, and Packman (2006) reported a case study of a preschool-aged child successfully treated using a parental model of paced speech for only a few minutes per day. The treatment was applied because the child was considered too young for Lidcombe therapy intervention (see discussion earlier in this chapter). After 16 weeks, stuttering was reduced to zero.

PHARMACEUTICAL TREATMENTS

History of Drug Treatments for Stuttering

A variety of pharmaceutical agents have been used from time to time in the treatment of stuttering. Wider interest in such therapy, however, began in the 1950s with the introduction of tranquilizers because of the central role that anxiety and tension have been assumed to play in the disorder. The results have been somewhat varied.[34] They have generally led to restrained optimism about the use of tranquilizers as an adjunct to other therapy. A frequent report is that the drug has more effect on the complexity or severity of stutters than on their frequency.

Following the introduction of haloperidol in 1960, a particularly large number of studies were done of its effect on stuttering.[35] These studies, including some carefully designed double-blind investigations making use of objective measures of stuttering and placebo groups or conditions, appear to show that the drug has a real though limited effect. In addition to finding that many subjects have received little or no benefit, the studies reveal that a large proportion of subjects have tended to drop out of treatment because of the side effects of the drug, especially drowsiness. Both Andrews and Dozsa (1977) and Murray, Kelly, et al. (1977) reported that few of the subjects whose stuttering was reduced wished to continue the medication after the experiment.

The reason for the ameliorative influence of haloperidol on stuttering is not known. The drug is thought to block dopamine receptors in the central nervous system. Burns, Brady, and Kuruvilla (1978) reasoned that the administration of apomorphine might therefore increase stuttering by dopamine receptor stimulation. They found that it did not, although most of their subjects responded to haloperidol with reduced stuttering.

Mechanisms of Action for Pharmacological Treatments

More recently, there has been systematic analysis of the potential mechanisms of action by which drugs might alleviate stuttering. Maguire, Yu, Franklin, and Riley (2004) and Ludlow (2006) have written overviews that delineate the various classes of pharmacological agents and their presumed mechanisms of action on the central nervous system. Ludlow notes that a variety of agents have been tried to date, including dopamine D2 receptor blockers (of

[34] Winkelman (1954), Maxwell and Paterson (1958), Di Carlo, Katz, and Batkin (1959), Holliday (1959), Kent and Williams (1959), Burr and Mullendore (1960), Yannatos (1960) Fish and Bowling (1962), Fujita et al. (1963), Kent (1963), Schilling (1963), Cacudi (1964), Aron (1965), Fish and Bowling (1965), Goldman and Guth (1965), Goldman (1966), Hommerich and Korzendorfer (1966), Leanderson and Levi (1967).

[35] Gattuso and Leocata (1962), Cozzo and Gabrielli (1965), Tapia (1969), Wells and Malcolm (1971), Quinn and Peachey (1973), Swift, Swift, and Arellano (1975), Rantalaka and Petri-Larmi (1976), Rosenberger, Wheelden, and Kalotkin (1976), Andrews and Dozsa (1977), Murray, Kelly, et al. (1977), Prins, Mandelkorn, and Cerf (1980). See also Ludlow (2006) for comparative details of these studies' designs and findings.

which, haloperidol is one; others include pimozide,[36] tiapride, risperidone, and olazapine),[37] norepinephrine reuptake inhibitors (e.g., desipramine), serotonin selective reuptake inhibitors (clomipraine, paroxotine, fluoxetine), and channel blockers (e.g., propanolol, verapamil).[38] Bothe, Davidow, Bramlett, Franic, and Ingham (2006) also note trials with clonodine (an alpha receptor agonist), and the anticonvulsive agent carbazepine.

Each of these classes of medication has primary uses in treating other conditions. For example, haloperidol is a conventional antipsychotic agent, and is also used to treat schizophrenia and Tourette Syndrome. Risperidone is also used as an antipsychotic. Channel blockers are used most conventionally to treat cardiovascular disorders, as well as situational anxiety. The reuptake inhibitors are typically used to treat depression, obsessive-compulsive disorder, panic and anxiety, and post-traumatic stress disorder, among a variety of conditions for which specific drugs in this category are approved. As noted, carbazepine is used to treat epileptic convulsions. Evidence regarding the effectiveness of each of these classes of drugs in treating stuttering will be discussed in turn.

Dopamine D2 Receptor Blockers

As noted, one of the possible reasons why haloperidol was considered as a treatment for stuttering was its known effects on the dopamine system. Maguire, Yu, et al. (2004) review the evidence that suggests that stuttering is associated with elevated dopamine activity, including cases in which stuttering has been induced or increased after administration of levodopa and other pharmacological treatments that increase dopamine levels. Wu, Maguire, Riley, Lee, Keator, Tang, Fallon, and Najafi (1997) had found elevated levels of dopamine in adults who stutter.[39]

Because, as noted, haloperidol has unacceptable side effects for the majority of people studied, some more selective agents thought to produce fewer side effects have been tried since the 1990s. However, Bloch et al. (1997) found serious depression and adverse motor symptoms among a group of eight adults studied in a trial of pimozide. More encouraging findings were reported by Rothenberger, Johannsen, Schulze, Amorosa, and Rommel (1994) for the use of tiapride with a group of 10 German adolescents; they found that stuttering was decreased by roughly 5 percent stuttered syllables from pre-intervention stuttering rate under drug administration.

Risperidone, a newer generation D2 blocker, also affects serotonin levels. More conventionally used to treat conditions such as bipolar disorder or schizophrenia, it has been trialed in two studies conducted by Gerald Maguire and his colleagues. In the first report, Maguire, Gottschalk, Riley, Franklin, Bechtel, and Ashurst (1999), 21 adults were randomized to treatment and no-treatment conditions; speech fluency was only slightly improved in the first group. In a follow-up double-blind, placebo-controlled study, Maguire, Riley, Franklin, and Gottschalk (2000) found more substantive fluency gains for eight adults, showing a roughly 50 percent reduction in percent stuttered syllables (percent SS) with few major side effects (although the mean pre-intervention rate was only about 10 percent SS). However, Maguire, Yu, et al. (2004) report that long-term compliance in taking risperidone was hampered by undesirable longer-term side effects that included sexual dysfunction, anxiety, and depression.

Finally, another drug in this category, olanzapine, was studied by Lavid, Frankin, and Maguire (1999) and Maguire, Yu, et al. (2004). The first study reported on improved fluency in three case studies of children treated with olanzapine. In the second study, 24 adults were enrolled in a three-month, double-blind, placebo-controlled trial. Participants'

[36] In the following discussions, the generic name of the drug is listed, rather than manufacturer-specific brand names.

[37] Curiously enough, Ludlow also notes that some drugs in this class (risperidone and clozapine) have been observed to induce stuttering in some case studies.

[38] She also provides a tutorial that details the methods of action for these classes of drugs.

[39] However, Goberman and Blomgren (2003) did not find that speech disfluencies of Parkinson's disease patients fluctuated under varying levels of l-dopa.

fluency was monitored for one month before the trial and they were followed for one year after the trial ended. Treatment resulted in a statistically significant improvement on three measures of stuttering severity, one of which was the *SSI-3*. The others included a clinician rating scale and a participant self-rating scale. Side effects were reported as minor, and included increased appetite, weight gain, and sedation. Maguire cautions that patients on such medication would need to be monitored, as both respiridone and olanzapine carry some known risk of lipid-level elevation and may trigger Type II diabetes. In spite of this, Maguire, Yu, et al. (2004) note that compliance was high with olanzapine, and that many patients opted to continue taking it over the year following the end of the trial, with some experiencing even greater improvement in their speech over time. Maguire, Yu, et al. (2004) conclude that drug trials may need to be longer in order to observe maximal benefits (or perhaps side effects) that accrue from the administration of medications to control stuttering.

Reuptake Inhibitors

The major drug that has been trialed in the norepinephrine reuptake inhibitor category is desipramine, typically used as an antidepressant. A pair of related studies, Stager, Ludlow, Gordon, Cotelingam, and Rapoport (1995) and Gordon, Cotelingam, Stager, Ludlow, Hamburger, and Rapoport (1995), compared desipramine to clomipramine, a serotonin selective reuptake inhibitor. No benefit was seen for those taking desipramine in either report, and Ludlow (2006) concluded that, "Given this poor result, it is unlikely that this class of medications will be proven beneficial in the treatment of stuttering."

As noted previously, clomipramine, a serotonin selective reuptake inhibitor, was evaluated by Stager et al. (1995) and Gordon et al. (1995) in comparison with desipramine, and produced more encouraging findings. The design in both reports, one of which included data from 16 participants and the other from 17 participants, included a baseline and placebo phase preceding random assignment to one medication for five weeks, a two-week washout period using inactive placebo, and then five weeks on the other medication. Clomipramine was significantly better than desipramine when judged on the basis of participant self-report of stuttering severity; observed fluency gains were more modest, although statistically significant. Ludlow (2006) reported that a number of participants chose to remain on the medication following the end of the trial, but that benefits 7 to 10 months later were even more modest than at trial end.

Paroxetine, another medication from this category, was trialed by Bloch, Stager, Braun, and Rubinow (1995), who compared it to pimozide. The study was terminated midway through its intended design for safety reasons after severe adverse psychiatric symptoms were observed following withdrawal from paroxetine. Similarly, pimozide was observed to induce depression (Bloch et al., 1997). Sertraline, another SSRI, was trialed by Costa and Kroll (1995). However, sertraline has been noted to induce stuttering in previously normally fluent individuals in a number of case reports.[40]

Other Categories of Medication

The beta blocker propanolol was studied by Bloch, Dalby, and Johannesen (1977). Propanolol, which has been found effective against essential tremor, had no statistically significant effect on stuttering, although a number of participants seemed to show improvement. In an uncontrolled case report by Cocores, Dackis, Davies, and Gold (1986), some benefits were seen, both in fluency and in anxiety. Oxprenolol, which has been found to improve skilled performance under stress (see Rustin, Kuhr, Cook, & James, 1981), also has shown little benefit in treating stuttering. Bethanecol chloride appeared to produce improvement in a study of two patients (Hays, 1987). Verapamil, which reduces calcium in smooth muscle cells, needed for muscle contraction, had no evident effect on stuttering in a study of 14 subjects by Brumfitt and Peake (1988),

[40] McCall (1994), Makela, Sullivan, and Taylor (1994), Makela and Sullivan (1996), Christensen, Byerly, and McElroy (1996), Brewerton, Markowitz, Keller, and Cochrane (1996).

while Brady, Price, McAllister, and Dietrich (1989) showed only modest decreases in stuttering while reading, but not conversation, for 10 adults treated with the drug.

The drug clonidine, which is used to control high blood pressure and treat migraine headaches, was studied by Althaus, Vink, Minderaa, Goorhuis-Brouwer, and Oosterhoff (1995) in a group of 25 stuttering children. The drug did not produce any measurable changes in fluency.

Pagoclone

The newest pharmaceutical agent to be trialed for stuttering treatment is pagoclone, a gamma amino butyric acid (GABA) selective receptor modulator. Originally developed to treat anxiety, it serendipitously reduced stuttering in some participants in the anxiety treatment trial. In late 2006, there was public announcement (not yet published in peer-reviewed journals at the time this text went to press), of an eight-week, placebo-controlled, double-blind, multi-center Phase II trial utilizing 132 patients randomized to treatment or placebo. The developing company (Indevus) reported significant improvement in behavioral indices of stuttering severity without any obvious side effects.[41] Clearly, we must examine the final data from this trial in order to reach any conclusion about its long-term benefits in treating stuttering.

Additional Pharmaceutical Agents

Over the years, favorable reports have also appeared about thiamin (Hale, 1951) and glutamic acid (Gutzmann, 1954), but information about their effectiveness is scanty. A survey by Kent (1961) of the use of carbon dioxide inhalation therapy with stutterers indicated varied and equivocal results.

Finally, botulinum toxin (better known as Botox, in its more popular current usage as a wrinkle-reducing cosmetic treatment) has been administered to reduce stuttering by weakening the vocal folds via bilateral injection (Brin, Stewart, Blitzer, & Diamond, 1994). Fourteen adults experienced modest gains in fluency, with relapse after 12 weeks. Speech produced under Botox was noticeably breathy in the case of one participant who was featured in an educational film about stuttering and its treatment.[42] There have been no long-term reports of its successful use by individuals who stutter.

Summary

As noted, Maguire, Yu, et al. (2004), Ludlow (2006), and Bothe, Davidow, Bramlett, Franic, and Ingham (2006) have all provided recent overviews of pharmacological treatments for stuttering. All emphasize that no medication has yet been shown to effectively improve fluency, and all express some concerns over risks of pharmacological treatments that may greatly exceed fluency benefit. All suggest that any pharmacological agent likely to be shown to improve fluency to some degree would have to be coupled with a behavioral treatment regimen in order to achieve meaningful increases in natural and fluent speech.

Bothe, Davidow, Bramlett, and Ingham (2006) also suggested additional criteria for the evaluation of pharmacological agents in the treatment of stuttering. Most of the published work in this area has appeared, as one might expect, in medical journals, where the design may meet expectations of appropriate drug trials (or be as uncontrolled as single case reports). However, such studies rarely employ evaluations of speech that would conform to best and meaningful practices in speech-language pathology. They suggest that studies should include random assignment to groups or appropriate single-subject design, include fluency measures computed by raters blind to condition and appropriately evaluated for reliability, compare pre- and post-treatment measures that go beyond in-clinic assessment, and provide additional data about speech rate, naturalness, and overall listener impression of stuttering severity. Few studies to date have provided such information, and those that have do not reveal any pharmacological agent to significantly improve fluency. Finally,

[41] www.Indevus.com (May 2006).

[42] "*The Doctor Is In: Stuttering*" (1992)

very few studies have addressed the safety or effectiveness of drug therapies for stuttering in children.

THE EFFECTIVENESS OF THERAPY

From this brief account of therapy approaches, it must be clear that we are as far as ever before in our history from any consensus about the best way to treat stuttering, a comment made in the last edition of the *Handbook* as well. Even the accumulating data on the effectiveness of some forms of therapy have fueled spirited discussion of the status of other therapies with lesser amounts of effectiveness data, particularly of the forms typically held in highest esteem by the medical professions when evaluating treatments (see the special issue of *Journal of Fluency Disorders, 28,* 3, 2003; and Bernstein Ratner, 2005).

At the same time, it is evident that we are able to offer many children and adults who stutter a considerable amount of help; many therapies are actually quite and almost equally effective, at least for some periods of time (Hancock, Craig, McCready, McCaul, Costello, Campbell, & Gilmore, et al., 1998; Herder, Howard, Nye, & Vanryckeghem, 2006). It is a challenge to try to arrive at a realistic notion of our actual therapeutic capacity. Clinical lore tends to hand down two conflicting impressions about the effectiveness of treatment. One is that stuttering is a relatively difficult problem to treat, at least in adults (Cooper & Cooper, 1995). The other is the impression that almost any kind of therapy is liable to work with the client who stutters, at least for a time. It is not a simple matter to reconcile these contradictory assumptions. Presumably, there may be something useful to be learned from the reports of clinicians who have tried to evaluate the results of their efforts systematically. A distillation of such reports is given in the Appendix, where we have listed in table form the outcomes of clinical studies based on groups of at least five participants, and assembled them thematically by basic approach as outlined in this chapter.

The data presented in the Appendix must be interpreted with caution. To try to use them for comparing one method of treatment with another would be futile. The studies we survey differed widely in their scientific rigor and sophistication. In order to present their results succinctly, we have been compelled to leave out many details. Finally, the various terms used for significant improvement (we have given the investigators' own words as far as possible) are likely to have such different meanings for different authors that, for that reason alone, the percentages in the table can have only the roughest kind of comparability. However, over time, even smaller and less well-controlled studies may provide some collective documentation of those therapy approaches most likely to merit larger and better-controlled clinical trials of effectiveness. It is to this end that we continue to provide reports of even small investigations of the effectiveness of particular therapies for stuttering. It should also be self-evident that use of an intervention not ever before reported in a peer-reviewed publication would be experimental at best, and poorly motivated at worst. Similarly, some interventions have been shown not to be effective in well-controlled investigations (e.g., acupuncture). Such findings should be taken seriously by clinicians and people who stutter and their families.

Despite some ambiguity, there is a remarkable message to be read in the table. It is unmistakable that a great variety of methods are capable of bringing about what a clinician may regard in good faith as a successful outcome of therapy in a large proportion of cases. Taking the table at face value, one would be inclined to infer that substantial improvement, as defined in these studies, typically occurs as a result of almost any kind of therapy in about 60 to 80 percent of cases.

Furthermore, the variety of methods that have some potential for eliminating stuttering in individual cases is even greater than one could guess from the table alone. The reference list of this book would have been much longer if it had included the multitude of published reports of success with single cases, sometimes accompanied by accounts of satisfactory carry-over outside the clinic and persistence of fluency for relatively long periods after the termination of treatment. We see such reports frequently at international conferences devoted to stuttering treatment, and they involve an almost limitless number of approaches. It would seem that therapy itself, apart from what is done in therapy, has considerable capacity for effecting change, particularly when clients are ready for such change (Zebrowski, 2007).

Why, then, is stuttering not universally regarded as the easiest of disorders to treat? We now come to the other side of the coin. The answer seems to be that few sophisticated clinicians of long experience are prepared to accept enthusiastic claims of success at face value. They have seen too many stutterers go from therapist to therapist achieving one ephemeral success after another. Many of them have also seen therapies once hailed for documented accomplishments fail to live up to their early promise and gradually fall into disuse. They would tend to be skeptical of many of the optimistic assertions about the outcome of therapy that we have gathered in the Appendix, and they would have a number of good reasons. For example, many of these reports, especially the older ones, are based on little more than subjective clinical impression. Most studies made little attempt to evaluate the stutterer's progress outside the clinic or to determine whether the benefits of treatment were lasting. We note that even programs with very good therapy outcomes have found it advisable to offer "refresher" sessions to maintain gains achieved during initial therapy (e.g., Block et al., 2005).

Various pertinent aspects of improvement besides fluency have been largely ignored in some studies (Bothe, Davidow, Bramlett, Franic, & Ingham 2006). As noted, attention has rarely been given to the part that spontaneous recovery may play in stuttering, especially in children. (Note, for example, Daskalov's preschool group, who were doing much better two years after therapy than at the end of treatment.) Waitlist controls (e.g., Jones et al., 2005) are making an important contribution to understanding this elemental problem in evaluating therapies for young children.

In short, the assessment of results of therapy is a process fraught with opportunities for error and self-delusion. The subject has been discussed extensively by Van Riper (1973, chap. 7), Andrews and Ingham (1972a), Ingham and Andrews (1973b), Ingham (1984b, chap. 12), and Sheehan (1984).

The Effectiveness of Stuttering Therapies: Systematic Review and Meta-Analysis

As may be clear from the preceding discussion, not all therapy outcome studies are equal in quality or rigor, nor in numbers of individuals followed, nor for how long. In medicine and other disciplines, this problem is being addressed by systematic reviews of the literature that apply evaluative criteria to the available studies for the treatment of a specific disorder. Such efforts are not only important because they sift and weight the available findings for the specialist; they are becoming critical for practicing professionals who often lack the time or means to follow each and every new study that appears in the literature.

A recent systematic review of non-pharmacological stuttering treatments was conducted by Bothe, Davidow, Bramlett, and Ingham (2006). They limited their selection criteria to treatments for developmental stuttering, published in English, in a peer-reviewed journal between 1970 and 2005, for which a methodology was provided. Their search identified 162 articles, reporting on 197 interventions. Of these, only 39 articles satisfied their set of methodological criteria for well-conducted studies. These included: either random assignment of clients to groups or appropriate single-subject design with either ABA or multiple baseline measurements, blinded or independent, reliable measurements of outcomes, both pre- and post-therapy measures for reported outcome variables, at least one beyond-clinic measurement for at least one targeted outcome, attempts to provide adjunct data on measures of speech rate or naturalness, as well as reliability for measures of stuttering severity.

The authors also established criteria for what they considered to be reasonable treatment outcomes. For fluency, these included the requirement, among others, that post-therapeutic percent stuttered syllables fall below 5 percent, and remain at that level for a minimum of one post-therapy assessment at least six months following termination of therapy. If affective and cognitive measures were taken prior to therapy, these measures had to improve as well.

Taken together, these two sets of requirements produced very few acceptable studies and even fewer acceptable outcomes. The average study of therapy fulfilled only half of the five design criteria, and only an average of one outcome criterion.[43] In brief, the authors concluded that the following treatments have shown some evidence of effectiveness in reducing stuttering frequency, although with widely varying degrees of empirical support: biofeedback (via EMG), Gradual Increase in Length and Complexity of Utterance (GILCU),[44] indirect management of stuttering in preschoolers using a Demands and Capacities Model, prolonged speech or other versions of fluency-shaped speech, response contingencies for stuttering, and self-modeling. The most robust data are available for approaches using fluency shaping and response contingencies. Prolonged/fluency-shaped speech has also, in some studies, shown improved affective and/or cognitive scores, while these features were not typically measured in studies utilizing response contingencies. Approaches that did not achieve acceptable outcomes, using the authors' criteria, even though they satisfied aspects of trial quality, were acupuncture, language training, metronome-paced speech, shadowing, and token economy. Results of regulated breathing therapies appeared mixed.

A slightly different approach was taken by Herder and colleagues at the University of Central Florida. Herder, Howard, Nye, and Vanryckeghem (2006) performed a systematic review and meta-analysis of behavioral stuttering treatments. Meta-analyses are able to combine results from smaller studies involving perhaps only a few individuals to estimate the likelihood that an intervention is in fact effective. In the analysis, the post-treatment results of 12 randomized-control trials (RCTs) that included both children and adults who stutter were aggregated in order to present an average effect size (a measure of effect that accounts for sample size). The results showed that, on average, the treated stutterers improved about one standard deviation when compared to those who were not treated. In addition, Herder and colleagues' analysis of the RCTs indicated that no single treatment demonstrated a statistically significant advantage over the others. In a subsequent study, Herder, Howard, Nye, Vanryckeghem, Schwartz, and Turner (2007) furthered the analysis by including four Quasi-Experimental Designed trials (QED, multiple group trials where subjects are not randomly allocated). Fifteen different treatments across the 16 studies were included. Results of this analysis showed that potential bias of the QEDs did not significantly affect the aggregated result. A continued analysis for the Campbell Collaboration, an international organization that collects and disseminates meta-analyses of medical, educational, and social research findings[45] (Herder, Howard, Nye, Vanryckeghem, Schwartz, & Turner, 2007), including only investigations of child treatments, showed similar results.

Beyond Specific Therapies: The Role of Common Factors in Therapy Outcomes

A certain amount of attention has been paid in recent years to factors beyond the specific therapeutic approach (e.g., fluency shaping vs. stuttering modification) to more global issues that might predict better therapy outcomes. One concept has been response cost (consequation of the client's response during the therapy session). In this regard, Bothe, Davidow, Bramlett, & Ingham (2006) note that therapies employing response contingencies have good outcome data. The notion of consequating the client's responses, however, can be broadly construed, and may have ramifications beyond those programs that describe themselves as operant. Other potential influences on therapy outcomes, such as whether therapies are best administered in an intensive format or weekly, less intensive sessions (more typical in American private practice, schools, and university clinics) have not attracted extensive research, despite suggestions by Andrews et al. (1983) that intensive programs fare better than non-intensive programs

[43] Studies eventually included in the review are detailed on pages 327–28 of the article.

[44] Although a troublingly high level of dropouts was reported.

[45] www.campbellcollaboration.org/

in producing fluency changes. A major question not answered in most areas of speech-language pathology, including stuttering, is whether group therapy differs from individual therapy in its effectiveness. A question clearly raised by the Lidcombe program is whether interventions for early stuttering are more effectively administered by parents, rather than clinicians. All of these questions illustrate the need for further research that transcends therapeutic techniques specific to methods for changing fluency, or speech attitudes and emotions. Finally, because the work we summarize here shows the tendency for specific therapies to be investigated by only a small number of sites potentially invested in the outcomes because they are associated with the developers of that particular therapeutic approach, we need therapy outcomes to be replicated across sites without obvious allegiance to the program developers (Bernstein Ratner, 2005).

Common Factors in Therapy Outcomes

In the field of clinical psychology, it has become increasingly evident that the contrasts between specific treatments do not account for all of the observed outcomes; in fact, in some cases, they account for relatively less than do what are sometimes called "common factors." These include the role of the clinician (expertise, knowledge of multiple therapy approaches, ability to problem-solve, ability to engage the client and establish therapeutic alliance) and the client (motivation, engagement, etc.). Bruce Wampold and his colleagues have been in the vanguard of such research in the psychology literature,[46] and their findings have relevance for our attempts to ascertain which therapies are most effective in treating stuttering. They have, for example, discovered that even drug therapies are more effective when administered by some clinicians than others (Wampold & Brown, 2005; McKay, Imel, & Wampold, 2006). In some studies that have been conducted in clinical psychology and psychiatry, the amount of variance accounted for by the therapy is in fact much less than the amount accounted for by the clinician (Wampold, Lichtenberg, & Waehler, 2005). For example, Wampold and Brown found that clinicians who were historically most successful in alleviating patients' symptoms actually obtained better results using a placebo medication than did poorer clinicians who administered an active pharmaceutical agent.[47]

Recent attention has also been paid to the role of the patient's mindset in approaching therapy. Patient "readiness for change" has been explored in other fields where treatment is sought for a chronic condition. Floyd, Zebrowski, and Flamme (2007) applied a "stages of change" model from clinical psychology to an analysis of responses by 44 adult and adolescent members of the National Stuttering Association to a questionnaire that probed readiness for change. They found clusters of responses that were a good statistical "fit" for differing stages of change among the respondents. They suggest, after examining the related literature from other therapies involving behavioral, cognitive, and affective change, that it might be appropriate to match therapies or therapy components to the stage that characterizes the client's current belief set. For example, clients at certain stages may do better with initial therapy components that address affect and cognition, while others may be more ready for behavioral change.

It is clear that the quest for a "best therapy" for stuttering is not likely to result in an unequivocal answer in the immediately foreseeable future, especially as we explore the contributions of these common factors to observed therapy outcomes. Models do not yet exist for stuttering that can combine an analysis of the best therapy to use with a particular client, although it is clear that researchers, especially in fields similar to ours, are beginning to understand the value of this question. What we can say is that we believe that therapies will need to be sensitive to patients' individual profiles, needs, values, motivations, and responses. Clinicians will need to be able to appraise best therapy "fit," establish therapeutic

[46]Some of their earlier work is summarized in Wampold (2001).

[47]The second author of that study made the observation in a personal communication to the second author of this text that she was wrong in stating in her 2005 article that "it doesn't matter who hands you a pill" when arguing against the use of medical models in assessing treatment efficacy. Apparently, it does.

alliance, and troubleshoot different patterns of response if they wish to achieve a positive and durable therapeutic outcome.

RELAPSE, PROGNOSIS, AND MAINTENANCE

Of all problems that limit the effectiveness of therapy, the one that has made the greatest claim on the attention of clinical researchers is relapse. In 1979, the problem of relapse in current programs of therapy was formally recognized by an international conference on the subject in Banff, Canada. In a paper reviewing objective studies of the long-term results of therapy, chiefly by some form of behavior modification, Martin concluded that roughly a third of stutterers appeared to achieve lasting fluency, about a third relapsed significantly after treatment, and about a third either dropped out of therapy before completing it or were not available for follow-up evaluation (Martin, 1981). Relapse is so common that "refresher" courses are routinely built in to many therapy programs.

Relatively little is known about the subject of relapse, and it is not entirely clear that it has even been adequately defined. As Craig (1998) notes, a definition that specifies any degree of stuttering following treatment is probably not reasonable. He suggests either "the recurrence of stuttering symptoms that were perceived as personally unacceptable after a time of improvement," or, as in Craig and Calver (1991), "stuttering to a degree which was not acceptable to yourself for at least a period of one week" (p. 50). Using such definitions, Craig and Hancock (1995) found that about 70 percent of 152 participants who had received fluency-shaping-type therapy could be considered to have relapsed, both by self-report and objective measures. Only around 28 percent did not experience relapse, a figure roughly consistent with Martin's estimates. However, most relapses were temporary, although frequent. Most of their respondents reported an average of three relapse episodes per year following treatment. Craig (1998) also notes that virtually identical profiles of relapse are very frequent in other complex conditions, both medical and psychological, including treatment for anxiety and substance addiction.

Some relapse figures are more positive, if taken in the short run. As measured clinically and by self-report, 28 percent of Dutch and 14 percent of Canadian adults who participated in the Comprehensive Stuttering Treatment Program (Langevin et al., 2006) could be considered to have relapsed if the proportion of gains seen at end of therapy are compared to follow-up values.

The nature of the process and its causes may differ with the type of treatment used, and we may not understand relapse well until we better understand why different kinds of therapy bring about reductions in stuttering in the first place. Although relapse plagues all forms of treatment, it is particularly distressing in the case of many of the most commonly used behavior therapies that appear to remove stuttering so rapidly and completely. Detractors argue that relapse is inevitable with such therapies. They assert that it is unreasonable to expect a lifelong problem such as stuttering to be permanently eradicated in the short time it takes to learn to speak fluently, for example, by talking in a slow manner by prolonging syllables, and they doubt that the stutterer has in any basic sense learned to speak normally in these cases.[48] Advocates sometimes lay the blame on what they regard as the stutterer's inherent proneness to disfluency. Thus, Andrews (1984b) noted: "Stuttering is a chronic disorder and many adults can only remain fluent by dint of constant effort." Such a notion is supported by a well-documented relationship between severity pre-treatment (as typically measured by percent stuttered syllables) and risk of relapse (Craig, 1998). Huinck, Langevin, Kully, Graamans, Peters, and Hulstijn (2006) also found that pre-treatment severity was predictive of relapse, with higher rates of stuttering associated with larger margin of behavioral progress, but also higher rate of relapse. Huinck et al. also suggested, given the outcomes of their therapy trial, that more mild stutterers might benefit more from therapeutic components that address attitudes and emotions, while

[48] See Sheehan (1984), Sheehan and Sheehan (1984).

more severe stutterers might require more attention to their speech fluency before such components could be meaningfully addressed.

Perkins (1979) suggested that for some individuals who stutter, the problem of maintaining fluency is largely one of identity. "When fluent, they feel like unwelcome strangers to themselves. . . . They wish to feel like themselves, and stuttering is part of that self-image." DiLollo and colleagues (DiLollo, Neimeyer, & Manning, 2002; DiLollo, Manning, & Neimeyer, 2003; DiLollo, Manning, and Neimeyer, 2005) agree with this perspective, which also is consistent with personal construct psychology. They suggest that narrative therapy may help to adjust the stutterer's identity to that of a fluent speaker.

In a long-term follow-up of clients who had undergone "smooth speech" therapy, Craig and Calver (1991) found that the majority of those who had suffered a relapse related it to feeling under pressure to talk faster. About 40 percent also imputed it to embarrassment about the speech pattern that they had been taught, such as prolongation.

For the most part, investigations of prognosis in stuttering therapy have been concerned chiefly with the influence of personality factors.[49] Although the results of these studies have been conflicting, a possible relationship has emerged between outcome of treatment and a measure of "locus of control of behavior" (LOC/LCB), the extent to which individuals perceive what happens to them to be a consequence of their own behavior (Craig & Andrews, 1985; Madison, Budd, & Itzkowitz, 1986). Studies by Guitar (1976), Guitar and Bass (1978), and Helps and Dalton (1979) suggest that stutterers with less favorable speech attitudes are less likely to obtain long-term benefit from a behavior therapy employing rate control techniques.[50] Results of locus of control investigations conducted more recently have not been as favorable: De Nil and Kroll (1995) did not find that LOC predicted either discharge fluency characteristics or those at long-term follow-up, although they did predict self-evaluation measures for 13 adults who had participated in an intensive precision fluency-shaping program. Notably, there had been a substantive degree of relapse after two years: while mean stuttering rates had decreased from a mean of 9 percent stuttered words to less than 1 percent immediately following therapy, rates increased to a mean of over 7 percent at long-term follow-up. Block, Onslow, Packman, and Dacakis (2006) did not find locus of control measures to predict long-term outcomes for 78 adults who participated in an intensive prolonged speech therapy program. In a review of predictive factors in relapse, Craig (1998) could not identify single factors that alone were reliable predictors of relapse. However, several, taken in combination, did appear to predict which clients were more or less likely to experience relapse, such as pre-treatment severity, speech attitudes, locus of control, and self-help activities.

Whatever factors underlie the relapse that dogs the use of artificial speech patterns, so seldom do such techniques result in genuinely spontaneous and automatic fluency that some advocates have come to believe the techniques should be taught essentially as an option for the person who stutters to use on occasions when normal-sounding speech is demanded, rather than as a standard manner of speaking to avoid stuttering altogether.[51] For example, Yaruss et al. (2002) found a statistically higher probability of self-reported relapse for members of a stuttering self-help group who had received fluency-shaping oriented therapies than those who had tried stuttering modification or avoidance-reduction therapies.

An increasing number of behavior therapy programs in recent years have incorporated so-called maintenance procedures in an effort to cope with the possibility of relapse following treatment. Examples of such procedures are periodic clinical contacts after the termination of treatment,[52] self-therapy

[49] Shames (1952), Sheehan, Frederick, Rosevear, and Spiegelman (1954), Prins and Miller (1973), Perkins, Rudas, Johnson, Michael, and Curlee (1974), Helps and Dalton (1979), Lanyon, Lanyon, and Goldsworthy (1979), Craig and Howie (1982), Craig, Franklin, and Andrews (1984), Craig and Andrews (1985), Madison, Budd, and Itzkowitz (1986), Kraaimaat, Janssen, and Brutten (1988).

[50] Controversy developed over the interpretation of the Guitar and Bass findings. See Young (1981) and Ulliana and Ingham (1984).

[51] Perkins (undated), Starkweather (1984).

[52] The term follow-up is sometimes used to refer to such contacts. They should not be confused with follow-up assessments some time after the termination of therapy.

assignments, and work on speech attitudes. Ingham (1980, 1982) conducted research on specific maintenance procedures. Boberg, Howie, and Woods (1979) reviewed the literature on the subject, and Ingham (1984a) offered a systematic description and classification of maintenance techniques. Many clinicians have come to believe that therapeutic gains are not likely to be maintained without changes in some of the feelings and attitudes of the person who stutters. Retrospective analysis of the recovery of seven adults who stuttered suggested that self-acceptance and fear reduction were among the consistent themes they identified (Plexico, Manning, & DiLollo, 2005).

To address the impact of work on feelings and attitudes, Hancock and Craig (2002) re-treated 12 teens who had relapsed six years following successful completion of three different therapy programs reported by Craig et al. (1996), discussed previously in this chapter. The follow-up intensive treatment (four days over two weeks) combined EMG feedback, smooth speech skill training, and a number of cognitive-behavioral components, including self-management, cognitive restructuring, and relaxation. The adolescents improved from a mean of 5 percent stuttered syllables to about 1 percent immediately and at two years post re-treatment. However, state and trait anxiety scores were unchanged over both sets of interventions, as were scores on the *CAT-R* (see Chapter 1). Thus, inspection of their speech improvement profiles (see Hancock & Craig, 2002, p.148) suggests that eventual fluency improvements might require continual and long-term follow-up. Because two-year follow-up was better with the second treatment that included psychological and cognitive-behavioral components, the authors suggested the value of addressing the psychological features of stuttering in treatment programs. In fact, the number of authors advocating attempts to combine behavior therapy with attention to speech attitudes indicates that such programs constitute a dominant trend,[53] and this emphasis can be expected to grow further.

[53] Perkins (1979), Guitar and Peters (1980), Shames and Florance (1980), Cooper (1984), Curlee (1984), Weiner (1984c), Evesham and Fransella (1985), Boberg (1984), Starkweather (1984).

SUMMARY AND CONCLUSIONS

The earliest methods for treating stuttering were based on suggestion, relaxation, and unusual modes of speaking. Since virtually all of these techniques tended to give effective and immediate relief from stuttering, they had undergone a long era of use by the earliest decades of the twentieth century. Relapse proved to be so frequent, however, that many professionals became disenchanted with the indiscriminate use of any measure that brought about immediate fluency.

The first reaction against these old forms of therapy came in the shape of the psychoanalytic approach to stuttering. As is usual with initial reactions, it was extreme. Those who hoped to help people who stutter were adjured to ignore the speech entirely and to give their attention to the "whole personality." A second wave of reaction produced what we have referred to in this book as Iowa therapy, shortly after the emergence of the profession of speech and language pathology in the United States. In fact, much of the impetus for the development of the new profession and scientific discipline came from growing opposition to outworn methods of treating stuttering used by commercial speech "specialists" and well-meaning professionals with little knowledge of speech disorders. To the inventors of Iowa therapy, it seemed that the trouble was not that it was so hard to help people who stutter, but that it was so easy to help them. These clinical researchers based their approach on a distrust of quick achievement of fluency. It seemed to them axiomatic that in the case of a problem such as stuttering, any gains so cheaply won were unlikely to be lasting. Consequently, they advocated gradual modification of the symptoms on the basis of the speakers' understanding of what they did when they stuttered and in the context of work designed to decrease their anxiety about stuttering.

Proponents of Iowa therapy believed it tended to achieve more stable gains than did the older methods. It also had certain limitations that the older methods did not. It tended to make relatively heavy demands on the time, skill, patience, and insight of both the stutterer and the clinician. In the hands of a poorly trained therapist, it could degenerate into little more than an attempt to teach people who stutter to live with their speech difficulty. At best, it almost never resulted in normal fluency.

By the 1960s, these limitations had become quite evident. Moreover, the professional climate of the 1930s had been all but forgotten. The time was ripe for a new development, and it came in the form of behavior therapies for stuttering. Some of these were based on conditioning, though not everyone agreed that all of their effects on stuttering were *bona fide* examples of conditioning. Behavior modification also lent a new respectability to slow speech, rhythmic speech, and other old devices. These emerged from the commercial "stammering schools" where, in the United States at least, they had been confined for 30 years and were taken up enthusiastically by new practitioners, often with the help of conditioning principles and electronic aids.

As a result of this development, the outcome of stuttering therapy began to be reported in more optimistic terms than it had been for some decades. At the same time, considerable skepticism was voiced by those to whom such claims seemed overenthusiastic and ill-informed. The soundness of methods that achieved quick fluency had hardly been an issue since these methods were challenged by Iowa therapy in the 1930s. Now it became an issue once more, with the roles of challenger and challenged reversed.

Although this debate is now of long standing, we believe that yet more time will have to elapse before the issue is resolved. At this writing it is possible to make some reasonable claims for either side. On the one hand, those who argued so vehemently against attempts at quick cures may have left an exaggerated impression of their futility on the generations of speech clinicians trained to be wary of them. The old methods certainly had their share of successes. On the other hand, some of the more extreme optimism about such methods has proved to be short-lived. It is interesting to note the assessment by Perkins (1973a) of eight years of clinical experience with behavior therapy based chiefly on rate control with the aid of DAF. He estimated that, while 70 percent of those treated acquired normal speech during therapy, more than half subsequently relapsed. Moreover, all felt they were still stutterers. "What became increasingly apparent," Perkins observed, "was that achievement of fluency was relatively easy, but that this was not tantamount to achieving normal speech."

A more recent development in the treatment of stuttering is the attempt to integrate aspects of Iowa therapy with elements of the behavioral or "fluency shaping" approach. In part, this means a return to preoccupation with the client's fears and avoidances from which there had been a broad retreat in the 1970s. In addition, a growing number of speech clinicians are equipping individuals who stutter both with techniques for acquiring immediate fluency and with methods of modifying stuttering in the Iowa tradition. Graduates of such programs, having learned both controlled fluency and acceptable stuttering, in the terminology of Guitar (2006), may proceed in several ways. They may use acceptable stuttering for every day and keep controlled fluency in reserve for special occasions. Or they may use acceptable stuttering when controlled fluency fails. Or they may use either, depending on what they feel most comfortable with in a given situation.

The growth of the stuttering self-help movement in recent years has added a new dimension to the outlook for people who stutter. Support groups for stutterers have grown in number worldwide, and there are now national organizations of such groups in the United States, Canada, Australia, Japan, and some 14 European countries. In the United States, the national organization is the National Stuttering Association (*nsastutter.org;* formerly the National Stuttering Project). The NSA establishes local self-help groups in all parts of the country, holds regional and national conferences, disseminates information, functions as a consumer advocate when issues affecting stutterers arise within the speech and hearing profession, and serves as an ombudsman for people who stutter, whether they are discriminated against as individuals in the workplace or denigrated as a class in the entertainment media. For the speech pathologist, the local self-help group, when one is available, is an invaluable resource. Self-help organizations encourage members to give up the struggle to hide their stuttering and to assert the right to speak without fear even though they stutter. And they generate the group spirit that provides the strength to do so. Speech pathologists possess nothing as powerful for changing stutterers' fearful and avoidant speech attitudes, and experience has shown many speech pathologists that self-help groups are, in turn, an important component of therapy (Klassen & Kroll, 2005). When participation in a self-help group is not a realistic possibility for some who stutter, a good alternative is the reading of the NSA's monthly publication, *Letting Go,* or the book-length gleanings from that periodical,[54] or their publication for children, *Letting Go, Jr.* A summary of the self-help movement in stuttering and a discussion of its documented benefits in other disciplines can be found in Reeves (2006). A self-help group specifically targeted for children and families (Friends; *Friendswhostutter.org*) was started in the 1990s and held its first annual convention in 1997. For speech-language pathologists, as well as people who stutter and their families, a long-standing resource is the Stuttering Foundation of America (formerly the Speech Foundation of America; *www.stutteringhelp.org*), which provides written materials as well as multimedia resources (demonstration videos of commonly employed diagnostic and therapy techniques) to enable better identification and intervention for fluency disorders, particularly those affecting children.

With the advent of the Internet age, additional self-help and public service resources have been developed and broadly utilized by people who stutter and their families.[55] These include websites, Listservs and chat rooms. The growing mismatch between demand for services and available, appropriately trained speech-language pathologists (Bernstein Ratner & Tetnowski, 2006) has also spawned changes in referral patterns and service delivery. For example, the growth of post-certification specialization among American Speech-Language Pathologists has led to an ASHA-approved specialty recognition plan and referral service for fluency specialists administered by the Specialty Board on Fluency Disorders (*www.stutteringspecialists.org*). The same shortage, even more evident in other countries, has led to as yet limited but reasonably successful experimentation with tele-health provision of fluency services. For example, both ISTAR and Lidcombe have reported acceptable outcomes from such distance treatment programs (Kully, 2000; Wilson, Onslow, & Lincoln, 2004). This trend will undoubtedly increase in the years to come as technological barriers to such vehicles for therapy delivery are progressively reduced.

THE NATURE OF RECOVERY

When we have said all that we must about the limitations of current therapies and the hazards that often make recovery more apparent than real, one fact of fundamental importance remains. It is that stuttering is remediable. We see evidence of this partly in the great number of children who recover from stuttering and partly in the observation that adults, too, make recoveries that meet all criteria for genuineness, although complete recovery in adulthood is far less common. Also, while no known therapy will help all who stutter, virtually all therapies, as we have seen, have the power to help some.

Recovery is a fact. It is the underlying nature of the recovery process that we do not yet fully understand. What is the necessary and irreducible factor that is common to all recoveries? Without the answer to this question, we are at a considerable disadvantage in our efforts to find a solution to the problem of therapy. Recognizing that it is a controversial question, we venture to suggest an answer. It is that the ultimate basis for essentially all true recovery from stuttering is to be found in the observation that if people could forget that they were stutterers, and in so doing forget to do all of the things that people who stutter think they have to do in order to talk, they would have no further difficulty with their speech.

Perhaps the most work to investigate "recovery" from stuttering has been done by Patrick Finn, who finds several themes in the self-reports of

[54] Ahlbach and Benson (1994).

[55] E.g., STUT-L, and STUT-HELP, Listservs for those who stutter and interested families and clinicians, and the Stuttering Home Page (www.stutteringhomepage.com), a hybrid consumer/professional site hosted by speech-language pathologist Judith Kuster. This site also hosts an annual "online conference" to address issues of interest and concern to stutterers, families, and clinicians. Instructions on how to access stuttering Listservs and self-help organizations around the world can be found at the Stuttering Home Page.

individuals describing themselves as recovered. First, some achieve this goal without any formal therapy whatsoever (Finn, 1996). Finn, Howard, and Kubala (2005) note that this group may be divided according to a number of distinctions. Self-reported recovered stutterers may include people whose speech is virtually indistinguishable from that of people who have never stuttered, and those whose speech can still be discriminated from typically fluent. Some individuals report never stuttering, while others report some tendency to stutter in some situations. Some report the necessity of monitoring, while others do not consciously monitor their speech. Many of these features overlap to create somewhat distinct profiles. By and large, what unites this group of speakers is that their attitudes toward speaking and stuttering have normalized to the point where stuttering no longer preoccupies and handicaps them.

In an important sense, this is what virtually all therapies appear to accomplish when they are successful. The hypnotist does it cheaply by a simple appeal to people to believe that they will not stutter. Many other therapists do much the same thing, more effectively on the whole by imbuing people who stutter with faith in a particular method. Some therapies make people who stutter forget about their speech difficulty by the use of bizarre speech patterns that compel them to masquerade as someone they are not. Others attempt it by measures for eliminating anxiety about stuttering. The chances are that permanent recovery can be plucked from any therapy if people become convinced that they will not stutter any more and have no need to be concerned about their speech.

Unfortunately, none of these methods is likely to accomplish this fully and permanently for a very large proportion of adult cases. To forget, for all practical purposes, that one is a stutterer in the face of every reminder is an extraordinarily difficult thing to do, especially when the problem is fully developed. Certain conditions seem to have great power to bring this about, but they are not always found in ordinary methods of therapy as we now know them. They are to be found in experiences so overwhelming that they shake people to their psychological roots. For example, one stutterer, according to a reliable report, recovered from stuttering after surviving an airplane crash. In a similar case related by Tawadros (1957), a young man got over his stuttering when his hand was battered in a machine-shop accident that almost cost him his life. The incident was said to have made his old problems and anxieties seem like trifles.

The lesson in these examples appears to be that recovery from stuttering may come from vicissitudes that reconfigure the stutterer's system of personal values so radically that fears or pressures involving speech no longer have a high priority. There are certainly other examples besides narrow escapes from death. Intense mystical or religious experiences appear to have this potentiality. A young woman of the first author's acquaintance stopped stuttering after she became a Christian Scientist. For a few who stutter, the potential for such vicissitudes is to be found in psychotherapy. For many, it may exist in personal development and maturation. Unfortunately, most such success stories fall within the category of less-than-reliable data, that of the single-subject retrospective report.

Perhaps the ultimate advances in our ability to cope with stuttering must await more adequate scientific theories of learning and cognition that will enable us to deal better with the commonplace irrationalities of everyday living. It may well be that to fully understand stuttering and its most effective treatment, particularly in older children and adults, we may need a much better understanding of human behavior. However, until that point, we are comfortable in saying that there are a large number of reasonably well-tested therapies for stuttering that have the good potential to help a large number of individuals. Some will work better for some than for others, and some clients may establish a better therapeutic alliance with some clinicians than others. In all this variety, there is continued hope for most who people stutter.

Appendix

APPENDIX[a,b]

Results of Treatment[c]

	Method	*N*	Age	Duration of Treatment	Results of Treatment	Follow-up Interval	Results of Follow-up[d]
THERAPIES PRIMARILY FOR ADULTS AND OLDER CHILDREN							
Cherry, Sayers, and Marland (1955)	Shadowing	5	Adults	2–4 weeks	100% showed striking improvement		
Kelham and McHale (1966)	Shadowing	38	4–43	5–70 sessions	74% improved or much improved		
Kondas (1967)	Shadowing	17	8–20	~3 weeks–9 months	71% much improved or cured	1–5 years	59% much improved or cured
Checiek (1983)	Hand-movement-timed speech	60	7–18	3–4 months	Positive results in 75%		
Andrews and Harris (1964)	Syllable-timed speech	10	21–30	11 weeks	100% stuttering inhibited for at least a few days	12 months	10% improved
Andrews and Harris (1964)	Syllable-timed speech and discussions of stuttering	10	19–44	11 weeks	100% stuttering inhibited for at least a few days	6 months	30% improved
Andrews and Harris (1964)	Syllable-timed speech	10	16–19	11 weeks	100% stuttering inhibited for at least a few days	9 months	20% improved
Andrews and Harris (1964)	Syllable-timed speech	5	11	11 weeks	100% stuttering inhibited for at least a few days	9 months	60% improved
Brandon and Harris (1964)	Syllable-timed speech	28		64% successful			

(Continues)

APPENDIX (Continued)

	Method	*N*	Age	Duration of Treatment	Results of Treatment	Follow-up Interval	Results of Follow-up[d]
Helps and Dalton (1979)	Syllable-timed speech	21	18–47	4 weeks	Mean %SW[e] fell from 20.7 to 11.7 in conversation	1 year	Mean %SW was 15.2 in conversation
Ingham, Andrews, and Winkler (1972)	Syllable-timed speech and group psychotherapy	20	Adults	2 weeks	Mean %SS[f] fell from 22.4 to 7.5		
Wohl (1968)	Electronic metronome	146	15–68	Up to 1 year	63% greatly improved or fluent		
Brady and Brady (1972)	Electronic metronome	26	12–53	Several months	81% showed substantial improvement	16–54 months	85% maintained increased fluency
Öst et al. (1976)	Shadowing or electronic metronome	15	14–46	3 months	Metronome group showed significant mean reduction in stuttering	14 months	Improvement was maintained
Mallard (1977)	Electronic metronome	5	Adults	1 month	Reduction of stuttering in 80%		
MacCulloch, Eaton, and Long (1970)	Auditory masking	8		24 weeks	100% improved		
Dewar, Dewar, Austin, and Brash (1979)	Edinburgh Masker	195	Adults		89% responded well	6–28 months	Of 67 tested, 82% reported great or considerable benefit
Adamczyk (1959)	Delayed auditory feedback	15	6–28	2–3 months	87% showed significant improvement		
Adamczyk (1965)	Delayed auditory feedback	60	6–45	4 months	60% showed significant or complete improvement		
Gross and Nathanson[g]	Delayed auditory feedback	8		4 weeks	100% significantly reduced stuttering	6 months	All maintained minimal stuttering in oral reading

Curlee and Perkins (1969)	Delayed auditory feedback	14	Adolescents and adults	30 hours	All achieved normal conversational speech		
Webster (1970)	Delayed auditory feedback	8	15–47	10–40 hours	Stuttering reduced essentially to zero in all subjects	10 months	Fluency persisted in all subjects
Perkins et al. (1974)	Delayed auditory feedback	27	12–52	90 hours	In 70% of subjects stuttering was reduced by at least 85%	6 months	In 30% of subjects stuttering was reduced by at least 85%
Perkins et al. (1974)	Delayed auditory feedback and speech training	17	19–51	91–184 hours	In 71% of subjects stuttering was reduced by at least 85%	6 months	In 53% of subjects stuttering was reduced by at least 85%
Ryan and Van Kirk (1974)	Delayed auditory feedback	50	9–66	Approx. 20 hours	SW per minute reduced from 9 to 0.1 on average	Mean of 4.8 years	Sample of 11 subjects had mean of 1.7 SW words per minute[h]
Van Borsel, Reunes, and Van den Bergh (2003)	Delayed auditory feedback	9	18–45	3 months (at roughly 20 minutes per day usage)	Initial exposure to DAF resulted in mean decrease from ~35% SW under NAF to ~13% in conversational speech[i]	3 months	After 3 months of wear, conversational fluency under DAF was still ~13%, but fluency under NAF had improved as well, to ~16.5%, suggesting carry-over to unaided speech; all other speaking conditions showed a similar trend
Stidham, Olson, Hllbratt, and Sinopoli (2006)	Delayed auditory feedback via bone conduction	9	18–58	4 weeks	Pre-fitting, 78% of subjects were rated very severe/severe, 22% as moderate, and 0% as mild/very mild. Immediate	2 weeks	At follow-up (without device), 33% rated very severe/severe, 56% moderate, and 11% mild/very mild; no

(*Continues*)

APPENDIX (Continued)

	Method	*N*	Age	Duration of Treatment	Results of Treatment	Follow-up Interval	Results of Follow-up[d]
					post-fitting ratings were 22% very severe/severe, 11% moderate, and 67% mild/very mild; *SSI-3* scores declined nonsignificantly at 2 weeks, but significantly at 4 weeks		significant difference between pre-fit and follow-up *SSI-3* scores
Stuart, Kalinowski, Rastatter, Saltuklaroglu, and Dayalu (2004)	Delayed auditory feedback plus frequency altered feedback (SpeechEasy©)	8	9–54		Under altered auditory feedback (AAF), mean of 81% reduction in SS during reading and monologue	4 and 12 months[j]	Very slight rise in %SS under AAF during monologue at 4 months,[k] no systematic change in fluency without device in place at follow-up. Behaviors under AAF were stable at 12 months, with improvement in *PSI* scores and judged speech naturalness
Stuart, Kalinowski, Saltuklaroglu, and Guntupalli (2006)	Delayed auditory feedback plus frequency altered feedback (SpeechEasy©)	9	13–41		Under AAF, mean %SS fell from ~19 in monologue to ~2.5%[l]	12 months	When not wearing device at 1-year follow up, mean %SS was ~17%; with device it was ~5%; *PSI* scores also were improved
Peins, McGough, and Lee (1972)	Slow, legato speech	12	Mean 21	6 months	92% showed reduction in severity	2-1/2 years	Of 7 cases, 6 had maintained improvement[m]
Spencer (1976)	Smooth motion speech	5	Adults and Children[n]	4 months	Stuttering was reduced to less than 1% SS		

Boberg (1976)	Prolonged speech	21	17–44	3 weeks	Stuttering decreased from mean of 21% SS to 1.3%	6–24 months	Sample of 13 subjects showed mean relapse of 22%[o]
Resick et al. (1978)	Prolonged speech	6	Adults	2 weeks		6 months	Improvement persisted in reading and conversation but not on the telephone
Helps and Dalton (1979)	Prolonged speech	44	18–43	4 weeks	Mean %SW fell from 24.3 to 7.8 in sample of conversation	1 year	Mean %SW was 7.1 in conversation
Franck (1980)	Prolonged speech	68	Mean of 20.2 years	1 year	93% increased fluency by 60% or more	6 months or more	Of 45 subjects, 55% maintained improvement of 60% or more
Boberg (1981)	Prolonged speech	16	16–46	3 weeks[p]	Mean %SS decreased from 16.55 to 1.41	12 months	Mean %SS of 8 subjects was 1.53 at end of 12-month maintenance period
Boberg (1981)	Prolonged speech	6		3 weeks	Mean %SS decreased from 29.89 to 2.33	2 years	Mean %SS of 3 subjects was 17.68; no maintenance was provided
Howie, Tanner, and Andrews (1981)	Prolonged speech	36	Adults	3 weeks[i]	Stuttering was virtually eliminated	2 months	After 2 months in maintenance program there was little significant deterioration
Howie, Tanner, and Andrews (1981)	Prolonged speech	43	Adults	3 weeks[i]		12–18 months	Of 43 subjects, 21 were at least 85% improved
Evesham and Huddleston (1983)	Prolonged speech	47	Adults	2 weeks	91% showed < 1% SS		
Boberg (1984)	Prolonged speech	12	18–47	3 weeks[i]	Mean %SS decreased from 18.9 to 0.9		
Evesham and Fransella (1985)	Prolonged speech	23	Adults	2 weeks[i]		18 months	Of 22 subjects, 21 were improved

(Continues)

APPENDIX (Continued)

	Method	*N*	Age	Duration of Treatment	Results of Treatment	Follow-up Interval	Results of Follow-up[d]
Evesham and Fransella (1985)	Prolonged speech and personal construct therapy	24	Adults	2 weeks[i]		18 months	Of 22 subjects, all were improved; relapse was less than in the prolonged speech–only group
Craig and Andrews (1985)	Smooth, slow speech	17	Adults	3 weeks	Mean %SS declined from 12.9 to 0.9	10 months	Mean %SS was 1.9
Andrews and Feyer (1985)	Smooth, slow speech	37	21–60	3 weeks	Mean %SS declined from 14.0 to 0.1	10–15 months	Mean %SS was 1.1
Jehle and Boberg (1987)	Slow speech, gentle onsets of phonation	8	17–30	3 weeks	Mean %SS declined from 18.0 to 0.7		
Jehle and Boberg (1987)	Slow speech, gentle onsets of phonation	7	13–16	3 weeks	Mean %SS declined from 21.6 to 4.1		
Boberg and Kully (1985)	Slow speech, gentle onsets of phonation	17	14–38	3 weeks	Mean %SS declined from 25.1 to 1.0		
Randoll (1988)	Slow speech	7	4–9	Mean of 6 months for most cases	In 4 cases, improvement in SW per minute		
Onslow, Costa, Andrews, Harrison, and Packman (1996)	Prolonged speech	12	10–41	2-week residential, followed by 12 weekly visits and 126-week maintenance assignments	Stuttering was reduced to < 1% SS for virtually all cases	12 months	Fluency was maintained for all but 2 participants, who still demonstrated < 5% SS and substantial improvement from pre-therapy baselines[q]
O'Brian, Onslow, Cream, and Packman (2003)	Prolonged Speech (Camperdown Program)	21	17–58	13–29 hours (mean = 20)	Mean %SS decreased from 7.9% to 0.4%	6 and 12 months	Mean %SS was 0.5 (*N*=18) at 6 months; 0.4% after 12 months (*N*=16)

Block, Onslow, Packman, Gray, and Dacakis (2005) and Block, Onslow, Packman, and Dacakis (2006)	Slow, smooth speech	78	16–70	5-day intensive with 2-hour follow-up sessions	Decrease in mean %SS within clinic from range of ~8–10% to 1–2% immediately following the program	3 and 12 months (not available for ~50% of cases), and 3.5–5 years (available for 87% of cases)	~2% SS at 3 months, ~4–5% SS at 12 months, and ~1.5% SS at 3.5–5 years
Craig, Hancock, Chang, McCready, Shepley, McCaul, et al. (1996) and Hancock, Craig, McCready, McCaul, Costello, Gilmore, et al. (1998; long-term follow-up)	Random assignment to intensive smooth speech, parent home smooth speech, and intensive electromyography (EMG) feedback	97 total 27 intensive smooth speech; 25 home-based smooth speech; 25 EMG feedback; 20 untreated controls	11–18	Intensive smooth speech, 1 week; Home smooth speech, 1x per week over 4 weeks; EMG Feedback, 1 week	Untreated stuttering did not change across time; all treatment groups' stuttering was decreased to very low levels post-treatment (less than 1% SS on average)	1 year post-treatment and 2–6 years post-treatment	Some relapse evident after one year; relative improvement of 75% for EMG feedback, 68% for intensive smooth speech, and 70% for the home-based smooth speech group 2–6 year follow-up results similar to those observed at 1 year. No single treatment showed superior efficacy
Ingham, Kilgo, Ingham, Moglia, Belknap, and Sanchez (2001)	Modification of Short Phonation Intervals (MPI)	5	18–28	12–19 months	All participants demonstrated reduced stuttering, increased speaking rate, and improved speech naturalness within and beyond the clinic environment[r]	12 months after completion	Changes were sustained; all participants showed levels of performance that were essentially identical to the levels reported at the completion of the maintenance phase

(*Continues*)

APPENDIX (Continued)

	Method	*N*	Age	Duration of Treatment	Results of Treatment	Follow-up Interval	Results of Follow-up[d]
De Nil, Kroll, Lafaille, and Houle (2003)	Precision Fluency Shaping[s]	13	20–40	3-week intensive, followed by 1 year of scheduled follow-up sessions	Percent disfluent speech during monologue fell from mean of 7.1% to 1.6%	1 year	Percent disfluent speech increased to 3.6%
Neumann, Preibisch, Euler, von Gudenberg, Lanfermann, Gall, et al. (2005)	Kassel Stuttering Therapy (a version of Precision Fluency Shaping)	9	24–41	3 weeks intensive inpatient treatment	Percent SS rates were reduced from a mean of approximately 10% to less than 1% following therapy		
Tasko, McClean, and Runyan (2007)	Group-based Precision Fluency Shaping	35	Mean age 24 years	1 month	*SSI-3* scores decreased from a mean of 26 to 9.3; mean percent reduction in scores = 60%; speech naturalness significantly reduced from a mean of 4.6 to 3.5		
Webster (1974)	Gentle phonatory onsets	20	8–52	3 weeks		4–33 months	45% stuttered on 1% of words or less in conversation
Webster (1975)	Gentle phonatory onsets	56	8–59	3 weeks	Significant differences in pre- and post-treatment measures of stuttering	2 years	70% retained significant gains in fluency
Schwartz and Webster (1977)	Gentle phonatory onsets	29	9–over 50	3 months	97% improved; 72% stuttered on 6% or less of words	Minimum of 45 days	Of 8 subjects followed up, 4 retained their gains or were improved

Webster (1979a)	Gentle phonatory onsets	200		3 weeks	Stuttering was reduced to a mean of 1.3% SW	Mean of 10 months	78% stuttered on 3% SW or less
Webster (1980)	Gentle phonatory onsets	200		3 weeks	Mean %SW decreased from 15.1 to 1.3	Mean of 10 months	Mean %SW was 3.2
Mallard and Kelley (1982)	Gentle phonatory onsets	50	14–50	3 weeks	Mean %SW fell from 20.05 to 2.92	At least 6 months	Mean %SW for 28 subjects was 9.74
Heller, Shulman, and Teryek (1983)	Gentle phonatory onsets	85	6–65	6 weeks	84% achieved normal or near-normal fluency in conversation	6 months–5 years	80% maintained their post-treatment fluency levels
Franken et al. (1992)	Gentle phonatory onsets	32	15–46	4 weeks	Mean %SS declined from 25.7 to 5.8	6 months	Mean %SS was 16.3
Hasbrouck et al. (1987)	Airflow, relaxation	6	10–16	4 weeks	Mean %SW declined from 9.7 to 0.2	6–7 months	Mean %SW was 3.5
Hasbrouck and Lowry (1989)	Airflow, relaxation	24	19–38	5 weeks	All had 1% or fewer SW	1–24 months	70% had 1% or fewer SW
Andrews and Tanner (1982b)	Airflow	6	Adults	5 days	Mean reduction in stuttering was 90%	12 months	Stuttering no longer differed significantly from level at intake
Azrin and Nunn (1974)	Regulated breathing	14	4–67	12–hour session[t]	All had at least 93% reduction in stuttering		
Azrin, Nunn, and Frantz (1979)	Regulated breathing	21	Adults	1 or 2 sessions[u]	Stuttering decreased by mean of 94%	16 months	11 subjects contacted reported a mean reduction in stuttering of 79%
Ladouceúr, Boudreau, and Théberge (1981)	Regulated breathing	16	15–47	2 hours	Reduction in stuttering averaged 50%	1 month	Reduction in stuttering averaged 50%
Côté and Ladouceúr (1982)	Regulated breathing	16	Adults	3 30-minute sessions	Subjects stuttered significantly less	6 months	Changes in stuttering were maintained
Greenberg and Marks (1982)	Regulated breathing	15	Adults	12 hours		6 months	Of 10 subjects, 8 were much improved, 1 slightly improved

(*Continues*)

APPENDIX (Continued)

	Method	*N*	Age	Duration of Treatment	Results of Treatment	Follow-up Interval	Results of Follow-up[d]
Andrews and Tanner (1982a)	Regulated breathing	6	Adults	2 6–hour sessions	5 subjects who completed therapy reduced stuttering by about 45%	3 months	Only 1 subject showed significant improvement
Ladouceúr, Côté, Leblond, and Bouchard (1982)	Regulated breathing	12	17–74	2 90–minute sessions	Average decrease from 11.5% to 5.6% SS	2 months	Average increase to 8.4% SS
Ladouceúr and Martineau (1982)	Regulated breathing	15	5–16	3 45–minute sessions		1 month	Average stuttering decreased 50% from baseline to follow-up, but did not differ from that of a control group
Wagaman, Miltenberger, and Arndorfer (1993); Wagaman, Miltenberger, and Woods (1995) (follow-up)	Regulated breathing	8	6–10	Initial 2-hour session plus up to 9 45-minute sessions	All met criterion of $< 3\%$ SW during implementation and 10–13 months post-treatment. Speech rates increased[v]	3.5 years	5 of the 8 children were at or below 3% SW at follow-up
Elliott, Miltenberger, Rapp, Long, and McDonald (1998)	Regulated breathing	5	5–11	Single 1-hour session and up to 5 30-minute booster sessions	4 of the 5 children met criterion of fewer than 3% stuttered words	6–9 months	3 children continued to meet criterion
Kuhr and Rustin (1985)	Relaxation and regulated breathing	8	22–54	3 weeks[i]	Average stuttering fell from 14.3% to 2.4% SS	25–61 months	Average of 5.9% SS

Weiner (1984c)	Vocal training	27		14–156 sessions	All achieved high levels of fluency	0–6 years	18 responding to questionnaire reported fluency of 80% to 100%, 60% to 100% under stress
Andrews and Ingham (1972a)	Token economy and prolonged or syllable-timed speech	23	Adults	20 days	Mean %SS reduced from 16.4 to 0.1	18 months	Mean %SS was 7.8
Ingham, Andrews, and Winkler (1972)	Token economy	9	Adults	2 weeks	Mean %SS reduced from 18.2 to 6.7		
Ingham, Andrews, and Winkler (1972)	Token economy, syllable-timed speech, and group psychotherapy	9	Adults	2 weeks	Mean %SS reduced from 17.4 to 0.2		
Guitar and Bass (1978)	Token economy and prolonged speech	20	Adults	3 weeks	Mean %SS reduced from 10 to 0	1 year	Mean %SS was 2.6
Elliott and Williamson (1973)	Token reward	10	Adolescents	12 days	100% improved markedly	6 months	Significant improvement in 7 of 8 cases
Mowrer (1975)	Reinforcement of fluency	20	8–43	3.5–46.5 hours	Mean %SW from 11.7 to 2.4		
Stocker and Gerstman (1983)	Reinforcement of fluency	24	Mean of 6.9	Mean of 7.4 months	75% were rated fluent or exceptionally fluent		
Ryan (1981)	Various programmed therapies	40	7–16	Mean of 15.6 hours	Mean SW per minute fell from 8.2 to 0.3[w]	Mean of 12.5 months	Average SW per minute for the 13 subjects followed up was 0.8
Ryan (2001a)	Monterey Fluency Program (MFP)[x]	294	4–66	~20 hours, including establishment, transfer, and maintenance	Mean SW per minute fell from 9.0 to 0.2		

(Continues)

APPENDIX (Continued)

	Method	*N*	Age	Duration of Treatment	Results of Treatment	Follow-up Interval	Results of Follow-up[d]
Rustin, Ryan, and Ryan (1987)	Verbal reward and punishment, DAF	107	6–45	Mean of 2.6 months	Mean SW per minute decreased from 10.9 to 0.2		
Mallard and Westbrook (1988)	Token and verbal reward and punishment	20	Grades K to 5	9 months	Mean %SS declined from 12.0 to 9.0	4 months	Mean %SS was 7.0
Hewat, Onslow, Packman, and O'Brian (2006)	Self-imposed time-out	22 (18 completed maintenance phase)	14–52	Single 8-hour day; group training	Mean reduction in %SS of 53%; however, half of participants did not improve to a clinically significant extent	6 months	y
Stang (1984)	Composite behavior therapy	78	8–17	4 to 6 months	49% were stutter-free, 19 usually fluent	22–64 months	Of 69 subjects, 17% were stutter-free, 48% usually fluent
Ladouceúr and Saint-Laurent (1986)	Composite therapy	8	18–36	4 weeks	Percent SS was significantly reduced	6 months	Percent SS did not differ significantly from that of 8 nonstutterers
Maxwell (1982)	Cognitive and behavioral self-control therapy	23	Mean of 24	12 months	Overall ratings fell from moderate to mild		
Purser and Rustin (1983)	Cognitive and behavioral therapy	32		10 weeks	The subjects were clearly improved, but did not differ from a control group		

Hancock and Craig (2002) See also Craig, Hancock, Chang, McCready, Shepley, McCaul, et al. (1996) Hancock, Craig, McCready, McCaul, Costello, Gilmore, et al. (1998; long-term follow-up)	Re-treatment of past participants, using cognitive behavioral therapy/self management including smooth speech and EMG feedback	12	11–17	4–5 sessions	Re-treatment showed an average improvement of almost 70%; mean %SS fell from 5% to 1%	Two years	Improvement reduced to about 50–60% after 3 months, but increased by the I2-year follow-up, at which time 75% of subjects demonstrated < 2% SS
Block, Onslow, Roberts, and White (2004)	EMG feedback	12	10–16	6 hours/ day over 5 consecutive days	Mean %SS fell from range of 7.1-7.6% to 4.4% SS immediately following therapy; %SS fell 36.7% during post-therapy conversation	3 months	Mean %SS at 3 months post-treatment was 4.9% for conversation and 5.5% for reading
Donath (1928)	Hypnosis	48	5–36		71% were improved or cured		
Lockhart and Robertson (1977)	Hypnosis	7	18–62	4–6 weeks	All achieved fluency		
Lockhart and Robertson (1977)	Hypnosis and speech therapy	23	15–43	12–54 weeks	10 achieved fluency; 8 were still in therapy		
Bryngelson[z]	Handedness change	127	6–16	16 months	90% had marked or normal speech		
Fishman (1937)	Negative practice	5	12–20	1 month	60% showed definite improvement		
Daskalov (1962)	Composite therapy	440	Adults		74% greatly improved or cured	2 years	54% greatly improved or cured
Kurth and Schmidt (1964)	Speech therapy and psychotherapy	32	6–13		67% significantly improved or cured		

(Continues)

APPENDIX (Continued)

	Method	*N*	Age	Duration of Treatment	Results of Treatment	Follow-up Interval	Results of Follow-up[d]
Zaliouk and Zaliouk (1965)	Relaxation, breathing and speech exercises	58	6–15	Mean of 6 months	81% had full recovery		
Lepsova (1965)	Speech training at summer camp	72	School children	3–4 weeks	60% showed significant or very good improvement		51% showed significant or very good improvement in the following school year
Novák (1975)	Composite therapy	25	17–35	6–8 weeks	Considerable improvement in practically 100%	2 years	Improvement in 44%
Fransella (1970)	Personal construct therapy	20	17–49	2 years	74% improved	9 months–3 years	Of 9 followed up, 8 maintained or bettered their improvement[aa]
Dalali and Sheehan (1974)	Assertion training	8	Adults	6 hours	No change in severity of stuttering		
Dalali and Sheehan (1974)	Feeling clarification	8	Adults	6 hours	No change in severity of stuttering		
Dalali and Sheehan (1974)	Avoidance reduction	8	Adults	6 hours	No change in severity of stuttering		
Haskell and Larr (1974)	Role training	6	Adults	11 hours	All improved considerably		
Moleski and Tosi (1976)	Rational-emotive therapy or systemic desensitization	20	Adults	8 sessions	Rational-emotive therapy was more effective than systemic desensitization		
Adams (1972)	Systematic desensitization	12	7–28	10–70 weeks	75% made at least some improvement	6 months–over 2 years	No loss of improvement
Gray and England (1972)	Systematic desensitization	30	14–45	1 year	50% of 15 who remained in therapy were improved, greatly improved, or cured		

Boudreau and Jeffrey (1973)	Systematic desensitization	8	16–22	2–3 months	5 subjects showed marked improvement	20 months	The 3 subjects who received no other speech therapy or home practice retained their gains
Burgraff (1974)	Systematic desensitization	9	Adults	7–8 weeks	Mean reduction in stuttering of 35 to 40%		
Helltoft Nilsén and Ramberg (1999)	Intensive non-avoidance-oriented treatment	13	13–17	21 days over a period of 6 months	5 subjects showed "major" positive change in stuttering severity; 6 showed no change, and 2 showed increased severity. Mean Locus of Control of Behavior was unchanged[bb]		
Gendelman (1977)	Confrontation	40	Adolescents	20 or more sessions	90% were normally fluent or improved	2 months–3 years	Prior level of fluency was maintained by 81% of 27 followed up
Rubin and Culatta (1971)	Commitment to fluency	15	13–40	½–18 months	60% had normal fluency outside clinic		
Bray and Kehle (2001)	Self-modeling	7[cc]	8–17			2 and 4 years	At 2 years, mean %SW declined from pre-treatment range of 6–9% to < 1–7% for 4 subjects (1998 study); at 4 years, decline was from 27–45% to 1–5% for 3 subjects (1996 study)
Irwin (1972)	Easy stammering	26	17–52	1–4 years	96% had good to complete improvement		
Peins, McGough, and Lee (1972)	Iowa therapy after Van Riper	12	Mean 22	6 months	67% showed a reduction in severity of stuttering		

(Continues)

APPENDIX (Continued)

	Method	*N*	Age	Duration of Treatment	Results of Treatment	Follow-up Interval	Results of Follow-up[d]
Prins (1970)	Residential Iowa therapy program	94	8–21 weeks	8 weeks		6 months–3.5 years	77% perceived themselves as making much or complete improvement
Gregory (1972)	Iowa therapy and relaxation	17	Mean of 28	9 months	There was a significant reduction in stuttering to a mild to moderate level of severity	9 months	A slight regressive trend was not statistically significant
Burgraff (1974)	Iowa therapy after Van Riper	9	Adults	7–8 weeks	Mean reduction in stuttering of 35–40%		
Prins and Nichols (1974)	Iowa therapy	9	11–15	6 weeks		5 months	48% perceived themselves as making much or complete improvement
Prins (1976)	Modified Iowa therapy	9	10–16	6 weeks		5 months	69% perceived themselves as making much or complete improvement
Mallard and Westbrook (1988)	Van Riper therapy	20	Grades K to 5	9 months	Mean percent of stuttered syllables declined from 12.0 to 1.0	4 months	Mean percent of stuttered syllables was 7.0
Laiho and Klippi (2007)	Van Riper therapy	21	6.8–14.0	14-18 days, total of 35–52 contact hours	Mean %SS declined significantly from 4.4 to 2.7; avoidance behavior declined from 13.1 to 9.5	9 months	For 12 adolescents, self-report of maintained improved fluency

Eichstadt, Watt, and Girson (1998)	Stuttering modification modeled after Successful Stuttering Management Program (SSMP)[dd]	5	16–33	3 weeks	Proportion of "clean stuttering" (stuttering without physical concomitants) increased for most participants	2 years	Substantial regression in proportion of "clean stuttering" was observed for 3 of the 5 participants; attitude gains were more durable
Kotby, Moussa, El-Sady, and Nabieh (2003)	Stuttering modification therapy (contrasted with three others)[ee]	120 (4 groups of 30)	15–35	2 times/week for 16 weeks	Significant difference between pre- and post-therapy for all therapeutic groups in comparison to a control group. No significant difference among results of all therapeutic groups		
Blomgren, Roy, Callister, and Merrill (2005)	Stuttering Modification treatment program (the Successful Stuttering Management Program [SSMP])	19	16–52	3 weeks	Statistically significant improvements observed on 6 of 14 behavioral measures. Mean %SS in monologue decreased from ~18% to ~12%; *PSI* decreased from ~11 in each section to ~2–4	6 months	Regression to 13.8% SS and ~3 to 9 on PSI scores; sustained improvements included self-perceived avoidance and expectancy of stuttering and measures of anxiety
Kully and Langevin (1999)	ISTAR Comprehensive Stuttering Program (CSP) (Mix of PFSP and Iowa therapies)	25	Adolescents	85 hours	Mean %SS declined from 14.3 to 1.75, with improvement in *S24* Scale Scores from 16.8 to 8.8	4 and 12 months	Mean %SS 3.65 at 4 months, 3.89 at 12 months. *S24* scores at 12 months averaged 11.57
Baumeister, Caspar, and Herziger (2003)	Integrated stuttering modification and fluency shaping summer camp	37	9–19		Stuttering frequency was reduced from 22.2% to 9.5%		

(*Continues*)

APPENDIX (Continued)

	Method	*N*	Age	Duration of Treatment	Results of Treatment	Follow-up Interval	Results of Follow-up[d]
Huinck, Langevin, Kully, Graamans, Peters, and Hulstijn (2006)	ISTAR Comprehensive Stuttering Program (CSP)	25	17–53	3-week intensive group therapy	"Severe" stutterers decreased %SS from mean of 16% to 2% post-therapy; milder stutterers decreased from about 4%SS to virtually no stuttering	1 and 2 years post treatment	Mean scores of all speech measures regressed at both follow-ups; at 1 and 2 years, severe group increased to a mean of ~12% SS and ~11%, respectively; milder group increased to ~2.5% and 2%; measures of emotional reactivity showed a similar pattern and did not correlate with %SS
Langevin, Huinck, Kully, Peters, Lomheim, and Tellers (2006)	ISTAR Comprehensive Stuttering Program (CSP)	25 stutterers from the Netherlands and 16 from Canada	Dutch: 17–53; Canadian: 15–42	3 weeks of intensive group therapy; 6 hours/day	Mean post-treatment %SS in beyond clinic conversation declined from 12 to 3.24 (Dutch) and ~12 to 0.9 (Canadian)	1 and 2 years post-treatment	At 1 year, stuttering rate increased slightly to 6.6/3.88% SS (Dutch/Canadian); at 2 years, rates were were ~7/4.4% SS. 71% of Dutch/86% of Canadian speakers were classified as maintaining clinically meaningful improvement at 2 years[ff]
Montgomery (2006)	Intensive group model; Modified Precision Fluency Shaping, combined with Iowa and cognitive/behavioral therapies	23	Mean = 22 years	3 weeks	Mean decrease in %SS from 13.7 to 0.4%; decrease in *PSI* scores from 29.9 to 8.5; in *WASSP* scores from 98.5 to 43.8; in *OASES* scores from 278 to 160.6		

TREATMENTS DESIGNED PRIMARILY FOR CHILDREN							
Petkov and Iosifov (1960)	Composite therapy	50	Grades 3–9	45 days	96% had significant improvement or recovery		
Jones-Prus (1980)	Slow rate, rhythmic speech	5	4–8	2–9 months	Children improved from moderate or severe to mild or very mild	7–18 months	Only 1 child showed a mild regression
Culp (1984)	Easy speech	14	2–5	15–70 hours	All had fluency within normal limits	2 years	Of 7 children, all but 1 had fluency within normal limits
Shine (1984)	Easy speaking voice	18	2–8	1–28 months	All were fluent	14–64 months	Of 14 children, 13 had maintained fluency
Ryan and Ryan (1995)	Gradual Increase in Length and Complexity of Utterance (GILCU)	9	Mean 12.2 years	Mean 7.9 hours	Decrease in mean SW per minute from 6.0 to 0.4	7 and 14 months (partial data)	For 6 children, mean SW per minute decreased from 5.9 (pre-treatment) to .6 at last visit; better long-term outcome than DAF
	Delayed Auditory Feedback (DAF)	11	Mean 11.4 years	Mean 8 hours	Decrease in mean SW per minute from 7.5 to 0.3		For 5 children, mean SW per minute decreased from 10.3 (pre-treatment) to 1.1 at last visit
Druce, Debney, and Byrt (1997)	Slowed speech/ GILCU[99]	15	6;9–8;1	Intensive: 5 days; with maintenance phase of 7 visits in 3 months (39.5 hours)	Reduction from 9.6% SS to 1.75% SS immediately following program; good rate and naturalness scores	18 months	Mean %SS was 3.83%, with increased rate and maintenance of naturalness scores; more severe stutterers had less good long-term outcomes

(*Continues*)

APPENDIX (Continued)

	Method	*N*	Age	Duration of Treatment	Results of Treatment	Follow-up Interval	Results of Follow-up[d]
Neaves (1970)	Child guidance clinic	93	8–12			1–3 years	44% responded successfully
Neaves (1970)	Child guidance clinic	72	13–17			1–3 years	60% responded successfully
Wyatt and Herzan (1962)	Psychotherapy with mother and child	8	7–15	4–12 months	63% showed marked improvement		
Mallard (1998)	Family-based problem solving[hh]	28	5–12	2 weeks	82% did not require therapy after program end	1 year	Only 5 of 28 children enrolled for therapy; 3 of these had other speech/language targets, rather than fluency
Lincoln, Onslow, Lewis, and Wilson (1996)	Lidcombe adapted for school-aged children	11	7–12	12 sessions	Less than 1.5% SS both in- and beyond clinic	1 year	Fluency gains maintained at follow-up
Shenker (2004)	Lidcombe	56;17 bilingual (BL) & 39 monolingual (ML)	3–10;3	Mean of 9.9 sessions (BL); 11.8 (ML) to end of Stage 1	Decrease in pretreatment from range of 1.5 to 33% SS to criterion (≤ 1%SS within clinic; ≤ 1.5%SS beyond clinic)		
Riley and Riley (1984)	Component-based therapy	44	3–12	Mean of 47.9 hours	82% had no or mild stuttering	2–4 years	Of 37 children, 81% had no or mild stuttering
Riley and Riley (1986)	Oral motor training	9	3–6	8–22 hours	Improvement percent ranged from 19 to 100, with a mean of 62		
Riley and Ingham (2000)	Speech Motor Training (SMT)	6	3–7	20–24 weeks	Mean %SS decreased from 7.8% to 4.6%; average decrease in %SS was 37%		

Ingham (1999)	Extended Length of Utterance (ELU)	5	3;6–9;1	20 hours	Stuttering reduced by 60%; stuttering eliminated in those under 6;0		
Riley and Ingham (2000)	Extended Length of Utterance (ELU)	6	3–8	20–24 weeks	Percent SS decreased from a mean of 4.25 to 1.89; average decrease in %SS was 64%		
Runyan and Runyan (1986)	Fluency Rules Program: Slow rate, light contacts, continuous phonation	9	3–7	1 year	Number of SW per minute decreased from 10–74 to 1.7–5	2 years	The subject evaluated stuttered on a mean of 1.7 to 3 words per minute
Runyan and Runyan (1999)	Fluency Rules Program	17	< 7 years	Mean of 9 months, 2–3 times per week for 30–40 minutes	All received scores within acceptable range of naturalness following therapy		
THERAPIES SPECIFICALLY FOR VERY YOUNG CHILDREN							
Johnson (1955a)	Parent counseling	46	2–9	5–51 months	72% had normal or nearly normal speech		
Johnson and Associates (1959)	Parent counseling	74	2–8	Varied from single interview to program of unspecified duration		Mean 28.5 months	45% had no problem[ii]
Daskalov (1962)	Speech exercises, improvement of home environment	123	Preschool	3–6 months or longer	69% greatly improved or cured	2 years	88% greatly improved or cured
Wyatt and Herzan (1962)	Psychotherapy with mother and child	12	2–6	4–12 months	83% showed marked improvement		

(*Continues*)

APPENDIX (Continued)

	Method	*N*	Age	Duration of Treatment	Results of Treatment	Follow-up Interval	Results of Follow-up[d]
Wyatt (1969)	Psychotherapy with parent and child	28	2–13	3–91 weeks	79% had improved or normal speech	3–11 years	58% had no stuttering
Conture and Melnick (1999)	Parent counseling (indirect therapy) plus direct treatment (stuttering modification)	> 200	3–5	Up to 4 cycles of 12 week blocks of once weekly 45-minute sessions	Over 70% demonstrated 3% or less stuttering 12–36 weeks after treatment onset		
Gottwald (2007)	Parent counseling plus direct treatment	30 "high-risk" children36	2;10–6;2 years; months	Mean of 13.7 sessions	Mean %SS decreased from ~9% to ~1.5%	1 year	96% were reported by parents to have normal fluency
Lincoln and Onslow (1997)	Lidcombe	43	3–6	Unspecified	Children were put on maintenance after achieving < 1% SS	1-4 years	All children demonstrated < 2% SS at follow-up from 1-4 years post-therapy
Jones, Onslow, Harrison, and Packman (2000)	Lidcombe program	250	27–71 months	45–60 minutes/week with a mean of 12.5 sessions to end of Stage 1 (< 1%SS)	Mean %SS decreased from 4.2 to "zero or near zero"		
Harris, Onslow, Packman, Harrison, and Menzies (2002)	Lidcombe program	23;10 randomized to treatment, 13 controls	2.0–4.11 years	12 weeks to end of Stage 1	Mean %SS for treated children decreased from 8.6% to ~3.5%; for untreated children, it decreased from 8.4% to 5.8% stuttered syllables		
Woods, Shearsby, Onslow, and Burnham (2002)	Lidcombe program	8	35–63 months	Mean of 12.5 clinic visits (range 4–33) to end of Stage 1	Mean %SS decreased from 4.2% to 0.7%		

Packman, Kingston, Huber, Onslow, and Jones (2003)	Lidcombe program	66 who met criterion for successful completion of program; 12 other children did not[kk]	32–71 months	Mean of 12 visits (range 3–32) to end of Stage 1	Mean %SS decreased from 5.8% to less than 1% for children who completed Stage 1		
Wilson, Onslow, and Lincoln (2004)	Lidcombe program (telehealth adaptation)	5	3.5–5.7 years old	11–40 weeks to end of Stage 1 3–34 consultations	All 5 participants reached clinical criteria for completion of Stage 1 (less than 1.0% SS). Larger numbers of consultations than in face-to-face practice suggests that telephone-based treatment may be less efficient	1 year	Post-treatment results were available for 4 children. 2 remained at less than 1.0% SS and 2 remained at below 2.0%. 1 child relapsed after Stage 1, but was managed successfully
Jones, Onslow, Packman, Williams, Ormond, Schwarz, et al. (2005)	Lidcombe program	47; 27 treated and 20 untreated controls	3–6 years: Mean age 3;9	9 months	Treated children decreased %SS from mean of 6.4% to 1.5%; untreated children decreased from mean of 6.8% SS to 3.9%; in treated children, numbers achieving < and > than 1%SS were 14/13, while numbers for untreated children were 3/17		
Shenker and Roberts (2007)	Lidcombe program	14 bilingual children	3–6 years		Percent SS for late bilinguals was 0.0–1.4 and for early bilinguals 0.2–1.0	2–7 years post-treatment	At follow-up, 11/14 children maintained a level < 1% SS. Residual stuttering was described as mild (< ~3%SS) without perceived tension

(*Continues*)

APPENDIX (Continued)

	Method	*N*	Age	Duration of Treatment	Results of Treatment	Follow-up Interval	Results of Follow-up[d]
Rousseau, Packman, Onslow, Harrison, and Jones (2007)	Lidcombe program	29	3;0–5;7	Median of 16 visits and 27 weeks to end of Stage 1	Mean %SS pretreatment ranged from 2.4–3.5 (across multiple samples); mean post-Stage 1 ranged from 0.9–1.2%SS	6, 12, and 24 months post Stage-1	Ranges of mean %SS were .8-1.1%SS, 0.6 – 1%SS and 0.1 to 0.4%SS, respectively
Miller and Guitar (2007)	Lidcombe program	15 children	2;5–5;9 (years; months)	Median of 17 visits to end of Stage 1	Mean %SS declined from 12.6 to 0.5 (96%). Mean *SSI*-3 declined from 24.9 to 3.5	Mean of 35 months	11 of 15 children were considered recovered at follow-up; 4 demonstrated mild residual stuttering
Franken, Kielstra-Van der Schalk, and Boelens (2005)	Lidcombe Program (LP)	11	Mean 4;3	12 weeks; mean 11.5 sessions	For LP, mean %SS decreased from 7.2% to 3.7%.		
	Demands and Capacities Model (DCM)	12	Mean 4;2	12 weeks; mean 11 sessions	For DCM, mean %SS decreased from 7.9% to 3.1%. No significant effect of treatment type		
Yaruss, Coleman, and Hammer (2006)	Family-focused treatment approach (parent counseling combined with integrated direct child therapy)[II]	17 (considered to be at high risk for persistence)	31–62 months	6–8 45-minute sessions	Mean decrease in %SS from 16.4 to 3.2%. 65% improved sufficiently following parent-focused training that they were dismissed without direct therapy	1–3 years	Of 11 dismissed following parent counseling, all were considered fluent on follow-up; of remaining 7 children, 6 were considered within normal limits for fluency on follow-up

DRUG THERAPIES					
Winkelman (1954)	Chlorpromazine	5	Adults	2–8 months	40% had moderate or marked improvement
Hackett et al.[mm]	Chlorpromazine	7	9–16	24 weeks	71% greatly improved[nn]
Mitchell[oo]	Reserpine and speech therapy	16	Adults	8 weeks	0% showed decreased frequency or severity of stuttering
Hollister[pp]	Reserpine and speech therapy	8	Adults	60 days	50% improved[qq]
Glasner[rr]	Reserpine	7	4–8	7 weeks	43% increased smoothness of speech pattern
Maxwell and Paterson (1958)	Meprobamate and speech therapy	18	18–50	8 months	78% showed good or very good improvement
Kent and Williams (1959)	Meprobamate and speech therapy	8	18–29	99 days	38% much improved[ss]
Di Carlo, Katz, and Batkin (1959)	Meprobamate	30	15–45	6 weeks	In the drug group (N=10) a substantial reduction occurred in stuttering in oral reading. Stuttering increased in the placebo group and showed no change in medication group
Holliday (1959)	Meprobamate	20	Adults	3 weeks	Neither the drug nor the placebo group showed significant change in frequency of stuttering, but clinicians' ratings of tension showed a decrease for the drug group

(Continues)

APPENDIX (Continued)

	Method	*N*	Age	Duration of Treatment	Results of Treatment	Follow-up Interval	Results of Follow-up[d]
Gattuso and Leocata (1962)	Haloperidol	50	5–12	1 month	80% of the children aged 5–8 had no symptoms; the remaining 20% improved		
Tapia (1969)	Haloperidol	12	8–16		2 subjects improved by count of stuttering		
Wells and Malcolm (1971)	Haloperidol	36	15–50	8 weeks	Of 12 in the drug group, 83% showed considerable improvement		
Quinn and Peachey (1973)	Haloperidol	18	15–39	3 weeks	22% showed more than a 50% decrease of stuttering in spontaneous speech		
Swift, Swift, and Arellano (1975)	Haloperidol	22	23–50	3 weeks	Of 7 in drug group who completed treatment, 6 showed improvement		
Plath and Caspers[tt]	Haloperidol and speech therapy	90	5–33	6 months	Substantial improvement and in some cases cures occurred		
Rantalaka and Petri-Larmi (1976)	Haloperidol	58	Adults and children	8 weeks	"Spasms" decreased more under drug than under placebo; decrease in repetitions was not significant		

Rosenberger, Wheelden, and Kalotkin (1976)	Haloperidol	8	20–32	6–12 weeks	No significant effect on mean frequency of stuttering; percent of time disfluent in spontaneous speech was less in the drug condition
Andrews and Dozsa (1977)	Haloperidol	15	19–29	At least 20 days	40% of subjects reduced their stuttering by at least half
Andrews and Dozsa (1977)	Haloperidol	15	16–46	At least 20 days	20% reduced stuttering by at least half; mean frequency of stuttering was not significantly less than under placebo
Murray, Kelly, et al. (1977)	Haloperidol	18	Adolescents and adults	3 months	61% were more improved on drug than on placebo
Prins, Mandelkorn, and Cerf (1980)	Haloperidol	14	7–41	8 weeks	The drug had a relatively small effect
Cozzo and Gabrielli (1965)	Haloperidol and Triperidol	48	4–14		33% showed marked improvement
Schilling (1963)	Bellergal	61	Children and adults	2–3 months	52% showed good or very good improvement
Aron (1965)	Trifluoperazine and amylobarbitone	46	Adults	3 weeks	80% showed varying degrees of improvement
Fish and Bowling (1965)	D-amphetamine and trifluoperazine	28	10–59	1–2 months	79% showed improvement
Fish and Bowling (1962)	Dexadrine	11	11–60	3 months	45% had dramatic improvement or no stuttering
Fujita et al. (1963)	Chlordiazepoxide	23	Children and adults		There was marked or moderate improvement in 65%

(Continues)

APPENDIX (Continued)

	Method	*N*	Age	Duration of Treatment	Results of Treatment	Follow-up Interval	Results of Follow-up[d]
Hommerich and Korzendorfer (1966)	Chlordiazepoxide	46	8 years–adulthood	3 months	74% were improved or cured[uu]		
Goldman and Guth (1965)	Thioridazine and chlordiazepoxide	8		6 weeks	75% were rated milder on thioridazine		
Cacudi (1964)	Thioridazine	21	4–14	2 months	Cure or marked improvement seen in 67%		
Goldman (1966)	Thioridazine and speech therapy	20	10–52	4 months	Drug group was rated less severe, but mean frequency of stuttering did not change		
Leanderson and Levi (1967)	Opipramol or diazepam	44	Adults	54 days	Neither drug had a marked effect; Opipramol reduced stuttering moderately		
Hale (1951)	Thiamin		2–8	1 month	55% had observable improvement		
Bloch et al. (1977)	Propanolol	26	Adults and children		No significant effect on the frequency of stuttering, but improvement was reported in individual cases		
Rustin, Kuhr, Cook, and James (1981)	Oxprenolol and speech therapy	31	18–55	12 weeks	The drug had no effect but speech therapy (slow rate and relaxation) resulted in a highly significant improvement		

Arthurs et al. (1954)	Carbon dioxide inhalation	14	21–36	30–70 administrations	0% showed improvement in fluency
Smith (1953)	Carbon dioxide inhalation	33	20–55	10–36 weeks	48% showed 50 to 100% improvement
Rothenberger et al. (1994)	Tiapride	10; no placebo control	10–17	20 weeks	Mean %SS fell roughly 5% (from mean of ~20 to ~15%) in conversation and description; more in reading
Maguire, Riley, Franklin, and Gottschalk (2000)	Risperidone	16	20–74	6 weeks	Significant reductions in scores on 3 of 4 measures, including %SS; the placebo group showed no significant change
Maguire, Riley, et al. (2004)	Olanzapine	24	18–55	3 months	Mean stuttering severity improved 33% on olanzapine and 14% on placebo. Notable side effects of treatment were mild sedation and weight gain
Stager, Calis, Grothe, Bloch, Berensen, Smith, et al. (2005)[vv]	Paroxetine and Pimozide	11	23–48	6 weeks	Improved percent fluent speaking time demonstrated with pimozide but not with paroxetine. However, pimozide was associated with a large number of side effects

(Continues)

APPENDIX (Continued)

	Method	*N*	Age	Duration of Treatment	Results of Treatment	Follow-up Interval	Results of Follow-up[d]
Inpharma Weekly (2006)[ww]	Pagoclone	132; 88 received drug, the rest placebo	Adults	8 weeks	*SSI-3* scores significantly improved at weeks 4 and 8, as well as other measures of severity and improvement; no adverse events were reported		

[a] The assistance of Joseph Grossman with portions of the Appendix appearing in prior editions is gratefully acknowledged.
[b] We have attempted to organize studies in this Appendix first in terms of general approach to treatment (recognizing that some treatments consist of multiple components), then by date (earliest to most recent), and then alphabetically by first author.
[c] Space does not allow full evaluation of therapies reviewed, or of individual treatment reports that included fewer than 5 participants. Entries should not be considered adequate by themselves for the purpose of selecting treatment approaches for patients/clients. For greater detail, readers should consult original articles and/or discussion in Chapter 14.
[d] Follow-up refers to reevaluation a specified time after termination of therapy.
[e] Percent stuttered words
[f] Percent stuttered syllables
[g] Cited by Soderberg (1969b).
[h] Follow-up data from Ryan (1981).
[i] Statistical analysis provided; but actual mean values must be abstracted from graphs in report; numerous speaking conditions are graphed.
[j] Twelve-month follow-up data from Stuart, Kalinowski, Saltuklaroglu, and Guntupalli (2006); most participants appear in both papers, with the exception of one who was seen at 4 months, but not 12 months, and one seen later but not earlier. Data on naturalness and consumer satisfaction also provided.
[k] Visual inspection of Figure 2, p. 103.
[l] Visual inspection of Figure 1, p. 760.
[m] Follow-up data from Peins, McGough, and Lee (1984).
[n] Members of the same family.
[o] Follow-up reported by Boberg and Sawyer (1977).
[p] Plus maintenance.
[q] Individual baseline data without group means.
[r] Multiple baselines across subjects and tasks design; individual results graphically displayed; pooled mean data not reported.
[s] See Webster (1974) for original conceptualization.
[t] Supplemented by 1–8 months of contacts by telephone.
[u] Supplemented by 3 months of contacts by telephone.
[v] Single-subject design; each participant's values plotted separately.
[w] For the 13 subjects who were followed up.
[x] Combination of DAF and Gradual Increase in Length and Complexity of Utterance; operant reinforcement. Data in these cells represent summary data from a number of MFP studies presented and published by Ryan from 1970–98.
[y] Difficult to extrapolate given subject attrition and method of data presentation.
[z] Cited by Travis (1931, p. 191).
[aa] Follow-up data from Fransella (1972).
[bb] Pre- and post-therapy fluency counts not provided.
[cc] Two 4-year combined follow-up of participants in Bray and Kehle (1996, 1998); the initial studies do not meet our inclusion criterion of at least 5 participants each.
[dd] Breitenfeldt and Lorenz (1989).
[ee] Other therapies were insufficiently well-described to permit contrast among approaches.
[ff] Extensive data on rate, naturalness, attitudes, and consumer satisfaction also provided.

[gg] Based on Ryan (1971).
[hh] Based on Rustin (1987); mix of family counseling and direct therapy with child.
[ii] This compared with 23% of those whose parents received no counseling.
[jj] Having negative prognostic indicators for recovery.
[kk] Authors provide detailed discussion of reasons why individual children did not complete program.
[ll] See details in Chapter 14, page 368
[mm] Reported by Kent (1963).
[nn] Of 6 stutterers treated with placebo, 50% were greatly improved.
[oo] Reported by Burr and Mullendore (1960).
[pp] Reported by Kent (1963).
[qq] 25% improved on placebo and speech therapy.
[rr] Reported by Kent (1963).
[ss] By judges' ratings. Other measures failed to show any improvement.
[tt] Cited by Wertenbroch (1976).
[uu] 77% of a placebo group were also reported improved or cured.
[vv] Study terminated early due to severe side effects in two participants during withdrawal from paroxetine.
[ww] Peer-reviewed report not yet available as Handbook went to press.

References

Abbeduto, L., & Hagerman, R. J. (1997). Language and communication in fragile X syndrome. *Mental Retardation and Developmental Disabilities Research Reviews, 3,* 313–22.

Abbott, J. A. (1947). Repressed hostility as a factor in adult stuttering. *Journal of Speech Disorders, 12,* 428–30.

Abwender, D. A., Trinidad, K. S., Jones, K. R., Como, P. G., Hymes, E., & Kurlan, R. (1998). Notes and discussion. Features resembling Tourette's syndrome in developmental stutterers. *Brain and Language, 62,* 455–64.

Accordi, M., Bianchi, R., Consolaro, C., Tronchin, F., DeFilippi, R., Pasqualon, L., Ugo, E., & Croatto, L. (1983). L'Eziopatogenesi della balbuzie: Studio stadstico su 2802 casi. *Acta Phoniatrica Latina, 5,* 171–80.

Adamczyk, B. (1959). Anwendung des Apparates für die Erzeugung von künstlichem Widerhall bei der Behandlung des Stotterns. *Folia Phoniatrica, 11,* 216–18.

Adamczyk, B. (1965). Die Ergebnisse der Behandlung des Stotterns durch das Telephonechosystem. *De Therapia Vocis et Loquelae, Vol. 1. XIII Congress of the. International Society Folia Phoniatrica et Logopedia.*

Adamczyk, B., & Kuniszyk-Jóźkowiak, W. (1987). Effect of echo and reverberation of a restricted information capacity on the speech process. *Folia Phoniatrica, 39,* 9–17.

Adamczyk, B., Kuniszyk-Jóźkowiak, W., & Smolka, E. (1979). Influence of echo and reverberation on the speech process. *Folia Phoniatrica, 31,* 70–81.

Adamczyk, B., Sadowska, E., & Kuniszyk-Jóźkowiak, W. (1975). Influence of reverberation on stuttering. *Folia Phoniatrica, 27,* 1–6.

Adams, L. H. (1955). A comparison of certain sound wave characteristics of stutterers and nonstutterers. In Johnson, W., & Leutenegger, R. R (Eds.), *Stuttering in children and adults.* Minneapolis: University of Minnesota Press.

Adams, M. R. (1972). The use of reciprocal inhibition procedures in the treatment of stuttering. *Journal of Communication Disorders, 5,* 59–66.

Adams, M. R. (1974). A physiologic and aerodynamic interpretation of fluent and stuttered speech. *Journal of Fluency Disorders, 1,* 35–47.

Adams, M. R. (1987). Voice onsets and segment durations of normal speakers and beginning stutterers. *Journal of Fluency Disorders, 12,* 133–39.

Adams, M. R. (1990). The demands and capacities model: I. Theoretical elaborations. *Journal of Fluency Disorders, 15,* 135–41.

Adams, M. R., & Brutten, G. J. (1970). An exploratory study of some learning-based procedures for modifying stuttering. *Journal of Communication Disorders, 3,* 123–32.

Adams, M. R., & Dietze, D. A. (1965). A comparison of the reaction times of stutterers and nonstutterers to items on a word association test. *Journal of Speech and Hearing Research, 8,* 195–202.

Adams, M. R., & Hayden, P. (1976). The ability of stutterers and nonstutterers to initiate and terminate phonation during production of an isolated vowel. *Journal of Speech and Hearing Research, 19,* 290–96.

Adams, M. R., & Hutchinson, J. (1974). The effects of three levels of auditory masking on selected vocal characteristics and the frequency of disfluency of adult stutterers. *Journal of Speech and Hearing Research, 17,* 682–88.

Adams, M. R., Lewis, J. I., & Besozzi, T. E. (1973). The effect of reduced reading rate on stuttering frequency. *Journal of Speech and Hearing Research, 16,* 671–75.

Adams, M. R., & Moore, W. H., Jr. (1972). The effects of auditory masking on the anxiety level, frequency of dysfluency, and selected vocal characteristics of stutterers. *Journal of Speech and Hearing Research, 15,* 572–78.

Adams, M. R., & Popelka, G. (1971). The influence of "time-out" on stutterers and their dysfluency. *Behavior Therapist, 2,* 334–39.

Adams, M. R., & Ramig, P. (1980). Vocal characteristics of normal speakers and stutterers during choral reading. *Journal of Speech and Hearing Research, 23,* 457–69.

Adams, M. R., & Reis, R. (1971). The influence of the onset of phonation on the frequency of stuttering. *Journal of Speech and Hearing Research, 14,* 639–44.

Adams, M. R., & Reis, R. (1974). Influence of the onset of phonation on the frequency of stuttering: A replication and reevaluation. *Journal of Speech and Hearing Research, 17,* 752–54.

Adams, M. R., & Reis, R. (1975). A reply to Martin Young. *Journal of Speech and Hearing Research, 18,* 602–05.

Adams, M. R., Riemenschneider, S., Metz, D., & Conture, E. (1975). Voice onset and articulatory constriction requirements in a speech segment and their relation to the amount of stuttering adaptation. *Journal of Fluency Disorders, 1,* 23–29.

Adams, M. R., & Runyan, C. M. (1981). Stuttering and fluency: Exclusive events or points on a continuum? *Journal of Fluency Disorders, 6,* 197–218.

Adams, M. R., Runyan, C.M., & Mallard, A. R. (1975). Air flow characteristics of the speech of stutterers and nonstutterers. *Journal of Fluency Disorders, 1,* 4–12.

Adams, M. R., Sears, R. L., & Ramig, P. R. (1982). Vocal changes in stutterers and nonstutterers during monotoned speech. *Journal of Fluency Disorder, 7,* 21–25.

Adams, S. (1932). A study of the growth of language between two and four years. *Journal of Juvenile Research, 16,* 269–77.

Adler, J. B., & Starkweather, C. W. (1979). Oral and laryngeal reaction times in stutterers [Abstract]. *ASHA, 21,* 769.

Agnello, J. (1962). The effects of manifest anxiety and stuttering adaptation: Implications for treatment [Abstract]. *ASHA, 4,* 377.

Agnello, J. G. (1975). Voice onset and voice termination features of stutterers. In L. M. Webster & L. C. Furst (Eds.), *Vocal tract dynamics and dysfluency.* New York: Speech and Hearing Institute.

Ahlbach, J., & Benson, V. (Eds.). (1994). *To say what is ours.* San Francisco: National Stuttering Project.

Aimard, P., Plantier, A., & Wittling, M. (1966). Le bégaiement: Contribution a l'étude de l'audition et l'intégration phonétique. *Rev. Laryng. Otol.-Rhinol., 87,* 254–56.

Ainsworth, S. (1939). Studies in the psychology of stuttering: XII. Empathetic breathing of auditors while listening to stuttering speech. *Journal of Speech Disorders, 4,* 149–56.

Alarcia, J., Pinard, G., Serrano, M., & Tetreault, L. (1982). Étude comparative de trois traitements du bégaiement: relaxation, désensibilisation, rééducation. *Revue de Psychologie Appliquée, 32*(1), 1–25.

Allen, A.V. (1948). The role of the Rh blood factor in the etiology of certain speech disorders [Abstract]. *Speech Monographs, 15,* 202–03.

Allen, C. P., & Daly, D. A. (1978). Effects of transcendental meditation and EMG biofeedback relaxation on stuttering. [Abstract]. *ASHA, 20,* 730.

Alm, P. A. (2004a). Stuttering and the basal ganglia circuits: A critical review of possible relations. *Journal of Communication Disorders, 37,* 325–96.

Alm, P. A. (2004b). Stuttring, emotions, and heart rate during anticipatory anxiety: A critical review. *Journal of Fluency Disorders, 29,* 123–33.

Alm, P. A. (2005). Copper in developmental stuttering. *Folia Phoniatrica, 57,* 216–22.

Alm, P. A. (2006). Stuttering and sensory gating: A study of acoustic startle prepulse inhibition. *Brain and Language, 97,* 317–21.

Alm, P. A., & Risberg, J. (2007). Stuttering in adults: The acoustic startle response, temperamental traits, and biological factors. *Journal of Communication Disorders, 40,* 1–41.

Althaus, M., Vink, H. J., Minderaa, R. B., Goorhuis-Brouwer, S. M., & Oosterhoff, M. D. (1995). Lack of effect of clonidine on stuttering in children. *The American Journal of Psychiatry, 152,* 1087–89.

Altrows, I. F., & Bryden, M. P. (1977). Temporal factors in the effects of masking noise on fluency of stutterers. *Journal of Communication Disorders, 10,* 315–29.

Ambrose, N. G., & Cox, N. J. (1997). The genetic basis of persistence and recovery in stuttering. *Journal of Speech, Language and Hearing Research, 40,* 567–80.

Ambrose, N. G., Cox, N. J., & Yairi, E. (1997). The genetic basis of persistence and recovery in stuttering. *Journal of Speech, Language, and Hearing Research, 40,* 567–80.

Ambrose, N. G., & Yairi, E. (1999). Normative disfluency data for early childhood stuttering. *Journal of Speech, Language and Hearing Research, 42,* 895–909.

Ambrose, N. G., & Yairi, E. (2002). The Tudor Study: Data and Ethics. *American Journal of Speech-Language Pathology, 11,* 190–204.

Ambrose, N. G., Yairi, E., & Cox, N. (1993). Genetic aspects of early childhood stuttering. *Journal of Speech and Hearing Research, 36,* 701–06.

Amir, O., & Yairi, E. (2002). The effect of temporal manipulation on the perception of disfluencies as normal or stuttering. *Journal of Communication Disorders, 35,* 63–82.

Amirov, R. Z. (1962). Daloneishie rezultaty izuchenia vysshei nervnoi deiatel'nosti pri zaikanii. *DSH Abstracts, 2,* 74–75.

Ammons, R., & Johnson, W. (1944). Studies in the psychology of stuttering: XVIII. The construction and application of a test of attitude toward stuttering. *Journal of Speech Disorders, 9,* 39–49.

Anderson, J. D., & Conture, E. G. (2000). Language abilities of children who stutter: A preliminary study. *Journal of Fluency Disorders, 25,* 283–304.

Anderson, J. D., & Conture, E. G. (2004). Sentence-structure priming in young children who do and do not stutter. *Journal of Speech, Language and Hearing Research, 47,* 552–71.

Anderson, J. D., Pellowski, M. W., & Conture, E. G. (2005). Childhood stuttering and dissociations across linguistic domains. *Journal of Fluency Disorders, 30,* 219–53.

Anderson, J. D., Pellowski, M. W., Conture, E. G., & Kelly, E. M. (2003). Temperamental characteristics of young children who stutter. *Journal of Speech, Language and Hearing Research, 46,* 1221–33.

Anderson, J. D., Wagovich, S. A., & Hall, N. E. (2006). Nonword repetition skills in young children who do and do not stutter. *Journal of Fluency Disorders, 31,* 177–99.

Anderson, J. M., Hood, S. B., & Sellers, D. E. (1988). Central auditory processing abilities of adolescent and preadolescent stuttering and nonstuttering children. *Journal of Fluency Disorders, 13,* 199–214.

Anderson, J. M., & Whealdon, M. L. (1941). A study of the blood group distribution among stutterers. *Journal of Speech Disorders, 6,* 23–28.

Anderson, L. O. (1923). Stuttering and allied disorders. *Comparative Psychology Monographs,* Vol. 1.

Anderson, T. K., & Felsenfeld, S. (2003). A thematic analysis of late recovery from stuttering. *American Journal of Speech-Language Pathology, 12,* 243–53.

Andrews, G. (1984a). Epidemiology of stuttering. In R. F. Curlee & W. H. Perkins (Eds.), *Nature and treatment of stuttering: New direction* (pp. 1–12). San Diego: College–Hill Press.

Andrews, G. (1984b). Evaluation of the benefits of treatment. In W. H. Perkins (Ed.), *Stuttering disorders.* New York: Thieme–Stratton.

Andrews, G., & Craig, A. (1982). Stuttering: Overt and covert measurement of the speech of treated subjects. *Journal of Speech and Hearing Disorders, 47,* 96–99.

Andrews, G., Craig, A., Feyer, A.-M., Hoddinott, S., Howie, P., & Neilson, M. (1983). Stuttering: A review of research findings and theories circa 1982. *Journal of Speech and Hearing Disorders, 48,* 226–46.

Andrews, G., & Cutler, J. (1974). Stuttering therapy: The relation between changes in symptom level and attitudes. *Journal of Speech and Hearing Disorders, 39,* 312–19.

Andrews, G., & Dozsa, M. (1977). Haloperidol and the treatment of stuttering. *Journal of Fluency Disorders, 2,* 217–24.

Andrews, G., & Feyer, A.-M. (1985). Does behavior therapy still work when the experimenters depart?

An analysis of a behavioral treatment program for stutterers. *Behavior Modification, 9,* 443–57.

Andrews, G., Guitar, B., & Howie, P. (1980). Meta–analysis of the effects of stuttering treatment. *Journal of Speech and Hearing Disorders, 45,* 287–307.

Andrews, G., & Harris, M. (1964). *The syndrome of stuttering. Clinics in Developmental Medicine,* No. 17. London: Spastics Society Medical Education and Information Unit in association with Wm. Heinemann Medical Books.

Andrews, G., & Harvey, R. (1981). Regression to the mean in pretreatment measures of stuttering. *Journal of Speech and Hearing Disorders, 46,* 204–07.

Andrews, G., Howie, P. M., Dozsa, M., & Guitar, B. E. (1982). Stuttering: Speech pattern characteristics under fluency-inducing conditions. *Journal of Speech and Hearing Research, 25,* 208–16.

Andrews, G., & Ingham, R. J. (1972a). An approach to the evaluation of stuttering therapy. *Journal of Speech and Hearing Research, 15,* 296–302.

Andrews, G., & Ingham, R. J. (1972b). Stuttering: An evaluation of follow-up procedures for syllable-timed speech/token system therapy. *Journal of Communication Disorders, 5,* 307–19.

Andrews, G., Morris-Yates, A., Howie, P., & Martin, N. G. (1991). Genetic factors in stuttering confirmed. *Archives of General Psychiatry, 48*(11), 1034–35.

Andrews, G., & Quinn, P. T. (1972). Stuttering and cerebral dominance. *Journal of Communication Disorders, 5,* 212.

Andrews, G., Quinn, P. T., & Sorby, W. A. (1972). Stuttering: An investigation into cerebral dominance for speech. *Journal of Neurology, Neurosurgery, & Psychiatry, 35,* 414–18.

Andrews, G., & Tanner, S. (l982a). Stuttering treatment: An attempt to replicate the regulated breathing method. *Journal of Speech and Hearing Disorders, 47,* 138–40.

Andrews, G., & Tanner, S. (1982b). Stuttering: The results of 5 days treatment with an airflow technique. *Journal of Speech and Hearing Disorders, 47,* 427–29.

Andrews, M. L., & Smith, R. G. (1976). Perceptions of auditory components of stuttered speech. *Journal of Communication Disorders, 9,* 121–28.

Andronico, M. P., & Blake, I. (1971). The application of filial therapy to young children with stuttering problems. *Journal of Speech and Hearing Disorders, 36,* 377–81.

Aram, D. M., Meyers, S. C., & Ekelman, B. L. (1990). Fluency of conversational speech in children with unilateral brain lesions. *Brain and Language, 38*(1), 105–21.

Archibald, L., & De Nil, L. F. (1999). The relationship between stuttering severity and kinesthetic acuity for jaw movements in adults who stutter. *Journal of Fluency Disorders, 24,* 25–42.

Ardila, A., Bateman, J. C., Niño, C. R., Pulido, E., Rivera, D. B., & Vanegas, C. J. (1994). An epidemiologic study of stuttering. *Journal of Communication Disorders, 27,* 37–48.

Ardila, A., & Lopez, M.V. (1986). Severe stuttering associated with right hemisphere lesion. *Brain and Language, 7,* 239–46.

Ardila, A., Rosselli, M. N., Bateman, J. R., & Guzmán, M. (2000). Neuropsychological profile of stuttering children. *Journal of Developmental and Physical Disabilities, 12,* 121–30.

Arend, R., Handzel, L., & Weiss, B. (1962). Dysphatic stuttering. *Folia Phoniatrica, 14,* 55–66.

Arends, N., Povel, D.-J., & Kolk, H. (1988). Stuttering as an attentional phenomenon. *Journal of Fluency Disorders, 13,* 141–51.

Armson, J., Foote, S., Witt, C., Kalinowski, J., & Stuart, A. (1997). Effect of frequency altered feedback and audience size on stuttering. *European Journal of Disorders of Communication, 32,* 359–66.

Armson, J., Jenson, S., Gallant, D., Kalinowski, J., & Fee, E. J. (1997). The relationship between degree of audible struggle and judgments of childhood disfluencies as stuttered or not stuttered. *American Journal of Speech-Language Pathology, 6,* 42–50.

Armson, J., & Kalinowski, J. (1994). Interpreting results of the fluent speech paradigm in stuttering research. Difficulties in separating cause from effect. *Journal of Speech and Hearing Research, 37,* 69–82.

Armson, J., Kiefte, M., Mason, J., & De Croos, D. (2006). The effect of SpeechEasy on stuttering frequency in laboratory conditions. *Journal of Fluency Disorders, 31,* 137–52.

Armson, J., & Stuart, A. (1998). Effect of extended exposure to frequency-altered feedback on stuttering during reading and monologue. *Journal of Speech, Language, and Hearing Research, 41,* 479–91.

Arndt, J., & Healey, E. C. (2001). Concomitant disorders in school-age children who stutter. *Language, Speech and Hearing Services in Schools, 32,* 68–79.

Arnold, G. E. (1958). Special features and new viewpoint of phoniatric practice in New York. *Folia Phoniatrica, 10,* 96–111.

Arnold, H. S., Conture, E. G., & Ohde, R. N. (2005). Phonological neighborhood density in the picture naming of young children who stutter: Preliminary study. *Journal of Fluency Disorders, 30,* 125–48.

Aron, M. L. (1962). The nature and incidence of stuttering among a Bantu group of school-going children. *Journal of Speech and Hearing Disorders, 27,* 116–28.

Aron, M. L. (1965). The effects of the combination of trifluoperazine and amylobarbitone on adult stutterers. *Medical Proceedings of the South African Journal of Advancement of Medical Science, 11,* 227–33.

Aron, M. L. (1967). The relationships between measurements of stuttering behavior. *Journal of the South African Logopedic Society, 14,* 15–34.

Arthurs, R. G. S., Cappon, D., Douglass, E., & Quarrington, B. (1954). Carbon dioxide therapy with stutterers. *Disorders of the Nervous System, 15,* 123–26.

Asp, C. W. (1968). Time-intensity trade and lateralized localization of interaural intensity differences by stutterers and non-stutterers. *Speech Monographs, 35,* 316–17.

Aten, J. L., & Blanchard, S. (1974). EMG biofeedback in the treatment of stuttering: Selected case studies. [Abstract]. *ASHA, 16,* 555.

Atkins, C. P. (1988). Perceptions of speakers with minimal eye contact: Implications for stutterers. *Journal of Fluency Disorders, 13,* 429–36.

Atkinson, L. (1983). Rational-emotive therapy versus systematic desensitization: A comment on Moleski and Tosi. *Journal of Consulting and Clinical Psychology, 51,* 776–78.

Au-Yeung, J., Gomez, I. V., & Howell, P. (2003). Exchange of disfluency with age from function words to content words in Spanish speakers who stutter. *Journal of Speech, Language and Hearing Research, 46,* 754–65.

Au-Yeung, J., & Howell, P. (1998a). Lexical and syntactic context and stuttering. *Clinical Linguistics and Phonetics, 12,* 67–78.

Au-Yeung, J., & Howell, P. (1998b). Phonological words and stuttering on function words. *Journal of Speech, Language and Hearing Research, 41,* 1019–31.

Au-Yeung, J., & Howell, P. (2002). Non-word reading, lexical retrieval and stuttering: Comments on Packman, Onslow, Coombes and Goodwin (2001). *Clinical Linguistics and Phonetics, 16,* 287–93.

Avari, D. N., & Bloodstein, O. (1974). Adjacency and prediction in school-age stutterers. *Journal of Speech and Hearing Research, 17,* 33–40.

Azrin, N., Jones, R. J., & Flye, B. (1968). A synchronization effect and its application to stuttering by a portable apparatus. *Journal of Applied Behavior Analysis, 1,* 283–95.

Azrin, N. H., & Nunn, R. G. (1974). A rapid method of eliminating stuttering by a regulated breathing approach. *Behavior Research Therapy, 12,* 279–86.

Azrin, N. H., Nunn, R. G., & Frantz, S. E. (1979). Comparison of regulated breathing versus abbreviated desensitization on reported stuttering episodes. *Journal of Speech and Hearing Disorders, 44,* 331–39.

Backus, O. (1938). Incidence of stuttering among the deaf. *Annals of Otology, Rhinology, and Laryngology, 47,* 632–35.

Bajaj, A., Hodson, B., & Schommer-Aikins, M. (2004). Performance on phonological and grammatical awareness metalinguistic tasks by children who stutter and their fluent peers. *Journal of Fluency Disorders, 29,* 63–78.

Bajaj, A., Hodson, B., & Westby, C. (2005). Communicative ability conceptions among children who stutter and their fluent peers: A qualitative exploration. *Journal of Fluency Disorders, 30,* 41–64.

Baken, R. J., McManus, D. A., & Cavallo, S. A. (1983). Prephonatory chest wall posturing in stutterers. *Journal of Speech and Hearing Research, 26,* 444–50.

Baker, B., Ross, E., & Girson, J. (1997). Attitudes of a group of South African speech-language pathologists towards stutterers and stuttering therapy. *The South African Journal of Communication Disorders. Die Suid-Afrikaanse Tydskrif vir Kommunikasieafwykings, 44,* 13–23.

Bakker, K. (1999). Clinical technologies for the reduction of stuttering and enhancement of speech fluency. *Seminars in Speech and Language, 20,* 271–79.

Bakker, K. (2006). Technical support for stuttering treatment. In N. Bernstein Ratner & J. Tetnowski (Eds.), *Current issues in stuttering research and practice* (pp. 205–38). Mahwah, NJ: Lawrence Erlbaum Associates.

Bakker, K., & Brutten, G. J. (1987). Labial and laryngeal reaction times of stutterers and nonstutterers. In H. F. M. Peters & W. Hulstijn (Eds.), *Speech motor dynamics in stuttering* (pp. 177–83). New York: Springer.

Bakker, K., & Brutten, G. J. (1989). A comparative investigation of the laryngeal premotor, adjustment, and reaction times of stutterers and nonstutterers. *Journal of Speech and Hearing Research, 32,* 239–44.

Bakker, K., Brutten, G. J., Janssen, P., & van der Meulen, S. (1991). An eyemarking study of anticipation and dysfluency among elementary school stutterers. *Journal of Fluency Disorders, 16,* 25–33.

Balaban, C. D., & Thayer, J. F. (2001). Neurological bases for balance-anxiety links. *Journal of Anxiety Disorders, 15,* 53–79.

Balasubramanian, V., Max, L., Van Borsel, J. V., Rayca, K. O., & Richardson, D. (2003). Acquired stuttering following right frontal and bilateral pontine lesion: A case study. *Brain and Cognition, 53,* 185–90.

Ballard, P. B. (1912). Sinistrality and speech. *Journal of Experimental Pedagogy, 1,* 298–310.

Bar, A. (1967). Effects of listening instructions on attention to manner and content of stutterers' speech. *Journal of Speech and Hearing Research, 10,* 87–92.

Bar, A. (1969). Analyses of roles, stuttering and interaction processes during interviews with stutterers. *Journal of Communication Disorders, 2,* 126–40.

Bar, A., & Jakab, I. (1969). Graphic identification of the stuttering episode as experienced by stutterers. In I. Jakab (Ed.), *Art Interpretation and Art Therapy. Psychiatry and Art,* Vol. 2. Fifth International Colloquium of Psychopathology of Expression. Basel: Karger.

Bar, A., Singer, J., & Feldman, R. G. (1969). Subvocal muscle activity during stuttering and fluent speech: A comparison. *Journal of the South African Logopedic Society, 16,* 9–14.

Bär, K. J., Häger, F., & Sauer, H. (2004). Olanzapine- and clozapine-induced stuttering. A case series. *Pharmacopsychiatry, 37,* 131–34.

Barasch, C. T., Guitar, B., McCauley, R. J., & Absher, R. G. (2000). Disfluency and time perception. *Journal of Speech, Language and Hearing Research, 43,* 1429–40.

Baratz, R., & Mesulam, M.-M. (1981). Adult-onset stuttering treated with anticonvulsants. *Archives of Neurology, 38,* 132.

Barbara, D. A. (1946). A psychosomatic approach to the problem of stuttering in psychotics. *American Journal of Psychiatry, 103,* 188–95.

Barbara, D. A. (1954). *Stuttering: A psychodynamic approach to its understanding and treatment.* New York: Julian Press.

Barber, V. (1939). Studies in the psychology of stuttering: XV. Chorus reading as a distraction in stuttering. *Journal of Speech Disorders, 4,* 371–83.

Barber, V. (1940). Studies in the psychology of stuttering: XVI. Rhythm as a distraction in stuttering. *Journal of Speech Disorder, 5,* 29–42.

Barr, D. F., & Carmel, N. R. (1969). Stuttering inhibition with high frequency narrow-band masking noise. *Journal of Auditory Research, 9,* 40–44.

Barr, H. (1940). A quantitative study of the specific phenomena observed in stuttering. *Journal of Speech Disorders, 5,* 277–80.

Barrett, K. H., Keith, R. W., Agnello, J. G., & Weiler, E. M. (1979). Central auditory processing of stutterers and nonstutterers. [Abstract]. *ASHA, 21,* 769.

Barrett, R. S., & Stoeckel, C. M. (1979). Unilateral eyelid movement control in stutterers and nonstutterers. [Abstract]. *ASHA, 21,* 769.

Baskin, T. W., Tierney, S. C., Minami, T., & Wampold, B. E. (2003). Establishing specificity in psychotherapy: A meta-analysis of structural equivalence of placebo controls. *Journal of Consulting and Clinical Psychology, 71,* 973–79.

Bastijens, P., Brutten, G. J., & Stés, R. (1978). The effect of punishment and reinforcement procedures on a stutterer's factor two avoidance response. *Journal of Fluency Disorders, 3,* 77–85.

Bates, E., Dale, P., & Thal, D. (1995). Individual differences and their implications for theories of language development. In P. Fletcher &

B. MacWhinney (Eds.), *Handbook of child language* (pp. 96–151). Oxford: Blackwell.

Baumeister, H., Caspar, F., & Herziger, F. (2003). [Treatment outcome study of the stuttering therapy summer camp 2000 for children and adolescents]. *Psychotherapie, Psychosomatik, Medizinische Psychologie, 53,* 455–63.

Baumgartner, J. M., & Brutten, G. J. (1983). Expectancy and heart rate as predictors of the speech performance of stutterers. *Journal of Speech and Hearing Research, 26,* 383–88.

Bearss, L. M. (1951). An investigation of conflict in stutterers and non-stutterers. [Abstract]. *Speech Monographs, 18,* 237–38.

Bearss, M. L. (1952). An investigation of the effect of penalty on the expectancy and frequency of stuttering. [Abstract]. *Speech Monographs, 19,* 189–90.

Bebout, L., & Arthur, B. (1997). Attitudes toward speech disorders: Sampling the views of Cantonese-speaking Americans. *Journal of Communication Disorders, 30,* 205–28.

Bebout, L., & Bradford, A. (1992). Cross–cultural attitudes toward speech disorders. *Journal of Speech and Hearing Research, 35,* 5–52.

Beech, H. R., & Fransella, F. (1968). *Research and experiment in stuttering.* New York: Pergamon.

Belyakova, L. I. (1973). Sravintelnaya kharakteristika elektromyogramm bolnikh s zaikaniem na fone organicheskovo porazhenia tsentralnoi nervnoi sistemi i nevroticheskikh reaktsii. *Zh. Nevropatol. Psikhiat., 73,* 715–20.

Bender, J. F. (1939). *The personality structure of stuttering.* New York: Pitman Publishing Corp.

Bender, J. F., & Kleinfeld, V. M. (1938). *Principles and practices of speech correction.* New York: Pitman Publishing Corp.

Bente, D., Schönhärl, E., & Krump, J. (1956). Elektroencephalographische Befunde bei Stotterern und ihre Bedeutung für die medikamentöse Therapie. *Arch. Ohr.-Nas.-Kehlk. Heilk., 169,* 513–19.

Bentin, S. (1989). Electrophysiological studies of visual word perception, lexical organization, and semantic processing: A tutorial review. *Language and Speech, 32,* 205–20.

Berecz, J. M. (1973). The treatment of stuttering through precision punishment and cognitive arousal. *Journal of Speech and Hearing Disorders, 38,* 256–67.

Berecz, J. M. (1976). Cognitive conditioning therapy in the treatment of stuttering. *Journal of Communication Disorders, 9,* 301–15.

Berger, E. M. (1952). The relation between expressed acceptance of self and expressed acceptance of others. *Journal of Abnormal Social Psychology, 47,* 778–82.

Bergmann, G. (1986). Studies in stuttering as a prosodic disturbance. *Journal of Speech and Hearing Research, 29,* 290–300.

Bergmann, G. (1987). Stuttering as a prosodic disturbance: A link between speech execution and emotional processes. In H. F. M. Peters & W. Hulstijn (Eds.), *Speech motor dynamics in stuttering* (pp. 393–407). New York: Springer.

Berko Gleason, J. & Bernstein Ratner, N. (Eds.). (1998). *Psycholinguistics* (2nd ed). Austin, TX: HBJ.

Berlin, A. J. (1955). An exploratory attempt to isolate types of stuttering. [Abstract]. *Speech Monographs, 22,* 196–97.

Berlini, C. I. (1960). Parents' diagnoses of stuttering. *Journal of Speech and Hearing Research, 3,* 372–79.

Berlinsky, S. L. (1955). A comparison of stutterers and non-stutterers in four conditions of induced anxiety. [Abstract]. *Speech Monographs, 22,* 197.

Berman Hakim, H. and Bernstein Ratner, N. (2004). Nonword repetition abilities of children who stutter. *Journal of Fluency Disorders, 29,* 179–99.

Bernhardt, R. B. (1954). Personality conflict and the act of stuttering. *Dissertation Abstracts, 14,* 709.

Bernstein, N. E. (1981). Are there constraints on childhood disfluency? *Journal of Fluency Disorders, 6,* 341–50.

Bernstein Ratner, N. (1988). On terminology in stuttering research: Reply to Quesal. *Journal of Speech and Hearing Disorders, 53,* 350–51.

Bernstein Ratner, N. (1992). Measurable outcomes of instructions to modify normal parent-child verbal interactions: Implications for indirect stuttering therapy. *Journal of Speech and Hearing Research, 35,* 14–20.

Bernstein Ratner, N. (1995). Treating the stuttering child with concomitant grammatical or phonological disorder. *Language, Speech and Hearing Services in Schools, 26,* 180–86.

Bernstein Ratner, N. (1997). Stuttering: A psycholinguistic perspective. In R. Curlee & G. Siegel (Eds.), *Nature and treatment of stuttering: New directions* (2nd ed.) (pp. 99–127). Needham, MA: Allyn & Bacon.

Bernstein Ratner, N. (1998). Linguistic and perceptual characteristics of children at stuttering onset. In E. C. Healey & H. F. M. Peters (Eds.), *Proceedings of the Second World Congress on Fluency Disorders* (pp. 3–6). Nijmegen: Nijmegen University Press.

Bernstein Ratner, N. (2000). Performance or capacity, the DCM model still requires definitions and boundaries it doesn't have. *Journal of Fluency Disorders, 25,* 337–46.

Bernstein Ratner, N. (2001). The phonology of early stuttering: Some reasons where there isn't one. In H.-G. Bosshardt, J. S. Yaruss, & H. F. M. Peters (Eds.), *Fluency disorders: theory, research, treatment and self-help* (pp. 203–05). Nijmegen: Nijmegen University Press.

Bernstein Ratner, N. (2004). Fluency and stuttering in bilingual children. In B. Goldstein (Ed.), *Bilingual language development and disorders in Spanish-English speakers* (pp. 287–308). Baltimore: Paul H Brookes Publishing.

Bernstein Ratner, N. (2005a). Is phonetic complexity a useful construct in understanding stuttering? *Journal of Fluency Disorders, 30,* 337–41.

Bernstein Ratner, N. (2005b). Evidence-based practice in stuttering: Some questions to consider. *Journal of Fluency Disorders, 30,* 163–88.

Bernstein Ratner, N. (2005c). Treating children with concomitant problems. In R. Lees (Ed.), *The treatment of stuttering in the young school aged child* (pp. 161–75). London: Whurr.

Bernstein Ratner, N. (2006). Setting the stage: Some thoughts about evidence-based practice. *Language, Speech and Hearing Services in Schools, 37,* 1–11.

Bernstein Ratner, N., & Benitez, M. (1985). Linguistic analysis of a bilingual stutterer. *Journal of Fluency Disorders, 10,* 211–19.

Bernstein Ratner, N. & Guitar, B. (2006). Treatment of very early stuttering and parent-administered therapy: The state of the art. In N. Bernstein Ratner & J. Tetnowski (Eds.), *Current issues in stuttering research and practice* (pp. 99–124). Mahwah, NJ: Lawrence Erlbaum Associates.

Bernstein Ratner, N., & Sih, C. C. (1987). Effects of gradual increases in sentence length and complexity on children's dysfluency. *Journal of Speech and Hearing Disorders, 52,* 278–87.

Bernstein Ratner, N., & Silverman, S. (2000). Parental perceptions of children's communicative development at stuttering onset. *Journal of Speech Language and Hearing Research,* 43, 1252–63.

Bernstein Ratner, N., & Tetnowski, J. (2006). Stuttering treatment in the new millennium: Changes in the traditional parameters of clinical focus. In N. Bernstein Ratner & J. Tetnowski (Eds.), *Current issues in stuttering research and practice* (pp. 1–16). Mahwah, NJ: Lawrence Erlbaum Associates.

Bernstein Ratner, N., & Wijnen, F. (2007). The Vicious Circle: Linguistic encoding, self-monitoring and stuttering. In J. Au-Yeung & M. Leahy (Eds.), *Research, treatment and self-help in fluency disorders: new horizons. Proceedings of the Fifth World Congress of the International Fluency Association* (pp. 84–90). International Fluency Association.

Berry, M. F. (1937a). The medical history of stuttering children. Ph.D. Dissertation, University of Wisconsin.

Berry, M. F. (1937b). Twinning in stuttering families. *Human Biology, 9,* 329–46.

Berry, M. F. (1938a). A common denominator in twinning and stuttering. *Journal of Speech Disorders, 3,* 51–57.

Berry, M. F. (1938b). Developmental history of stuttering children. *Journal of Pediatrics, 12,* 209–17.

Berry, M. F. (1938c). A study of the medical history of stuttering children. *Speech Monographs, 5,* 97–114.

Berry, M. F., & Eisenson, J. (1956). *Speech disorders.* New York: Appleton-Century Crofts.

Berry, R. C., & Silverman, F. H. (1972). Equality of intervals on the Lewis-Sherman scale of stuttering severity. *Journal of Speech and Hearing Research, 15,* 185–88.

Berryman, J. D., & Kools, J. A. (1975). Disfluency of nonstuttering children in relation to specific measures of language, reading, and mental maturity. *Journal of Fluency Disorders, 1,* 18–24.

Berwick, N. H. (1955). Stuttering in response to photographs of selected listeners. In W. Johnson & R. R. Leutenegger (Eds.), *Stuttering in children and adults.* Minneapolis: University of Minnesota Press.

Besozzi, T. E., & Adams, M. R. (1969). The influence of prosody on stuttering adaptation. *Journal of Speech and Hearing Research, 12,* 818–24.

Biermann-Ruben, K., Salmelin, R., & Schnitzler, A. (2005). Right rolandic activation during speech perception in stutterers: A MEG study. *NeuroImage, 25,* 793–801.

Biggs, B., & Sheehan, J. (1969). Punishment or distraction? Operant stuttering revisited. *Journal of Abnormal Psychology, 74,* 256–62.

Bijleveld, H., Lebrun, Y., & van Dongen, H. (1994). A case of acquired stuttering. *Folia Phoniatrica, 46,* 250–53.

Bills, A. G. (1934). The relation of stuttering to mental fatigue. *Journal of Experimental Psychology, 17,* 574–84.

Bilto, E. W. (1941). A comparative study of certain physical abilities of children with speech defects and children with normal speech. *Journal of Speech Disorders, 6,* 187–203.

Bishop, D. V. M. (1986). Is there a link between handedness and hypersensitivity? *Cortex, 22,* 289–96.

Bishop, D. V. M., North, T., & Donlan, C. (1996). Nonword repetition as a behavioural marker for inherited language impairment: Evidence from a twin study. *Journal of Child Psychology and Psychiatry and Allied Disciplines, 37,* 391–403.

Bishop, J. H., Williams, H. G., & Cooper, W. A. (1991a). Age and task complexity variables in motor performance of stuttering and nonstuttering children. *Journal of Fluency Disorders, 16,* 207–17.

Bishop, J. H., Williams, H. G., & Cooper, W. A. (1991b). Age and task complexity variables in motor performance of children with articulation-disordered, stuttering, and normal speech. *Journal of Fluency Disorders, 16,* 219–28.

Bjerkan, B. (1980). Word fragmentations and repetitions in the spontaneous speech of 2–6-year-old children. *Journal of Fluency Disorders, 5,* 137–48.

Black, J. A. (1937). A comparative study of the perception of freedom-in-leisure between stuttering and nonstuttering individuals. *Journal of Fluency Disorders, 12,* 239–43.

Blackburn, B. (1931). Voluntary movements of the organs of speech in stutterers and non-stutterers. *Psychology Monographs, 41,* 1–13.

Blankenship, J. (1964). "Stuttering" in normal speech. *Journal of Speech and Hearing Research, 7,* 95–96.

Blankenship J., & Kay, C. (1964). Hesitation phenomena in English speech: A study in distribution. *Word, 20,* 360–72.

Blanton, S. (1916). A survey of speech defects. *Journal of Educational Psychology, 7,* 581–92.

Blanton, S. (1931). Stuttering. *Mental Hygiene, 15,* 271–82.

Blanton, S., & Blanton, M. G. (1936). *For stutterers.* New York: D. Appleton-Century.

Blitzer, A., & Sulica, L. (2001). Botulinum toxin: Basic science and clinical uses in otolaryngology. *The Laryngoscope, 111,* 218–26.

Bloch, E. L., & Goodstein, L. D. (1971). Functional speech disorders and personality: A decade of research. *Journal of Speech and Hearing Disorders, 36,* 295–314.

Bloch, M., Stager, S., Braun, A., Calis, K. A., Turcasso, N. M., Grothe, D. R., et al. (1997). Pimozide-induced depression in men who stutter. *The Journal of Clinical Psychiatry, 58,* 433–36.

Bloch, M., Stager, S. V., Braun, A. R., & Rubinow, D. R. (1995). Severe psychiatric symptoms associated with paroxetine withdrawal. *Lancet, 346,* 57.

Bloch, V., Dalby, M., & Johannesen, E. (1977). Effekten af propanolol (inderal) på stammen. *DSH Abstracts, 17,* 226.

Block, S., Ingham, R. J., & Bench, R. J. (1996). The effects of the Edinburgh Masker on stuttering. *Australian Journal of Human Communication Disorders, 24,* 11–18.

Block, S., Onslow, M., Packman, A., & Dacakis, G. (2006). Connecting stuttering management and measurement: IV. Predictors of outcome for a behavioural treatment for stuttering. *International Journal of Language and Communication Disorders, 41,* 395–406.

Block, S., Onslow, M., Packman, A., Gray, B., & Dacakis, G. (2005). Treatment of chronic stuttering: Outcomes from a student training clinic. *International Journal of Language & Communication Disorders, 40,* 455–66.

Block, S., Onslow, M., Roberts, R., & White, S. (2004). Control of stuttering with EMG feedback. *Advances in Speech Language Pathology, 6,* 100–06.

Blomgren, M., Nagarajan, S. S., Lee, J. N., Li, T., & Alvord, L. (2003). Preliminary results of a functional

MRI study of brain activation patterns in stuttering and nonstuttering speakers during a lexical access task. *Journal of Fluency Disorders, 28,* 337–57.

Blomgren, M., & Robb, M. (1998). A note on vowel centralization in stuttering and nonstuttering individuals. *Journal of Speech, Language and Hearing Research, 41,* 1042–52.

Blomgren, M., Roy, N., Callister, T., & Merrill, R. M. (2005). Intensive stuttering modification therapy: A multidimensional assessment of treatment outcomes. *Journal of Speech, Language and Hearing Research, 48,* 509–23.

Blood, G. W. (1985). Laterality differences in child stutterers: Heterogeneity, severity levels, and statistical treatments. *Journal of Speech and Hearing Disorders, 50,* 66–72.

Blood, G. W. (1995). POWER(2): Relapse management with adolescents who stutter—Permission, Ownership, Well-being, Esteem, Resilience, and Responsibility. *Language, Speech, and Hearing Services in Schools, 26,* 169–79.

Blood, G. W., & Blood, I. M. (1984). Central auditory function in young stutterers. *Perceptual and Motor Skills, 59,* 699–705.

Blood, G. W., & Blood, I. M. (1989a). Laterality preferences in adult female and male stutterers. *Journal of Fluency Disorders, 14,* 1–10.

Blood, G. W., & Blood, I. M. (1989b). Multiple data analysis of dichotic listening advantages of stutterers. *Journal of Fluency Disorders, 14,* 97–107.

Blood, G. W., & Blood, I. M. (1994). Subjective anxiety measures and cortisol responses in adults who stutter. *Journal of Speech and Hearing Research, 37,* 760–69.

Blood, G. W., & Blood, I. M. (1997). Cortisol responses in adults who stutter: Coping preferences and apprehension about communication. *Perceptual & Motor Skills, 84,* 883–90.

Blood, G. W., Blood, I. M., Bennett, S., Simpson, K. C., & Susman, E. J. (1994). Subjective anxiety measurements and cortisol responses in adults who stutter. *Journal of Speech and Hearing Research, 37,* 760–68.

Blood, G. W., Blood, I. M., Frederick, S. B., Wertz, H. A., & Simpson, K. C. (1997). Cortisol responses in adults who stutter: Coping preferences and apprehension about communication. *Perceptual and Motor Skills, 84,* 883–89.

Blood, G. W., Blood, I. M., & Hood, S. B. (1987). The development of ear preferences in stuttering and nonstuttering children: A longitudinal study. *Journal of Fluency Disorders, 12,* 119–31.

Blood, G. W., Blood, I. M., Tellis, G. M., & Gabel, R. M. (2003). A preliminary study of self-esteem, stigma, and disclosure in adolescents who stutter. *Journal of Fluency Disorders, 28,* 143–60.

Blood, G. W., & Hood, S. B. (1978). Elementary school–aged stutterers' disfluencies during oral reading and spontaneous speech. *Journal of Fluency Disorders, 3,* 155–65.

Blood, G. W., Ridenour, V. J., Jr., Qualls, C. D., & Hammer, C. S. (2003). Co-occurring disorders in children who stutter. *Journal of Communication Disorders, 36,* 427–49.

Blood, G. W., & Seider, R. (1981). The concomitant problems of young stutterers. *Journal of Speech and Hearing Disorders, 46,* 31–33.

Blood, I. M. (1996). Disruptions in auditory and temporal processing in adults who stutter. *Perceptual and Motor Skills, 82,* 272–74.

Blood, I. M., & Blood, G. W. (1984). Relationship between stuttering severity and brainstem-evoked response testing. *Perceptual and Motor Skills, 59,* 935–38.

Blood, I. M., & Blood, G. W. (1986). Relationship between disfluency variables and dichotic listening in stutterers. *Perceptual and Motor Skills, 62,* 37–38.

Blood, I. M., & Wertz, H. (1997). The effects of life stressors and daily stressors on stuttering. *Journal of Speech, Language and Hearing Research, 40,* 134–44.

Blood, I. M., Wertz, H., Blood, G. W., Bennett, S., & Simpson, K. C. (1997). The effects of life stressors and daily stressors on stuttering. *Journal of Speech, Language, and Hearing Research, 40,* 134–43.

Bloodstein, O. (1944). Studies in the psychology of stuttering: XIX. The relationship between oral reading rate and severity of stuttering. *Journal of Speech Disorders, 9,* 161–73.

Bloodstein, O. (1949). Conditions under which stuttering is reduced or absent: A review of literature. *Journal of Speech and Hearing Disorders, 14,* 295–302.

Bloodstein, O. (1950a). Hypothetical conditions under which stuttering is reduced or absent. *Journal of Speech and Hearing Disorders, 15,* 142–53.

Bloodstein, O. (1950b). A rating scale study of conditions under which stuttering is reduced or absent. *Journal of Speech and Hearing Disorders, 15,* 29–36.

Bloodstein, O. (1958). Stuttering as an anticipatory struggle reaction. In J. Eisenson (Ed.), *Stuttering: A symposium.* New York: Harper & Row.

Bloodstein, O. (1960a). The development of stuttering: I. Changes in nine basic features. *Journal of Speech and Hearing Disorders, 25,* 219–37.

Bloodstein, O. (1960b). The development of stuttering: II. Developmental phases. *Journal of Speech and Hearing Disorders, 25,* 366–76.

Bloodstein, O. (1961a). The development of stuttering: III. Theoretical and clinical implications. *Journal of Speech and Hearing Disorders, 26,* 67–82.

Bloodstein, O. (1961b). Stuttering in families of adopted stutterers. *Journal of Speech and Hearing Disorders, 26,* 395–96.

Bloodstein, O. (1970). Stuttering and normal nonfluency—A continuity hypothesis. *British Journal of Disorders of Communication, 5,* 30–39.

Bloodstein, O. (1972). The anticipatory struggle hypothesis; Implications of research on the variability of stuttering. *Journal of Speech and Hearing Research, 15,* 487–99.

Bloodstein, O. (1974). The rules of early stuttering. *Journal of Speech and Hearing Disorders, 39,* 379–94.

Bloodstein, O. (1975). Stuttering as tension and fragmentation. In J. Eisenson (Ed.), *Stuttering: A second symposium* (pp. 1–95). New York: Harper & Row.

Bloodstein, O. (1981). *A handbook on stuttering* (3rd ed.). Chicago, IL: National Easter Seals Society.

Bloodstein, O. (1984). Stuttering as an anticipatory struggle disorder. In R. F. Curlee & W. H. Perkins (Eds.), *Nature and treatment of stuttering: New directions* (pp. 167–81). San Diego: College–Hill Press.

Bloodstein, O. (1993). *Stuttering: The search for a cause and cure.* Boston: Allyn & Bacon.

Bloodstein, O. (1995). *A handbook on stuttering* (5th ed.). Clifton Park, NY: Thomson-Delmar.

Bloodstein, O. (2000). Genes versus cognitions in stuttering: A needless dichotomy . . . commentary on A. Packman, R. G. Menzies, & M. Onslow (2000). Anxiety and the anticipatory struggle hypothesis. *American Journal of Speech-Language Pathology, 9,* 358–59.

Bloodstein, O. (2001). Incipient and developed stuttering as two distinct disorders: Resolving a dilemma. *Journal of Fluency Disorders, 26,* 67–73.

Bloodstein, O. (2002). Early stuttering as a type of language difficulty. *Journal of Fluency Disorders, 27,* 163–66.

Bloodstein, O. (1993). Communication attitudes of school-age stutterers. *Journal of Fluency Disorders, 18*(4), 403–05.

Bloodstein, O. (2006). Some empirical observations about early stuttering: A possible link to language development. *Journal of Communication Disorders, 39,* 185–91.

Bloodstein, O., Alper, J., & Zisk, P. K. (1965). Stuttering as an outgrowth of normal disfluency. In D. A. Barbara (Ed.), *New directions in stuttering.* Springfield, IL: Charles C. Thomas.

Bloodstein, O., & Bloodstein, A. (1955). Interpretations of facial reactions to stuttering. *Journal of Speech and Hearing Disorders, 20,* 148–55.

Bloodstein, O., & Gantwerk, B. F. (1967). Grammatical function in relation to stuttering in young children. *Journal of Speech and Hearing Research, 10,* 786–89.

Bloodstein, O., & Grossman, M. (1981). Early stutterings: Some aspects of their form and distribution. *Journal of Speech and Hearing Research, 24,* 298–302.

Bloodstein, O., Jaeger, W., & Tureen, J. (1952). A study of the diagnosis of stuttering by parents of stutterers and non-stutterers. *Journal of Speech and Hearing Disorders, 17,* 308–15.

Bloodstein, O., & Schreiber, L. R. (1957). Obsessive-compulsive reactions in stutterers. *Journal of Speech and Hearing Disorders, 22,* 33–39.

Bloodstein, O., & Shogan, R. L. (1972). Some clinical notes on forced stuttering. *Journal of Speech and Hearing Disorders, 37,* 177–86.

Bloodstein, O., & Smith, S. M. (1954). A study of the diagnosis of stuttering with special reference to the sex ratio. *Journal of Speech and Hearing Disorders, 19,* 459–66.

Bloom, C. M., & Silverman, F. H. (1973). Do all stutterers adapt? *Journal of Speech and Hearing Research, 16,* 518–21.

Bloom, C., & Silverman, F. (1979). Stability of performances of individual stutterers on oral reading adptation tasks. *Journal of Fluency Disorders, 4,* 39–44.

Bloom, J. (1959). Child training and stuttering. [Abstract]. *Speech Monographs, 26,* 132–33.

Bloom, L. (1978). Notes for a history of speech pathology. *Psychoanalysis Review, 65,* 433–63.

Bluemel, C. S. (1932). Primary and secondary stammering. *Quarterly Journal of Speech, 18,* 187–200.

Bluemel, C. S. (1933). The dominant gradient in stuttering. *Quarterly Journal of Speech, 19,* 233–42.

Bluemel, C. S. (1935). *Stammering and allied disorders.* New York: Macmillan.

Bluemel, C. S. (1957). *The riddle of stuttering.* Danville, IL: Interstate Publishing Co.

Blum, G. S., & Hunt, H. F. (1952). The validity of the Blacky Pictures. *Psychological Bulletin, 49,* 238–50.

Boberg, E. (1976). Intensive group therapy program for stutterers. *Human Communication, 1,* 29–42.

Boberg, E. (1981). Maintenance of fluency: An experimental program. In E. Boberg (Ed.), *Maintenance of fluency: Proceedings of the Banff conference* (pp. 71–112). New York: Elsevier.

Boberg, E. (1984). Intensive adult/teen therapy program. In W. H. Perkins (Ed.), *Stuttering disorders.* New York: Thieme-Stratton.

Boberg, E. (Ed.). (1993). *Neuropsychology of stuttering* (pp. 161–72). Edmonton, Alberta: University of Alberta Press.

Boberg, E., Ewart, B., Mason, G., Lindsay, K., & Wynn, S. (1978). Stuttering in the retarded: II. Prevalence of stuttering in EMR and TMR children. *Mental Retardation Bulletin, 6,* 67–76.

Boberg, E., Howie, P., & Woods, L. (1979). Maintenance of fluency: A review. *Journal of Fluency Disorders, 4,* 93–116.

Boberg, E., & Kully, D. (1985). *Comprehensive stuttering program.* San Diego: College-Hill Press.

Boberg, E., & Kully, D. (1994). Long-term results of an intensive treatment program for adults and adolescents who stutter. *Journal of Speech and Hearing Research, 37,* 1050–60.

Boberg, E., & Sawyer, L. (1977). The maintenance of fluency following intensive therapy. *Human Communication, 2,* 21–28.

Boberg, E., Yeudall, L. T., Schopflocher, D., & Bo-Lassen, P. (1983). The effect of an intensive behavioral program on the distribution of EEG alpha power in stutterers during the processing of verbal and visuospatial information. *Journal of Fluency Disorders, 8,* 245–63.

Bodenhamer, B. G. (2004). Can hypnotherapy assist people who stammer? *European Journal of Clinical Hypnosis, 5,* 2–11.

Boehmler, R. M. (1958). Listener responses to non-fluencies. *Journal of Speech and Hearing Research, 1,* 132–41.

Bohland, J. W., & Guenther, F. H. (2006). An fMRI investigation of syllable sequence production. *NeuroImage, 32,* 821–41.

Böhme, G. (1968). Stammering and cerebral lesions in early childhood. Examinations of 802 children and adults with cerebral lesions. *Folia Phoniatrica, 20,* 239–49.

Boland, J. L. (1950). An investigation of certain birth factors as they relate to stuttering. [Abstract]. *Speech Monographs, 17,* 287.

Boland, J. L. (1951). Type of birth as related to stuttering. *Journal of Speech and Hearing Disorders, 16,* 40–43.

Boland, J. L. (1953). A comparison of stutterers and non-stutterers on several measures of anxiety. [Abstract]. *Speech Monographs, 20,* 144.

Bonelli, P., Dixon, M., Bernstein Ratner, N., & Onslow, M. (2000). Pre- and post-treatment characteristics of adult-child interactions of Lidcombe stuttering program participants. *Clinical Linguistics and Phonetics, 14,* 427–46.

Bonfanti, B. H., & Culatta, R. (1977). An analysis of the fluency patterns of institutionalized retarded adults. *Journal of Fluency Disorders, 2,* 117–28.

Bonin, B., Ramig, P., & Prescott, T. (1985). Performance differences between stuttering and nonstuttering subjects on a sound fusion task. *Journal of Fluency Disorders, 10,* 291–300.

Boome, E. J., & Richardson, M. A. (1931). *The nature and treatment of stuttering.* London: Methuen.

Borack, S. A. (1969). A study of disfluency in children with articulation defects. M. S. Thesis, Brooklyn College.

Borden, G. J. (1983). Initiation versus execution time during manual and oral counting by stutterers. *Journal of Speech and Hearing Research, 26,* 389–96.

Borden, G. J., Baer, T., & Kenney, M. K. (1985). Onset of voicing in stuttered and fluent utterances. *Journal of Speech and Hearing Research, 28,* 363–72.

Borden, G. J., Dorman, M. F., Freeman, F. J., & Raphael, L. J. (1977). Electromyographic changes with delayed auditory feedback of speech. *Journal of Phonetics, 5,* 1–8.

Borden, G. J., Kim., D. H., & Spiegler, K. (1987). Acoustics of stop consonant-vowel relationships during fluent and stuttered utterances. *Journal of Fluency Disorders, 12,* 175–84.

Boscolo, B., Bernstein Ratner, N., & Rescorla, L. (2002). Fluency characteristics of children with a history of Specific Expressive Language Impairment (SLI-E). *American Journal of Speech-Language Pathology, 11,* 41–49.

Bosshardt, H.-G. (1990). Subvocalization and reading rate differences between stuttering and nonstuttering children and adults. *Journal of Speech and Hearing Research, 33,* 776–85.

Bosshardt, H.-G. (1993). Differences between stutterers' and nonstutterers' short-term recall and recognition performance. *Journal of Speech and Hearing Research, 36,* 286–93.

Bosshardt, H.-G. (1999). Effects of concurrent mental calculation on stuttering, inhalation and speech timing. *Journal of Fluency Disorders, 24,* 43–72.

Bosshardt, H.-G. (2002). Effects of concurrent cognitive processing on the fluency of word repetition: comparison between persons who do and do not stutter. *Journal of Fluency Disorders, 27,* 93–113.

Bosshardt, H.-G. (2006). Cognitive processing load as a determinant of stuttering: Summary of a research programme. *Clinical Linguistics and Phonetics, 20,* 371–85.

Bosshardt, H.-G., Ballmer, W., & De Nil, L. F. (2002). Effects of category and rhyme decisions on sentence production. *Journal of Speech, Language and Hearing Research, 45,* 844–58.

Bosshardt, H.-G., & Fransen, H. (1996). Online sentence processing in adults who stutter and adults who do not stutter. *Journal of Speech and Hearing Research, 39,* 785–98.

Bosshardt, H.-G., & Nandyal, I. (1988). Reading rates of stutterers and nonstutterers during silent and oral reading. *Journal of Fluency Disorders, 13,* 407–20.

Bosshardt, H. G., Sappok, C., Knipschild, M., & Hölscher, C. (1997). Spontaneous imitation of fundamental frequency and speech rate by nonstutterers and stutterers. *Journal of Psycholinguistic Research, 26,* 425–48.

Bothe, A. K. (2004). *Evidence-based treatment of stuttering: Empirical bases and clinical applications.* Mahwah, NJ: Lawrence Erlbaum Associates.

Bothe, A. K., & Andreatta, R. D. (2004). Quantitative and qualitative research paradigms: Thoughts on the quantity and the creativity of stuttering research. *Advances in Speech Language Pathology, 6,* 167–73.

Bothe, A. K., Davidow, J. H., Bramlett, R. E., Franic, D. M., & Ingham, R. J. (2006). Stuttering treatment research 1970–2005: II. Systematic review incorporating trial quality assessment of pharmacological approaches. *American Journal of Speech-Language Pathology, 15,* 342–52.

Bothe, A. K., Davidow, J. H., Bramlett, R. E., & Ingham, R. J. (2006). Stuttering treatment research 1970–2005: I. Systematic review incorporating trial quality assessment of behavioral, cognitive, and related approaches. *American Journal of Speech-Language Pathology, 15,* 321–41.

Boucher, V. J. (2001). A stumbling block in the development of motor theories of speech: relating EMG to force-related changes in articulation. *Clinical Linguistics & Phonetics, 15,* 123–27.

Boudreau, L. A., & Jeffrey, C. J. (1973). Stuttering treated by desensitization. *Journal of Behavior Therapy and Experimental Psychiatry, 4,* 209–12.

Bourdon, K. H., & Silber, D. E. (1970). Perceived parental behavior among stutterers and nonstutterers. *Journal of Abnormal Psychology, 75,* 93–97.

Boutsen, F. R., Brutten, G. J., & Watts, C. R. (2000). Timing and intensity variability in the metronomic speech of stuttering and nonstuttering speakers. *Journal of Speech, Language and Hearing Research, 43,* 513–20.

Boysen, A. E., & Cullinan, W. L. (1971). Object-naming latency in stuttering and nonstuttering children. *Journal of Speech and Hearing Research, 14,* 728–38.

Bradberry, A. (1997). The role of support groups and stuttering therapy. *Seminars in Speech and Language, 18,* 391–99.

Brady, J. P. (1968). A behavioral approach to the treatment of stuttering, *American Journal of Psychiatry, 125,* 843–48.

Brady, J. P. (1969). Studies on the metronome effect on stuttering. *Behavior Research Therapy, 7,* 197–204.

Brady, J. P. (1971). Metronome-conditioned speech retraining for stuttering. *Behavior Therapist, 2,* 129–50.

Brady, J. P. (1991). The pharmacology of stuttering: A critical review. *American Journal of Psychiatry, 148,* 1309–16.

Brady, J. P. (1998). Drug-induced stuttering: A review of the literature. *Journal of Clinical Psychopharmacology, 18,* 50–54.

Brady, J. P., & Ali, Z. (2000). Alprazolam, citalopram, and clomipramine for stuttering. *Journal of Clinical Psychopharmacology, 20,* 287.

Brady, J. P., & Berson, J. (1975). Stuttering, dichotic listening, and cerebral dominance. *Archives of General Psychiatry, 32,* 1449–52.

Brady, J. P., & Brady, C. N. (1972). Behavior therapy of stuttering. *Folia Phoniatrica, 24,* 355–59.

Brady, J., Price, T., McAllister, T., & Dietrich, K. (1989). A trial of verapamil in the treatment of stuttering in adults. *Biological Psychiatry, 25,* 626–30.

Brady, W. A., & Hall, D. E. (1976). The prevalence of stuttering among school-age children. *Language and Speech and Hearing Services in Schools, 7,* 75–81.

Brady, W. A., Sommers, R. K., & Moore, W. H., Jr. (1973). Cerebral speech processing in stuttering children and adults. [Abstract]. ASHA, 15, 472.

Bramlett, R. E., Bothe, A. K., & Franic, D. M. (2006). Using preference-based measures to assess quality of life in stuttering. *Journal of Speech, Language and Hearing Research, 49,* 381–94.

Brandon, S., & Harris, M. (1967). Stammering—An experimental treatment programme using syllable-timed speech. *British Journal of Disorders of Communication, 2,* 64–68.

Brandt, D. E., & Wilde, G. J. S. (1977). A technique for controlling speech disfluencies induced by delayed auditory feedback. *Journal of Fluency Disorders, 2,* 149–56.

Brankel, O. (1961). Pneumotachographische Studien bei Stotterern. *Folia Phoniatrica, 13,* 136–43.

Brankel, O. (1963). Die Bedeutung der synchronen Erfassung von akustischen, pneumotachographischen, myographischen und elektromyographischen Symptomenbildern beim Stottern. *Folia Phoniatrica, 15,* 177–88.

Branscom, M. E., Hughes, J., & Oxtoby, E. T. (1955). Studies of nonfluency in the speech of preschool children. In W. Johnson & R. R. Leutenegger (Eds.), *Stuttering in children and adults* (pp. 157–80). Minneapolis: University of Minnesota Press.

Braun, A. R., Varga, M., Stager, S., Schulz, G., Selbie, S., Maisog, J. M., et al. (1997). Altered patterns of cerebral activity during speech and language production in developmental stuttering: An H215O positron emission tomography study. *Brain, 120,* 761–84.

Braun, O. (1974). Probleme and Möglichkeiten der Lernmotivierung sprachbehinderte Kinder in Unterricht und Therapie in Schulen für Sprachbehinderte. *Sprachheilarbeit, 19,* 47–62.

Bray, M. A., & Kehle, T. J. (1996). Self-modeling as an intervention for stuttering. *School Psychology Review, 25,* 358–70.

Bray, M. A., & Kehle, T. J. (1998). Self-modeling as an intervention for stuttering. *School Psychology Review, 27,* 587–99.

Bray, M. A., & Kehle, T. J. (2001). Long-term follow-up of self-modeling as an intervention for stuttering. *School Psychology Review, 30,* 135–42.

Bray, M. A., Kehle, T. J., Lawless, K. A., & Theodore, L. A. (2003). The relationship of self-efficacy and depression to stuttering. *American Journal of Speech-Language Pathology, 12,* 425–31.

Bray, M. A., Lawless, K. A., & Theodore, L. A. (2003). The relationship of self-efficacy and depression to stuttering. *American Journal of Speech-Language Pathology, 12,* 425.

Brayton, E. R., & Conture, E. G. (1978). Effects of noise and rhythmic stimulation on the speech of stutterers. *Journal of Speech and Hearing Research, 21,* 285–94.

Breitenfeldt, D., & Lorenz, D. (1989). *Successful stuttering management program.* Cheney, WA: Eastern Washington University School of Health Sciences.

Brenner, N. C., Perkins, W. H., & Soderberg, G. A. (1972). The effect of rehearsal on frequency of stuttering. *Journal of Speech and Hearing Research, 15,* 483–86.

Brewerton, T. D., Markowitz, J. S., Keller, S. G., & Cochrane, C. E. (1996). Stuttering with sertraline. *The Journal of Clinical Psychiatry, 57,* 90–91.

Bright, C. M. (1948). The development of a test of listening ability of stutterers. [Abstract]. *Speech Monographs, 15,* 214–15.

Brill, A. A. (1923). Speech disturbances in nervous and mental diseases. *Quarterly Journal of Speech Education, 9,* 129–35.

Brin, M. F., Stewart, C., Blitzer, A., & Diamond, B. (1994). Laryngeal botulinum toxin injections for disabling stuttering in adults. *Neurology, 44,* 2262–66.

Brindle, B. R., & Dunster, J. R. (1984). Prevalence of communication disorders in an institutionalized mentally retarded population. *Human Communication, 8,* 72–80.

Brisk, D. J., Healey, E. C., & Hux, K. A. (1997). Clinicians' training and confidence associated with treating school-age children who stutter: A national survey. *Language, Speech, and Hearing Services in Schools, 28,* 164–76.

Broida, H. (1963). An empirical study of sex-role identification and sex-role preference in stuttering. [Abstract]. *Speech Monographs, 30,* 242–43.

Bronfenbrenner, U., & Ceci, S. (1994). Nature-nurture reconceptualized in developmental perspective: A bioecological model. *Psychologial Review, 101,* 568–86.

Brookshire, R. H. (1969). Effects of random and response contingent noise upon disfluencies of normal speakers. *Journal of Speech and Hearing Research, 12,* 126–34.

Brookshire, R. H., & Eveslage, R. A. (1969). Verbal punishment of disfluency following augmentation of disfluency by random delivery of aversive stimuli. *Journal of Speech and Hearing Research, 12,* 383–88.

Brookshire, R. H., & Martin, R. R. (1967). The differential effects of three verbal punishers on the disfluencies of normal speakers. *Journal of Speech and Hearing Research, 10,* 496–505.

Brosch, S., Häge, A., & Johannsen, H. S. (2002). Prognostic indicators for stuttering: The value of computer-based speech analysis. *Brain and Language, 82,* 75–87.

Brosch, S., Häge, A., Kalehne, P., & Johannsen, H. S. (1999). Stuttering children and the probability of remission-the role of cerebral dominance and speech production. *International Journal of Pediatric Otorhinolaryngology, 47,* 71–76.

Brown, C. J., Zimmermann, G. N., Linville, R. N., & Hegmann, J. P. (1990). Variations in self-paced behaviors in stutterers and nonstutterers. *Journal of Speech and Hearing Research, 33,* 317–23.

Brown, S., Ingham, R. J., Ingham, J. C., Laird, A. R., & Fox, P. T. (2005). Stuttered and fluent speech production: an ALE meta-analysis of functional neuroimaging studies. *Human Brain Mapping, 25,* 105–17.

Brown, S. F. (1937). The influence of grammatical function on the incidence of stuttering. *Journal of Speech Disorders, 2,* 207–15.

Brown, S. F. (1938a). A further study of stuttering in relation to various speech sounds. *Quarterly Journal of Speech, 24,* 390–97.

Brown, S. F. (1938b). Stuttering with relation to word accent and word position. *Journal of Abnormal Social Psychology, 33,* 112–20.

Brown, S. F. (1938c). The theoretical importance of certain factors influencing the incidence of stuttering. *Journal of Speech Disorders, 3,* 223–30.

Brown, S. F. (1945). The loci of stutterings in the speech sequence. *Journal of Speech Disorders, 10,* 181–92.

Brown, S. F., & Hull, H. C. (1942). A study of some social attitudes of a group of 59 stutterers. *Journal of Speech Disorders, 7,* 323–24.

Brown, S. F., & Moren, A. (1942). The frequency of stuttering in relation to word length during oral reading. *Journal of Speech Disorders, 7,* 153–59.

Brown, S. F., & Shulman, E. E. (1940). Intramuscular pressure in stutterers and non-stutterers. *Speech Monographs, 7,* 63–74.

Brown, S. L., & Colcord, R. D. (1987). Perceptual comparisons of adolescent stutterers' and nonstutterers' fluent speech. *Journal of Fluency Disorders, 12,* 419–27.

Bruce, M. C., & Adams, M. R. (1978). Effects of two types of motor practice on stuttering adaptation. *Journal of Speech and Hearing Research, 21,* 421–28.

Brumfitt, S. M., & Peake, M. D. (1988). A double-blind study of verapamil in the treatment of stuttering. *British Journal of Disorders of Communication, 23,* 35–40.

Brundage, S. B., & Bernstein Ratner, N. (1989). The measurement of stuttering frequency in children's speech. *Journal of Fluency Disorders, 14,* 351–58.

Brundage, S. B., Bothe, A. K., Lengeling, A. N., & Evans, J. J. (2006). Comparing judgments of stuttering made by students, clinicians, and highly experienced judges. *Journal of Fluency Disorders, 31,* 271–83.

Brunner, W., & Frank, F. (1975). Vergleichende pulstelemetrische Undersuchungen an Stotterern. *Folia Phoniatrica, 27,* 325–36.

Brunner, W., & Frank, F. (1976). Das pulstelemetrische Verhalten von Stotterern, geheilten Stotterern und Sprachgesunden. *Folia Phoniatrica, 28,* 174–81.

Bruno, G., Camarda, V., & Curi, L. (1965). Contributo allo studio dei fattori causali organici nella patogenesi della balbuzie. *Bol. Mal. Or. Gola Naso, 83,* 753–58.

Brutten, E. J. (1951). Anxiety as a personality factor among stutterers. M. A. Thesis, Brooklyn College.

Brutten, E. J. (1959). Colorimetric measurement of anxiety: A clinical and experimental procedure. *Speech Monographs, 26,* 282–87.

Brutten, E. J. (1963). Palmar sweat investigation of disfluency and expectancy adaptation. *Journal of Speech and Hearing Research, 6,* 40–48.

Brutten, E. J., & Gray, B. B. (1961). Effect of word cue removal on adaptation and adjacency: A clinical paradigm. *Journal of Speech and Hearing Disorders, 26,* 385–89.

Brutten, E. J., & Shoemaker, D. J. (1967). *The modification of stuttering.* Englewood Cliffs, NJ: Prentice-Hall.

Brutten, G. J. (1975). Stuttering: Topography, assessment and behavior change strategies. In J. Eisenson (Ed.), *Stuttering: A second symposium* (pp. 199–262). New York: Harper & Row.

Brutten, G. J. (1980). The effect of punishment on a Factor I stuttering behavior. *Journal of Fluency Disorders, 5,* 77–85.

Brutten, G. J., Bakker, K., Janssen, P., & van der Meulen, S. (1984). Eye movements of stuttering and nonstuttering children during silent reading. *Journal of Speech and Hearing Research, 27,* 562–66.

Brutten, G. J., & Dancer, J. E. (1980). Stuttering adaptation under distributed and massed conditions. *Journal of Fluency Disorders, 5,* 1–10.

Brutten, G. J., & Dunham, S. L. (1989). The *Communication Attitude Test:* A normative study of grade school children. *Journal of Fluency Disorders, 14,* 371–77.

Brutten, G. J., & Janssen, P. (1979). An eye-marking investigation of anticipated and observed stuttering. *Journal of Speech and Hearing Research, 22,* 20–28.

Brutten, G. J., & Janssen, P. (1981). A normative and factor analysis study of the responses of Dutch and American stutterers to the Speech Situations Checklist. *Proceedings of the 18th Congress of the International Association of Logopedics and Phoniatrics.* Washington, DC: American Speech and Language Hearing Association.

Brutten, G. J., & Miller, R. (1988). The disfluencies of normally fluent black first graders. *Journal of Fluency Disorders, 13,* 291–99.

Brutten, G. J., & Shoemaker, D. J. (1969). Stuttering: The disintegration of speech due to conditioned negative emotion. In B. B. Gray & G. England (Eds.), *Stuttering and the conditioning therapies.* Monterey, CA: Monterey Institute Speech Hearing.

Brutten, G. J., & Trotter, A. C. (1985). Hemispheric interference: A dual-task investigation of youngsters who stutter. *Journal of Fluency Disorders, 10,* 77–85.

Brutten, G. J., & Trotter, A. C. (1986). A dual-task investigation of young stutterers and nonstutterers. *Journal of Fluency Disorders, 11,* 275–84.

Brutten, G. J., & Vanryckeghem, M. (2006). *Behavior assessment battery for children who stutter.* San Diego: Plural Publishing, Inc.

Brutten, G. J., & Vanryckeghem, M. (2007). *Behavior assessment battery for school-aged children who stutter.* San Diego: Plural Publishing.

Bryden, M. P., McManus, I. C., & Bulman-Fleming, M. B. (1994). Evaluating the empirical support for the Geschwind-Behan-Galaburda model of cerebral lateralization. *Brain and Cognition, 26,* 103–67.

Bryngelson, B. (1932). A photophonographic analysis of the vocal disturbances in stuttering. *Psychology Monographs, 43,* 1–30.

Bryngelson, B. (1935). Sidedness as an etiological factor in stuttering. *Journal of Genetic Psychology, 47,* 204–17.

Bryngelson, B. (1939). A study of laterality of stutterers and normal speakers. *Journal of Speech Disorders, 4,* 231–34.

Bryngelson, B., & Brown, S. F. (1939). Season of birth of speech defectives in Minnesota. *Journal of Speech Disorders, 4,* 319–22.

Bryngelson, B., & Rutherford, B. (1937). A comparative study of laterality of stutterers and non-stutterers. *Journal of Speech Disorders, 2,* 15–16.

Büchel, C., & Sommer, M. (2004, February). What causes stuttering? *PloS Biology, 2*(2 (Electronic)), E46. http://biology.plosjournals.org

Buck, S. M., Lees, R., & Cook, F. (2002). The influence of family history of stuttering on the onset of stuttering in young children. *Folia Phoniatrica, 54,* 117–24.

Bullen, A. K. (1945). A cross-cultural approach to the problem of stuttering. *Child Development, 16,* 1–88.

Burdin, L. G. (1940). A survey of speech defectives in the Indianapolis primary grades. *Journal of Speech Disorders, 5,* 247–58.

Burger, R., & Wijnen, F. (1999). Phonological encoding and word stress in stuttering and nonstuttering subjects. *Journal of Fluency Disorders, 24,* 91–106.

Burgraff, R. I. (1974). The efficacy of systematic desensitization via imagery as a therapeutic technique with stutterers. *British Journal of Disorders of Communication, 9,* 134–39.

Burke, B. D. (1969). Reduced auditory feedback and stuttering. *Behavior Research Therapy, 7,* 303–08.

Burke, B. D. (1975). Variables affecting stutterers' initial reactions to delayed auditory feedback. *Journal of Communication Disorders, 8,* 141–55.

Burleson, D. E. (1951). A personality study of fourth, fifth and sixth grade stutterers and non-stutterers based on the *Bender Visual Motor Gestalt Test.* [Abstract]. *Speech Monographs, 18,* 238.

Burley, P. M., & Morely, R. (1987). Self-monitoring processes in stutterers. *Journal of Fluency Disorders, 12,* 71–78.

Burley, P. M., & Rinaldi, W. (1986). Effects of sex of listener and of stutterer on ratings of stuttering speakers. *Journal of Fluency Disorders, 11,* 329–33.

Burns, D., Brady, J. P., & Kuruvilla, K. (1978). The acute effect of haloperidol and apomorphine on the severity of stuttering. *Biological Psychiatry, 13,* 255–64.

Burr, H. G., & Mullendore, J. M. (1960). Recent investigations on tranquilizers and stuttering. *Journal of Speech and Hearing Disorders, 25,* 33–37.

Buscaglia, L. F. (1963). An experimental study of the *Sarbin-Hardyck Test* as indexes of role perception for adolescent stutterers. [Abstract]. *Speech Monographs, 30,* 243.

Busse, E. W., & Clark, R. M. (1957). The use of the electroencephalogram in diagnosing speech disorders in children. *Folia Phoniatrica, 9,* 182–87.

Butcher, C., McFadden, D., Quinn, B., & Ryan, B. P. (2003). The effects of language training on stuttering in young children, without and with contingency management. *Journal of Developmental and Physical Disabilities, 15,* 255–80.

Byrd, K., & Cooper, E. B. (1989a). Apraxic speech characteristics in stuttering, developmentally apraxic, and normal speaking children. *Journal of Fluency Disorders, 14,* 215–29.

Byrd, K., & Cooper, E. B. (1989b). Expressive and receptive language skills in stuttering children. *Journal of Fluency Disorders, 14,* 121–26.

Cabañas, R. (1954). Some findings in speech and voice therapy among mentally deficient children. *Folia Phoniatrica, 6,* 34–39.

Cacudi, G. (1964). Effeti di un psicofarmaco (tioridazina) nella practica pedopsichiatrica. Turbe funzionali del linguaggio. *Infanz. Anorm., 60,* 861–68.

Cali, G., Pisana, F., and Tagliareni, F. (1965). Balbuzie e rilievi elettroencefalografici. *Clin. ORL, 17,* 316–28.

Canter, G. J. (1971). Observations on neurogenic stuttering: A contribution to differential diagnosis. *British Journal of Disorders of Communication, 6,* 139–43.

Caplan, L. (1972). An investigation of some aspects of stuttering-like speech in adult dysphasic subjects. *Journal of the South African Speech and Hearing Association, 19,* 52–66.

Card, R. E. (1939). A study of allergy in relation to stuttering. *Journal of Speech Disorders, 4,* 223–30.

Carlo, E. J., & Watson, J. B. (2003). Disfluencies of 3- and 5-year old Spanish-speaking children. *Journal of Fluency Disorders, 28,* 37–54.

Carlson, J. J. (1946). Psychosomatic study of fifty stuttering children: III. Analysis of responses on the *Revised Stanford-Binet. American Journal of Orthopsychiatry, 16,* 120–26.

Carp, F. M. (1962). Psychosexual development of stutterers. *Journal of Projective Techniques, 26,* 388–91.

Carpenter, M., & Sommers, R. K. (1987). Unisensory and bisensory perceptual and memory processing in stuttering adults and normal speakers. *Journal of Fluency Disorders, 12,* 291–304.

Caruso, A. J., Abbs, J. H., & Gracco, V. L. (1988). Kinematic analysis of multiple movement coordination during speech in stutterers. *Brain, 111,* 439–55.

Caruso, A. J., Chodzko-Zajko, W. J., Bidinger, D. A., & Sommers, R. K. (1994). Adults who stutter: Responses to cognitive stress. *Journal of Speech and Hearing Research, 37,* 746–54.

Caruso, A. J., Conture, E. G., & Colton, R. H. (1988). Selected temporal parameters of coordination associated with stuttering in children. *Journal of Fluency Disorders, 13,* 57–82.

Caruso, A. J., Gracco, V. L., & Abbs, J. H. (1987). A speech motor control perspective on stuttering: Preliminary observations. In H. F. M. Peters & W. Hulstijn (Eds.), *Speech motor dynamics in stuttering* (pp. 245–258). New York: Springer.

Castellini, V., Salami, A., & Ottoboni, A. (1972). Ricerche elettronistagmografiche in soggetti balbuzienti. *Minerva ORL,* 22, 119–25.

Cecconi, C. P., Hood, S. B., & Tucker, R. K. (1977). Influence of reading level difficulty on the disfluencies of normal children. *Journal of Speech and Hearing Research, 20,* 475–84.

Cerf, A., & Prins, D. (1974). Stutterers' ear preference for dichotic syllables. [Abstract]. *ASHA, 16,* 566–67.

Chaney, C. F. (1969). Loci of disfluencies in the speech of nonstutterers. *Journal of Speech and Hearing Research, 12,* 667–68.

Chapman, A. H., & Cooper, E. B. (1973). Nature of stuttering in a mentally retarded population. *American Journal of Mental Deficiency, 78,* 153–57.

Chang, S.-E., Erickson, K., & Ambrose, N. (2005). *Regional white and gray matter volumetric growth differences in children with persistent versus recovered stuttering: An MRI (VBM) study* Society for Neuroscience, Washington, DC.

Chang, S.-E., Erickson, K., Ambrose, N., Hasegawa-Johnson, M., & Ludlow, C. (2006). *Deficient white matter development in left hemisphere speech-language regions in children who stutter.* Paper presented at the Society for Neuroscience, Atlanta, GA.

Chase, R. A. (1958). Effect of delayed auditory feedback on the repetition of speech sounds. *Journal of Speech and Hearing Disorders, 23,* 583–90.

Chase, R. A., & Sutton, S. (1968). Reply to: "Masking of auditory feedback in stutterers' speech." *Journal of Speech and Hearing Research, 11,* 222–23.

Chase, R. A., Sutton, S., & Rapin, I. (1961). Sensory feedback influences on motor performance. *Journal of Auditory Research, 1,* 212–23.

Checiek, M. S. (1983). Ergebnisse der psychophysiologischen Therapiemethode bei stotternden Kindern und Jugendlichen im Alter von 7–18 Jahren. [Abstract]. *Folia Phoniatrica, 35,* 115.

Cherry, C., & Sayers, B. (1956). Experiments upon the total inhibition of stammering by external control and some clinical results. *Journal of Psychosomatic Research, 1,* 233–46.

Cherry, C., Sayers, B., & Marland, P. M. (1955). Experiments on the complete suppression of stammering. *Nature,* 176, 874–75.

Chmelová, A., Kujalová, V., Sedláčková, E., & Zelený, A. (1975). Neurohumorale Reaktionen bei Stotterern und Polterern. *Folia Phoniatrica, 27,* 283–86.

Christensen, A. H. (1952). A quantitative study of personality dynamics in stuttering and nonstuttering siblings. [Abstract]. *Speech Monographs, 19,* 144–145.

Christensen, J. E., & Lingwall, J. B. (1982). Verbal contingent stimulation of stuttering in laboratory and home settings. *Journal of Fluency Disorders, 7,* 359–68.

Christensen, J. E., & Lingwall, J. B. (1983). The relationship between treatment exposure times and changes in stuttering frequency during contingent stimulation. *Journal of Fluency Disorders, 8,* 275–81.

Christensen, R. C., Byerly, M. J., & McElroy, R. A. (1996). A case of sertraline-induced stuttering. *Journal of Clinical Psychopharmacology, 16,* 92–93.

Christman, S. S., Boutsen, F. R., & Buckingham, H. W. (2004). Perseveration and other repetitive verbal behaviors: Functional dissociations. *Seminars in Speech and Language, 25,* 295–307.

Chung, S. J., Im, J.-H., Lee, J.-H., & Lee, M. C. (2004). Stuttering and gait disturbance after supplementary motor area seizure. *Movement Disorders, 19,* 1106–09.

Chworowski, C. R. (1952). A comparative study of the diadochokinetic rates of stutterers and nonstutterers in speech related and non-speech related movements. [Abstract]. *Speech Monographs, 19,* 192.

Ciabarra, A. M., Elkind, M. S., Roberts, J. K., & Marshall, R. S. (2000). Subcortical infarction resulting in acquired stuttering. *Journal of Neurology, Neurosurgery, and Psychiatry, 69,* 546–49.

Ciambrone, S. W., Adams, M. R., & Berkowitz, M. (1983). A correlational study of stutterers' adaptation and voice initiation times. *Journal of Fluency Disorders, 8,* 29–37.

Cimorell-Strong, J. M., Gilbert, H. R., & Frick, J. V. (1983). Dichotic speech perception: A comparison between stuttering and nonstuttering children. *Journal of Fluency Disorders, 8,* 77–91.

Civier, O., & Guenther, F. (2005). Simulations of feedback and feedforward control in stuttering. *Proceedings of the 7th Oxford Dysfluency Conference.* Retrieved from http://speechlab.bu.edu/publications/Civier_Guenther_2005_ODC.pdf

Clifford, S., Twitchell, M., & Hull, R. H. (1965). Stuttering in South Dakota Indians. *Central States Speech Journal, 16,* 59–60.

Cocores, J. A., Dackis, C. A., Davies, R. K., & Gold, M. S. (1986). Propranolol and stuttering. *The American Journal of Psychiatry, 143,* 1071–72.

Code, C., Lincoln, M., & Dredge, R. (2005). Asymmetries in mouth opening during word generation in male stuttering and non-stuttering participants. *Laterality: Asymmetries of Body, Brain and Cognition, 10,* 471–86.

Cohen, E. (1953). A comparison of oral [reading] and spontaneous speech of stutterers with special reference to the adaptation and consistency effects. [Abstract]. *Speech Monographs, 20,* 144–45.

Cohen, L. R., Thompson, P. F., Ruppel, R. W., & Flaherty, R. P. (1975). Assertive training: An adjunct to fluency shaping. *Journal of Fluency Disorders, 1,* 10–25.

Cohen, M. S., & Hanson, M. L. (1975). Intersensory processing efficiency of fluent speakers and stutterers. *British Journal of Disorders of Communication, 10,* 111–22.

Colburn, N. (1985). Clustering of disfluency in nonstuttering children's early utterances. *Journal of Fluency Disorders, 10,* 51–58.

Colburn, N., & Mysak, E. D. (1982a). Developmental disfluency and emerging grammar. I. Disfluency characteristics in early syntactic utterances. *Journal of Speech and Hearing Research, 25,* 414–20.

Colburn, N., & Mysak, E. D. (1982b). Developmental disfluency and emerging grammar. II. Co-occurrence of disfluency with specified semantic-syntactic structures. *Journal of Speech and Hearing Research, 25,* 421–27.

Colcord, R. D., & Adams, M. R. (1979). Voicing duration and vocal SPL changes associated with stuttering reduction during singing. *Journal of Speech and Hearing Research, 22,* 468–79.

Colcord, R. D., & Gregory, H. H. (1987). Perceptual analyses of stuttering and nonstuttering children's fluent speech productions. *Journal of Fluency Disorders, 12,* 185–95.

Collins, C. R., & Blood, G. W. (1990). Acknowledgment and severity of stuttering as factors influencing nonstutterers' perceptions of stuttering. *Journal of Speech and Hearing Disorders, 55,* 75–81.

Comas, R. C. (1974). Tartamudez o espasmofemia funcional. Relato y aportes conceptuales. *Rev. Cubana Pediat., 46,* 595–605.

Comas, R. C. (1975). Incidencia de espasmofemia functional (tartamudez) durante la rehabilitación del fisurado palatino. *DSH Abstracts, 15,* 393.

Comings, D. E., & MacMurray, J. P. (2006). Maternal age at the birth of the first child as an epistatic factor in polygenic disorders. *American Journal of Medical Genetics. Part B, Neuropsychiatric Genetics, 141,* 1–6.

Commodore, R. W. (1980). Communicative stress and stuttering frequency during normal, whispered and articulation-without-phonation speech modes: A further study. *Human Communication, 5,* 143–50.

Commodore, R. W., & Cooper, E. B. (1978). Communicative stress and stuttering frequency during normal, whispered, and articulation-without-phonation speech modes. *Journal of Fluency Disorders, 3,* 1–12.

Connett, M. H. (1955). Experimentally induced changes in the relative frequency of stuttering on a specified speech sound. In W. Johnson & R. R. Leutenneger (Eds.), *Stuttering in children and adults* (pp. 268–274). Minneapolis: University of Minnesota Press.

Conradi, E. (1904). Psychology and pathology of speech development in the child. *Pedagogical Seminar, 11,* 328–80.

Conradi, E. (1912). Speech defects and intellectual progress. *Journal of Educational Psychology, 3,* 35–38.

Conture, E. G. (1974). Some effects of noise on the speaking behavior of stutterers. *Journal of Speech and Hearing Research, 17,* 714–23.

Conture, E. G., & Brayton, E. R. (1975). The influence of noise on stutterers' different disfluency types. *Journal of Speech and Hearing Research, 18,* 381–84.

Conture, E. G., Colton, R. H., & Gleason, J. R. (1988). Selected temporal aspects of coordination during fluent speech of young stutterers. *Journal of Speech and Hearing Research, 31,* 640–53.

Conture, E. G., & Kelly, E. M. (1991). Young stutterers' nonspeech behavior during stuttering. *Journal of Speech and Hearing Research, 34,* 1041–56.

Conture, E. G., McCall, G. N., & Brewer, D. W. (1977). Laryngeal behavior during stuttering. *Journal of Speech and Hearing Research, 20,* 661–68.

Conture, E. G., & Melnick, K. S. (1999). Parent-child group approach to stuttering in preschool and school-age children. In M. Onslow & A. Packman (Eds.), *The handbook of early stuttering intervention* (pp. 17–51). San Diego: Singular.

Conture, E. G., Rothenberg, M., & Molitar, R. D. (1986). Electroglottographic observations of young stutterers' fluency. *Journal of Speech and Hearing Research, 29,* 384–93.

Conture, E. G., Schwartz, H. D., & Brewer, D. W. (1985). Laryngeal behavior during stuttering: A further study. *Journal of Speech and Hearing Research, 28,* 233–40.

Conture, E. G., & van Naerssen, E. (1977). Reading abilities of school-age stutterers. *Journal of Fluency Disorders, 2,* 295–300.

Conture, E. G., Walden, T., Graham, C., Arnold, H., Hartfield, H., Karrass, J., et al. (2006). Communication-emotional model of stuttering. In N. Bernstein Ratner & J. Tetnowski (Eds.), *Stuttering research and practice: Contemporary issues and approaches* (pp. 17–46). Mahwah, NJ: Lawrence Erlbaum Associates.

Conway, J. K., & Quarrington, B. (1963). Positional effects in the stuttering of contextually organized verbal material. *Journal of Abnormal Social Psychology, 67,* 299–303.

Cook, F., & Fry, J. (2006). Connecting stuttering measurement and management: III. Accountable therapy. *International Journal of Language & Communication Disorders, 41,* 379–94.

Cook, R. D., & Cook, D. R. (1987). Measuring shame: The internalized shame scale. *Alcoholism Treatment Quarterly, 4*(2), 197–215.

Cookson, I. B., & Wells, P. G. (1973). Haloperidol in the treatment of stutterers. *British Journal of Psychiatry, 123,* 491.

Cooper, C. S., & Cooper, E. B. (1969). Variations in adult stutterer attitudes towards clinicians during therapy. *Journal of Communication Disorders, 2,* 141–53.

Cooper, E. B. (1966). Client-clinician relationships and concomitant factors in stuttering therapy. *Journal of Speech and Hearing Research, 9,* 194–207.

Cooper, E. B. (1968). A therapy process for the adult stutterer. *Journal of Speech and Hearing Disorders, 33,* 246–60.

Cooper, E. B. (1971). Integrating behavior therapy and traditional insight treatment procedures with stutterers. *Journal of Communication Disorders, 4,* 40–43.

Cooper, E. B. (1972). Recovery from stuttering in a junior and senior high school population. *Journal of Speech and Hearing Research, 15,* 632–38.

Cooper, E. B. (1984). Personalized fluency control therapy: A status report. In M. Peins (Ed.), *Contemporary approaches in stuttering therapy* (pp. 1–38). Boston: Little, Brown.

Cooper, E. B., Cady, B. B., & Robbins, C. J. (1970). The effect of the verbal stimulus words wrong, right, and tree on the disfluency rates of stutterers and nonstutterers. *Journal of Speech and Hearing Research, 13,* 239–44.

Cooper, E. B., & Cooper, C. S. (1996). Clinician attitudes towards stuttering: Two decades of change. *Journal of Fluency Disorders, 21,* 119–35.

Cooper, E. B., Parris, R., & Wells, M. T. (1974). Prevalence of and recovery from speech disorders in a group of freshmen at the University of Alabama. [Abstract]. *ASHA, 16,* 359–60.

Cooper, M. H., & Allen, G. D. (1977). Timing control accuracy in stutterers and non-stutterers. *Journal of Speech and Hearing Research, 20,* 55–71.

Coppa, A., & Bar, A. (1974). Use of questions to elicit adaptation in the spontaneous speech of stutterers and nonstutterers. *Folia Phoniatrica, 26,* 378–88.

Coppola, V. A., & Yairi, E. (1982). Rhythmic speech training with preschool stuttering children: An experimental study. *Journal of Fluency Disorders, 7,* 447–57.

Corbera, S. L, Corral, M., Escera, C., & Idiazábal, M. (2005). Abnormal speech sound representation in persistent developmental stuttering. *Neurology, 65,* 1246–52.

Corcoran, J. A., Jr. (1980). Effects of neutral and positive stimuli on stuttering: "Calling attention to stuttering" revisited. *Journal of Fluency Disorders, 5,* 99–114.

Cordes, A. K., & Ingham, R. J. (1994). Time-interval measurement of stuttering: Effects of interval duration. *Journal of Speech and Hearing Research, 37,* 779–88.

Cordes, A. K., & Ingham, R. J. (1996). Time-interval measurement of stuttering: Establishing and modifying judgment accuracy. *Journal of Speech and Hearing Research, 39,* 298–311.

Cordes, A. K., & Ingham, R. J. (1999). Effects of time-interval judgment training on real-time measurement of stuttering. *Journal of Speech, Language and Hearing Research, 42,* 862–79.

Cordes, A. K., Ingham, R. J., Frank, P., & Costello Ingham, J. (1992). Time-interval analysis of interjudge and intrajudge agreement for stuttering event judgments. *Journal of Speech and Hearing Research, 35,* 483–94.

Cords, T. (1936). Untersuchung der lautdauer innerhalb eines Satzes bei Stottern mit Hilfe der kymographischen Aufnahme. *Vox, 22,* 70–75.

Coriat, I. H. (1928). Stammering. A psychoanalytic interpretation. *Nervous and Mental Disease Monographs, 47,* 1–68.

Coriat, I. H. (1943). The psychoanalytic conception of stammering. *Nervous Child, 2,* 167–71.

Costa, A. D., & Kroll, R. M. (1995). Sertraline in stuttering. *Journal of Clinical Psychopharmacology, 15,* 443–44.

Costello, J. (1975). The establishment of fluency with time-out procedures: Three case studies. *Journal of Speech and Hearing Disorders, 409,* 216–31.

Costello, J. M. (1983). Current behavioral treatments for children. In D. Prins & R. J. Ingham (Eds.), *Treatment of stuttering in early childhood* (pp. 69–112). San Diego: College-Hill Press.

Costello, J. M., & Hurst, M. R. (1981). An analysis of the relationship among stuttering behaviors. *Journal of Speech and Hearing Research, 24,* 247–56.

Côté, C., & Ladouceúr, R. (1982). Effects of social aids and the regulated breathing method in the treatment of stutterers. *Journal of Consulting and Clinical Psychology, 50,* 450.

Coull, J. T., Vidal, F., Nazarian, B., & Macar, F. (2004). Functional anatomy of the attentional modulation of time estimation. *Science, 303*(5663), 1506–08.

Cox, M. D. (1982). The stutterer and stuttering: Neuropsychological correlates. *Journal of Fluency Disorders, 7,* 129–40.

Cox, N. J., & Kidd, K. K. (1983). Can recovery from stuttering be considered a genetically milder subtype of stuttering? *Behavior Genetics, 13,* 129–39.

Cox, N. J., Kramer, P. L., & Kidd, K. K. (1984). Segregation analyses of stuttering. *Genetic Epidemiology, 1,* 245–53.

Cox, N. J., Seider, R. A., & Kidd, K. K. (1984). Some environmental factors and hypotheses for stuttering in families with several stutterers. *Journal of Speech and Hearing Research, 27,* 543–48.

Coyle, M. M., & Mallard, A. R. (1979). Word-by-word analysis of observer agreement utilizing audio and audiovisual techniques. *Journal of Fluency Disorders, 4,* 23–28.

Cozzo, G., & Gabrielli, L. (1965). La therapie du begayement avec les butyrophenones. *De Therapia Vocis et Loquelae, Vol. I. of the XIII Congress of the International Society of Logopedics and Phoniatrics.*

Craig, A. (1990). An investigation into the relationship between anxiety and stuttering. *Journal of Speech and Hearing Disorders, 55,* 290–94.

Craig, A. (1994). Anxiety levels in persons who stutter: Comments on the research of Miller and Watson (1992). *Journal of Speech and Hearing Research, 37,* 90–95.

Craig, A. (1998). Relapse following treatment for stuttering: A critical review and correlative data. *Journal of Fluency Disorders, 23,* 1–30.

Craig, A. (2007). Smooth speech and cognitive behaviour therapy for the treatment of older children and adolescents who stutter In B. Guitar & R. J. McCauley (Eds.). *Stuttering treatment: Established and emerging approaches.* Baltimore, MD: Lippincott, Williams and Wilkins.

Craig, A., & Andrews, G. (1985). The prediction and prevention of relapse in stuttering. The value of self-control techniques and locus of control measures. *Behavior Modification, 9,* 427–42.

Craig, A. R., & Calver, P. (1991). Following up on treated stutterers: Studies of perceptions of fluency and job status. *Journal of Speech and Hearing Research, 34,* 279–84.

Craig, A. R., & Cleary, P. J. (1982). Reduction of stuttering by young male stutterers using EMG feedback. *Biofeedback and Self-Regulation, 7,* 241–55.

Craig, A. R., Franklin, J. A., & Andrews, G. (1984). A scale to measure locus of control behavior. *British Journal of Medical Psychology, 57,* 173–80.

Craig, A. & Hancock, K. (1995). Self-reported factors related to relapse following treatment for stuttering. *Australian Journal of Human Communication Disorders, 23,* 48–60.

Craig, A., Hancock, K., Chang, E., McCready, C., Shepley, A., McCaul, A., et al. (1996). A controlled clinical trial for stuttering in persons aged 9 to 14 years. *Journal of Speech and Hearing Research, 39,* 808–26.

Craig, A., Hancock, K., Tran, Y., & Craig, M. (2003). Anxiety levels in people who stutter: A randomized population study. *Journal of Speech, Language and Hearing Research, 46,* 1197–206.

Craig, A., Hancock, K., Tran, Y., Craig, M., & Peters, K. (2002). Epidemiology of stuttering in the community across the entire life span. *Journal of Speech, Language and Hearing Research, 45,* 1097–106.

Craig, A., & Howie, P. M. (1982). Locus of control and maintenance of behavioral therapy skills. *British Journal of Clinical Psychology, 21,* 65–66.

Craig, A. R., & Kearns, M. (1995). Results of a traditional acupuncture intervention for stuttering. *Journal of Speech and Hearing Research, 38,* 572–78.

Craig, A., & Tran, Y. (2005). The epidemiology of stuttering: The need for reliable estimates of prevalence and anxiety levels over the lifespan. *Advances in Speech Language Pathology, 7,* 41–46.

Craig, A., Tran, Y., & Craig, M. (2003). Stereotypes towards stuttering for those who have never had direct contact with people who stutter: a randomized and stratified study. *Perceptual and Motor Skills, 97,* 235–45.

Craven, D. C., & Ryan, B. P. (1984). The use of a portable delayed auditory feedback unit in stuttering therapy. *Journal of Fluency Disorders, 9,* 237–43.

Cream, A., Onslow, M., Packman, A., & Llewellyn, G. (2003). Protection from harm: The experience of adults after therapy with prolonged-speech. *International Journal of Language and Communication Disorders, 38,* 379–96.

Cream, A., Packman, A., & Llewellyn, G. (2004). The playground rocker: A metaphor for communication after treatment for adults who stutter. *Advances in Speech Language Pathology, 6,* 182–87.

Crichton-Smith, I. (2002). Communicating in the real world: accounts from people who stammer. *Journal of Fluency Disorders, 27,* 333–53.

Crichton-Smith, I., Wright, J., & Stackhouse, J. (2003). Attitudes of speech and language therapists towards stammering: 1985 and 2000. *International Journal of Language and Communication Disorders, 38,* 213–34.

Cross, D. E. (1977). Effects of false increasing, decreasing, and true electromyographic biofeedback on the frequency of stuttering. *Journal of Fluency Disorders, 2,* 109–16.

Cross, D. E. (1978). Finger reaction time of stuttering and nonstuttering children and adults. [Abstract]. *ASHA, 20,* 730.

Cross, D. E. (1987). Comparison of reaction time and accuracy measures of laterality for stutterers and normal speakers. *Journal of Fluency Disorders, 12,* 271–86.

Cross, D. E., & Cooper, E. B. (1976). Self-versus investigator-administered presumed fluency reinforcing stimuli. *Journal of Speech and Hearing Research, 19,* 241–46.

Cross, D. E., & Luper, H. L. (1979). Voice reaction time of stuttering and nonstuttering children and adults. *Journal of Fluency Disorders, 4,* 59–77.

Cross, D. E., & Luper, H. L. (1983). Relation between finger reaction time and voice reaction time in stuttering and nonstuttering children and adults. *Journal of Speech and Hearing Research, 26,* 356–61.

Cross, D. E., & Olson, P. L. (1987a). Articulatory-laryngeal interaction in stutterers and normal speakers: Effects of a bite-block on rapid voice initiation. *Journal of Fluency Disorders, 12,* 407–18.

Cross, D. E., & Olson, P. (1987b). Interaction between jaw kinematics and voice onset for stutterers and nonstutterers in a VRT task. *Journal of Fluency Disorders, 12,* 367–80.

Cross, D. E., Shadden, B. B., & Luperr, H. L. (1979). Effects of stimulus ear presentation on the voice reaction time of adult stutterers and nonstutterers. *Journal of Fluency Disorders, 4,* 45–58.

Cross, H. M. (1936). The motor capacities of stutterers. *Archives of Speech, 7,* 112–32.

Cross, J., & Cooke, P. A. (1979). Vocal and manual reaction times of adult stutterers and nonstutterers. [Abstract]. *ASHA, 21,* 693.

Crowe, K. M., & Kroll, R. M. (1991). Response latency and response class for stutterers and nonstutterers as measured by a word-association task. *Journal of Fluency Disorders, 16,* 35–54.

Crowe, T. A., & Cooper, E. B. (1977). Parental attitudes toward and knowlege of stuttering. *Journal of Communication Disorders, 10,* 343–57.

Crowe, T. A., & Walton, J. H. (1981). Teacher attitudes toward stuttering. *Journal of Fluency Disorders, 6,* 163–74.

Cuadrado, E. M., & Weber-Fox, C. M. (2003). Atypical syntactic processing in individuals who stutter: Evidence from event-related brain potentials and behavioral measures. *Journal of Speech, Language and Hearing Research, 46,* 960–76.

Cucchiarini, C., Strik, H., & Boves, L. (2000). Quantitative assessment of second language learners' fluency by means of automatic speech recognition technology. *Journal of the Acoustical Society of America, 107,* 989–99.

Culatta, R., Bader, J., McCaslin, A., & Thomason, N. (1985). Primary-school stutterers: Have attitudes changed? *Journal of Fluency Disorders, 10,* 87–91.

Culatta, R., & Sloan, A. (1977). The acquisition of the label "stuttering" by primary level schoolchildren. *Journal of Fluency Disorders, 2,* 29–34.

Cullinan, W. L. (1963a). Stability of adaptation in the oral performance of stutterers. *Journal of Speech and Hearing Research, 6,* 70–83.

Cullinan, W. L. (1963b). Stability of consistency measures in stuttering. *Journal of Speech and Hearing Research, 6,* 134–38.

Cullinan, W. L. (1988). Consistency measures revisited. *Journal of Fluency Disorders, 13,* 1–9.

Cullinan, W. L., & Prather, E. M. (1968). Reliability of "live" ratings of the speech of stutterers. *Perceptual and Motor Skills, 27,* 403–09.

Cullinan, W. L., Prather, E. M., & Williams, D. E. (1963). Comparison of procedures for scaling severity of stuttering. *Journal of Speech and Hearing Research, 6,* 187–94.

Cullinan, W. L., & Springer, M. T. (1980). Voice initiation times in stuttering and nonstuttering children. *Journal of Speech and Hearing Research, 23,* 344–60.

Culp, D. M. (1984). The preschool fluency development program: Assessment and treatment. In M. Peins (Ed.), *Contemporary approaches in stuttering therapy* (pp. 39–72). Boston: Little, Brown.

Culton, G. L. (1986). Speech disorders among college freshmen: A 13-year survey. *Journal of Speech and Hearing Disorders, 51,* 3–7.

Curlee, R. F. (1981). Observer agreement on disfluency and stuttering. *Journal of Speech and Hearing Research, 24,* 595–600.

Curlee, R. F. (1984). Counseling with adults who stutter. In W. H. Perkins (Ed.), *Stuttering disorders* (pp. 153–60). New York: Thieme-Stratton.

Curlee, R. F., & Perkins, W. H. (1968). The effect of punishment of expectancy to stutter on the frequencies of subsequent expectancies and stuttering. *Journal of Speech and Hearing Research, 11,* 787–95.

Curlee, R. F., & Perkins, W. H. (1969). Conversational rate control therapy for stuttering. *Journal of Speech and Hearing Disorders, 34,* 245–50.

Curlee, R. F., & Perkins, W. H. (1973). Effectiveness of a DAF conditioning program for adolescent and adult stutterers. *Behavior Research Therapy, 11,* 395–401.

Curran, M. F., & Hood, S. B. (1977a). The effect of instructional bias on listener ratings of specific disfluency types in children. *Journal of Fluency Disorders, 2,* 99–107.

Curran, M. F., & Hood, S. B. (1977b). Listener ratings of severity for specific disfluency types in children. *Journal of Fluency Disorders, 2,* 87–97.

Curry, F. K. W., & Gregory, H. H. (1969). The performance of stutterers on dichotic listening tasks thought to reflect cerebral dominance. *Journal of Speech and Hearing Research, 12,* 73–82.

Curtis, J. F. (1942). A study of the effect of muscular exercise upon stuttering. *Speech Monographs, 9,* 61–74.

Curtis, J. F. (1967). Disorders of articulation. In W. Johnson, S. F. Brown, J. F. Curtis, C. W. Edney, &

J. Keaster (Eds.), *Speech handicapped school children* (3rd ed.). New York: Harper & Row.

Cypreansen, L. (1948). Group therapy for adult stutterers. *Journal of Speech and Hearing Disorders, 13,* 313–19.

Cyprus, S., Hezel, R. T., Rossi, D., & Adams, M. R. (1984). Effects of simulated stuttering on listener recall. *Journal of Fluency Disorders, 9,* 191–97.

Dabul, B., & Perkins, W. H. (1973). The effects of stuttering on systolic blood pressure. *Journal of Speech and Hearing Research, 16,* 586–91.

Dahlstrom, W. G., & Craven, D. D. (1952). The *MMPI* and stuttering phenomena in young adults. [Abstract]. *American Psychologist, 7,* 341.

Dalali, I. D., & Sheehan, J. G. (1974). Stuttering and assertion training. *Journal of Communication Disorders, 7,* 97–111.

Dale, P. (1977). Factors related to dysfluent speech in bilingual Cuban-American adolescents. *Journal of Fluency Disorders, 2,* 311–13.

Dale, P. S., Dionne, G., Eley, T. C., & Plomin, R. (2000). Lexical and grammatical development: A behavioural genetic perspective. *Journal of Child Language, 27,* 619–42.

Daly, D. A., & Cooper, E. B. (1967). Rate of stuttering adaptation under two electroshock conditions. *Behavior Research Therapy, 5,* 49–54.

Daly, D. A., & Frick, J. V. (1970). The effects of punishing stuttering expectations and stuttering utterances: A comparative study. *Behavior Therapist, 1,* 228–39.

Daly, D. A., & Kimbarow, M. L. (1978). Stuttering as operant behavior: Effects of the verbal stimuli *wrong, right,* and *tree* on the disfluency rates of school-age stutterers and nonstutterers. *Journal of Speech and Hearing Research, 21,* 589–97.

Daniels, D. E., & Gabel, R. M. (2004). The impact of stuttering on identity construction. *Topics in Language Disorders, 24,* 200–15.

Daniels, E. M. (1940). An analysis of the relation between handedness and stuttering with special reference to the Orton-Travis theory of cerebral dominance. *Journal of Speech Disorders, 5,* 309–26.

Danzger, M., & Halpern, H. (1973). Relation of stuttering to word abstraction, part of speech, word length, and word frequency. *Perceptual and Motor Skills, 37,* 959–62.

Darley, F. L. (1940). A normative study of oral reading rate. M. A. Thesis, University of Iowa.

Darley, F. L. (1955). The relationship of parental attitudes and adjustments to the development of stuttering. In W. Johnson & R. R. Leutenegger (Eds.), *Stuttering in children and adults* (pp. 74–153). Minneapolis: University of Minnesota Press.

Darley, F. L., & Spriestersbach, D. C. (1978). *Diagnostic methods in speech pathology* (2nd ed.). New York: Harper & Row.

Daskalov, D. D. (1962). K voprosu ob osnovnikh printsipakh i metodakh preduprezhdenia lechenia zaikania. *Zh. Nevropatol. Psikhiat., 62,* 1047–52.

Davenport, R. W. (1979). Dichotic listening in four severity levels of stuttering. [Abstract]. *ASHA, 21,* 769.

Davis, D. M. (1939). The relation of repetitions in the speech of young children to certain measures of language maturity and situational factors: Part I. *Journal of Speech Disorders, 4,* 303–18.

Davis, D. M. (1940). The relation of repetitions in the speech of young children to certain measures of language maturity and situational factors: Parts II & III. *Journal of Speech Disorders, 5,* 235–46.

Davis, S., Howell, P., & Cooke, F. (2002). Sociodynamic relationships between children who stutter and their non-stuttering classmates. *Journal of Child Psychology and Psychiatry and Allied Disciplines, 43,* 939–47.

Dayalu, V. N., Kalinowski, J., & Stuart, A. (2005). Stuttering frequency on meaningful and nonmeaningful words in adults who stutter. *Folia Phoniatrica, 57,* 193–201.

Dayalu, V. N., Kalinowski, J., Stuart, A., Holbert, D., & Rastatter, M. P. (2002). Stuttering frequency on content and function words in adults who stutter: A concept revisited. *Journal of Speech, Language and Hearing Research, 45,* 871–79.

Deal, J. L. (1982). Sudden onset of stuttering: A case report. *Journal of Speech and Hearing Disorders, 47,* 301–03.

Dean, C. R., & Brown, R. A. (1977). A more recent look at the prevalence of stuttering in the United States. *Journal of Fluency Disorders, 2,* 157–66.

de Andrade, C. R. F., Cervone, L. M., & Sassi, F. C. (2003). Relationship between the stuttering severity index and speech rate. *São Paulo Medical Journal, 121,* 81–84.

de Carle, A. J., & Pato, M. T. (1996). Social phobia and stuttering. *The American Journal of Psychiatry, 153,* 1367–68.

Decker, T. N., Healey, E. C., & Howe, S. W. (1982). Brainstem auditory electrical response characteristics of stutterers and nonstutterers: A preliminary report. *Journal of Fluency Disorders, 7,* 385–401.

de Houwer, A. (1999). Two or more languages in early childhood: Some general points and practical recommendations. Retrieved July 15, 2007, from http://www.cal.org/resources/Digest/RaiseBilingChild.html

DeJoy, D. A., & Gregory, H. H. (1973). The relationship of children's disfluencies to the syntax, length, and vocabulary of their sentences. [Abstract]. *ASHA, 15,* 472.

DeJoy, D. A., & Gregory, H. H. (1976). The relationship of preschoolers' syntactic maturity to the frequency of specific disfluency types in their spontaneous speech. [Abstract]. *Folia Phoniatrica, 28,* 219–20.

DeJoy, D. A., & Gregory, H. H. (1985). The relationship between age and frequency of disfluency in preschool children. *Journal of Fluency Disorders, 10,* 107–22.

DeJoy, D. A., & Jordan, W. J. (1988). Listener reactions to interjections in oral reading versus spontaneous speech. *Journal of Fluency Disorders, 13,* 11–25.

Delaney, C. M. (1979). The function of the middle ear muscles in stuttering. *South African Journal of Communication Disorders, 26,* 20–34.

Dembrowski, J., & Watson, B. C. (1991a). An instrumented method for assessment and remediation of stuttering: A single-subject case study. *Journal of Fluency Disorders, 16,* 241–73.

Dembrowski, J., & Watson, B. C. (1991b). Preparation time and response complexity effects on stutterers' and nonstutterers' acoustic LRT. *Journal of Speech and Hearing Research, 34,* 49–59.

Dempsey, G. L., & Granich, M. (1978). Hypnobehavioral therapy in the case of a traumatic stutterer: A case study. *International Journal of Clinical Experimental Hypnosis, 26,* 125–33.

De Nil, L. F. (1999). Stuttering: A neurophysiological perspective. In N. Bernstein Ratner & E.Charles Healey (Eds.), *Stuttering research and practice: Bridging the gap* (pp. 85–102). Mahwah, NJ: Lawrence Erlbaum Associates.

De Nil, L. (2004). Recent developments in brain imaging research in stuttering. In B. Maassen, H. Peters, & R. Kent (Eds.), *Speech motor control in normal and disordered speech* (pp. 113–37). Oxford: Oxford University Press.

De Nil, L. F., & Abbs, J. H. (1991). Kinaesthetic acuity of stutterers and nonstutterers for oral and non-oral movements. *Brain, 114,* 2145–58.

De Nil, L., & Brutten, G. J. (1986). Stutterers and nonstutterers: A preliminary investigation of children's speech-associated attitudes. *Tijdschrift voor Logopedie en Audiologie, 16,* 85–90.

De Nil, L. F., & Brutten, G. J. (1991a). Speech-associated attitudes of stuttering and nonstuttering children. *Journal of Speech and Hearing Research, 34,* 60–66.

De Nil, L. F., & Brutten, G. J. (1991b). Voice onset times of stuttering and nonstuttering children: The influence of externally and linguistically imposed time pressure. *Journal of Fluency Disorders, 16,* 143–58.

De Nil, L., Jokel, R., & Rochon, E. (2007). Etiology, symptomology, and treatment of neurogenic stuttering. In E. G. Conture & R. Curlee (Eds.), *Stuttering and related disorders of fluency* (3rd ed.) (pp. 326–43). New York: Thieme.

De Nil, L. F., & Kroll, R. M. (1995). The relationship between locus of control and long-term stuttering treatment outcome in adult stutterers. *Journal of Fluency Disorders, 20,* 345–64.

De Nil, L. F., & Kroll, R. M. (2001). Searching for the neural basis of stuttering treatment outcome: recent neuroimaging studies. *Clinical Linguistics and Phonetics, 15,* 163–68.

De Nil, L. F., Kroll, R. M., & Houle, S. (2001). Functional neuroimaging of cerebellar activation during single word reading and verb generation in stuttering and nonstuttering adults. *Neuroscience Letters, 302,* 77–80.

De Nil, L. F., Kroll, R. M., Kapur, S., & Houle, S. (2000). A positron emission tomography study of silent and oral single word reading in stuttering and nonstuttering adults. *Journal of Speech, Language and Hearing Research, 43,* 1038–54.

De Nil, L. F., Kroll, R. M., Lafaille, S. J., & Houle, S. (2003). A positron emission tomography study of short- and long-term treatment effects on functional brain activation in adults who stutter. *Journal of Fluency Disorders, 28,* 357–81.

De Nil, L. F., Sasisekaran, J., Van Lieshout, P. H. H. M., & Sandor, P. (2005). Speech disfluencies in individuals with Tourette syndrome. *Journal of Psychosomatic Research, 58,* 97–102.

Denny, M., & Smith, A. (1992). Gradations in a pattern of neuromuscular activity associated with stuttering. *Journal of Speech and Hearing Research, 35,* 1216–29.

Denny, M., & Smith, A. (2000). Respiratory control in stuttering speakers: Evidence from respiratory high-frequency oscillations. *Journal of Speech, Language, and Hearing Research, 43,* 1024–37.

DePlatero, D. M. (1969). La prueba del dibujo de la figura humana en el níno tardamudo. *DSH Abstracts, 9,* 94–95.

Derazne, J. (1966). Speech pathology in the U.S.S.R. In R. W. Rieber & R. S. Brubaker (Eds.), *Speech pathology* (pp. 611–18). Amsterdam: North Holland.

Despert, J. L. (1946). Psychosomatic study of fifty stuttering children: I. Social, physical and psychiatric findings. *American Journal of Orthopsychiatry, 16,* 100–13.

Devenny, D. A., & Silverman, W. P. (1990). Speech dysfluency and manual specialization in Down's syndrome. *Journal of Mental Deficiency Research, 34,* 253–60.

Devore, J. E., Nandur, M. S., & Manning, W. H. (1984). Projective drawings and children who stutter. *Journal of Fluency Disorders, 9,* 217–26.

Dewar, A., Dewar, A. D., & Anthony, J. F. K. (1976). The effect of auditory feedback masking on concomitants of stammering. *British Journal of Disorders of Communication, 11,* 95–102.

Dewar, A., Dewar, A. D., Austin, W. T. S., & Brash, H. M. (1979) The long term use of an automatically triggered auditory feedback masking device in the treatment of stammering. *British Journal of Disorders of Communication, 14,* 219–29.

Dewar, A., Dewar, A. D., & Barnes, H. E. (1976). Automatic triggering of auditory feedback masking in stammering and cluttering. *British Journal of Disorders of Communication, 11,* 19–26.

Di Carlo, L. M., Katz, J., & Batkin, S. (1959). An exploratory investigation of the effect of meprobamate on stuttering behavior. *Journal of Nervous and Mental Disorders, 128,* 558–61.

Dickson, S. (1954). An application of the Blacky Test of a study of the psychosexual development of stutterers. M. A. Thesis, Brooklyn College.

Dickson, S. (1971). Incipient stuttering and spontaneous remission of stuttered speech. *Journal of Communication Disorders, 4,* 99–110.

Dietrich, S., & Roaman, M. H. (2001). Physiologic arousal and predictions of anxiety by people who stutter. *Journal of Fluency Disorders, 26,* 207–25.

DiLollo, A., Manning, W. H., & Neimeyer, R. A. (2005). Cognitive complexity as a function of speaker role for adult persons who stutter. *Journal of Constructivist Psychology, 18,* 215–36.

DiLollo, A., Neimeyer, R. A., & Manning, W. H. (2002). A personal construct psychology view of relapse: indications for a narrative therapy component to stuttering treatment. *Journal of Fluency Disorders, 27,* 19–43.

Dingwall, W. O. (1998). The biological bases of human communicative behavior. In J. Berko Gleason & N. Bernstein Ratner (Eds.), *Psycholinguistics* (2nd ed.) (pp. 51–106). Fort Worth, TX: Harcourt Brace.

Dinnan, J. A., McGuiness, E., & Perrin, L. (1970). Auditory feedback—Stutterers versus nonstutterers. *Journal of Learning Disabilities, 3,* 209–13.

Di Simoni, F. G. (1974). Preliminary study of certain timing relationships in the speech of stutterers. *Journal of the Acoustical Society of America, 56,* 695–96.

Dixon, C. C. (1955). Stuttering adaptation in relation to assumed level of anxiety. In W. Johnson & R. R. Leutenegger (Eds.), *Stuttering in children and adults* (pp. 181–88). Minneapolis: University of Minnesota Press.

Dixon, C. C. (1957). The effect of interjected non-propositional verbalization during oral reading on stuttering frequency. *Journal of Educational Research, 51,* 153–55.

Dmitrieva, E. S., & Zaĭtseva, K. A. (1998). [Features of the lateralization of speech function in stutterers as a function of the sex of the subjects]. *Fiziologiia cheloveka, 24,* 45–50.

Doi, M., Nakayasu, H., Soda, T., Shimoda, K., Ito, A., & Nakashima, K. (2003). Brainstem infarction presenting with neurogenic stuttering. *Internal Medicine, 42,* 884–87.

Dollaghan, C. A. (2004). Taxometric analyses of Specific Language Impairment in 3- and 4-year-old children. *Journal of Speech, Language and Hearing Research, 47,* 464–75.

Doms, M. C., & Lissens, D. (1973). Stuttering and the laryngectomee. In Y. Lebrun & R. Hoops (Eds.), *Neurolinguistic approaches to stuttering.* The Hague: Mouton.

Donath, J. (1928). Heilung des Stotterns mittels Hypnose. *Med. Welt, 2,* 1532–33.

Donnan, G. A. (1979). Stuttering as a manifestation of stroke. *Medical Journal of Australia, 66,* 44–45.

Donohue, I. R. (1955). Stuttering adaptation during three hours of continuous oral reading. In W. Johnson & R. R. Leutenegger (Eds.), *Stuttering in children and adults* (pp. 264–67). Minneapolis: University of Minnesota Press.

Donovan, G. (1971). A new device for the treatment of stammering. *British Journal of Disorders of Communication, 6,* 86–88.

Doody, I., Kalinowski, J., Armson, J., & Stuart, A. (1993). Stereotypes of stutterers and nonstutterers in three rural communities in Newfoundland. *Journal of Fluency Disorders, 18,* 363–73.

Dorman, M. F., & Porter, R. J., Jr. (1975). Hemispheric lateralization for speech perception in stutterers. *Cortex, 11,* 181–85.

Douglass, E., & Quarrington, B. (1952). The differentiation of interiorized and exteriorized secondary stuttering. *Journal of Speech and Hearing Disorders, 17,* 377–85.

Douglass, L. C. (1943). A study of bilaterally recorded electroencephalograms of adult stutterers. *Journal of Experimental Psychology, 32,* 247–65.

Douglass, R. L. (1952). An experimental electroencephalographic study of stimulus reaction in stutterers. [Abstract]. *Speech Monographs, 19,* 146.

Dowrick, P. W. (1999). A review of self modeling and related interventions. *Applied & Preventive Psychology, 8*(1), 23–39.

Dowrick, P. W., & Raeburn, J. M. (1977). Video editing and medication to produce a therapeutic self model. *Journal of Clinical and Consulting Psychology, 45,* 1156–58.

Drayna, D. T. (1997). Genetic linkage studies of stuttering: ready for prime time? *Journal of Fluency Disorders, 22,* 237–41.

Drayna, D., Kilshaw, J., & Kelly, J. (1999). The sex ratio in familial persistent stuttering. *American Journal of Human Genetics, 65,* 1473–75.

Druce, T., Debney, S., & Byrt, T. (1997). Evaluation of an intensive treatment program for stuttering in young children. *Journal of Fluency Disorders, 22*(3), 169–86.

Duffy, R. J., Hunt, M. F., Jr., & Giolas, T. G. (1975). Effects of four types of disfluency on listener reactions. *Folia Phoniatrica, 27,* 106–15.

Duggal, H. S., Jagadheesan, K., & Nizamie, S. H. (2002). Clozapine-induced stuttering and seizures. *The American Journal of Psychiatry, 159,* 315.

Duncan, M. H. (1949). Home adjustment of stutterers versus nonstutterers. *Journal of Speech and Hearing Disorders, 14,* 255–59.

Dunlap, K. (1932). *Habits: Their making and unmaking.* New York: Liveright.

Dworzynski, K., & Howell, P. (2004). Predicting stuttering from phonetic complexity in German. *Journal of Fluency Disorders, 29,* 149–73.

Dworzynski, K., Howell, P., & Natke, U. (2003). Predicting stuttering from linguistic factors for German speakers in two age groups. *Journal of Fluency Disorders, 28,* 95–114.

Ebeling, T. A., Compton, A. D., & Albright, D. W. (1997). Clozapine-induced stuttering. *The American Journal of Psychiatry, 154,* 1473.

Edgren, B., Leanderson, R., & Levi, L. (1970). A research programme on stuttering and stress. *Acta Oto-Laryngolica, Supplement No. 263,* 113–18.

Egland, G. O. (1955). Repetitions and prolongations in the speech of stuttering and nonstuttering children. In W. Johnson & R. R. Leutenegger (Eds.), *Stuttering in children and adults* (pp. 181–88). Minneapolis: University of Minnesota Press.

Egolf, D. B., Shames, G. H., Johnson, P. R., & Kasprisin-Burrelli, A. (1972). The use of parent-child interaction patterns in therapy for young stutterers. *Journal of Speech and Hearing Disorders, 37,* 222–32.

Egolf, D. B., Shames, G. H., and Seltzer, H. N. (1971). The effects of time-out on the fluency of stutterers in group therapy. *Journal of Communication Disorders, 4,* 111–18.

Eichstadt, A., Watt, N., & Girson, J. (1998). Evaluation of the efficacy of a stutter modification program with particular reference to two new measures of secondary behaviors and control of stuttering. *Journal of Fluency Disorders, 23,* 231–46.

Einarsdöttir, J. & Ingham, R. J. (2005). Have disfluency-type measures contributed to the understanding and treatment of developmental stuttering? *American Journal of Speech-Language Pathology, 14,* 260–73.

Eisenberg, S. L., Fersko, T. M., & Lundgren, C. (2001). The use of MLU for identifying language impairment in preschool children: A review. *American Journal of Speech-Language Pathology, 10,* 323–42.

Eisenson, J. (1937). Some characteristics of the written speech of stutterers. *Pedagogical Seminars, 50,* 457–58.

Eisenson, J. (1958). A perseverative theory of stuttering. In J. Eisenson (Ed.), *Stuttering: A symposium (pp. 223–72).* New York: Harper & Row.

Eisenson, J. (1966). Observations of the incidence of stuttering in a special culture. *ASHA, 8,* 391–94.

Eisenson, J. (1975). Stuttering as perseverative behavior. In J. Eisenson (Ed.), *Stuttering: A second symposium (pp. 401–52).* New York: Harper & Row.

Eisenson, J., & Horowitz, E. (1945). The influence of propositionality on stuttering. *Journal of Speech Disorders, 10,* 193–97.

Eisenson, J., & Pastel, E. (1936). A study of the perseverating tendency in stutterers. *Quarterly Journal of Speech, 22,* 626–31.

Eisenson, J., & Wells, C. (1942). A study of the influence of communicative responsibility in a choral speech situation for stutterers. *Journal of Speech Disorders, 7,* 259–62.

Eisenson, J., & Winslow, C. N. (1938). The perseverating tendency in stutterers in a perceptual function. *Journal of Speech Disorders, 3,* 195–98.

Eldridge, K. A., & Felsenfeld, S. (1998). Differentiating mild and recovered stutterers from nonstutterers. *Journal of Fluency Disorders, 23,* 173–94.

Elgar, F. J., McGrath, P. J., Waschbusch, D. A., Stewart, S. H., & Curtis, L. J. (2004). Mutual influences on maternal depression and child adjustment problems. *Clinical Psychology Review, 24,* 441–59.

Elliott, A. J., Miltenberger, R. G., Rapp, J., Long, E. S., & McDonald, R. (1998). Brief application of simplified habit reversal to treat stuttering in children. *Journal of Behavior Therapy and Experimental Psychiatry, 29,* 289–302.

Elliott, S., & Williamson, C. (1973). An evaluation of a token reward system in the treatment of adolescent stammerers. *DSH Abstracts, 13,* 296.

Emerick, L. L. (1960). Extensional definition and attitude toward stuttering. *Journal of Speech and Hearing Research, 3,* 181–86.

Enger, N. C., Hood, S. B., & Shulman, B. B. (1988). Language and fluency variables in the conversational speech of linguistically advanced preschool and school-aged children. *Journal of Fluency Disorders, 13,* 173–98.

Erickson, R. L. (1969). Assessing communication attitudes among stutterers. *Journal of Speech and Hearing Research, 12,* 711–24.

Ervin, S. (1961). Changes with age in the verbal determinants of word-association. *American Journal of Psychology, 74,* 361–72.

Everhart, R. W. (1949). An investigation of stuttering in an individual as related to genetically transmitted factors. [Abstract]. *Speech Monographs, 16,* 316.

Evesham, M., & Fransella, F. (1985). Stuttering relapse: The effect of a combined speech and psychological reconstruction programme. *British Journal of Disorders of Communication, 20,* 237–48.

Evesham, M., & Huddleston, A. (1983). Teaching stutterers the skill of fluent speech as a preliminary to the study of relapse. *British Journal of Disorders of Communication, 18,* 31–38.

Ezrati-Vinacour, R., & Levin, I. (2001). Time estimation by adults who stutter. *Journal of Speech, Language and Hearing Research, 44,* 144–57.

Ezrati-Vinacour, R., & Levin, I. (2004). The relationship between anxiety and stuttering: A multidimensional approach. *Journal of Fluency Disorders, 29,* 135–48.

Ezrati-Vinacour, R., Platzky, R., & Yairi, E. (2001). The young child's awareness of stuttering-like Disfluency. *Journal of Speech, Language and Hearing Research, 44,* 368.

Fagan, L. B. (1931). The relation of dextral training to the onset of stuttering. *Quarterly Journal of Speech, 17,* 73–76.

Fagan, L. B. (1932). A clinico-experimental approach to the reeducation of the speech of stutterers. *Psychology Monographs, 43,* 53–66.

Fairbanks, G. (1937). Some correlates of sound difficulty in stuttering. *Quarterly Journal of Speech, 23,* 67–69.

Fairbanks, G. (1954). Systematic research in experimental phonetics: 1. A theory of the speech mechanism as a servosystem. *Journal of Speech and Hearing Disorders, 19,* 133–39.

Fairbanks, G. (1955). Selective vocal effects of delayed auditory feedback. *Journal of Speech and Hearing Disorders, 20,* 333–46.

Fairbanks, G., & Guttman, N. (1958). Effects of delayed auditory feedback upon articulation. *Journal of Speech and Hearing Research, 1,* 12–22.

Falck, F. J. (1956). Interrelationships among certain behavioral characteristics, age, sex, and duration of therapy in a group of stutterers. [Abstract]. *Speech Monographs, 23,* 141–42.

Falck, F. J., Lawler, P. S., & Yonovitz, A. (1985). Effects of stuttering on fundamental frequency. *Journal of Fluency Disorders, 10,* 123–35.

Farber, S. (1981). *Identical twins reared apart: a reanalysis.* New York: Basic Books.

Farmer, A., & Brayton, E. R. (1979). Speech characteristics of fluent and dysfluent Down's syndrome adults. *Folia Phoniatrica, 31,* 284–90.

Fein, L. I. (1970). Stuttering as a cue related to the precipitation of moments of stuttering. [Abstract]. *ASHA, 12,* 456.

Feinberg, A. Y., Griffin, B. P., & Levey, M. (2000). Psychological aspects of chronic tonic and clonic stuttering: suggested therapeutic approaches. *American Journal of Orthopsychiatry, 70,* 465–73.

Feldman, R. L. (1976). Self-disclosure in parents of stuttering children. *Journal of Communication Disorders, 9,* 227–34.

Felsenfeld, S. (1996). Progress and needs in the genetics of stuttering. *Journal of Fluency Disorders, 21,* 77–103.

Felsenfeld, S. (2002). Finding susceptibility genes for developmental disorders of speech: The long and winding road. *Journal of Communication Disorders, 35,* 329–45.

Felsenfeld, S., & Broen, P. A. (1994). A 28-year follow-up of adults with a history of moderate phonological disorder: Educational and occupational results. *Journal of Speech and Hearing Research, 37,* 1341–54.

Felsenfeld, S., Kirk, K. M., Zhu, G., Statham, D. J., Neale, M. C., & Martin, N. G. (2000). A study of the genetic and environmental etiology of stuttering in a selected twin sample. *Behavior Genetics, 30,* 359–66.

Felstein, J. (1950). Language analysis of stutterers. [Abstract]. *Speech Monographs, 17,* 290.

Fenichel, O. (1945). *The psychoanalytic theory of neurosis.* New York: W. W. Norton.

Ferber, R. (1991). Slip of the tongue or slip of the ear? On the perception and transcription of naturalistic slips of the tongue. *Journal of Psycholinguistic Research, 20,* 105–22.

Ferrand, C. T., Gilbert, H. R., & Blood, G. W. (1991). Selected aspects of central processing and vocal motor function in stutterers and nonstutterers. *Journal of Fluency Disorders, 16,* 101–15.

Few, L. R., & Lingwall, J. B. (1972). A further analysis of fluency within stuttered speech. *Journal of Speech and Hearing Research, 15,* 356–63.

Fiedler, F. E., & Wepman, J. M. (1951). An exploratory investigation of the self-concept of stutterers. *Journal of Speech and Hearing Disorders, 16,* 110–14.

Fierman, E. Y. (1955). The roles of cues in stuttering adaptation. In W. Johnson & R. R. Leutenegger (Eds.), *Stuttering in children and adults* (pp. 256–63). Minneapolis: University of Minnesota Press.

Finitzo, T., Pool, K. D., Freeman, F. J., Devous, M. D., & Watson, B. C. (1991). Cortical dysfunction in developmental stutterers. In H. F. M. Peters, W. Hulstijn, & C. W. Starkweather (Eds.), *Speech motor control and stuttering* (pp. 251–62). Amsterdam: Elsevier.

Finkelstein, P., & Weisberger, S. E. (1954). The motor proficiency of stutterers. *Journal of Speech and Hearing Disorders, 19,* 52–58.

Finn, P. (1996). Establishing the validity of recovery from stuttering without formal treatment. *Journal of Speech and Hearing Research, 39,* 1171–82.

Finn, P. (1997). Adults recovered from stuttering without formal treatment: Perceptual assessment of speech normalcy. *Journal of Speech, Language and Hearing Research, 40,* 821–33.

Finn, P., Bothe, A. K., & Bramlett, R. E. (2005). Science and pseudoscience in communication disorders: Criteria and applications. *American Journal of Speech-Language Pathology, 14,* 172–86.

Finn, P., & Felsenfeld, S. (2004). Recovery from stuttering: the contributions of the qualitative research approach. *Advances in Speech-Language Pathology, 6,* 159–66.

Finn, P., Howard, R., & Kubala, R. (2005). Unassisted recovery from stuttering: Self-perceptions of current speech behavior, attitudes, and feelings. *Journal of Fluency Disorders, 30,* 281–305.

Finn, P., & Ingham, R. J. (1994). Stutterers' self-ratings of how natural speech sounds and feels. *Journal of Speech and Hearing Research, 37,* 326–41.

Finn, P., & Ingham, R. J. (1997). Children recovered from stuttering without formal treatment: Perceptual assessment of speech. *Journal of Speech, Language and Hearing Research, 40,* 867–76.

Fish, C. H., & Bowling, E. (1962). Effect of amphetamines on speech defects in the mentally retarded. *California Medicine, 96,* 109–11.

Fish, C. H., & Bowling, E. (1965). Stuttering: The effect of treatment with d-amphetamine and a tranquilizing agent, trifluoperazine. A preliminary report on an uncontrolled study. *California Medicine, 103,* 337–39.

Fisher, M. N. (1970), Stuttering: A psychoanalytic view. *Journal of Contemporary Psychotherapy, 2,* 124–27.

Fisher, M. S. (1932), Language patterns of pre-school children. *Journal of Experimental Education, 1,* 70–85.

Fisher, S. E., Plomin, R., DeFries, J. C., Craig, I. W., & McGuffin, P. (2003). Isolation of the genetic factors underlying speech and language disorders. In *Behavioral genetics in the postgenomic era* (pp. 205–26). Washington, DC: American Psychological Association.

Fishman, H. C. (1937). A study of the efficacy of negative practice as a corrective for stammering. *Journal of Speech Disorders, 2,* 67–72.

Fitch, J. L., & Batson, E. A. (1989). Hemispheric asymmetry of alpha wave suppression in stutterers and nonstutterers. *Journal of Fluency Disorders, 14,* 47–55.

Fitzgerald, H. E., Cooke, P. A., & Greiner, J. R. (1984). Speech and bimanual hand organization in adult stutterers and nonstutterers. *Journal of Fluency Disorders, 9,* 51–65.

Fitzgerald, H. E., Djurdjic, S. D., & Maguin, E. (1992). Assessment of sensitivity to interpersonal stress in stutterers. *Journal of Communication Disorders, 25,* 31-42.

Fitzpatrick, J. A. (1960). An investigation of the body image in secondary stutterers revealed through self-drawings. [Abstract]. *Speech Monographs, 27,* 240.

Flanagan, B., Goldiamond, I., & Azrin, N. (1958). Operant stuttering: The control of stuttering behavior through response-contingent consequences. *Journal of Experimental Analysis of Behavior, 1,* 173–77.

Flanagan, B., Goldiamond, I., & Azrin, N. H. (1959). Instatement of stuttering in normally fluent individuals through operant procedures. *Science, 130,* 979–81.

Fleischman, B. L. (1946). Stuttering and delinquency. [Abstract]. *Speech Monographs, 13,* 110–11.

Fletcher, J. M. (1914). An experimental study of stuttering. *American Journal of Psychology, 25,* 201–55.

Floyd, J., Zebrowski, P. M., & Flamme, G. A. (2007). Stages of change and stuttering: A preliminary view. *Journal of Fluency Disorders, 32,* 95–120.

Floyd, S., & Perkins, W. H. (1974). Early syllable dysfluency in stutterers and nonstutterers: A preliminary report. *Journal of Communication Disorders, 7,* 279–82.

Flügel, F. (1979). Erhebungen von Persönlichkeitsmerkmalen an Müttern stotternder Kinder und Jugendlicher. *DSH Abstracts, 19,* 226.

Fodor, J., Bever, T., & Garrett, M. (1974). *The psychology of language: An introduction to psycholinguistics and generative grammar.* New York: McGraw-Hill.

Font, M. M. (1955). A comparison of the free associations of stutterers and nonstutters. In W. Johnson & R. R. Leutenegger (Eds.), *Stuttering in children and adults.* Minneapolis: University of Minnesota Press.

Forster, D. C., & Webster, W. G. (1991). Concurrent task interference in stutterers: dissociating hemispheric specialization and activation. *Canadian Journal of Psychology, 45,* 321–35.

Forster, D. C., & Webster, W. G. (2001). Speech-motor control and interhemispheric relations in recovered and persistent stuttering. *Developmental Neuropsychology, 19,* 125–45.

Forte, M., & Schlesinger, I. M. (1972). Stuttering as a function of time of expectation. *Journal of Communication Disorders, 5,* 347–58.

Fossler, H. R. (1930). Disturbances in breathing during stuttering. *Psychology Monographs, 40,* 1–32.

Foundas, A. L., Bollich, A. M., Corey, D. M., Hurley, M., & Heilman, K. M. (2001). Anomalous anatomy of speech-language areas in adults with persistent developmental stuttering. *Neurology, 57,* 207–15.

Foundas, A. L., Bollich, A. M., Corey, D. M., Hurley, M., Heilman, K. M., Salmelin, R., et al. (2003). Cortical connectivity and stuttering. *Neuroscientist, 9,* 2–3.

Foundas, A. L., Bollich, A. M., Feldman, J., Corey, D. M., Hurley, M., Lemen, L. C., et al. (2004). Aberrant auditory processing and atypical planum temporale in developmental stuttering. *Neurology, 63,* 1640–46.

Foundas, A. L., Corey, D. M., Angeles, V., Bollich, A. M., Crabtree-Hartman, E., & Heilman, K. M. (2003). Atypical cerebral laterality in adults with persistent developmental stuttering. *Neurology, 61,* 1378–85.

Foundas, A. L., Corey, D. M., Hurley, M. M., & Heilman, K. M. (2004). Verbal dichotic listening in developmental stuttering: subgroups with atypical auditory processing. *Cognitive and Behavioral Neurology, 17,* 224–32.

Fowler, S., & Ingham, R. (1986). Stuttering treatment rating recorder. Santa Barbara, CA: University of California, Santa Barbara.

Fowlie, G. M., & Cooper, E. B. (1978). Traits attributed to stuttering and nonstuttering children by their mothers. *Journal of Fluency Disorders, 3,* 233–46.

Fox, D. R. (1966). Electroencephalographic analysis during stuttering and nonstuttering. *Journal of Speech and Hearing Research, 9,* 488–97.

Fox, P. T. (2003). Brain imaging in stuttering: where next? *Journal of Fluency Disorders, 28,* 265–72.

Fox, P. T., Ingham, R. J., Ingham, J. C., Hirsch, T. B., Downs, J. H., Martin, C., et al. (1996). A PET study of the neural systems of stuttering. *Nature, 382,* 158–61.

Fox, P. T., Ingham, R. J., Ingham, J. C., Zamarripa, F., Xiong, J. H., & Lancaster, J. L. (2000). Brain correlates of stuttering and syllable production. A PET performance-correlation analysis. *Brain, 123,* 1985–2004.

Franck, A. L., Jackson, R. A., Pimentel, J. T., & Greenwood, G. S. (2003). School-age children's perceptions of a person who stutters. *Journal of Fluency Disorders, 28,* 1–15.

Franck, R. (1980). Integration of an intensive program for stutterers within the normal activities of a major acute hospital. *Australian Journal of Human Communication Disorders, 8,* 4–15.

Franco, E., Casado, J. L., López Domínguez, J. M., Díaz Espejo, C., Blanco, A., & Robledo, A. (2000). [Stuttering as the only manifestation of a cerebral infarct]. *Neurologĩa 15,* 414–16.

Frank, A., & Bloodstein, O. (1971). Frequency of stuttering following repeated unison readings. *Journal of Speech and Hearing Research, 14,* 519–24.

Franke, U. (1983). Geschlechter Verhältnis und Geschwisterposition bei sprachauffälligen Kindern. *Sprachheilarb., 28,* 8–16.

Franken, M. C., Boves, L., Peters, H. F. M., & Webster, R. L. (1991). Prosodic features in the speech of post-therapy stutterers compared with the speech of nonstutterers. In H. F. M. Peters, W. Hulstijn, & C. W. Starkweather (Eds.), *Speech motor control and stuttering.* Amsterdam: Elsevier.

Franken, M. C., Boves, L., Peters, H. F. M., & Webster, R. L. (1992). Perceptual evaluation of the speech before and after fluency shaping stuttering therapy. *Journal of Fluency Disorders, 17,* 223–41.

Franken, M. C., Boves, L., Peters, H. F. M., & Webster, R. L. (1995). Perceptual rating instrument for speech evaluation of stuttering treatment. *Journal of Speech and Hearing Research, 38,* 280–88.

Franken, M. J., Kielstra-Van der Schalk, C. J., & Boelens, H. (2005). Experimental treatment of early stuttering: A preliminary study. *Journal of Fluency Disorders, 30,* 189–99.

Fransella, F. (1965). An experimental evaluation of the speech correction semantic differential. *Speech Monographs, 32,* 488–51.

Fransella, F. (1967). Rhythm as a distractor in the modification of stuttering. *Behavior Research Therapy, 5,* 253–55.

Fransella, F. (1968). Self concepts and the stutterer. *British Journal of Psychiatry, 114,* 1531–35.

Fransella, F. (1970). Stuttering: Not a symptom but a way of life. *British Journal of Disorders of Communication, 5,* 22–29.

Fransella, F. (1971). The "rhythm effect" in stuttering as a function of predictability of utterance. *Behavior Research Therapy, 9,* 265–71.

Fransella, F. (1972). *Personal change and reconstruction.* London: Academic.

Fransella, F., & Beech, H. R. (1965). An experimental analysis of the effect of rhythm on the speech of stutterers. *Behavior Research Therapy, 3,* 195–201.

Frasier, J. (1955). An exploration of stutterers' theories of their own stuttering. In W. Johnson & R. R. Leutenegger (Eds.), *Stuttering in children and adults (pp. 325–44).* Minneapolis: University of Minnesota Press.

Frayne, H., Coates, S., & Marriner, N. (1977). Evaluation of post treatment fluency by naive subjects. *Australian Journal of Human Communication Disorders, 5,* 48–54.

Freeman, F. J. (1979). Phonation in stuttering: A review of current research. *Journal of Fluency Disorders, 4,* 78–89.

Freeman, F. J. (1984). Laryngeal muscle activity of stutterers. In R. F. Curlee & W. H. Perkins (Eds.), *Nature and treatment of stuttering: New directions* (pp. 104–16). San Diego: College-Hill Press.

Freeman, F. J., & Rosenfield, D. B. (1982). "Source" in dysfluency. *Journal of Fluency Disorders, 7,* 295–96.

Freeman, F. J., & Ushijima, T. (1975). Laryngeal activity accompanying the moment of stuttering: A preliminary report of EMG investigations. *Journal of Fluency Disorders, 1,* 36–45.

Freeman, F. J., & Ushijima, T. (1978). Laryngeal muscle activity during stuttering. *Journal of Speech and Hearing Research, 21,* 538–62.

Freeman, K., & Armson, J. (1998). Extent and stability of stuttering reduction during choral reading. *Journal of Speech-Language Pathology and Audiology, 22,* 188–202.

Freeman, K. A., & Friman, P. C. (2004). Using simplified regulated breathing with an adolescent stutterer: Application of effective intervention in a residential context. *Behavior Modification, 28,* 247–60.

Freestone, N. W. (1942). An electroencephalographic study of the moment of stuttering. *Speech Monographs, 9,* 28–60.

Freund, H. (1934a). Über inneres Stottern. *Zeitschr. Ges. Neurology Psychiat., 151,* 585–98.

Freund, H. (1934b). Zur Frage der Beziehungen zwischen Stottern und Poltern. *Monatsschr. Ohrenheilk. Laryngol. Rhinol., 68,* 1446–57.

Freund, H. (1955). Psychosis and stuttering. *Journal of Nervous and Mental Disorders, 122,* 161–72.

Freund, H. (1966). *Psychopathology and the problems of stuttering.* Springfield, IL: Charles C. Thomas.

Frick, J. V. (1951). An exploratory study of the effect of punishment (electric shock) upon stuttering behavior. Ph.D. Dissertation, University of Iowa.

Frick, J. V. (1955). Spontaneous recovery of the stuttering response as a function of the degree of adaptation. In W. Johnson & R. R. Leutenegger (Eds.), *Stuttering in children and adults.* Minneapolis: University of Minnesota Press.

Frick, J. V. (1965). Evaluation of motor planning techniques for the treatment of stuttering. [Abstract]. *ASHA,* 7, 377.

Friedman, S. (1955). Diadochocinesis of the breathing mechanism of stutterers and nonstutterers. M.A. Thesis, Brooklyn College.

Fritzell, B. (1976). The prognosis of stuttering in schoolchildren: A 10-year longitudinal study. In *Proceedings of the XVI Congress of the International Society of Logopedics and Phoniatrics.* Basel: Karger.

Fritzell, B., Petersén, I., & Selldén, U. (1965). An EEG study of stuttering and nonstuttering school children. *De Therapia Vocis et Loquelae, Vol. I. of the XIII Congress International Society of Logopedics and Phoniatrics.*

Froeschels, E. (1921). Beitrage zur Symptomatologie des Stotterns. *Monatsschr. Ohrenheilk., 55,* 1109–12.

Froeschels, E. (1943). Pathology and therapy of stuttering. *Nervous Child, 2,* 148–61.

Froeschels, E. (1950). A technique for stutterers—"ventriloquism." *Journal of Speech and Hearing Disorders, 15,* 336–37.

Froeschels, E., & Rieber, R. W. (1963). The problem of auditory and visual imperceptivity in stutterers. *Folia Phoniatrica, 15,* 13–20.

Fruewald, E. (1936). Intelligence rating of severe college stutterers compared with that of others entering universities. *Journal of Speech Disorders, 1,* 47–51.

Fucci, D., Leach, E., McKenzie, J., & Gonzales, M. D. (1998). Comparison of listeners' judgments of simulated and authentic stuttering using magnitude estimation scaling. *Perceptual and Motor Skills, 87,* 1103–06.

Fucci, D., Petrosino, L., Gorman, P., & Harris, D. (1985). Vibrotactile magnitude production scaling: A method for studying sensory-perceptual responses of stutterers and fluent speakers. *Journal of Fluency Disorders, 10,* 69–75.

Fujita, K., Eguchi, C., Hirose, H., Shigeki, S., & Sakai, Y. (1963). [Clinical and experimental studies on the effectiveness of chlordiazepoxide in speech disorders.] [English Abstract]. *Otolaryngol.* (Tokyo), *35,* 89–97.

Fukawa, T., Yoshioka, H., Ozawa, E., & Yoshida, S. (1988). Difference of susceptibility to delayed auditory feedback between stutterers and nonstutterers. *Journal of Speech and Hearing Research, 31,* 475–79.

Furnham, A., & McDermott, M. R. (1994). Lay beliefs about the efficacy of self-reliance, seeking help and external control as strategies for overcoming obesity, drug addiction, marital problems, stuttering and insomnia. *Psychology and Health, 9,* 397–406.

Gabel, R. M., Colcord, R. D., & Petrosino, L. (2002). Self-reported anxiety of adults who do and do not stutter. *Perceptual and Motor Skills, 94,* 775–84.

Gaines, N. D., Runyan, C. M., & Meyers, S. C. (1991). A comparison of young stutterers' fluent versus stuttered utterances on measures of length and complexity. *Journal of Speech and Hearing Research, 34,* 37–42.

Galamon, T., Szulc-Kuberska, J., & Tronczyńska, J. (1969). The disturbances of histidine metabolism in hereditary stammering. *Folia Phoniatrica, 21,* 449–53.

Garber, S. F., & Martin, R. R. (1974). The effects of white noise on the frequency of stuttering. *Journal of Speech and Hearing Research, 17,* 73–79.

Garber, S. F., & Martin, R. R. (1977). Effects of noise and increased vocal intensity on stuttering. *Journal of Speech and Hearing Research, 20,* 233–40.

Gardner, W. H. (1937). Study of the pupillary reflex with special reference to stuttering. *Psychology Monographs, 49,* 1–31.

Garite, T. J., Clark, R. H., Elliott, J. P., & Thorp, J. A. (2004). Twins and triplets: The effect of plurality and growth on neonatal outcome compared with singleton infants, twins and triplets. *American Journal of Obstetrics and Gynecology, 191,* 700–07.

Gately, W. G. (1967). The effects of generalized anxiety on listeners' responses to dysfluent speech. [Abstract]. *Speech Monographs, 34,* 302–03.

Gattuso, R., & Leocata, A. (1962). L'Haloperidol nella terapia della balbuzie. *Clin. ORL, 14,* 227–34.

Gautheron, B., Liorzou, A., Even, C., & Vallancien, B. (1973). The role of the larynx in stuttering. In Y. Lebrun & R. Hoops (Eds.), *Neurolinguistic approaches to stuttering.* The Hague: Mouton.

Gemelli, R. J. (1982a). Classification of child stuttering: Part I. Transient developmental, neurogenic acquired, and persistent child stuttering. *Child Psychiatry and Human Development, 12,* 220–53.

Gemelli, R. J. (1982b). Classification of child stuttering: Part II. Persistent late onset male stuttering, and treatment issues for persistent stutterers—psychotherapy or speech therapy, or both? *Child Psychiatry and Human Development, 13,* 3–34.

Gendelman, E. G. (1977). Confrontation in the treatment of stuttering. *Journal of Speech and Hearing Disorders, 42,* 85–89.

Geniesse, H. (1935). Stuttering. *Science, 82,* 518.

Gens, G. W. (1950). Correlation of neurological findings, psychological analyses and speech disorders among institutionalized epileptics. *Training School Bulletin, 47,* 3–18.

Geschwind, N., & Behan, P. (1982). Left-handedness: Association with immune disease, migraine, and developmental learning disorder. *Proceedings of the National Academy of Sciences, 79,* 5097–5100.

Geschwind, N., & Behan, P. O. (1984). Laterality, hormones, and immunity. In N. Geschwind & A. M. Galaburda (Eds.), *Cerebral dominance: The biological foundations.* Cambridge, MA: Harvard University Press.

Geschwind, N., & Galaburda, A. M. (1985). Cerebral lateralization: Biological mechanisms, associations, and pathology: I. A hypothesis and a program for research. *Archives of Neurology, 42,* 429–59.

Gibney, N. J. (1973). Delayed auditory feedback: Changes in the volume intensity and the delay interval as variables affecting the fluency of stutterers' speech. *British Journal of Psychology, 64,* 55–63.

Gifford, M. F. (1940). *Correcting nervous speech disorders.* New York: Prentice-Hall.

Gildston, P. (1959). Stuttering and delinquency: A study of the possible relationship between repressed hostility and stuttering. M. A. Thesis, Queens College.

Gildston, P. (1967). Stutterers' self-acceptance and perceived parental acceptance. *Journal of Abnormal Psychology, 72,* 59–64.

Gilger, J. W. (1995). Behavioral genetics: concepts for research and practice in language development and disorders. *Journal of Speech and Hearing Research, 38,* 1126–42.

Gilger, J. W., & Rice, M. L. (1996). How can behavioral genetic research help us understand language development and disorders? In M. Rice (Ed.), *Toward a genetics of language* (pp. 77–110). Mahwah, NJ: Lawrence Erlbaum Associates.

Gillespie, S. K., & Cooper, E. B. (1973). Prevalence of speech problems in junior and senior high schools. *Journal of Speech and Hearing Research, 16,* 739–43.

Gilman, M., & Yaruss, J. S. (2000). Stuttering and relaxation: Applications for somatic education in stuttering treatment. *Journal of Fluency Disorders, 25,* 59–76.

Ginsberg, A. P. (2000). Shame, self-consciousness, and locus of control in people who stutter. *Journal of Genetic Psychology, 161,* 389–400.

Giolas, T. G., & Williams, D. E. (1958). Children's reactions to nonfluencies in adult speech. *Journal of Speech and Hearing Research, 1,* 86–93.

Girone, D., & Bruno, G. (1957). Some characteristics of the glycemic curve in stutterers. *Folia Phoniatrica, 9,* 87–91.

Gladstien, K. L., Seider, R. A., & Kidd, K. K. (1981). Analysis of the sibship patterns of stutterers. *Journal of Speech and Hearing Research, 24,* 460–62.

Glasner, P. J., & Rosenthal, D. (1957). Parental diagnosis of stuttering in young chidren. *Journal of Speech and Hearing Disorders, 22,* 288–95.

Glassmann, D. M. (1967). Personality characteristics of the stutterer as revealed through projective figure drawings. M. A. Thesis, Brooklyn College.

Glauber, I. P. (1958). The psychoanalysis of stuttering. In J. Eisenson (Ed.), *Stuttering: A symposium (pp. 71–120).* New York: Harper & Row.

Glogowski, K. (1976). Ist das Stottern erbbedingt? [Abstract]. *Folia Phoniatrica, 28,* 235–36.

Glover, H., Kalinowski, J., Rastatter, M., & Stuart, A. (1996). Effect of instruction to sing on stuttering frequency at normal and fast rates. *Perceptual and Motor Skills, 83,* 511–22.

Goberman, A. M., & Blomgren, M. (2003). Parkinsonian speech disfluencies: Effects of l-dopa-related fluctuations. *Journal of Fluency Disorders, 28,* 55–71.

Godai, U., Tatarelli, R., & Bonanni, G. (1976). Stuttering and tics in twins. *Acta Geneticae Medicae et Gemellologiae, 25,* 369–75.

Godinho, T., Ingham, R. J., Davidow, J., & Cotton, J. (2006). The distribution of phonated intervals in the speech of individuals who stutter. *Journal of Speech, Language and Hearing Research, 49,* 161–71.

Gold, C. (1994). Frequency of stuttering following repeated unison readings: A replication of Frank and Bloodstein (1971). M.A. Project, University of Minnesota.

Goldberg, S. A. & Culata, R. A. (1991). The demise of stuttering therapy: An indictment. Presentation at the American Speech-Language-Hearing Association annual convention, San Antonio, TX.

Goldfarb, R. (2006). *Ethics: A case study from fluency.* San Diego: Plural Publishing.

Goldiamond, I. (1965). Stuttering and fluency as manipulatable operant response classes. In L. Krasner & L. P. Ullmann (Eds.), *Research in behavior modification.* New York: Holt, Rinehart & Winston.

Goldman, R. (1966). The use of Mellaril as an adjunct to the treatment of stuttering. *Excerpta Medica. International Congress Series No. 150. Proceedings of the IV World Congress of Psychiatry.*

Goldman, R. (1967). Cultural influences on the sex ratio in the incidence of stuttering. *American Anthropologist, 69,* 78–81.

Goldman, R., & Guth, P. (1965). The effects of psychotherapeutic drugs on stuttering. *De Therapia Vocis et Loquelae, Vol. I. of the XIII Congress of the International Society of Logopedics and Phoniatrics.*

Goldman, R., & Shames, G. H. (1964a). Comparisons of the goals that parents of stutterers and parents of nonstutterers set for their children. *Journal of Speech and Hearing Disorders, 29,* 381–89.

Goldman, R., & Shames, G. H. (1964b). A study of goal-setting behavior of parents of stutterers and parents of nonstutterers. *Journal of Speech and Hearing Disorders, 29,* 192–94.

Goldman-Eisler, F. (1958a). The predictability of words in context and the length of pauses in speech. *Language and Speech, 1,* 226–31.

Goldman-Eisler, F. (1958b). Speech production and the predictability of words in context. *Quarterly Journal of Experimental Psychology, 10,* 96–106.

Goldman-Eisler, F. (1961). A comparative study of two hesitation phenomena. *Language and Speech, 4,* 18–26.

Goldsand, J. G. (1944). Sensory perseveration in stutterers and nonstutterers. [Abstract]. *Journal of Speech Disorders, 9,* 180.

Golub, A. (1955). The cumulative effect of constant and varying reading material on stuttering adaptation. In W. Johnson & R. R. Leutenegger (Eds.), *Stuttering in children and adults (pp. 237–44).* Minneapolis: University of Minnesota Press.

Golub, A. J. (1953). The heart rates of stutterers and nonstutterers in relation to frequency of stuttering during a series of oral readings. [Abstract]. *Speech Monographs, 20,* 146–47.

Goodall, H. B., & Brobby, G. W. (1982). Stuttering, sickling, and cerebral malaria: A possible organic basis for stuttering. *Lancet, 1* (8284), 1279–81.

Goodstein, L. D. (1956). *MMPI* profiles of stutterers' parents: A follow-up study. *Journal of Speech and Hearing Disorders, 21,* 430–35.

Goodstein, L. D. (1958). Functional speech disorders and personality: A survey of the research. *Journal of Speech and Hearing Research, 1,* 359–76.

Goodstein, L. D., & Dahlstrom, W. G. (1956). *MMPI* differences between parents of stuttering and nonstuttering children. *Journal of Consulting Psychology, 20,* 365–70. Reproduced, with editorial adaptations, as Chapter 7 in Johnson, W. and Associates, *The onset of stuttering.* Minneapolis: University of Minnesota Press.

Goodyer, I. (1981). Hysterical conversion reactions in childhood. *Journal of Child Psychology and Psychiatry and Allied Disciplines, 22,* 179–88.

Gordon, C. T., Cotelingam, G. M., Stager, S., Ludlow, C. L., Hamburger, S. D., & Rapoport, J. L. (1995). A double-blind comparison of clomipramine and desipramine in the treatment of developmental stuttering. *The Journal of Clinical Psychiatry, 56,* 238–42.

Gordon, E., Gordon, A., Gordon, L., Shapiro, M., Mentis, M., & Suchet, M. (1981). Biofeedback and stuttering. *South African Journal of Communication Disorders, 28,* 105–12.

Gordon, I. (1942). Allergy, enuresis, and stammering. *British Medical Journal,* March 14, 357–58.

Gordon, N. (2002). Stuttering: Incidence and causes. *Developmental Medicine and Child Neurology, 44,* 278–81.

Gordon, P. A. (1991). Language task effects: A comparison of stuttering and nonstuttering children. *Journal of Fluency Disorders, 16,* 275–87.

Gordon, P. A., & Luper, H. L. (1989). Speech disfluencies in nonstutterers: Syntactic complexity and production task effects. *Journal of Fluency Disorders, 14,* 429–45.

Gordon, P. A., Luper, H. L., & Peterson, H. A. (1986), The effects of syntactic complexity on the occurrence of disfluencies in 5 year old stutterers. *Journal of Fluency Disorders, 11,* 151–64.

Goss, A. E. (1952). Stuttering behavior and anxiety theory: I. Stuttering behavior and anxiety as a function of the duration of stimulus words. *Journal of Abnormal Social Psychology, 47,* 38–50.

Goss, A. E. (1956). Stuttering behavior and anxiety as a function of experimental taining. *Journal of Speech and Hearing Disorders, 21,* 343–51.

Gottsleben, R. H. (1955). The incidence of stuttering in a group of mongoloids. *Training School Bulletin, 51,* 209–18.

Gottwald, S. (2007). Stuttering prevention and early Intervention: A multidimensional approach. In B. Guitar & R. J. McCauley (Eds.), *Stuttering Treatment: Established and Emerging Approaches.* Baltimore, MD: Lippincott, Williams and Wilkins.

Gottwald, S. R., & Starkweather, C. W. (1995). Fluency intervention for preschoolers and their families in the public schools. *Language, Speech, and Hearing Services in Schools, 26,* 117–26.

Gould, E., & Sheehan, J. (1967). Effect of silence on stuttering. *Journal of Abnormal Psychology, 72,* 441–45.

Gow, M. L., & Ingham, R. J. (1992). Modifying electroglottograph-identified intervals of phonation: The effect on stuttering. *Journal of Speech and Hearing Research, 35,* 495–511.

Graf, O. I. (1955). Incidence of stuttering among twins. In W. Johnson & R. Leutenegger (Eds.), *Stuttering in children and adults* (pp. 381–88). Minneapolis: University of Minnesota Press.

Graham, J. K. (1966). A neurologic and electroencephalographic study of adult stutterers and matched normal speakers. [Abstract]. *Speech Monographs, 33,* 290.

Gray, B. B. (1965a). Theoretical approximations of stuttering adaptation. *Behavior Research Therapy, 3,* 171–85.

Gray, B. (1965b). Theoretical approximations of stuttering adaptation: Statement of predictive accuracy. *Behavior Research Therapy, 3,* 221–27.

Gray, B. B., & Brutten, E. J. (1965). The relationship between anxiety, fatigue and spontaneous recovery in stuttering. *Behavior Research Therapy, 2,* 251–59.

Gray, B. B., & England, G. (1972). Some effects of anxiety deconditioning upon stuttering frequency. *Journal of Speech and Hearing Research, 15,* 114–22.

Gray, B. B., & Karmen, J. L. (1967). The relationship between nonverbal anxiety and stuttering adaptation. *Journal of Communication Disorders, 1,* 141–51.

Gray, K. C., and Williams, D. E. (1969). Anticipation and stuttering: A pupillographic study. *Journal of Speech and Hearing Research, 12,* 833–39.

Gray, M. (1940). The X family: A clinical and laboratory study of a "stuttering" family. *Journal of Speech Disorders, 5,* 343–48.

Green, T. (1998). The reactions of elementary school children who stutter to social speech interactions. *Logopedics Phoniatrics Vocology, 23,* 3–10.

Green, T. (1999). The relationship of self-conception to perceived stuttering severity in children and adults who stutter. *Journal of Fluency Disorders, 24,* 281–92.

Greenberg, D., & Marks, I. (1982). Behavioural psychotherapy of uncommon referrals. *British Journal of Psychiatry, 141,* 148–53.

Greenberg, J. B. (1970). The effect of a metronome on the speech of young stutterers. *Behavior Therapist, 1,* 240–44.

Greene, J. S., & Small, S. M. (1944). Psychosomatic factors in stuttering. *Medical Clinics of North America, 28,* 615–28.

Gregg, B. A., & Yairi, E. (2007) Phonological skills and disfluency levels in preschool children who stutter. *Journal of Communication Disorders, 40,* 97–115.

Gregory, H. H. (1964). Stuttering and auditory central nervous system disorder. *Journal of Speech and Hearing Research, 7,* 335–41.

Gregory, H. H. (1972). An assessment of the results of stuttering therapy. *Journal of Communication Disorders, 5,* 320–34.

Gregory, H. H. (1997). The speech-language pathologist's role in stuttering self-help groups. *Seminars in Speech and Language, 18,* 401–09.

Gregory, H. H., & Hill, D. (1984). Stuttering therapy for children. In W. H. Perkins (Ed.), *Stuttering disorders* (pp. 77–94). New York: Thieme-Stratton.

Gregory, H. H., & Mangan, J. (1982). Auditory processes in stutterers. In N. J. Lass (Ed.), *Speech and language: Advances in basic research and practice,* Vol. 7. New York: Academic Press.

Greiner, J. R., Fitzgerald, H. E., & Cooke, P. A. (1986a). Bimanual hand writing in right-handed and left-handed stutterers and nonstutterers. *Neuropsychologia, 24,* 441–47.

Greiner, J. R., Fitzgerald, H. E., & Cooke, P. A. (1986b). Speech fluency and hand performance on a sequential tapping task in left- and right-handed stutterers and nonstutterers. *Journal of Fluency Disorders, 11,* 55–69.

Greiner, J. R., Fitzgerald, H. E., Cooke, P. A., & Djurdíc, S. D. (1985). Assessment of sensitivity to interpersonal stress in stutterers and nonstutterers. *Journal of Communication Disorders, 18,* 215–25.

Griggs, S., & Still, A. W. (1979). An analysis of individual differences in words stuttered. *Journal of Speech and Hearing Research, 22,* 572–80.

Gronhovd, K. D. (1977). A comparison of the fluent oral reading rates of stutterers and nonstutterers. *Journal of Fluency Disorders, 2,* 247–52.

Gross, M. S. (1969). A study of the effects of punishment and reinforcement on the dysfluencies of stutterers. [Abstract]. *Speech Monographs, 36,* 281.

Gross, M. S., & Holland, A. L. (1965). The effects of response contingent electroshock upon stuttering. [Abstract]. *ASHA, 7,* 376.

Grossman, D. J. (1952). A study of the parents of stuttering and non-stuttering children using the *Minnesota Multiphasic Personality Inventory* and the *Minnesota Scale of Parents' Opinions.* [Abstract]. *Speech Monographs, 19,* 193–94.

Gruber, L., & Powell, R. L. (1974). responses of stuttering and nonstuttering children to a dichotic listening task. *Perceptual and Motor Skills, 38,* 263–64.

Guitar, B. (1975). Reduction of stuttering frequency using analog electromyographic feedback. *Journal of Speech and Hearing Research, 18,* 672–85.

Guitar, B. (1976). Pretreatment factors associated with the outcome of stuttering therapy. *Journal of Speech and Hearing Research, 19,* 590–60.

Guitar, B. (1982). Fluency shaping with young stutterers. *Journal of Childhood Communication Disorders, 6,* 50–59.

Guitar, B. (2003). Acoustic startle responses and temperament in individuals who stutter. *Journal of Speech, Language and Hearing Research, 46,* 233–41.

Guitar, B. (2006). *Stuttering: an integrated approach to its nature and treatment* (3rd ed.). Baltimore: Williams and Wilkins.

Guitar, B., & Bass, C. (1978). Stuttering therapy: The relation between attitude change and long-term outcome. *Journal of Speech and Hearing Disorders, 43,* 392–400.

Guitar, B., & Grims, S. (1979). Assessing attitudes of children who stutter. [Abstract]. *ASHA, 21,* 763.

Guitar, B., Guitar, C., Neilson, P., O'Dwyer, N., & Andrews, G. (1988). Onset sequencing of selected lip muscles in stutterers and nonstutterers. *Journal of Speech and Hearing Research, 31,* 28–35.

Guitar, B., & Marchinkoski, L. (2001). Influence of mothers' slower speech on their children's speech rate. *Journal of Speech, Language and Hearing Research, 44,* 853–61.

Guitar, B., & Peters, T. J. (1980). *Stuttering: An integration of contemporary therapies.* Memphis: Speech Foundation of America.

Guitar, B., Schaefer, H. K., Donahue-Kilburg, G., & Bond, L. (1992). Parent verbal interactions and speech rate: A case study in stuttering. *Journal of Speech and Hearing Research, 35,* 742–54.

Guntupalli, V. K., Kalinowski, J., Saltuklaroglu, T., & Nanjundeswaran, C. (2005). The effects of temporal modification of second speech signals on stuttering inhibition at two speech rates in adults. *Neuroscience Letters, 385,* 7–12.

Guttman, N. (1960). Speech correction in the U.S.S.R. *Journal of Speech and Hearing Disorders, 25,* 306.

Gutzmann, H. (1898). *Das stottern.* Frankfurt am Main: J. Rosenheim.

Gutzmann, H. (1908). Die Atembewegung in ihrer Beziehung zu dem Sprachstörungen. *Monatsschr. Sprachheilk., 18,* 179–201.

Gutzmann, H. (1954). Versuche mit Glutamin-Behandlung bei Sprachstörungen aller Art. *Folia Phoniatrica, 6,* 1–8.

Hafford, J. (1941). A comparative study of the salivary pH of the normal speaker and stutterer. *Journal of Speech Disorders, 6,* 173–84.

Hage, A. (2001). Is there a link between the development of cognitive-linguistic abilities in children and the course of stuttering? In H.-G. Bosshardt, J. S. Yaruss, & H. F. M. Peters (Eds.), *Fluency disorders: Theory, research, treatment and self-help. Proceedings of the Third World Congress on Fluency Disorders* (pp. 192–94). Nijmegen: Nijmegen University Press.

Hageman, C. F., & Greene, P. N. (1989). Auditory comprehension of stutterers on a competing message task. *Journal of Fluency Disorders, 14,* 109–20.

Hahn, E. F. (1940). A study of the relationship between the social complexity of the oral reading situation and the severity of stuttering. *Journal of Speech Disorders, 5,* 5–14.

Hahn, E. F. (1942a). A study of the relationship between stuttering occurrence and grammatical factors in oral reading. *Journal of Speech Disorders, 7,* 329–35.

Hahn, E. F. (1942b). A study of the relationship between stuttering occurrence and phonetic factors in oral reading. *Journal of Speech Disorders, 7,* 143–51.

Hakim, H. Berman, & Bernstein Ratner, N. (2004). Nonword repetition abilities of children who stutter: An exploratory study. *Journal of Fluency Disorders, 29,* 179–99.

Hale, L. L. (1951). A consideration of thiamin supplement in prevention of stuttering in preschool children. *Journal of Speech and Hearing Disorders, 16,* 327–33.

Hall, J. W., & Jerger, J. (1978). Central auditory function in stutterers. *Journal of Speech and Hearing Research, 21,* 324–37.

Hall, K. D., Amir, O., & Yairi, E. (1999). A longitudinal investigation of speaking rate in preschool children who stutter. *Journfal of Speech, Language, and Hearing Research, 42,* 1367–77.

Hall, K. D., & Yairi, E. (1992). Fundamental frequency, jitter, and shimmer in preschoolers who stutter.

Journal of Speech and Hearing Research, 35, 1002–08.

Hall, N. E. (1999). Speech disruptions in pre-school children with specific language impairment and phonological impairment. *Clinical Linguistics and Phonetics, 13,* 295–307.

Hall, N., Wagovich, S., & Bernstein Ratner, N. (2007). Language considerations in childhood stuttering. In R. Curlee & E. G. Conture (Eds.), *Stuttering and related disorders of fluency* (3rd ed.) (pp.153–67). New York: Thieme.

Hall, N. E., Yamashita, T. S., & Aram, D. M. (1993). Relationship between language and fluency in children with developmental language disorders. *Journal of Speech and Hearing Research, 36,* 568–79.

Hall, P. K. (1977). The occurrence of disfluencies in language-disordered school-age children. *Journal of Speech and Hearing Disorders, 42,* 364–69.

Halle, F. (1900). Über Störungen der Atmung bei Stotterern. *Monatsschr. Sprachheilk., 10,* 225–36.

Halvorson, J. A. (1971). The effects on stuttering frequency of pairing punishment (response cost) with reinforcement. *Journal of Speech and Hearing Research, 14,* 356–64.

Ham, R. (1986). *Techniques of stuttering therapy.* Englewood Cliffs, NJ: Prentice-Hall.

Ham, R. (1990a). Clinician preparation: Experiences with pseudostuttering. *Journal of Fluency Disorders, 15,* 305–15.

Ham, R. E. (1990b). *Therapy of stuttering: preschool through adolescence.* Englewood Cliffs, NJ: Prentice-Hall.

Ham, R. E. (1990c). What is stuttering: Variations and stereotypes. *Journal of Fluency Disorders, 15,* 259–73.

Ham, R., & Steer, M. D. (1967). Certain effects of alterations in auditory feedback. *Folia Phoniatrica, 19,* 53–62.

Hamano, T., Hiraki, S., Kawamura, Y., Hirayama, M., Mutoh, T., & Kuriyama, M. (2005). Acquired stuttering secondary to callosal infarction. *Neurology, 64,* 1092–93.

Hamilton, P. G. (1940). The visual characteristics of stutterers during silent reading. Ph.D. Dissertation, Columbia University Teachers College.

Hamre, C. E., & Wingate, M. E. (1973). Stuttering consistency in varied contexts. *Journal of Speech and Hearing Research, 16,* 238–47.

Hancock, K., & Craig, A. (1998). Predictors of stuttering relapse one year following treatment for children aged 9 to 14 years. *Journal of Fluency Disorders, 23,* 31–48.

Hancock, K., & Craig, A. (2002). The effectiveness of re-treatment for adolescents who stutter. *Asia Pacific Journal of Speech, Language and Hearing, 7,* 138–56.

Hancock, K., Craig, A., McCready, C., McCaul, A., Costello, D., Gilmore, G., et al. (1998). Two- to six-year controlled-trial stuttering outcomes for children and adolescents. *Journal of Speech, Language, and Hearing Research, 41,* 1242–52.

Hand, C. R., & Haynes, W. O. (1983). Linguistic processing and reaction time differences in stutterers and nonstutterers. *Journal of Speech and Hearing Research, 26,* 181–85.

Hanna, R., & Morris, S. (1977). Stuttering, speech rate, and the metronome effect. *Perceptual and Motor Skills, 44,* 452–54.

Hanna, R., & Owen, N. (1977). Facilitating transfer and maintenance of fluency in stuttering therapy. *Journal of Speech and Hearing Disorders, 42,* 65–76.

Hanna, R., Wilfling, F., & McNeil, B. (1975). A biofeedback treatment for stuttering. *Journal of Speech and Hearing Disorders, 40,* 270–73.

Hannah, E. P., & Gardner, J. G. (1968). A note on syntactic relationships in nonfluency. *Journal of Speech and Hearing Research, 11,* 853–60.

Hannley, M., and Dorman, M. F. (1982). Some observations on auditory function and stuttering. *Journal of Fluency Disorders, 7,* 93–108.

Hansen, H. P. (1956). The effect of a measured audience reaction on stuttering behavior patterns. [Abstract]. *Speech Monographs, 23,* 144.

Hansen, K. (1927). Objektive Untersuchungen über Atembewegungen bei stotternden Schulkindern. Vol, 13, 25–29.

Hanson, B. R. (1978). The effects of a contingent lightflash on stuttering and attention to stuttering. *Journal of Communication Disorders, 11,* 451–58.

Hanson, B. R., Gronhovd, K. D., & Rice, P. L. (1981), A shortened version of the *Southern Illinois University Speech Situation Checklist* for the identification of speech-related anxiety. *Journal of Fluency Disorders, 6,* 351–60.

Hardin, C. B., Pindzola, R. H., & Haynes, W. O. (1992). A tachistoscopic study of hemispheric processing in stuttering and nonstuttering children. *Journal of Fluency Disorders, 17,* 265–81.

Hargrave, S., Kalinowski, J., Stuart, A., Armson, J., & Jones, K. (1994). Effect of frequency-altered feedback on stuttering frequency at normal and fast speech rates. *Journal of Speech and Hearing Research, 37*(6), 1313–19.

Harms, M. A., & Malone, J. Y. 70 (1939). The relationship of hearing acuity to stammering. *Journal of Speech Disorders, 4,* 363.

Haroldson, S. K., Martin, R. R., & Starr, C. D. (1968). Time-out as a punishment for stuttering. *Journal of Speech and Hearing Research, 11,* 560–66.

Harrington, J. (1987). Coarticulation and stuttering: An acoustic and electropalatographic study. In H. F. M. Peters, & W. Hulstijn (Eds.), *Speech motor dynamics in stuttering* (pp. 381–92). New York: Springer.

Harrington, J. (1988). Stuttering, delayed auditory feedback, and linguistic rhythm. *Journal of Speech and Hearing Research, 31,* 36–47.

Harris, C. M., Martin, R. R., & Haroldson, S. K. (1971). Punishment of expectancy responses by stutterers. *Journal of Speech and Hearing Research, 14,* 710–17.

Harris, D., Fucci, D., & Petrosino, L. (1991). Magnitude estimation and cross-modal matching of auditory and lingual vibrotactile sensation by normal speakers and stutterers. *Journal of Speech and Hearing Research, 34,* 177–82.

Harris, R. (1955). The effect of amplification of the stutterer's voice on the frequency of stuttering. M. A. Thesis, Brooklyn College.

Harris, V., Onslow, M., Packman, A., Harrison, E., & Menzies, R. (2002). An experimental investigation of the impact of the Lidcombe Program on early stuttering. *Journal of Fluency Disorders, 27,* 203–15.

Harris, W. E. (1942). Studies in the psychology of stuttering: XVII. A study of the transfer of the adaptation effect in stuttering. *Journal of Speech Disorders, 7,* 209–21.

Harrison, E., & Onslow, M. (1999). Early intervention for stuttering: The Lidcombe Program. In R. Curlee (Ed.), *Stuttering and related disorders of fluency* (2nd ed.) (pp. 65–79). New York: Thieme.

Harrison, E., Onslow, M., Andrews, C., Packman, A., & Webber, M. J. (1998). Control of stuttering with prolonged speech: Development of a one-day instatement program. In A. K. Cordes & R. Ingham (Eds.), *Treatment efficacy in stuttering: A search for empirical bases* (pp. 191–212). San Diego: Singular.

Harrison, E., Onslow, M., & Menzies, R. (2004). Dismantling the Lidcombe Program of early stuttering intervention: verbal contingencies for stuttering and clinical measurement. *International Journal of Language and Communication Disorders, 39,* 257–67.

Harrison, H. S. (1947). A study of the speech of sixty institutionalized epileptics. [Abstract]. *Speech Monographs, 14,* 210.

Hartfield, K. N., & Conture, E. G. (2006). Effects of perceptual and conceptual similarity in lexical priming of young children who stutter: Preliminary findings. *Journal of Fluency Disorders, 31*(4), 303–24.

Hartwell, E. M. (1893). Application of the laws of physical training for the prevention and cure of stuttering. *Proceedings of the International Congress of Education of the World's Columbian Exposition,* 739–49.

Hartz, G. (1970). Zur Frage des Zusammenhangs zwischen Intelligenz und Stottern. *Sprachheilarb., 15,* 109–16.

Hasbrouck, J. M. (1992). FAMC Intensive Stuttering Treatment Program: Ten years of implementation. *Military Medicine, 157,* 244–47.

Hasbrouck, J. M., Doherty, J., Mehlmann, M. A., Nelson, R., Randle, B., & Whitaker, R. (1987). Intensive stuttering therapy in a public school setting. *Language Speech and Hearing Services in Schools, 18,* 330–43.

Hasbrouck, J. M., Graham, N. L., & Brooks, R. S. (1976). The effect of manipulation of speech disfluency on stuttering frequency. [Abstract]. *ASHA, 18,* 610.

Hasbrouck, J. M., & Lowry, F. (1989). Elimination of stuttering and maintenance of fluency by means of airflow, tension reduction, and discrimination stimulus control procedures. *Journal of Fluency Disorders, 14,* 165–83.

Hasbrouck, J. M., & Martin, R. R. (1974). Further comparison of two different schedules of time-out for disfluency. [Abstract]. *ASHA, 16,* 514.

Haskell, R. J., & Larr, A. L. (1974). Psychodramatic role training with stutterers. *Group Psychotherapy and Psychodrama, 27,* 30–36.

Hawkins, R. T., & Brutten, E. J. (1964). The effect of stimulus strength on stuttering adjacency. [Abstract]. *ASHA, 6,* 416.

Hayden, P. A., Adams M. R., & Jordahl, N. (1982). The effects of pacing and masking on stutterers' and nonstutterers' speech initiation times. *Journal of Fluency Disorders, 7,* 9–19.

Hayden, P. A., Jordahl, N., & Adams, M. R. (1982). Stutterers' voice initiation times during conditions of novel stimulation. *Journal of Fluency Disorders, 7,* 1–7.

Hayden, P. A., Scott, D. A., & Addicott, J. (1977). The effects of delayed auditory feedback on the overt behaviors of stutterers. *Journal of Fluency Disorders, 2,* 235–46.

Hayhow, R., Cray, A. M., & Enderby, P. (2002). Stammering and therapy views of people who stammer. *Journal of Fluency Disorders, 27,* 1–17.

Hayhow, R., Kingston, M., & Ledzion, R. (1998). The use of clinical measures in the Lidcombe Programme for children who stutter. *International Journal of Language and Communication Disorders, 33,* 364–70.

Haynes, W. O., & Hood, S. B. (1977). Language and disfluency variables in normal speaking children from discrete chronological age groups. *Journal of Fluency Disorders, 2,* 57–74.

Haynes, W. O., & Hood, S. B. (1978). Disfluency changes in children as a function of the systematic modification of linguistic complexity. *Journal of Communication Disorders, 11,* 79–93.

Hays, P. (1987). Bethanecol chloride in treatment of stuttering. *Lancet,* January 31; (8527), 271.

Haywood, H. C. (1963). Differential effects of delayed auditory feedback on palmar sweating, heart rate, pulse pressure. *Journal of Speech and Hearing Research, 6,* 181–86.

Healey, E. C. (1982). Speaking fundamental frequency characteristics of stutterers and nonstutterers. *Journal of Communication Disorders, 15,* 21–29.

Healey, E. C. (1984). Fundamental frequency contours of stutterers' vowels following fluent stop consonant productions. *Folia Phoniatrica, 36,* 145–51.

Healey, E. C., & Adams, M. R. (1981). Speech timing skills of normally fluent and stuttering children and adults. *Journal of Fluency Disorders, 6,* 233–46.

Healey, E. C., & Bernstein, B. (1991). Acoustic analyses of young stutterers' and nonstutterers' disfluencies. In H. F. M. Peters, W. Hulstijn, & C. W. Starkweather (Eds.), *Speech motor control and stuttering.* Amsterdam: Elsevier.

Healey, E. C., & Gutkin, B. (1984). Analysis of stutterers' voice onset times and fundamental frequency contours during fluency. *Journal of Speech and Hearing Research, 27,* 219–25.

Healey, E. C., & Howe, S. W. (1987). Speech shadowing characteristics of stutterers under diotic and dichotic conditions. *Journal of Communication Disorders, 20,* 493–506.

Healey, E. C., Mallard, A. R. III, & Adams, M. R. (1976). Factors contributing to the reduction of stuttering during singing. *Journal of Speech and Hearing Research, 19,* 475–80.

Healey, E. C., & Ramig, P. R. (1986). Acoustic measures of stutterers' and nonstutterers' fluency in two speech contexts. *Journal of Speech and Hearing Research, 29,* 325–31.

Healey, E. C., & Reid, R. (2003). ADHD and stuttering: a tutorial. *Journal of Fluency Disorders, 28,* 79–94.

Healey, E. C., & Scott, L. A. (1995). Strategies for treating elementary school-age children who stutter: an integrative approach. *Language, Speech, and Hearing Services in Schools, 26,* 151–61.

Hedges, D., Umar, F., Mellon, C. D., Herrick, L., Hanson, M., & Wahl, M. (1995). Direct comparison of the family history method and the family study method using a large stuttering pedigree. *Journal of Fluency Disorders, 20,* 25–33.

Hegde, M. N. (1970). Propositional speech and stuttering. *Journal of the All India Institute for Speech and Hearing, 1,* 21–24.

Hegde, M. N. (1971a). The effect of shock on stuttering. *Journal of the All India Institute for Speech and Hearing, 2,* 104–10.

Hegde, M. N. (1971b). The short and long term effects of contingent aversive noise on stuttering. *Journal of the All India Institute for Speech and Hearing, 2,* 7–14.

Hegde, M. N. (1971c). Stuttering adaptation, reactive inhibition and spontaneous recovery. *Journal of the All India Institute for Speech and Hearing, 2,* 40–47.

Hegde, M. N. (1972). Stuttering, neuroticism and extraversion. *Behavior Research Therapy, 10,* 395–97.

Hegde, M. N. (1978). Fluency and fluency disorders: Their definition, measurement, and modification. *Journal of Fluency Disorders, 3,* 51–71.

Hegde, M. N. (1982). Antecedents of fluent and dysfluent oral reading: A descriptive analysis. *Journal of Fluency Disorders, 7,* 323–41.

Hegde, M. N., & Brutten, G. J. (1977). Reinforcing fluency in stutterers: An experimental study. *Journal of Fluency Disorders, 2,* 315–28.

Hegde, M. N., & Hartman, D. E. (1979a). Factors affecting judgments of fluency: I. Interjections. *Journal of Fluency Disorders, 4,* 1–11.

Hegde, M. N., & Hartman, D. E. (1979b). Factors affecting judgments of fluency: II. Word repetitions. *Journal of Fluency Disorders,* 4, 13–22.

Heinzel, J., & Ubricht, W. (1983). Untersuchung zur intellektuellen Struktur stotternder Kinder. *Sprachheilarb., 28,* 229–33.

Heitmann, R. R., Asbjørnsen, A., & Helland, T. (2004). Attentional functions in speech fluency disorders. *Logopedics Phoniatrics Vocology, 29,* 119–27.

Hejna, R. F. (1955). A study of the loci of stuttering in spontaneous speech. Ph.D. Dissertation, Northwestern University.

Hejna, R. F. (1963). Stuttering frequency in relation to word frequency usage. [Abstract]. *ASHA, 5,* 781.

Hejna, R. F. (1972). The relationship between accent or stress and stuttering during spontaneous speech. [Abstract]. *ASHA, 14,* 479.

Heller, J. C., Shulman, A. T., & Teryek, J. (1983). Short- and long-term outcome of intensive stuttering therapy: Factors affecting results. [Abstract]. *Folia Phoniatrica, 34,* 133–34.

Hellige, J. (2001). *Hemispheric Asymmetry: What's Right and What's Left?* Cambridge, MA: Harvard University Press.

Helltoft Nilsén, C., & Ramberg, C. (1999). Evaluation of a Scandinavian intensive program for stuttering in adolescence. *Logopedics Phoniatrics Vocology, 24,* 66–75.

Helm, N. A., & Butler, R. B. (1977). Transcutaneous nerve stimulation in acquired speech disorders. *Lancet,* No. 8049, Vol. II, 1177–78.

Helm, N. A., Butler, R. B., & Benson, D. F. (1978). Acquired stuttering. *Neurology, 28,* 1159–65.

Helm, N. A., Butler, R. B., & Canter, G. J. (1980). Neurogenic acquired stuttering. *Journal of Fluency Disorders, 5,* 269–79.

Helm-Estabrooks, N., & Hotz, G. (1998). Sudden onset of "stuttering" in an adult: neurogenic or psychogenic? *Seminars in Speech and Language, 19,* 23–34.

Helmreich, H. G., & Bloodstein, O. (1973). The grammatical factor in childhood disfluency in relation to the continuity hypothesis. *Journal of Speech and Hearing Research, 16,* 731–38.

Helps, R., & Dalton, P. (1979). The effectiveness of an intensive group speech therapy programme for adult stammerers. *British Journal of Disorders of Communication, 14,* 17–30.

Heltman, H. J. (1943). *First aid for stutterers.* New York: Expression Co.

Heltman, H. J., & Peacher, G. M. (1943). Misarticulation and diadokokinesis in the spastic paralytic. *Journal of Speech Disorders, 8,* 137–45.

Hendel, D., & Bloodstein, O. (1973). Consistency in relation to inter-subject congruity in the loci of stutterings. *Journal of Communication Disorders, 6,* 37–43.

Henrikson, E. H. (1936). Simultaneously recorded breathing and vocal disturbances of stutterers. *Archives of Speech, 1,* 133–49.

Herder, C., Howard, C., Nye, C., & Vanryckeghem, M. (2006). Effectiveness of behavioral stuttering treatment: A systematic review and meta-analysis. *Contemporary Issues in Communication Sciences and Disorders, 33,* 61–73.

Herder, C., Howard, C., Nye, C., Vanryckeghem, M., Schwartz, M., & Turner, H. (2007). Behavioral-based interventions for stuttering in children and adolescents. from http://www.cochrane.org.

Herndon, G.Y. (1967). A study of the time discrimination abilities of stutterers and nonstutterers. *Speech Monographs, 34,* 303–04.

Herren, R.Y. (1931). The effect of stuttering on voluntary movement. *Journal of Experimental Psychology, 14,* 289–98.

Herren, R.Y. (1932). The relation of stuttering and alcohol to certain tremor rates. *Journal of Experimental Psychology, 15,* 87–96.

Hertzman, J. (1948). High school mental hygiene survey. *American Journal of Orthopsychiatry, 18,* 238–56.

Heuer, R. J., & Sataloff, R. T. (1996). Neurogenic stuttering: Further corroboration of site of lesion. *Ear, Nose & Throat Journal, 75,* 161–69.

Hewat, S., Onslow, M., Packman, A., & O'Brian, S. (2006). A phase II clinical trial of self-imposed time-out treatment for stuttering in adults and adolescents. *Disability and Rehabilitation, 28,* 33–42.

Hill, D. (1999). Evaluation of child factors related to early stuttering: A descriptive study. In N. Bernstein Ratner & E. Charles Healey (Eds.), *Stuttering research and practice: Bridging the gap* (pp. 145–74). Mahwah, NJ: Lawrence Erlbaum Associates.

Hill, H. (1944a). Stuttering: I. A critical review and evaluation of biochemical investigations. *Journal of Speech Disorders, 9,* 245–61.

Hill, H. (1944b). Stuttering: II. A review and integration of physiological data. *Journal of Speech Disorders, 9,* 289–324.

Hill, H. E. (1954). An experimental study of disorganization of speech and manual responses in normal subjects. *Journal of Speech and Hearing Disorders, 19,* 295–305.

Hillman, R. E., & Gilbert, H. R. (1977). Voice onset time for voiceless stop consonants in the fluent reading of stutterers and nonstutterers. *Journal of the Acoustical Society of America, 61,* 610–11.

Hirschberg, J. (1965). A dadogásról. *Orvosi Hetilap, 106,* 780–84.

Hogewind, F. (1940). Medical treatment of stuttering. *Journal of Speech Disorders, 5,* 203–08.

Hohmeier, J. (1987). Zur beruflichen Situation von Stotternden. *Sprachheilarb., 32,* 25–31.

Holliday, A. R. (1959). Effect of meprobamate on stuttering. *Northwest Medicine, 58,* 837–41.

Hommerich, K. W., & Korzendorfer, M. (1966). Untersuchung über die Anwendung von Chlordiazepoxyd (Librium) in der Stottertherapie. *HNO, 14,* 211–18.

Homzie, M. J., Lindsay, J. S., Simpson, J., & Hasenstab, S. (1988). Concomitant speech, language, and learning problems in adult stutterers and in members of their families. *Journal of Fluency Disorders, 13,* 261–77.

Hood, S. B. (1975). Effect of communicative stress on the frequency and form-types of disfluent behavior in adult stutterers. *Journal of Fluency Disorders, 1,* 36–47.

Hoops, R., & Wilkinson, P. (1973). Group ratings of stuttering severity. In Y. Lebrun & R. Hoops (Eds.), *Neurolinguistic approaches to stuttering.* The Hague: Mouton.

Horan, M. C. (1968). An improved device for inducing rhythmic speech in stutterers. *Australian Psychology, 3,* 19–25.

Horii, Y., & Ramig, P. R. (1987). Pause and utterance durations and fundamental frequency characteristics of repeated oral readings by stutterers and nonstutterers. *Journal of Fluency Disorders, 12,* 257–70.

Horlick, R. S., & Miller, M. H. (1960). A comparative personality study of a group of stutterers and hard of hearing patients. *Journal of General Psychology, 63,* 259–66.

Horner, J., & Massey, W. (1983). Progressive dysfluency associated with right hemisphere disease. *Brain and Language, 18,* 71–85.

Horovitz, L. J., Johnson, S. B., Pearlman, R. C., Schaffer, E. J., & Hedin, A. K. (1978). Stapedial reflex and anxiety in fluent and disfluent speakers. *Journal of Speech and Hearing Research, 21,* 762–67.

Horowitz, E. (1965). Effects of parental criticism of defective articulation. *De Therapia Vocis et Loquelae, Vol. I. of the XIII Congress of the International Society of Logopedics and Phoniatrics.*

Horsely, I. A., & Fitzgibbon, C. T. (1987). Stuttering children: Investigation of a stereotype. *British Journal of Disorders of Communication, 22,* 19–35.

Howell, P. (1990). Changes in voice level caused by several forms of altered feedback in fluent speakers and stutterers. *Language and Speech, 33,* 325–38.

Howell, P. (2004). Assessment of some contemporary theories of stuttering that apply to spontaneous speech. *Contemporary Issues in Communication Sciences and Disorders, 31,* 123–40.

Howell, P., & Au-Yeung, J. (1995). Syntactic determinants of stuttering in the spontaneous speech of normally fluent and stuttering children. *Journal of Fluency Disorders, 20,* 317–30.

Howell, P., & Au-Yeung, J. (2002). The EXPLAN theory of fluency control applied to the diagnosis of stuttering. In E. Fava (Ed.), *Pathology and therapy of speech disorders* (pp. 75–94). Amsterdam: John Benjamins.

Howell, P., Au-Yeung, J., & Pilgrim, L. (1999). Utterance rate and linguistic properties as determinants of lexical dysfluencies in children who stutter. *The Journal of the Acoustical Society of America, 105,* 481–90.

Howell, P., Au-Yeung, J., & Rustin, L. (1997). Clock and motor variance in lip tracking: A comparison between children who stutter and those who do not. In W. Hulstijn, H. F. M. Peters, & P. H. H. M. v. Lieshout (Eds.), *Speech production: Motor control, brain research and fluency disorders* (pp. 573–78). Amsterdam: Elsevier.

Howell, P., Au-Yeung, J., & Sackin, S. (1999). Exchange of stuttering from function words to content words with age. *Journal of Speech, Language and Hearing Research, 42,* 345–54.

Howell, P., Davis, S., & Au-Yeung, J. (2003). Syntactic development in fluent children, children who stutter, and children who have English as an additional language. *Child Language Teaching and Therapy, 19,* 311–37.

Howell, P., Davis, S., & Williams, S. M. (2006). Auditory abilities of speakers who persisted, or recovered, from stuttering. *Journal of Fluency Disorders, 31*(4), 257–70.

Howell, P., & Dworzynski, K. (2005). Reply to letter to the editor: Planning and execution processes in speech control by fluent speakers and speakers who stutter. *Journal of Fluency Disorders, 30,* 343–54.

Howell, P., & El-Yaniv, N. (1987). The effects of presenting a click in syllable-initial position on the speech of stutterers: Comparison with a metronome click. *Journal of Fluency Disorders, 12,* 249–56.

Howell, P., El-Yaniv, N., & Powell, D. J. (1987). Factors affecting fluency in stutterers when speaking under altered auditory feedback. In H. F. M. Peters, & W. Hulstijn (Eds.), *Speech motor dynamics in stuttering* (pp. 361–70). New York: Springer.

Howell, P., Marchbanks, R. J., & El-Yaniv, N. (1986). Middle ear muscle activity during vocalization in normal speakers and stutterers. *Acta Otolaryngologica, 102,* 396–402.

Howell, P., Rosen, S., Hannigan, G., & Rustin, L. (2000). Auditory backward-masking performance by children who stutter and its relation to dysfluency rate. *Perceptual and Motor Skills, 90,* 355–63.

Howell, P., Sackin, S., & Glenn, K. (1997). Development of a two-stage procedure for the automatic recognition of dysfluencies in the speech of children who stutter: II. ANN recognition of repetitions and prolongations with supplied word segment markers. *Journal of Speech, Language, and Hearing Research, 40,* 1085–96.

Howell, P., Sackin, S., & Williams, R. (1999). Differential effects of frequency-shifted feedback between child and adult stutterers. *Journal of Fluency Disorders, 24,* 127–36.

Howell, P., & Vause, L. (1986). Acoustic analysis and perception of vowels in stuttered speech. *Journal of the Acoustical Society of America, 79,* 1571–79.

Howell, P., & Williams, M. (1988). The contribution of the excitatory source to the perception of neutral vowels in stuttered speech. *Journal of the Acoustical Society of America, 84,* 80–89.

Howell, P., & Williams, M. (1992). Acoustic analysis and perception of vowels in children's and teenagers' stuttered speech. *Journal of the Acoustical Society of America, 91,* 1697–1706.

Howell, P., & Williams, S. M. (2004). Development of auditory sensitivity in children who stutter and fluent children. *Ear and Hearing, 25,* 265–74.

Howell, P., Williams, M., & Vause, L. (1987). Acoustic analysis of repetitions in stutterers' speech. In H. F. M. Peters, & W. Hulstijn (Eds.), *Speech motor dynamics in stuttering* (pp. 371–80). New York: Springer.

Howell, P., Williams. M., & Young, K. (1991). Production of vowels by stuttering children and teenagers. In H. F. M. Peters, W. Hulstijn, & C. W. Starkweather (Eds.), *Speech motor control and stuttering.* Amsterdam: Elsevier.

Howell, P., & Wingfield, T. (1990). Perceptual and acoustic evidence for reduced fluency in the vicinity of stuttering episodes. *Language and Speech, 33,* 31–46.

Howie, P. (1976). The identification of genetic components in speech disorders. *Australian Journal of Human Communication Disorders, 4,* 155–63.

Howie, P. M. (1981a). Concordance for stuttering in monozygotic and dizygotic twin pairs. *Journal of Speech and Hearing Research, 24,* 317–21.

Howie, P. M. (1981b). Intrapair similarity in frequency of disfluency in monozygotic and dizygotic twin pairs containing stutterers. *Behavioral Genetics, 11,* 227–37.

Howie, P., & Andrews, G. (1984). Treatment of adult stutterers: Managing fluency. In R. F. Curlee & W. H. Perkins (Eds.), *Nature and treatment of stuttering: New directions* (pp. 425–46). San Diego: College-Hill Press.

Howie, P. M., Tanner, S., & Andrews, G. (1981). Short- and long-term outcome in an intensive treatment program for adult stutterers. *Journal of Speech and Hearing Disorders, 46,* 104–09.

Howie, P. M., & Woods, C. L. (1982). Token reinforcement during the instatement and shaping of fluency in the treatment of stuttering. *Journal of Applied Behavior Analysis, 15,* 55–64.

Howie, P. M., Woods, C. L., & Andrews, G. (1982). Relationship between covert and overt speech measures immediately before and immediately after stuttering treatment. *Journal of Speech and Hearing Disorders, 47,* 419–22.

Hubbard, C. P. (1998a). Reliability of judgments of stuttering and disfluency in young children's speech. *Journal of Communication Disorders, 31,* 245–60.

Hubbard, C. P. (1998b). Stuttering, stressed syllables, and word onsets. *Journal of Speech, Language and Hearing Research, 41,* 802–09.

Hubbard, C. P., & Prins, D. (1994). Word familiarity, syllabic stress pattern, and stuttering. *Journal of Speech and Hearing Research, 37,* 564–71.

Hubbard, C. P., & Yairi, E. (1988). Clustering of disfluencies in the speech of stuttering and nonstuttering preschool children. *Journal of Speech and Hearing Research, 31,* 228–33.

Huffman, E. S., & Perkins, W. H. (1974). Dysfluency characteristics identified by listeners as "stuttering" and "stutterer." *Journal of Communication Disorders, 7,* 89–96.

Hugh-Jones, S., & Smith, P. K. (1999). Self-reports of short- and long-term effects of bullying on children who stammer. *British Journal of Educational Psychology, 69,* 141–58.

Hugo, R. (1972). 'n Kommunikatiefgefundeerde ondersoek na bepaalde waarnemingsverskynsels by disfemie. *Journal of the South African Speech and Hearing Association, 19,* 39–51.

Huinck, W. J., Langevin, M., Kully, D., Graamans, K., Peters, H. F., & Hulstijn, W. (2006). The relationship between pre-treatment clinical profile and treatment outcome in an integrated stuttering program. *Journal of Fluency Disorders, 31,* 43–63.

Huinck, W. J., & Rietveld, T. (2007). The validity of a simple outcome measure to assess stuttering therapy. *Folia Phoniatrica, 59,* 91–99.

Huinck, W. J., van Lieshout, P. H. H. M., Peters, H. F. M., & Hulstijn, W. (2004). Gestural overlap in consonant clusters: effects on the fluent speech of stuttering and non-stuttering subjects. *Journal of Fluency Disorders, 29,* 3–26.

Hulit, L. M. (1976). Effects of nonfluencies on comprehension. *Perceptual and Motor Skills, 42,* 1119–22.

Hull, F. M. (1969). National Speech and Hearing Survey. U.S. Dept. Health, Educ., Welfare, Project No. 50978, Grant No. OE-32-15-0050-5010.

Hulstijn, W., Summers, J. J., Van Lieshout, P. H., & Peters, H. F. (1992). Timing in finger tapping and speech: A comparison between stutterers and fluent speakers. *Human Movement Science, 11,* 113–24.

Hunsley, Y. L. (1937). Dysintegration in the speech musculature of stutterers during the production of a non-vocal temporal pattern. *Psychology Monographs, 49,* 32–49.

Hurford, D. P., & Webster, R. L. (1985). Decreases in simple reaction time as a function of stutterers' participation in a behavioral therapy. *Journal of Fluency Disorders, 10,* 301–10.

Hurst, M. A., & Cooper, E. B. (1983a). Vocational rehabilitation counselors' attitudes toward stuttering. *Journal of Fluency Disorders, 8,* 13–27.

Hurst, M. I., & Cooper, E. B. (1983b). Employer attitudes toward stuttering. *Journal of Fluency Disorders, 8,* 1–12.

Hurwitz, T. A. (2004). Somatization and Conversion Disorder. *Canadian Journal of Psychiatry, 49,* 172–78.

Hutchinson, E. C., & Mackay, G. R. (1973). Conditioning speech nonfluencies through the use of an aversive stimulus. *Folia Phoniatrica, 25,* 373–82.

Hutchinson, J. M. (1975). Aerodynamic patterns of stuttered speech. In L. M. Webster & L. C. Furst (Eds.), *Vocal tract dynamics and dysfluency.* New York: Speech and Hearing Institute.

Hutchinson, J. M., & Brown, D. (1978). The Adams and Reis observations revisited. *Journal of Fluency Disorders, 3,* 149–54.

Hutchinson, J. M., & Burk, K. W. (1973). An investigation of the effects of temporal alterations in auditory feedback upon stutterers and clutterers. *Journal of Communication Disorders, 6,* 193–205.

Hutchinson, J. M., & Navarre, B. M. (1977). The effect of metronome pacing on selected aerodynamic patterns of stuttered speech: Some preliminary observations and interpretations. *Journal of Fluency Disorders, 2,* 189–204.

Hutchinson, J. M., & Norris, G. M. (1977). The differential effect of three auditory stimuli on the frequency of stuttering behaviors. *Journal of Fluency Disorders, 2,* 283–93.

Hutchinson, J. M., & Ringel, R. L. (1975). The effect of oral sensory deprivation on stuttering behavior. *Journal of Communication Disorders, 8,* 249–58.

Hutchinson, J. M., & Watkin, K. L. (1974). A preliminary investigation of lip and jaw coarticulation in stutterers. [Abstract]. *ASHA, 16,* 533.

Hutchinson, J. M., & Watkin, K. L. (1976). Jaw mechanics during release of the stuttering moment: Some initial observations and interpretations. *Journal of Communication Disorders, 9,* 269–79.

Iacono, T. A. (1984). The effect of pre-information on naive listeners' judgements of post treatment stutterers. *Australian Journal of Human Communication Disorders, 12,* 25–34.

Ickes, W. K. (1975). A palmar sweat measure of the effect of drugs on stuttering behavior. *Journal of Fluency Disorders, 1,* 2–9.

Ickes, W. K., & Pierce, S. (1973). The stuttering moment: A plethysmographic study. *Journal of Communication Disorders, 6,* 155–64.

Ilg, F., Learned, J., Lockwood, A., & Ames, L. B. (1949). The three-and-a-half-year old. *Journal of Genetic Psychology, 75,* 21–31.

Indefrey, P., & Levelt, W. J. M. (2004). The spatial and temporal signatures of word production components. *Cognition, 92,* 101–45.

Ingebregtsen, E. (1936). Some experimental contributions to the psychology and psychopathology of stutterers. *American Journal of Orthopsychiatry, 6,* 630–50.

Ingham, J. C. (1999). Behavioral treatment of young children who stutter. In R. F. Curlee (Ed.), *Stuttering and related disorders of fluency* (2nd ed.) (pp. 80–109). New York: Thieme.

Ingham, J. C., & Riley, G. (1998). Guidelines for documentation of treatment efficacy for young children who stutter. *Journal of Speech, Language and Hearing Research, 41,* 753–70.

Ingham, R. J. (1975). A comparison of covert and overt assessment procedures in stuttering therapy outcome evaluation. *Journal of Speech and Hearing Research, 18,* 346–54.

Ingham, R. J. (1976). Onset, prevalence, and recovery from stuttering: A reassessment of findings from the Andrews and Harris study. *Journal of Speech and Hearing Disorders, 41,* 280–81.

Ingham, R. J. (1980). Modification of maintenance and generalization during stuttering treatment. *Journal of Speech and Hearing Research, 23,* 732–45.

Ingham, R. J. (1982). The effects of self-evaluation training on maintenance and generalization during stuttering treatment. *Journal of Speech and Hearing Disorders, 47,* 271–80.

Ingham, R. J. (1984a). Generalization and maintenance of treatment. In R. F. Curlee & W. H. Perkins (Eds.), *Nature and treatment of stuttering: New directions* (pp. 447–71). San Diego: College-Hill Press.

Ingham, R. J. (1984b). *Stuttering and behavior therapy.* San Diego: College-Hill Press.

Ingham, R. J. (2001). Brain imaging studies of developmental stuttering. *Journal of Communication Disorders, 34,* 493–520.

Ingham, R. J. (2003). Brain imaging and stuttering: some reflections on current and future developments. *Journal of Fluency Disorders,* 411.

Ingham, R. J. (2004). Emerging controversies, findings and directions in neuroimaging and developmental stuttering: on avoiding petard hoisting in Athens, Georgia. In A. C. Bothe (Ed.), *Evidence-based treatment of stuttering: empirical bases and clinical applications* (pp. 27–64). Mahwah, New Jersey: Lawrence Erlbaum Associates.

Ingham, R. J., & Andrews, G. (1971a). The relation between anxiety reduction and treatment. *Journal of Communication Disorders, 4,* 289–301.

Ingham, R. J., & Andrews, G. (1971b). Stuttering: The quality of fluency after treatment. *Journal of Communication Disorders, 4,* 279–88.

Ingham, R. J., & Andrews, G. (1973a). An analysis of a token economy in stuttering therapy. *Journal of Applied Behavior Analysis, 6,* 219–29.

Ingham, R. J., & Andrews, G. (1973b). Behavior therapy and stuttering: A review. *Journal of Speech and Hearing Disorders, 38,* 405–41.

Ingham, R. J., Andrews, G., & Winkler, R. (1972). Stuttering; A comparative evaluation of the short-term effectiveness of four treatment techniques. *Journal of Communication Disorders, 5,* 91–117.

Ingham, R. J., & Carroll, P. J. (1977). Listener judgment of differences in stutterers' nonstuttered speech during chorus- and nonchorus-reading conditions. *Journal of Speech and Hearing Research, 20,* 293–302.

Ingham, R. J., & Cordes, A. K. (1992). Interclinic differences in stuttering-event counts. *Journal of Fluency Disorders, 17,* 171–76.

Ingham, R. J., Cordes, A. K., & Finn, P. (1993). Time-interval measurement of stuttering: Systematic replication of Ingham, Cordes, and Gow (1993). *Journal of Speech and Hearing Research, 36,* 1168–76.

Ingham, R. J., Cordes, A. K., & Gow, M. L. (1993). Time-interval measurement of stuttering: Modifying interjudge agreement. *Journal of Speech and Hearing Research, 36,* 503–15.

Ingham, R. J., Finn, P., & Belknap, H. (2001). The modification of speech naturalness during rhythmic stimulation treatment of stuttering. *Journal of Speech, Language and Hearing Research, 44,* 841–52.

Ingham, R. J., Finn, P., & Bothe, A. K. (2005). "Roadblocks" revisited: Neural change, stuttering treatment, and recovery from stuttering. *Journal of Fluency Disorders, 30,* 91–107.

Ingham, R. J., Fox, P. T., Ingham, J. C., Jinhu, X., Zamarripa, F., Hardies, L. J., et al. (2004). Brain correlates of stuttering and syllable production: gender comparison and replication. *Journal of Speech, Language and Hearing Research, 47,* 321–41.

Ingham, R. J., Fox, P. T., Ingham, J. C., & Zamarripa, F. (2000). Is overt stuttered speech a prerequisite for the neural activations associated with chronic developmental stuttering? *Brain and Language, 75,* 163–94.

Ingham, R. J., Fox, P. T., Ingham, J. C., Zamarripa, F., Martin, C., Jerabek, P., et al. (1996). Functional-lesion investigation of developmental stuttering with positron emission tomography. *Journal of Speech, Language and Hearing Research, 39,* 1208–27.

Ingham, R. J., Gow, M., & Costello, J. M. (1985). Stuttering and speech naturalness: Some additional data. *Journal of Speech and Hearing Disorders, 50,* 217–19.

Ingham, R. J., Ingham, J. C., Cordes, A. K., Moglia, R., & Frank, P. (1998). The effects of frequency-altered feedback on stuttering. *Journal of Speech, Language and Hearing Research, 41,* 513–16.

Ingham, R. J., Ingham, J. C., Finn, P., & Fox, P. T. (2003). Towards a functional neural systems model of developmental stuttering. *Journal of Fluency Disorders, 28,* 297–319.

Ingham, R. J., Ingham, J. C., Onslow, M., & Finn, P. (1989). Stutterers' self-ratings of speech naturalness: Assessing effects and reliability. *Journal of Speech and Hearing Research, 32,* 419–31.

Ingham, R. J., Kilgo, M., Ingham, J. C., Moglia, R., Belknap, H., & Sanchez, T. (2001). Evaluation of a stuttering treatment based on reduction of short phonation intervals. *Journal of Speech, Language, and Hearing Research, 44,* 1229–44.

Ingham, R. J., Martin, R. R., Haroldson, S. K., Onslow, M., & Leney, M. (1985). Modification of listener-judged naturalness in the speech of stutterers. *Journal of Speech and Hearing Research, 28,* 495–504.

Ingham, R. J., Martin, R. R., & Kuhl, P. (1974). Modification and control of rate of speaking by stutterers. *Journal of Speech and Hearing Research, 17,* 489–96.

Ingham, R. J., & Moglia, R. A. (1997). Experimental investigation of the effects of frequency-altered auditory feedback on the speech of adults who stutter. *Journal of Speech, Language and Hearing Research, 40,* 361–73.

Ingham, R. J., Moglia, R. A., Frank, P., Ingham, J. C., & Cordes, A. K. (1997). Experimental investigation of the effects of frequency-altered auditory feedback on the speech of adults who stutter. *Journal of Speech, Language, and Hearing Research, 40,* 361–72.

Ingham, R. J., Montgomery, J., & Ulliana, L. (1983). The effect of manipulating phonation duration on stuttering. *Journal of Speech and Hearing Research, 26,* 579–87.

Ingham, R. J., & Onslow, M. (1985). Measurement and modification of speech naturalness during stuttering therapy. *Journal of Speech and Hearing Disorders, 50,* 261–18.

Ingham, R. J., & Onslow, M. (1987). Generalization and maintenance of treatment benefits of children who stutter. *Seminars in Speech and Language, 8,* 303–26.

Ingham, R. J., & Packman, A. C. (1978). Perceptual assessment of normalcy of speech following stuttering therapy. *Journal of Speech and Hearing Research, 21,* 63–73.

Ingham, R. J., & Packman, A. (1979). A further evaluation of the speech of stutterers during chorus-and nonchorus reading conditions. *Journal of Speech and Hearing Research, 22,* 784–93.

Ingham, R. J., Southwood, H., & Horsburgh, G. (1981). Some effects of the Edinburgh masker on stuttering during oral reading and spontaneous speech. *Journal of Fluency Disorders, 6,* 135–54.

Ingham, R. J., Warner, A., Byrd, A., & Cotton, J. (2006). Speech effort measurement and stuttering: Investigating the chorus reading effect. *Journal of Speech, Language and Hearing Research, 49,* 660–70.

Inglis, A. L. (1979). Neurological stammer-A case study. *Australian Journal of Human Communication Disorders, 7,* 58–62.

Irving, R. W., & Webb, M. W. (1961). Teaching esophageal speech to a pre-operative severe stutterer. *Annals of Otology, Rhinology, and Laryngology, 70,* 1069–79.

Irwin, A. (1972). The treatment and results of "easy-stammering." *British Journal of Disorders of Communication, 7,* 151–56.

Ito, T. (1986). Speech dysfluency and acquisition of syntax in children 2–6 years old. *Folia Phoniatrica, 38,* 310. [Abstract].

Jacoby, B. (1947). An investigation of the carotid sinus reflex in stutterers. *Speech Monographs, 14,* 201–02. [Abstract].

Jakobovits, L. A. (1966). Utilization of semantic satiation in stuttering: A theoretical analysis. *Journal of Speech and Hearing Disorders, 31,* 105–14.

James, J. E. (1976). The influence of duration on the effects of time-out from speaking. *Journal of Speech and Hearing Research, 19,* 206–15.

James, J. E. (1981a). Punishment of stuttering: Contingency and stimulus parameters. *Journal of Communication Disorders, 14,* 375–86.

James, J. E. (1981b). Self-monitoring of stuttering: Reactivity and accuracy. *Behavior Research Therapy, 19,* 291–96.

James, J. E. (1983). Parameters of the influence of self-initiated time-out from speaking on stuttering. *Journal of Communication Disorders, 16,* 123–32.

James, J. E., & Ingham, R. J. (1974). The influence of stutterers' expectancies of improvement upon response to time-out. *Journal of Speech and Hearing Research, 17,* 86–93.

James, J. E., Ricciardelli, L. A., Rogers, P., & Hunter, C. E. (1989). A preliminary analysis of the ameliorative effects of time-out from speaking on stuttering. *Journal of Speech and Hearing Research, 32,* 604–10.

Jamison, D. J. (1955). Spontaneous recovery of the stuttering response as a function of the time following adaptation. In W. Johnson & R. R. Leutenegger (Eds.), *Stuttering in children and adults* (pp. 245–48). Minneapolis: University of Minnesota Press.

Jäncke, L. (1991). The 'audio-phoniatric coupling' in stuttering and nonstuttering adults: Experimental contributions. In H. F. M. Peters, W. Hulstijn & C. W. Starkweather (Eds.), *Speech motor control and stuttering.* Amsterdam: Elsevier.

Jäncke, L. (1994). Variability and duration of voice onset time and phonation in stuttering and nonstuttering adults. *Journal of Fluency Disorders, 19,* 21–37.

Jäncke, L., Bauer, A., Kaiser, P., & Kalveram, K. T. (1997). Timing and stiffness in speech motor control of stuttering and nonstuttering adults. *Journal of Fluency Disorders, 22,* 309–21.

Jäncke, L., Bauer, A., & Kalveram, K. T. (1996). Duration of phonation under changing stress conditions in stuttering and non-stuttering adults. *Clinical Linguistics and Phonetics, 10,* 225–34.

Jäncke, L., Hänggi, J. & Steinmetz, H. (2004). Morphological brain differences between adult stutterers and non-stutterers. *BMC Neurology, 4,* 23.

Jankelowitz, D. L., & Bortz, M. A. (1996). The interaction of bilingualism and stuttering in an adult. *Journal of Communication Disorders, 29,* 223–34.

Janssen, P., & Brutten, G. J. (1973). The differential effects of punishment of oral prolongations. In Y. Lebrun & R. Hoops (Eds.), *Neurolinguistic approaches to stuttering* (pp. 337–44), The Hague: Mouton.

Janssen, P., & Brutten, G. J. (1981). Pupillometric responses of young stutterers. *Proceedings of the 18th Congress of the International Association of Logopedics and Phoniatrics.* Washington, DC: American Speech and Language Hearing Association.

Janssen, P., Kloth, S., Kraaimaat, F., & Brutten, G. J. (1996). Genetic factors in stuttering: a replication of Ambrose, Yairi, and Cox's (1993) study with adult probands. *Journal of Fluency Disorders, 21,* 105–08.

Janssen, P., & Kraaimaat, F. (1980). Disfluency and anxiety in stuttering and nonstuttering adolescents. *Behavior Analysis and Modification, 4,* 116–26.

Janssen, P., & Kraaimaat, F. (1986). Onset and termination of accessory facial movements during stuttering. *Perceptual and Motor Skills, 63,* 11–17.

Janssen, P., Kraaimaat, F., & Brutten, G. (1990). Relationship between stutterers' genetic history and speech associated variables. *Journal of Fluency Disorders, 15,* 39–48.

Janssen, P., Kraaimaat, F., & van der Meulen, S. (1983). Reading ability and disfluency in stuttering and nonstuttering elementary school children. *Journal of Fluency Disorders, 8,* 39–53.

Janssen, P., & Wieneke, G. (1987). The effects of fluency inducing conditions on the variability in the duration of laryngeal movements during stutterers' fluent speech. In H. F. M. Peters & W. Hulstijn (Eds.), *Speech motor dynamics in stuttering* (pp. 337–44). New York: Springer.

Janssen P., Wieneke, G., & Vaane, E. (1983). Variability in the initiation of articulatory movements in the speech of stutterers and normal speakers. *Journal of Fluency Disorders, 8,* 341–58.

Jasper, H. H. (1932). A laboratory study of diagnostic indices of bilateral neuromuscular organization in stutterers and normal speakers. *Psychology Monographs, 43,* 72–1744.

Jasper, H. H., & Murray, E. (1932). A study of the eye-movements of stutterers during oral reading. *Journal of Experimental Psychology, 15,* 528–38.

Jayaram, M. (1983). Grammatical factors in stuttering in monolingual and bilingual stutterers. *Journal of Communication Disorders, 16,* 287–97.

Jayaram, M. (1984). Distribution of stuttering in sentences: Relationship to sentence length and clause position. *Journal of Speech and Hearing Research, 27,* 338–41.

Jehle, P., & Boberg, E. (1987). Intensivbehandlung für jugendliche und erwachsene Stotternde von Boberg und Kully. *Folia Phoniatrica, 39,* 256–68.

Jehle, P., Kühn, T., & Renner, J. A. (1989). Einstellungen Stotternder und Nicht-Stotternder zur Kommunikation: Einige Ergebnisse aus der Anwendung der Skala "S24" von Erickson und Andrews/Cutler. *Sprachheilarb., 34,* 121–28.

Jensen, P. J., Markel, N. N., & Beverung, J. W. (1986). Evidence of conversational disrhythmia in stutterers. *Journal of Fluency Disorders, 11,* 183–200.

Jensen, P. J., Sheehan, J. G., Williams, W. N., & LaPointe, L. L. (1975). Oral sensory-perceptual integrity of stutterers. *Folia Phoniatrica, 27,* 38–45.

Jerger, J. (1973). Diagnostic audiometry. In J. Jerger (Ed.), *Modern developments in audiology* (2nd ed.). New York: Academic.

Jerger, J. (1975). Diagnostic use of impedance measures. In J. Jerger (Ed.), *Manual of impedance audiometry.* New York: American Electromedics.

Johannsen, H. S., & Victor, C. (1986). Visual information processing in the left and right hemispheres during unilateral tachistoscopic stimulation of stutterers. *Journal of Fluency Disorders, 11,* 285–91.

Johnson, L. (1984). Facilitating parental involvement in therapy of the preschool difluent child. In W. H. Perkins (Ed.), *Stuttering disorders* (pp. 29–40). New York: Thieme-Stratton.

Johnson, W. (1932). *The influence of stuttering on the personality.* University of Iowa Studies in Child Welfare, Vol. 5, No. 5. Iowa City: University of Iowa.

Johnson, W. (1933). An interpretation of stuttering. *Quarterly Journal of Speech, 19,* 70–76.

Johnson, W. (1934a). The influence of stuttering on the attitudes and adaptations of the stutterer. *Journal of Social Psychology, 5,* 415–20.

Johnson, W. (1934b). Stutterers' attitudes toward stuttering. *Journal of Abnormal Social Psychology, 29,* 32–44.

Johnson, W. (1937). The dominant thumb in relation to stuttering, eyedness and handedness. *American Journal of Psychology, 49,* 293–97.

Johnson, W. (1938). The role of evaluation in stuttering behavior. *Journal of Speech Disorders, 3,* 85–89.

Johnson, W. (1944). The Indians have no word for it. I. Stuttering in children. *Quarterly Journal of Speech, 30,* 330–37.

Johnson, W. (1955a). A study of the onset and development of stuttering. In W. Johnson & R. R. Leutenegger (Eds.), *Stuttering in children and adults* (pp. 37–73). Minneapolis: University of Minnesota Press.

Johnson, W. (1955b). The time, the place, and the problem. In W. Johnson & R. R. Leutenegger

(Eds.), *Stuttering in children and adults* (pp. 3–24). Minneapolis: University of Minnesota Press.

Johnson, W. (1961a). Measurements of oral reading and speaking rate and disfluency of adult male and female stutterers and nonstutterers. *Journal of Speech and Hearing Disorders,* Monograms Supplement No. 7, 1–20.

Johnson, W. (1961b). *Stuttering and what you can do about it.* Minneapolis: University of Minnesota Press.

Johnson, W., & Ainsworth, S. (1938). Studies in the psychology of stuttering: X. Constancy of loci of expectancy of stuttering. *Journal of Speech Disorders, 3,* 101–04.

Johnson, W., et al. (1942). A study of the onset and development of stuttering. *Journal of Speech Disorders, 7,* 251–57. (Published in more complete form in Johnson, 1955a.)

Johnson, W., et al. (1956). *Speech handicapped school children* (rev. ed.). New York: Harper & Row.

Johnson, W., et al. (1967). *Speech handicapped school children* (3rd ed.). New York: Harper & Row.

Johnson, W. & Associates (1959). *The onset of stuttering.* Minneapolis: University of Minnesota Press.

Johnson, W., & Brown, S. F. (1935). Stuttering in relation to various speech sounds. *Quarterly Journal of Speech, 21,* 481–96.

Johnson, W., & Colley, W. H. (1945). The relationship between frequency and duration of moments of stuttering. *Journal of Speech Disorders, 10,* 35–38.

Johnson, W., Darley, F. L., & Spriestersbach, D. C. (1963). *Diagnostic methods in speech pathology.* New York: Harper & Row.

Johnson, W., & Innes, M. (1939). Studies in the psychology of stuttering: XIII. A statistical analysis of the adaptation and consistency effects in relation to stuttering. *Journal of Speech Disorders, 4,* 79–86.

Johnson, W., & King, A. (1942). An angle board and hand usage study of stutterers and non-stutterers. *Journal of Experimental Psychology, 31,* 293–311.

Johnson, W., & Knott, J. R. (1936). The moment of stuttering. *Journal of Genetic Psychology, 48,* 475–79.

Johnson, W., & Knott, J. R. (1937). Studies in the psychology of stuttering: I. The distribution of moments of stuttering in successive readings of the same material. *Journal of Speech Disorders, 2,* 17–19.

Johnson, W., Larson, R. P., & Knott, J. R. (1937). Studies in the psychology of stuttering: VI. The role of cues representative of stuttering moments during oral reading. *Journal of Speech Disorders, 2,* 101–04.

Johnson, W., & Millsapps, L. S. (1937). Studies in the psychology of stuttering: VI. The role of cues representative of stuttering moments during oral reading. *Journal of Speech Disorders, 2,* 101–04.

Johnson, W., & Rosen, L. (1937). Studies in the psychology of stuttering: VII. Effect of certain changes in speech pattern upon frequency of stuttering. *Journal of Speech Disorders, 2,* 105–09.

Johnson, W., & Sinn, A. (1937). Studies in the psychology of stuttering: V. Frequency of stuttering with expectation of stuttering controlled. *Journal of Speech Disorders, 2,* 98–100.

Johnson, W., & Solomon, A. (1937). Studies in the psychology of stuttering: IV. A quantitative study of expectation of stuttering as a process involving a low degree of consciousness. *Journal of Speech Disorders, 2,* 95–97.

Johnson, W., Stearns, G., & Warweg, E. (1933). Chemical factors and the stuttering spasm. *Quarterly Journal of Speech, 19,* 409–15.

Johnson, W., Young, M. A., Sahs, A. L., & Bedell, G. N. (1959). Effects of hyperventilation and tetany on the speech fluency of stutterers and nonstutterers. *Journal of Speech and Hearing Research, 2,* 203–15.

Johnston, S. J., Watkin, K. L., & Macklem, P. T. (1993). Lung volume changes during relatively fluent speech in stutterers. *Journal of Applied Physiology, 75,* 696–703.

Jones, E. L. (1955). Explorations of experimental extinction and spontaneous recovery in stuttering. In W. Johnson & R. R. Leutenegger (Eds.), *Stuttering in children and adults* (pp. 226–31). Minneapolis: University of Minnesota Press.

Jones, M. J. (1949). An electroencephalographic study of stutterers and normal speakers during silence. [Abstract]. *Speech Monographs, 16,* 310–11.

Jones, M., Gebski, V., Onslow, M., & Packman, A. (2002). Statistical power in stuttering research: A tutorial. *Journal of Speech, Language and Hearing Research, 45,* 243–55.

Jones, M., Onslow, M., Harrison, E., & Packman, A. (2000). Treating stuttering in young children: predicting treatment time in the Lidcombe Program.

Journal of Speech, Language and Hearing Research, 43, 1440–51.

Jones, M., Onslow, M., Packman, A., Williams, S., Ormond, T., Schwarz, I., et al. (2005). Randomised controlled trial of the Lidcombe programme of early stuttering intervention. *British Medical Journal, 331,* 659–61.

Jones, P. H., & Ryan, B. P. (2001). Experimental analysis of the relationship between speaking rate and stuttering during mother-child conversation. *Journal of Developmental and Physical Disabilities, 13,* 279–305.

Jones, R. D., White, A. J., Lawson, K. H. C., & Anderson, T. J. (2002). Visuoperceptual and visuomotor deficits in developmental stutterers: An exploratory study. *Human Movement Science, 21,* 603–20.

Jones, R. J., & Azrin, N. H. (1969). Behavioral engineering: Stuttering as a function of stimulus duration during speech synchronization. *Journal of Applied Behavior Analysis, 2,* 223–29.

Jones, R. K. (1966). Observations on stammering after localized cerebral injury. *Journal of Neurology, Neurosurgery and Psychiatry, 29,* 192–95.

Jones-Prus, D. (1980). Training fluency as a motor skill in the treatment of dysfluent children. *Human Communication, 5,* 75–86.

Juste, F., & de Andrade, C. R. F. (2006). [Typology of speech disruptions and grammatical classes in stuttering and fluent children]. *Pró-Fono: Revista De Atualização Cientifica, 18,* 129–40.

Kaasin, K., & Bjerkan, B. (1982). Critical words and the locus of stuttering in speech. *Journal of Fluency Disorders, 7,* 433–46.

Kadi-Hanifi, K., & Howell, P. (1992). Syntactic analysis of the spontaneous speech of normally fluent and stuttering children. *Journal of Fluency Disorders, 17,* 151–70.

Kalinowski, J., Armson, J., Roland-Mieszkowski, M., Stuart, A., & Gracco, V. L. (1993). Effects of alterations in auditory feedback and speech rate on stuttering frequency. *Language and Speech, 36,* 1–16.

Kalinowski, J. S., Lerman, J. W., & Watt, J. (1987). A preliminary examination of the perceptions of self and others in stutterers and others. *Journal of Fluency Disorders, 12,* 317–31.

Kalinowski, J., Noble, S., Armson, J., & Stuart, A. (1994). Pretreatment and posttreatment speech naturalness ratings of adults with mild and severe stuttering. *American Journal of Speech-Language Pathology, 3,* 61–66.

Kalinowski, J., & Saltuklaroglu, T. (2003a). Choral speech: the amelioration of stuttering via imitation and the mirror neuronal system. *Neuroscience and Biobehavioral Reviews, 27,* 339–47.

Kalinowski, J., & Saltuklaroglu, T. (2003b). Speaking with a mirror: engagement of mirror neurons via choral speech and its derivatives induces stuttering inhibition. *Medical Hypotheses, 60,* 538–43.

Kalinowski, J., Saltuklaroglu, T., Dayalu, V. N., & Guntupalli, V. (2005). Is it possible for speech therapy to improve upon natural recovery rates in children who stutter? *International Journal of Language & Communication Disorders, 40,* 349–58.

Kalinowski, J., Saltuklaroglu, T., Guntupalli, V., & Stuart, A. (2004). Gestural recovery and the role of forward and reversed syllabic repetitions as stuttering inhibitors in adults. *Neuroscience Letters, 363,* 144–49.

Kalinowski, J., Stuart, A., Wamsley, L., & Rastatter, M. P. (1999). Effects of monitoring condition and frequency-altered feedback on stuttering frequency. *Journal of Speech, Language and Hearing Research, 42,* 1347–55.

Kalotkin, M., Manschreck, T., and O'Brien, D. (1979). Electromyographic tension levels in stutterers and normal speakers. *Perceptual and Motor Skills, 49,* 109–10.

Kamhi, A. G., Lee, R. F., and Nelson, L. K. (1985). Word, syllable, and sound awareness in language-disordered children. *Journal of Speech and Hearing Disorders, 50,* 207–12.

Kamhi, A. G., & McOsker, T. G. (1982). Attention and stuttering: Do stutterers think too much about speech? *Journal of Fluency Disorders, 7,* 309–21.

Kamiyama, G. (1964). A comparative study of stutterers and nonstutterers in respect to critical flicker frequency and sound localization. [Abstract]. *Speech Monographs, 31,* 291.

Kaplan, B. J., & Crawford, S. G. (1994). The GBG model: is there more to consider than handedness? *Brain and Cognition, 26,* 291–99.

Kapos, E., & Standlee, L. S. (1958). Behavioral rigidity in adult stutterers. *Journal of Speech and Hearing Research, 1,* 294–96.

Karlin, I. W., & Sobel, A. E. (1940). A comparative study of the blood chemistry of stutterers and nonstutterers. *Speech Monographs, 7,* 75–84.

Karlin, I. W., & Strazzulla, M. (1952). Speech and language problems of mentally deficient children. *Journal of Speech and Hearing Disorders, 17,* 286–94.

Karniol, R. (1995). Stuttering, language, and cognition: A review and a model of stuttering as suprasegmental sentence plan alignment (SPA). *Psychological Bulletin, 117,* 104–24.

Karr, G. M. (1977). The performance of stutterers on central auditory tests. *South African Journal of Communication Disorders, 24,* 100–09.

Karrass, J., Walden, T. A., Conture, E. G., Graham, C. G., Arnold, H. S., Hartfield, K. N., et al. (2006). Relation of emotional reactivity and regulation to childhood stuttering. *Journal of Communication Disorders, 32,* 402–23.

Kasprisin-Burrelli, A., Egolf, D. B., & Shames, G. H. (1972). A comparison of parental verbal behavior with stuttering and nonstuttering children. *Journal of Communication Disorders, 5,* 335–46.

Kathard, H. (2001). Sharing stories: life history narratives in stuttering research. *International Journal of Language and Communication Disorders, 36,* 52–58.

Kathard, H., Pillay, M., Samuel, M., & Reddy, V. (2004). Genesis of self-identity as disother: life histories of people who stutter. *The South African Journal Of Communication Disorders., 51,* 4–14.

Katz, J. (1962). The use of staggered spondiac words for assessing the integrity of the central auditory nervous system. *Journal of Auditory Research, 2,* 327–37.

Katz, L. (1966). Dependency and immaturity in stuttering children. M. A. Thesis, Brooklyn College.

Kazdin, A. E. (1973). The effect of response cost and aversive stimulation in suppressing punished and nonpunished speech disfluencies. *Behavior Therapist, 4,* 73–82.

Keane, V. E. (1972). The incidence of speech and language problems in the mentally retarded. *Mental Retardation, 10,* 3–8.

Keating, D., Keating, D., Turrell, G., & Ozanne, A. (2001). Childhood speech disorders: Reported prevalence, comorbidity and socioeconomic profile. *Journal of Paediatrics and Child Health, 37,* 431–36.

Keele, S. W. (1972). Attention demands of memory retrieval. *Journal of Experimental Psychology, 93,* 245–48.

Keese, A., & Fischer, U. (1976). Das Zielsetzungsverhalten stotternder Schüler. *Sprachheilarb., 21,* 39–47.

Keisman, I. B. (1958). Stuttering and anal fixation. Ph.D. Dissertation, New York. University.

Kelham, R., & McHale, A. (1966). The application of learning theory to the treatment of stammering. *British Journal of Disorders of Communication, 1,* 114–18.

Kelly, E. M. (1994). Speech rates and turn-taking behaviors of children who stutter and their fathers. *Journal of Speech and Hearing Research, 37,* 1284–94.

Kelly, E. M., & Conture, E. G. (1988). Acoustic and perceptual correlates of adult stutterers' typical and imitated stuttering. *Journal of Fluency Disorders, 13,* 233–52.

Kelly, E. M., & Conture, E. G. (1992). Speaking rates, response time latencies, and interrupting behaviors of young stutterers, nonstutterers, and their mothers. *Journal of Speech and Hearing Research, 35,* 1256–67.

Kelly, E. M., Martin, J. S., Baker, K. E., Rivera, N. I., Bishop, J. E., Krizizke, C. B., et al. (1997). Academic and clinical preparation and practices of school speech-language pathologists with people who stutter. *Language, Speech, and Hearing Services in Schools, 28,* 195–212.

Kelly, E. M., & Smith, A. (1995). Orofacial muscle activity of children who stutter: A preliminary study. *Journal of Speech and Hearing Research, 38,* 1025–37.

Kelly, E. M., Smith, A., & Goffman, L. (1995). Orofacial muscle activity of children who stutter: A preliminary study. *Journal of Speech and Hearing Research, 38,* 1025–37.

Kelly, G. A. (1932). Some common factors in reading and speech disabilities. *Psychology Monographs, 43,* 175–201.

Kelly, J. C. (1935). A study of the suggestibility of stammerers and normals. M. A. Thesis, Northwestern University.

Kennedy, A. M., & Williams, D. A. (1938). Association of stammering and the allergic diathesis. *British Medical Journal,* Dec. 24, No. 4068, 1306–09.

Kent, L. R. (1961). Carbon dioxide therapy as a medical treatment for stuttering. *Journal of Speech and Hearing Disorders, 26,* 268–71.

Kent, L. R. (1963). The use of tranquilizers in the treatment of stuttering. *Journal of Speech and Hearing Disorders, 28,* 288–94.

Kent, L. R., & Williams, D. E. (1959). Use of meprobamate as an adjunct to stuttering therapy. *Journal of Speech and Hearing Disorders, 24,* 64–69.

Kent, L. R., & Williams, D. E. (1963). Alleged former stutterers in grade two. [Abstract]. *ASHA, 5,* 772.

Kent, R. D. (1984). Stuttering as a temporal programming disorder. In R. F. Curlee & W. H. Perkins (Eds.), *Nature and treatment of stuttering: new directions.* San Diego: College-Hill Press.

Kent, R. D. (2000). Research on speech motor control and its disorders: A review and prospective. *Journal of Communication Disorders, 33,* 391–427.

Kenyon, E. L. (1942). The etiology of stammering: Fundamentally a wrong psycho-physiologic habit in the control of the vocal cords for the production of an individual speech sound. *Journal of Speech Disorders, 7,* 97–104.

Kern, A. (1932). Der Einfluss des Hörens auf das Stottern. *Arch. Psychiat. Nervenk., 97,* 429–50.

Kerr, S. H. (1976). Phonatory adjustment times in stutterers and nonstutterers. [Abstract]. *ASHA, 18,* 664.

Khedr, E., El-Nasser, W. A., Abdel Haleem, E. K., Bakr, M. S., & Trakhan, M. N. (2000). Evoked potentials and electroencephalography in stuttering. *Folia phoniatrica, 52,* 178–86.

Kidd, K. K. (1977). A genetic perspective on stuttering. *Journal of Fluency Disorders, 2,* 259–69.

Kidd, K. K., Heimbuch, R. C., & Records, M. A. (1981). Vertical transmission of susceptibility to stuttering with sex-modified expression. *Proceedings of the National Academy of Science, 78,* 606–10.

Kidd, K. K., Heimbuch, R. C., Records, M. A., Oehlert, G., & Webster, R. L. (1980). Familial stuttering patterns are not related to one measure of severity. *Journal of Speech and Hearing Research, 23,* 539–45.

Kidd, K. K., Kidd, J. R., & Records, M. A. (1978). The possible causes of the sex ratio in stuttering and its implications. *Journal of Fluency Disorders, 3,* 13–23.

Kidd, K. K., Reich, T., & Kessler, S. (1973). *Genetics,* 74, No. 2, Part 2: s137.

Kidd, K. K., Reich, T., & Kessler, S. (1974). Genetic analyses of stuttering. Unpublished manuscript.

Kiehn, E. (1935). Untersuchungen über die Fähigkeit zu feinabgemessenen Bewegungen (Feinmotorick) bei stammelnden, stotternden und normalen Volksschülern. *Vox, 21,* 32–35.

Kimmell, M. (1938). Studies in the psychology of stuttering: IX. The nature and effect of stutterers' avoidance reactions. *Journal of Speech Disorders, 3,* 95–100.

Kimura, D. (1961). Cerebral dominance and the perception of verbal stimuli. *Canadian Journal of Psychology, 15,* 156–65.

King, P. T. (1961). Perseveration in stutterers and nonstutterers. *Journal of Speech and Hearing Research, 4,* 346–57.

Kingston, M., Huber, A., Onslow, M., Jones, M., & Packman, A. (2003). Predicting treatment time with the Lidcombe Program: Replication and meta-analysis. *International Journal of Language and Communication Disorders, 38,* 165–77.

Kinstler, D. B. (1961). Covert and overt maternal rejection in stuttering. *Journal of Speech and Hearing Disorders, 26,* 145–55.

Kirk, L. (1977). Stuttering and quasi-stuttering in Ga. *Journal of Communication Disorders, 10,* 109–26 (1977). Reprinted in R. W. Rieber (Ed.), *The problem of stuttering: Theory and therapy.* New York: Elsevier North-Holland.

Klaniczay, S. (2001). Über kindliches Stottern und die Theorie der "Anklammerung." (Childhood stuttering and the theory of "clinging."). *Kinderanalyse, 9,* 60–80.

Klassen, T. R. (2002). Social distance in the negative stereotype of people who stutter. *Journal of Speech-Language Pathology and Audiology, 26,* 90–99.

Klassen, T. R., & Kroll, R. M. (2005). Opinions on stuttering and its treatment: A follow-up survey and cross-cultural comparison. *Journal of Speech-Language Pathology and Audiology, 29,* 73–82.

Klein, J. F., & Hood, S. B. (2004). The impact of stuttering on employment opportunities and job performance. *Journal of Fluency Disorders, 29,* 255–73.

Kleinow, J., & Smith, A. (2000). Influences of length and syntactic complexity on the speech motor stability of the fluent speech of adults who stutter. *Journal of Speech, Language and Hearing Research, 43,* 548–60.

Klich, R. J., & May, G. M. (1982). Spectrographic study of vowels in stutterers' fluent speech. *Journal of Speech and Hearing Research, 25,* 364–70.

Kline, D. F. (1959). An experimental study of the frequency of stuttering in relation to certain goal-activity drives in basic human behavior. [Abstract]. *Speech Monographs, 26,* 137.

Kline, M. L., & Starkweather, C. W. (1979). Receptive and expressive language performance in young stutterers. [Abstract]. *ASHA, 21,* 797.

Kloth, S. A., Janssen, P., Kraaimaat, F. W., & Brutten, G. J. (1995a). Communicative behavior of mothers of stuttering and nonstuttering high-risk children prior to the onset of stuttering. *Journal of Fluency Disorders, 20,* 365–77.

Kloth, S. A., Janssen, P., Kraaimaat, F. W., & Brutten, G. J. (1995b). Speech-motor and linguistic skills of young stutterers prior to onset. *Journal of Fluency Disorders, 20,* 157–70.

Kloth, S. A., Janssen, P., Kraaimaat, F., & Brutten, G. J. (1998). Child and mother variables in the development of stuttering among high-risk children: a longitudinal study. *Journal of Fluency Disorders, 23,* 217–30.

Kloth, S. A., Kraaimaat, F. W., Janssen, P., & Brutten, G. J. (1999). Persistence and remission of incipient stuttering among high-risk children. *Journal of Fluency Disorders, 24,* 253–65.

Klouda, G. V., & Cooper, W. E. (1987). Syntactic clause boundaries, speech timing, and stuttering frequency in adult stutterers. *Language and Speech, 30,* 263–76.

Klouda, G. V., & Cooper, W. E. (1988). Contrastive stress, intonation, and stuttering frequency. *Language and Speech, 31,* 3–20.

Knabe, J. M., Nelson, L. A., & Williams, F. (1966). Some general characteristics of linguistic output: Stutterers versus nonstutterers. *Journal of Speech and Hearing Disorders, 31,* 178–82.

Knepflar, K. J. (1965). Speaking fluency in the parents of stutterers and nonstutterers. [Abstract]. *ASHA, 7,* 391.

Knott, J. R. (1935). A study of stutterers' stuttering and nonstuttering experiences on the basis of pleasantness and unpleasantness. *Quarterly Journal of Speech, 21,* 328–31.

Knott, J. R., Correll, R. E., & Shephard, J. N. (1959). Frequency analysis of electroencephalograms of stutterers and nonstutterers. *Journal of Speech and Hearing Research, 2,* 74–80.

Knott, J. R., & Johnson, W. (1936). The factor of attention in relation to the moment of stuttering. *Journal of Genetic Psychology, 48,* 479–80.

Knott, J. R., Johnson, W., & Webster, M. J. (1937). Studies in the psychology of stuttering: II. A quantitative evaluation of expectation of stuttering in relation to the occurrence of stuttering. *Journal of Speech Disorders, 2,* 20–22.

Knott, J. R., & Tjossem, T. D. (1943). Bilateral electroencephalograms from normal speakers and stutterers. *Journal of Experimental Psychology, 32,* 357–62.

Knower, F. H. (1938). A study of speech attitudes and adjustments. *Speech Monographs, 5,* 130–203.

Knox, J. A. (1976). Acoustic analysis of stuttering behavior within the context of fluent speech. *Dissertation Abstracts International, Section B,* Vol. 36, No. 12, Part I.

Knudsen, T. A. (1939). A study of the oral recitation problems of stutterers. *Journal of Speech Disorders, 4,* 235–39.

Knura, G. (1970). Experimentelle Untersuchung des Lernerfolgs bei stotternden und nichtstotternden Volksschulkindern. *Sprachheilarb.,* 15, 1–12.

Kolk, H., & Postma, A. (1997). Stuttering as a covert repair phenomenon. In R. Curlee & G. Siegel (Eds.), *Nature and treatment of stuttering: new directions* (2nd ed.) (pp. 182–203). Boston: Allyn & Bacon.

Koller, W. C. (1983). Dysfluency (stuttering) in extrapyramidal disease. *Archives of Neurology, 40,* 175–77.

Kondas, O. (1967). The treatment of stammering in children by the shadow method. *Behavior Research Therapy, 5,* 325–29.

Kondas, O. (1971). Experiment of the shadowing method with children stammerers. *DSH Abstracts, 11,* 338.

Kools, J. A., & Berryman, J. D. (1971). Differences in disfluency behavior between male and female nonstuttering children. *Journal of Speech and Hearing Research, 14,* 125–30.

Koopmans, M., Slis, I., & Rietveld, T. (1991). The influence of word position and word type on the incidence of stuttering. In H. F. M. Peters, W. Hulstijn, & C. W. Starkweather (Eds.), *Speech motor control and stuttering.* Amsterdam: Elsevier.

Koopmans, M. L., Slis, I. H., & Rietveld, A. C. (1992). Is stuttering due to a deficient comprehension of linguistic structures? *Perceptual and Motor Skills, 75,* 1347–50.

Kopp, G. A. (1934). Metabolic studies of stutterers: I. Biochemical study of blood composition. *Speech Monographs, 1,* 117–32.

Kopp, H. (1946). Psychosomatic study of fifty stuttering children: II. Ozeretzky tests. *American Journal of Orthopsychiatry, 16,* 114–19.

Kopp, H. G. (1963). Eye movements in reading as related to speech dysfunction in male stutterers. [Abstract]. *Speech Monographs, 30,* 248.

Korzybski, A. (1941). *Science and sanity: an introduction to non-Aristotelian systems and general semantics* (2nd ed.). New York: Int. Non-Aristotelian Library Publishing Co.

Kotby, M., Moussa, A., El-Sady, S., & Nabieh, A. (2003). A comparative study between certain behavioral methods in treatment of stuttering. *International Congress Series, 1240,* 1243–49.

Kraaimaat, F., & Janssen, P. (1981). Relation between specific types of dysfluencies and autonomic and cognitive indices of anxiety in stuttering and nonstuttering adolescents. *Proceedings of the 18th Congress of the International Association of Logopedics and Phoniatrics.* Washington, DC: American Speech and Language Hearing Association.

Kraaimaat, F., & Janssen, P. (1985). Are the accessory facial movements of the stutterer learned behaviors? *Perceptual and Motor Skills, 60,* 11–17.

Kraaimaat, F., Janssen, P., & Brutten, G. J. (1988). The relationship between stutterers' cognitive and autonomic anxiety and therapy outcome. *Journal of Fluency Disorders, 13,* 107–13.

Kraaimaat, F. L., Janssen, P., & van Dam-Baggen, R. (1991). Social anxiety and stuttering. *Perceptual and Motor Skills, 72,* 766.

Kraaimaat, F. W., Vanryckeghem, M., & van Dam-Baggen, R. (2002). Stuttering and social anxiety. *Journal of Fluency Disorders, 27,* 319.

Kramer, M. B., Green, D., & Guitar, B. (1987). A comparison of stutterers and nonstutterers on masking level differences and synthetic sentence identification tasks. *Journal of Communication Disorders, 20,* 379–90.

Krause, R. (1978). Nonverbales interaktives Verhalten von Stotterern und ihren Gesprächspartnern. *Schweiz. Zeitschr. Psychol. Anwend., 37,* 177–201.

Krause, R. (1982). A social psychological approach to the study of stuttering. In C. Fraser, & K. R. Scherer (Eds.), *Advances in the social psychology of language* (pp. 77–122). Maison des Sciences de l'Homme and Cambridge University Press.

Krikorian, C. M., & Runyan, C. M. (1983). A perceptual comparison: Stuttering and nonstuttering children's nonstuttered speech. *Journal of Fluency Disorders, 8,* 283–90.

Kroll, R. M., & De Nil, L. F. (1998). Positron emission tomography studies of stuttering: Their relationship to our theoretical and clinical understanding of the disorder. *Journal of Speech-Language Pathology and Audiology, 22,* 261–70.

Kroll, R. M., & Hood, S. B. (1974). Differences in stuttering adaptation between oral reading and spontaneous speech. *Journal of Communication Disorders, 7,* 227–37.

Kroll, R. M., & Hood, S. B. (1976). The influence of task presentation and information load on the adaptation effect in stutterers and normal speakers. *Journal of Communication Disorders, 9,* 95–110.

Kroll, R. M., & O'Keefe, B. M. (1985). Molecular self-analysis of stuttered speech via speech time expansion. *Journal of Fluency Disorders, 10,* 93–105.

Kroll, R. M., & Scott-Sulsky, L. (2007). The Fluency Plus Program: An integration of fluency shaping and cognitive restructuring procedures for adolescents and adults who stutter. In B. Guitar & R. J. McCauley (Eds.), *Stuttering treatment: Established and emerging Approaches.* Baltimore, MD: Lippincott, Williams & Wilkins.

Krugman, M. (1946). Psychosomatic study of fifty stuttering children: IV. Rorschach study. *American Journal of Orthopsychiatry, 16,* 127–33.

Kuhr, A. (1994). The rise and fall of operant treatments for the treatment of stammering. *Folia Phoniatrica, 46,* 232–40.

Kuhr, A., & Rustin, L. (1985). The maintenance of fluency after intensive in-patient therapy: Long-term follow-up. *Journal of Fluency Disorders, 10,* 229–36.

Kully, D. (2000). Telehealth in speech pathology: applications to the treatment of stuttering. *Journal of Telemedicine and Telecare, 6 Suppl 2,* S39–41.

Kully, D., & Boberg, E. (1988). An investigation of interclinic agreement in the identification of fluent and stuttered syllables. *Journal of Fluency Disorders, 13,* 309–18.

Kully, D., & Langevin, M. (1999). Intensive behavioral treatment for stuttering adolescents. In R. Curlee (Ed.), *Stuttering and related disorders of fluency* (2nd ed.) (pp. 139–59). New York: Thieme.

Kully, D., Langevin, M., & Lomheim, H. (2007). Intensive treatment of adolescents and adults who stutter. In E. G. Conture & R. F. Curlee (Eds.), *Stuttering and related disorders of fluency* (3rd ed.) (pp. 213–32). New York: Thieme.

Kuniszyk-Józkowiak, W., Smolka, E., & Adamczyk, B. (1996). Effect of acoustical, visual and tactile echo on speech fluency of stutterers. *Folia Phoniatrica, 48,* 193–200.

Küppers, B., & Wünschmann, G. (1985). Neue Entwicklungen auf dem Gebiet Elektroakustischer Sprech- and Therapiehilfen für Stotterer. *Sprachheilarb., 30,* 261–72.

Kurshev, V. A. (1968a). Emotsionalnye reaktsii pri zaikanii po dannym pletizmografii. *Zh. Vyssh. Nerv. Deiatel., 18,* 517–18.

Kurshev, V. A. (1968b). Issledovanie vnerechenovo dykhaniya u zaikayuschikhsya. *Zh. Nevropatol. Psikhiat., 68,* 1840–41.

Kurshev, V. A. (1969). O neosoznannykh reaktsiyakh u zaikayuschikhsya. *Zh. Nevropatol. Psikhiat., 69,* 1075–77.

Kurth, E., & Schmidt, E. (1964). Mehrdimensionale Untersuchungen an stotternden Kindern. *Probleme Ergebnisse Psychol.,* 12, 49–58.

Kuster, J., Lundberg, A., DiGrande, A., & Andrews, L. (2000). A picture is worth one thousand words. Paper for the Third Annual International Stuttering Awareness Day Conference. http://www.mnsu.edu/comdis/ISAD3/papers/gallery/albumindex.html

LaCroix, Z. E. (1973). Management of disfluent speech through self-recording procedures. *Journal of Speech and Hearing Disorders, 38,* 272–74.

Laczkowska, M. (1965). Painting in stuttering children. *De Therapia Vocis et Loquelae, Vol. I. of the XIII Congress of the International Society of Logopedics and Phoniatrics.*

Laczkowski, A. (1965). Urine investigations in children with speech defects. *De Therapia Vocis et Loquelae, Vol. I. of the XIII Congress of the International Society of Logopedics and Phoniatrics.*

Ladouceúr, R., Boudreau, L., & Théberge, S. (1981). Awareness training and regulated-breathing method in modification of stuttering. *Perceptual and Motor Skills, 53,* 187–94.

Ladouceúr, R., Côté, C., Leblond, G., & Bouchard, L. (1982). Evaluation of regulated-breathing method and awareness training in the treatment of stuttering. *Journal of Speech and Hearing Disorders, 47,* 422–26.

Ladouceúr, R., & Martineau, G. (1982). Evaluation of regulated-breathing method with and without parental assistance in the treatment of child stutterers. *Journal of Behavior Therapy and Experimental Psychiatry, 13,* 301–06.

Ladouceúr, R., & Saint-Laurent, L. (1986). Stuttering: A multidimensional treatment and evaluation package. *Journal of Fluency Disorders, 11,* 93–103.

LaFollette, A. C. (1956). Parental environment of stuttering children. *Journal of Speech and Hearing Disorders, 21,* 202–07.

Laiho, A., & Klippi, A. (2007). Long- and short-term results of children's and adolescents' therapy courses for stuttering. *International Journal of Language and Communication Disorders, 42,* 367–82.

Laird, A. R., Fox, P. M., Price, C. J., Glahn, D. C., Uecker, A. M., Lancaster, J. L., et al. (2005). ALE meta-analysis: controlling the false discovery rate and performing statistical contrasts. *Human Brain Mapping, 25,* 155–64.

Lambeck, A. (1925). Objektive Untersuchungen an Stotterern zur Festellung der Beziehungen der Mitbewegung zur Sprechatmung. *Vox, 11,* 25–26.

Langer, R. M. (1969). A clinical study of the reactions of preschool children to stuttered and non-stuttered speech in another child. [Abstract]. *Speech Monographs, 36,* 286.

Langevin, M., Huinck, W. J., Kully, D., Peters, H. F. M., Lomheim, H., & Tellers, M. (2006). A cross-cultural, long-term outcome evaluation of the ISTAR

Comprehensive Stuttering Program across Dutch and Canadian adults who stutter. *Journal of Fluency Disorders, 31,* 229–56.

Langevin, M., & Kully, D. (2003). Evidence-based treatment of stuttering: III. Evidence-based practice in a clinical setting. *Journal of Fluency Disorders, 28,* 219–337.

Langlois, A., Hanrahan, L. L., & Inouye, L. L. (1986). A comparison of interactions between stuttering children, nonstuttering children, and their mothers. *Journal of Fluency Disorders, 11,* 263–73.

Langlois, A., & Long, S. H. (1988). A model for teaching parents to facilitate fluent speech. *Journal of Fluency Disorders, 13,* 163–72.

Langová, J., & Morávek, M. (1964). Some results of experimental examinations among stutterers and clutterers. *Folia Phoniatrica, 16,* 290–96.

Langová, J., Morávek, M., Novák, A., & Petřík, M. (1970). Experimental interference with auditory feedback. *Folia Phoniatrica, 22,* 191–96.

Langová, J., Morávek, M., Široký, A., & Šváb, L. (1975). Einfluss der Sprechaktivität auf den evozierten Vestibularnystagmus bei Stotterern. *Folia Phoniatrica, 27,* 287–91.

Langová, J., Široký, A., Šváb, L., & Morávek, M. (1979). Odraz neuróz rěčive funkci vestibulárnihó ústroji. *DSH Abstracts,* 19, 490.

Langová, J., & Šváb, L. (1973). Reduction of stuttering under experimental social isolation. The role of the adaptation effect. *Folia Phoniatrica, 25,* 17–22.

Lankford, S. D., & Cooper, E. B. (1974). Recovery from stuttering as viewed by parents of self-diagnosed recovered stutterers. *Journal of Communication Disorders, 7,* 171–80.

Lanyon, R. I. (1965). The relationship of adaptation and consistency to improvement in stuttering therapy. *Journal of Speech and Hearing Research, 8,* 263–69.

Lanyon, R. I. (1967). The measurement of stuttering severity. *Journal of Speech and Hearing Research, 10,* 836–43.

Lanyon, R. I. (1968). Some characteristics of nonfluency in normal speakers and stutterers. *Journal of Abnormal Psychology, 73,* 550–55.

Lanyon, R. I. (1977). Effect of biofeedback-based relaxation on stuttering during reading and spontaneous speech. *Journal of Consulting and Clinical Psychology, 45,* 860–66.

Lanyon, R. I., & Barocas, V. S. (1975). Effects of contingent events on stuttering and fluency. *Journal of Consulting and Clinical Psychology, 43,* 786–93.

Lanyon, R. I., Barrington, C. C., & Newman, A. C. (1976). Modification of stuttering through EMG biofeedback: A preliminary study. *Behavior Therapist, 7,* 96–103.

Lanyon, R. I., & Duprez, D. A. (1970). Nonfluency, information, and word length. *Journal of Abnormal Psychology, 76,* 93–97.

Lanyon, R. I., Goldsworthy, R. J., & Lanyon, B. P. (1978). Dimensions of stuttering and relationship to psychopathology. *Journal of Fluency Disorders, 3,* 103–13.

Lanyon, R. I., Lanyon, B. P., & Goldsworthy, R. J. (1979). Outcome predictors in the behavioral treatment of stuttering. *Journal of Fluency Disorders, 4,* 131–39.

LaSalle, L. R., & Conture, E. G. (1991). Eye contact between young stutterers and their mothers. *Journal of Fluency Disorders, 16,* 173–99.

LaSalle, L. R., & Conture, E. G. (1995). Disfluency clusters of children who stutter: relation of stutterings to self-repairs. *Journal of Speech and Hearing Research, 38,* 965–77.

Lass, N. J., Ruscello, D. M., Pannbacker, M., & Schmitt, J. F. (1995). The perceptions of stutterers by people who stutter. *Folia Phoniatric, 47,* 247–51.

Lass, N. J., Ruscello, D. M., Pannbacker, M. D., Schmitt, J. F., & Everly-Myers, D. S. (1989). Speech-language pathologists' perceptions of child and adult female and male stutterers. *Journal of Fluency Disorders, 14,* 127–34.

Laštovka, M. (1970). The monosynaptic spinal cord reflex activity changes in stuttering. *Folia Phoniatrica, 22,* 129–38.

Laštovka, M. (1978). Tetanická pohotovost u koktavých a brebtavých. *DSH Abstracts, 18,* 464.

Laštovka, M. (1979a). Influence of some psychopharmaca on the increase of the amplitude of electrically induced monosynaptic spinal cord reflex during the paroxysm of stuttering: 1. Effect of diazepam. *Folia Phoniatrica, 31,* 15–20.

Laštovka, M. (1979b). Influence of some psychopharmaca on the increase of the amplitude of electrically induced monosynaptic spinal cord reflex during the paroxysm of stuttering: 2. Effect of chlorpromazine. *Folia Phoniatrica, 31,* 21–26.

Laštovka, M. (1979c). Pokus o sledováni cásti motorické zpetná vazby u koktavých pomoci elektricky evokavané inervacni pauzy [tzv. silent period]. *DSH Abstracts, 19,* 490.

Laštovka, M. (1995). Tremor in stutterers. *Folia Phoniatrica, 47,* 318–23.

Lattermann, C., & Shenker, R. C. (2005). Bilingualism and early stuttering-do we really have to sacrifice one language? [German]. *Forum Logopadie, 19,* 12–16.

Lattermann, C., Shenker, R. C., & Thordardottir, E. (2005). Progression of language complexity during treatment with the Lidcombe Program for early stuttering intervention. *American Journal of Speech-Language Pathology, 14,* 242–53.

Lavid, N., Franklin, D. L., & Maguire, G. A. (1999). Management of child and adolescent stuttering with olanzapine: Three case reports. *Annals of Clinical Psychiatry, 11,* 233–36.

Lavie, N., Hirst, A., de Fockert, J. W., & Viding, E. (2004). Load theory of selective attention and cognitive control. *Journal of Experimental Psychology: General, 133,* 339–54.

Leach, E. (1967). Stuttering: Clinical application of response-contingent procedures. In B. B. Gray & G. England (Eds.) (1969). *Stuttering and the conditioning therapies.* Monterey, CA: Monterey Institute of Speech and Hearing.

Leach, E. A., Wolfolk, W. B., Fucci, D., & Gonzales, M. D. (1995). Simulations of stuttered speech: numbers and types of dysfluencies. *Perceptual and Motor Skills, 81,* 367–70.

Leanderson, R., and Levi, L. (1967). A new approach to the experimental study of stuttering and stress. *Acta Oto-Laryngolica, Supplement 224,* 311–16.

Leavitt, R. R. (1974). *The Puerto Ricans: Culture change and language deviance.* Tucson: University of Arizona Press.

Lebrun, Y., Bijleveld, H., & Rousseau, J.-J. (1990). A case of persistent neurogenic stuttering following a missile wound. *Journal of Fluency Disorders, 15,* 251–85.

Lebrun, Y., & Leleux, C. (1985). Acquired stuttering following right brain damage in dextrals. *Journal of Fluency Disorders, 10,* 137–41.

Lebrun, Y., Leleux, C., Rousseau, J.-J., & Devreaux, F. (1983). Acquired stuttering. *Journal of Fluency Disorders, 8,* 323–30.

Lebrun, Y., Rétif, J., & Kaiser, G. (1983). Acquired stuttering as a forerunner of motorneuron disease. *Journal of Fluency Disorders, 8,* 161–67.

Lechner, B. K. (1979). The effects of delayed auditory feedback and masking on the fundamental frequency of stutterers and nonstutterers. *Journal of Speech and Hearing Research, 22,* 343–53.

Lee, B. S. (1950a). Some effects of side-tone delay. *Journal of the Acoustical Society of America, 22,* 639–40.

Lee, B. S. (1950b). Effects of delayed speech feedback. *Journal of the Acoustical Society of America, 22,* 824–26.

Lee, B. S. (1951). Artificial stutter. *Journal of Speech and Hearing Disorders, 16,* 53–55.

Lee, B. S., McGough, W. E., & Peins, M. (1976). Automated desensitization of stutterers to use of the telephone. *Behavior Therapy, 7,* 110–12.

Lee, H.-J., Lee, H.-S., Kim, L., Lee, M. S., Suh, K.-Y., & Kwak, D.-I. (2001). A case of risperidone-induced stuttering. *Journal of Clinical Psychopharmacology, 21,* 115–16.

Lees, R. M. (1988). The effect of foreperiod length on the acoustic voice reaction times of stutterers. *Journal of Fluency Disorders, 13,* 157–62.

Leith, W. R., & Mims, H. A. (1975). Cultural influences in the development and treatment of stuttering: A preliminary report on the black stutterer. *Journal of Speech and Hearing Disorders, 40,* 459–66.

Leith, W. R., & Timmons, J. L. (1983). The stutterer's reaction to the telephone as a speaking situation. *Journal of Fluency Disorders, 8,* 233–43.

Lemert, E. M. (1953). Some Indians who stutter. *Journal of Speech and Hearing Disorders, 18,* 168–74.

Lemert, E. M. (1962). Stuttering and social structure in two Pacific societies. *Journal of Speech and Hearing Disorders, 27,* 3–10.

Lepsova, M. (1965). Ein Ferienlager für stotternde Kinder. *De Therapia Vocis et Loquelae, Vol. I. of the XIII Congress of the International Society of Logopedics and Phoniatrics.*

Lerea, L. (1955). An exploratory study of the effects of experimentally induced success and failure upon the oral reading performances and the levels of aspiration of stutterers. [Abstract]. *Speech Monographs, 22,* 202–03.

Lerman, J. W., Powers, G. R., & Rigrodsky, S. (1965). Stuttering patterns observed in a sample of mentally retarded individuals. *Training School Bulletin, 62,* 27–32.

Lerman, J. W., & Shames, G. H. (1965). The effect of situational difficulty difficulty on stuttering. *Journal of Speech and Hearing Research, 8,* 271–80.

Leske, M. C. (1981). Prevalence estimates of communicative disorders in the U.S.: Speech disorders. *ASHA, 23,* 217–25.

Leutenegger, R. R. (1957). Adaptation and recovery in the oral reading of stutterers. *Journal of Speech and Hearing Disorders, 22,* 276–87.

Levelt, W. J. M., Indefrey, P., Marantz, A., Miyashita, Y., & O'Neil, W. (2000). The speaking mind/brain: Where do spoken words come from? In *Image, language, brain: papers from the first mind- articulation project symposium.* (pp. 77–93). Cambridge, MA: The MIT Press.

Levelt, W. J., Roelofs, A., & Meyer, A. S. (1999). A theory of lexical access in speech production. *The Behavioral and Brain Sciences, 22,* 1–49.

Levis, B., Ricci, D., Lukong, J., & Drayna, D. (2004). *Genetic linkage studies of stuttering in a large West African kindred.* Paper presented at the Abstracts of the Annual Meeting of the American Society of Human Genetics.

Lev-Wiesel, R., Shabat, A., & Tsur, A. (2005). Stuttering as reflected in adults' self-figure drawings. *Journal of Developmental and Physical Disabilities, 17,* 85–93.

Lewis, B. A. (1992). Pedigree analysis of children with phonology disorders. *Journal of Learning Disabilities, 25,* 586–97.

Lewis, D., & Sherman, D. (1951). Measuring the severity of stuttering. *Journal of Speech and Hearing Disorders, 16,* 320–26.

Lewis, J. I., Ingham, R. J., & Gervens, A. (1979). Voice initiation and termination times in stutterers and normal speakers. [Abstract]. *ASHA, 21,* 693.

Lewis, K. E. (1991). The structure of disfluency behaviors in the speech of adult stutterers. *Journal of Speech and Hearing Research, 34,* 492–500.

Lewis, K. E. (1995). Do SSI-3 scores adequately reflect observations of stuttering behaviors? *American Journal of Speech-Language Pathology, 4,* 46–59.

Lewis, K. E., & Golberg, L. L. (1997). Measurements of temperament in the identification of children who stutter. *European Journal of Disorders of Communication, 32,* 441–48.

Lickley, R. J., Hartsuiker, R. J., Corley, M., Russell, M., & Nelson, R. (2005). Judgment of disfluency in people who stutter and people who do not stutter: Results from magnitude estimation. *Language & Speech, 48*(3), 299–312.

Liebetrau, R. M., & Daly, D. A. (1981). Auditory processing and perceptual abilities of "organic" and "functional" stutterers. *Journal of Fluency Disorders, 6,* 219–31.

Lightfoot, C. (1948). Serial identification of colors by stutterers. *Journal of Speech and Hearing Disorders, 13,* 193–208.

Lincoln, M. A., & Onslow, M. (1997). Long-term outcome of early intervention for stuttering. *American Journal of Speech-Language Pathology, 6,* 51–58.

Lincoln, M., Onslow, M., Lewis, C., & Wilson, L. (1996). A clinical trial of an operant treatment for school-age children who stutter. *American Journal of Speech-Language Pathology, 5,* 73–85.

Lincoln, M., Onslow, M., & Menzies, R. G. (1996). Beliefs about stuttering and anxiety: Research and clinical implications. *Australian Journal of Human Communication Disorders, 24,* 3–10.

Lincoln, M. A., Onslow, M., & Reed, V. (1997). Social validity of the treatment outcomes of an early intervention program for stuttering. *American Journal of Speech-Language Pathology, 6,* 77–84.

Lincoln, M., Packman, A., & Onslow, M. (2006). Altered auditory feedback and the treatment of stuttering: A review. *Journal of Fluency Disorders, 31,* 71–89.

Lindsay, J. S. (1989). Relationship of developmental disfluency and episodes of stuttering to the emergence of cognitive stages in children. *Journal of Fluency Disorders, 14,* 271–84.

Lindsley, D. B. (1940). Bilateral differences in brain potentials from the two cerebral hemispheres in relation to laterality and stuttering. *Journal of Experimental Psychology, 26,* 211–25.

Lingwall, J. B., & Bergstrand, G. G. (1979). Perceptual boundaries for judgments of "normal," "abnormal" and "stuttered" prolongations. [Abstract]. *ASHA, 21,* 733.

Liotti, M., Ingham, R., Ingham, J. C., Kothmann, D., Perez, R., & Fox, P. (2001). Abnormal event-related potentials to spoken and replayed vowels in stuttering. *Neuroimage, 13*(Part 2 Supplement), S560.

Liu, Y., Shi, W., Ding, B., Li, X., Xiao, K., Wang, X., et al. (2001). Analysis of correlates in the SAS, the SDS, and the MMPI of stutterers. *Chinese Journal of Clinical Psychology, 9,* 133–34.

Livingston, L. A., Flowers, Y. E., Hodor, B. A., & Ryan, B. P. (2000). The experimental analysis of interruption during conversation for three children who stutter. *Journal of Developmental and Physical Disabilities, 12,* 235–66.

Lockhart, M. S., & Robertson, A. W. (1977). Hypnosis and speech therapy as a combined therapeutic approach to the problem of stammering: A study of thirty patients. *British Journal of Disorders of Communication, 12,* 97–108.

Logan, K. J. (2001). The effect of syntactic complexity upon the speech fluency of adolescents and adults who stutter. *Journal of Fluency Disorders, 26,* 85–106.

Logan, K. J. (2003a). The effect of syntactic structure upon speech initiation times of stuttering and nonstuttering speakers. *Journal of Fluency Disorders, 28,* 17–36.

Logan, K. J. (2003b). Language and fluency characteristics of preschoolers' multiple-utterance conversational turns. *Journal of Speech, Language and Hearing Research, 46,* 178–89.

Logan, K. J., & Conture, E. G. (1997). Selected temporal, grammatical, and phonological characteristics of conversational utterances produced by children who stutter. *Journal of Speech, Language, and Hearing Research, 40,* 107–20.

Logan, K. J., & LaSalle, L. R. (1999). Grammatical characteristics of children's conversational utterances that contain disfluency clusters. *Journal of Speech, Language and Hearing Research, 42,* 80–92.

Logan, K. J., Roberts, R. R., Pretto, A. P., & Morey, M. J. (2002). Speaking slowly: Effects of four self-guided training approaches on adults' speech rate and naturalness. *American Journal of Speech-Language Pathology, 11,* 163–75.

Long, E. S., Miltenberger, R. G., & Rapp, J. T. (1998). A survey of habit behaviors exhibited by individuals with mental retardation. *Behavioral Interventions, 13,* 79–80.

Long, K. M., & Pindzola, R. H. (1985). Manual reaction time to linguistic stimuli in child stutterers and nonstutterers. *Journal of Fluency Disorders, 10,* 143–49.

Lotzmann, G. (1961). Zur Anwendung variierter Verzögerungszeiten bei Balbuties. *Folia Phoniatrica, 13,* 276–312.

Loucks, T. M. J., & De Nil, L. F. (2006a). Anomalous sensorimotor integration in adults who stutter: A tendon vibration study. *Neuroscience Letters, 402,* 195–200.

Loucks, T. M. J., & De Nil, L. F. (2006b). Oral kinesthetic deficit in adults who stutter: A target-accuracy study. *Journal of Motor Behavior, 38,* 238–46.

Loucks, T. M. J., De Nil, L. F., & Sasisekaran, J. (2007). Jaw-phonatory coordination in chronic developmental stuttering. *Journal of Communication Disorders, 40,* 257–72.

Louis, E. D., Winfield, L., Fahn, S., & Ford, B. (2001). Speech dysfluency exacerbated by levodopa in Parkinson's disease. *Movement Disorders, 16,* 562–65.

Louko, L. J., Edwards, M. L., & Conture, E. G. (1990) Phonological characteristics of young stutterers and their normally fluent peers: Preliminary observations. *Journal of Fluency Disorders, 15,* 191–210.

Lounsbury, F. G. (1954). Pausal, juncture and hesitation phenomena. In C. E. Osgood & T. A. Sebeok (Eds.), *Psycholinguistics: A survey of theory and research* (pp. 93–101). Baltimore: Waverly Press.

Louttit, C. M., & Halls, E. C. (1936). Survey of speech defects among public school children of Indiana. *Journal of Speech Disorders, 1,* 73–80.

Love, L. R., & Jeffress, L. A. (1971). Identification of brief pauses in the fluent speech of stutterers and nonstutterers. *Journal of Speech and Hearing Research, 14,* 229–40.

Love, W. R. (1955). The effect of pentobarbital sodium (Nembutal) and amphetamine sulphate (Benzedrine) on the severity of stuttering. In W. Johnson & R. R. Leutenegger (Eds.), *Stuttering in children and adults* (pp. 298–312). Minneapolis: University of Minnesota Press.

Lovett Doust, J. W. (1956). Stress and psychopathology in stutterers. *Canadian Journal of Psychology, 10,* 31–37.

Lovett Doust, J. W., & Coleman, L. I. M. (1955). The psychophysics of communication: III. Discriminatory awareness in stutterers and its measurement by the critical flicker fusion threshold. *Archives of Neurology and Psychiatry, 74,* 650–52.

Lowinger, L. (1952). The psychodynamics of stuttering: An evaluation of the factors of aggression and guilt feelings in a group of institutionalized children. *Dissertation Abstracts, 12,* 725.

Lubman, C. G. (1955). Speech program for severely retarded children. *American Journal of Mental Deficiency, 60,* 297–300.

Luchsinger, R. (1943). Untersuchungen des vegetativen Nervensystems bei Stotterern. *Schweiz. Med. Wochenschr., 73,* 868–870.

Luchsinger, R. (1954). Gibt es organisch bedingte Stottererfälle? *Arch. Ohr.-Nas.-Kehlk. Heilk., 165,* 612–18.

Luchsinger, R. (1959). Die Vererbung von Spach- und Stimmstörungen. *Folia Phoniatrica, 11,* 7–64.

Luchsinger, R., & Dubois, C. (1963). Ein Vergleich der Sprachmelodie- und Lautstärkekurve bei Normalen, Gehirnkranken und Stotterern. *Folia Phoniatrica, 15,* 21–41.

Luchsinger, R., & Landolt, H. (1955). Uber das Poltern, das sogenannte "Stottern mit Polterkomponente," und deren Beziehung zu den Aphasien. *Folia Phoniatrica, 7,* 12–43.

Ludlow, C. (2006). Neuropharmacology of stuttering. In N. Bernstein Ratner & J. Tetnowski (Eds.), *Current issues in stuttering research and practice* (pp 239–54). Mahwah, NJ: Lawrence Erlbaum Associates.

Ludlow, C. L., & Loucks, T. (2003). Stuttering: a dynamic motor control disorder. *Journal of Fluency Disorders, 28,* 273–96.

Ludlow, C., Siren, K., & Zikria, M. (1997). Speech production learning in adults with chronic developmental stuttering. In W. Hulstijn, H. M. F. Peters, & P. H. H. M. v. Lieshout (Eds.), *Speech production: Motor control, brain research and fluency disorders. Proceedings from the 3rd international conference on speech motor production and fluency disorders* (pp. 221–30). Nijmegen: Nijmegen University Press.

Luessenhop, A. J., Boggs, J. S., LaBorwit, L. J., & Walle, E. L. (1973). Cerebral dominance in stutterers determined by Wada testing. *Neurology, 23,* 1190–92.

Luper, H. L. (1956). Consistency of stuttering in relation to the goal gradient hypothesis. *Journal of Speech and Hearing Disorders,* 21, 336–42.

Luper, H. L., & Chambers, J. L. (1962). An analysis of stutterers' responses to the *Picture Identification Test.* [Abstract]. *ASHA, 4,* 377.

Lybolt, J. T. (1986). Language disability and dysfluent speech in elementary school children. [Abstract]. *Folia Phoniatrica, 38,* 326–27.

MacCulloch, M. J., & Eaton, R. (1971). A note on reduced auditory pain threshold in 44 stuttering children. *British Journal of Disorders of Communication, 6,* 148–53.

MacCulloch, M. J., Eaton, R., & Long, E. (1970). The long term effect of auditory masking on young stutterers. *British Journal of Disorders of Communication, 5,* 165–73.

MacDonald, J. D., & Martin, R. R. (1973). Stuttering and disfluency as two reliable and unambiguous response classes. *Journal of Speech and Hearing Research, 16,* 691–99.

MacFarlane, W. B., Hanson, M., Walton, W., & Mellon, C. D. (1991). Stuttering in five generations of a single family. *Journal of Fluency Disorders, 16,* 117–23.

Macioszek, G. (1973). Die verzögerte akustische Rückmeldung bei Stotterern mit unterschied lichem Ausmass der Störung. *Zeitschr. für Klinische Psychol., 2,* 278–99.

MacKay, D. G. (1969). Effects of ambiguity on stuttering: Towards a theory of speech production at the semantic level. *Kybernetik, 5,* 195–208.

MacKay, D. G., & MacDonald, M. C. (1984). Stuttering as a sequencing and timing disorder. In R. F. Curlee & W. H. Perkins (Eds.), *Nature and treatment of stuttering: New directions* (pp. 261–82). San Diego: College-Hill Press.

Mackey, L. S., Finn, P., & Ingham, R. J. (1997). Effect of speech dialect on speech naturalness ratings: a systematic replication of Martin, Haroldson, and Triden (1984). *Journal of Speech, Language, and Hearing Research, 40,* 349–60.

Maclay, H., & Osgood, C. E. (1959). Hesitation phenomena in spontaneous English speech. *Word, 15,* 19–44.

MacLeod, J., Kalinowski, J., Stuart, A., & Armson, J. (1995). Effect of single and combined altered auditory feedback on stuttering frequency at two speech rates. *Journal of Communication Disorders, 28,* 217–28.

Maddox, J. (1938). Studies in the psychology of stuttering: VIII. The role of visual cues in the precipitation of moments of stuttering. *Journal of Speech Disorders, 3,* 90–94.

Madison, L. S., Budd, K. S., & Itzkowitz, J. S. (1986). Changes in stuttering in relation to children's locus of control. *Journal of Genetic Psychology, 147,* 233–40.

Madison, L., & Norman, R. D. (1952). A comparison of the performance of stutterers and nonstutterers on the *Rosenzweig Picture Frustration Test. Journal of Clinical Psychology, 8,* 179–83.

Maguire, G. A., Gottschalk, L. A., Riley, G. D., Franklin, D. L., Bechtel, R. J., & Ashurst, J. (1999). Stuttering: neuropsychiatric features measured by content analysis of speech and the effect of risperidone on stuttering severity. *Comprehensive Psychiatry, 40,* 308–14.

Maguire, G. A., Riley, G. D., Franklin, D. L., & Gottschalk, L. A. (2000). Risperidone for the treatment of stuttering. *Journal of Clinical Psychopharmacology, 20,* 479–82.

Maguire, G. A., Riley, G. D., Franklin, D. L., Maguire, M. E., Nguyen, C. T., & Brojeni, P. H. (2004). Olanzapine in the treatment of developmental stuttering: A double-blind, placebo-controlled trial. *Annals of Clinical Psychiatry, 16,* 63–67.

Maguire, G. A., Riley, G. D., & Yu, B. P. (2002). A neurological basis of stuttering? *Lancet, 1,* 407.

Maguire, G. A., Yu, B. P., Franklin, D. L., & Riley, G. D. (2004). Alleviating stuttering with pharmacological interventions. *Expert Opinion on Pharmacotherapy, 5,* 1565–71.

Mahl, G. F. (1956). Disturbances and silences in the patient's speech in psychotherapy. *Journal of Abnormal Social Psychology, 53,* 1–15.

Mahl, G. F. (1961). Measures of two expressive aspects of a patient's speech in two psychotherapeutic interviews. In L. A. Gottschalk (Ed.), *Comparative psycholinguistic analysis of two psychotherapeutic interviews.* New York: International University Press.

Mahr, G., & Leith, W. (1992). Psychogenic stuttering of adult onset. *Journal of Speech and Hearing Research, 35,* 283–86.

Mahr, G. C., & Torosian, T. (1999). Anxiety and Social Phobia in Stuttering. *Journal of Fluency Disorders, 24*(2), 119–26.

Makela, E. H., & Sullivan, P. (1996). "A case of sertraline-induced stuttering": Reply. *Journal of Clinical Psychopharmacology, 16,* 93.

Makela, E. H., Sullivan, P., & Taylor, M. (1994). Sertraline and speech blockage. *Journal of Clinical Psychopharmacology, 14,* 432–33.

Mallard, A. R. (1977). The effects of syllable-timed speech on stuttering behavior: An audiovisual analysis. *Behavior Therapist, 8,* 947–52.

Mallard, A. R. (1998). Using problem-solving procedures in family management of stuttering. *Journal of Fluency Disorders, 23,* 127–35.

Mallard, A. R., Hicks, D. M., & Riggs, D. E. (1982). A comparison of stutterers and nonstutterers in a task of controlled voice onset. *Journal of Speech and Hearing Research, 25,* 287–90.

Mallard, A. R., & Kelley, J. S. (1982). The precision fluency shaping program: Replication and evaluation. *Journal of Fluency Disorders, 7,* 287–94.

Mallard, A. R., & Meyer, L. A. (1979). Listener preferences for stuttered and syllable-timed speech production. *Journal of Fluency Disorders,* 4, 117–21.

Mallard, A. R., & Webb, W. G. (1980). The effects of auditory and visual "distractors" on the frequency of stuttering. *Journal of Communication Disorders, 13,* 207–12.

Mallard, A. R., & Westbrook, J. B. (1985). Vowel duration in stutterers participating in Precision Fluency Shaping. *Journal of Fluency Disorders,* 10, 221–28.

Mallard, A. R., & Westbrook, J. B. (1988). Variables affecting stuttering therapy in school settings. *Language Speech and Hearing Services Schools, 19,* 362–70.

Manaut-Gil, E. (2005). [Developmental stuttering and acquired stuttering: resemblances and differences]. *Revista de neurologia., 40,* 587–94.

Mann, M. B. (1955). Nonfluencies in the oral reading of stutterers and nonstutterers of elementary school age. In W. Johnson & R. R. Leutenegger (Eds.), *Stuttering in children and adults* (pp. 189–98). Minneapolis: University of Minnesota Press.

Manning, W. (2001). *Clinical decision-making in fluency disorders* (2nd ed.). Clifton Park, NY: Thomson-Delmar.

Manning, W. (2004). Review: Programmed therapy for stuttering in children and adults. *Journal of Fluency Disorders, 29,* 343–49.

Manning, W., Emal, K., & Jamison, W. (1975). Listener judgments of fluency: The effect of part word CV repetitions and neutral vowel substitutions. *Journal of Fluency Disorders, 1,* 18–23.

Manning, W. H., Burlison, A. E., & Thaxton, D. (1999). Listener response to stuttering modification techniques. *Journal of Fluency Disorders, 24,* 267–80.

Manning, W. H., & Cooper, E. B. (1969). Variations in attitudes of the adult stutterer toward his clinician related to progress in therapy. *Journal of Communication Disorders, 2,* 154–62.

Manning, W. H., & Coufal, K. J. (1976). The frequency of disfluencies during phonatory transitions in stuttered and nonstuttered speech. *Journal of Communication Disorders, 9,* 75–81.

Manning, W. H., Dailey, D., & Wallace, S. (1984). Attitude and personality characteristics of older stutterers. *Journal of Fluency Disorders, 9,* 207–15.

Manning, W. H., Lee, B. A., & Lass, N. J. (1978). The use of time-expanded speech in the identification of part-word repetitions of stutterers. *Journal of Communication Disorders, 11,* 11–15.

Manning, W. H., & Riensche, L. (1976). Auditory assembly abilities of stuttering and nonstuttering children. *Journal of Speech and Hearing Research, 19,* 77–83.

Manning, W. H., Trutna, P. A., & Shaw, C. K. (1976). Verbal versus tangible reward for children who stutter. *Journal of Speech and Hearing Disorders, 41,* 52–62.

Månsson, H. (2000). Childhood stuttering: incidence and development. *Journal of Fluency Disorders, 25,* 47–57.

Maraist, J. A., & Hutton, C. (1957). Effects of auditory masking upon the speech of stutterers. *Journal of Speech and Hearing Disorders, 22,* 385–89.

Market, K. E., Montague, J. C., Jr., Buffalo, M.D., & Drummond, S. S. (1990). Acquired stuttering: Descriptive data and treatment outcome. *Journal of Fluency Disorders, 15,* 21–33.

Marshall, R. C., & Neuburger, S. I. (1987). Effects of delayed auditory feedback on acquired stuttering following head injury. *Journal of Fluency Disorders, 12,* 355–65.

Martens, C. F., & Engel, D. C. (1986). Measurement of the sound-based word avoidance of persons who stutter. *Journal of Fluency Disorders, 11,* 241–50.

Martin, R. R. (1962). Stuttering and perseveration in children. *Journal of Speech and Hearing Research, 5,* 332–39.

Martin, R. R. (1965). Direct magnitude-estimation judgments of stuttering severity using audible and audible-visible speech samples. *Speech Monographs, 32,* 169–77.

Martin, R. R. (1981). Introduction and perspective: Review of published studies. In E. Boberg (Ed.), *Maintenance of fluency: Proceedings of the Banff Conference* (pp. 1–30). New York: Elsevier North-Holland.

Martin, R., & Gaviser, J. (1971). Time-out as a punishment for button pushing. *Journal of Speech and Hearing Research, 14,* 144–48.

Martin, R. R., & Haroldson, S. K. (1967). The relationship between anticipation and consistency of stuttered words. *Journal of Speech and Hearing Research, 10,* 323–27.

Martin, R. R., & Haroldson, S. K. (1969). The effects of two treatment procedures on stuttering. *Journal of Communication Disorders, 2,* 115–25.

Martin, R. R., & Haroldson, S. K. (1971). Time-out as a punishment for stuttering during conversation. *Journal of Communication Disorders, 4,* 15–19.

Martin, R. R., & Haroldson, S. K. (1975). Disfluencies of young children in private speech and in conversation. *Human Communication, 3,* 21–25.

Martin, R., & Haroldson, S. (1977). Effect of vicarious punishment on stuttering frequency. *Journal of Speech and Hearing Research, 20,* 21–26.

Martin, R., & Haroldson, S. K. (1979). Effects of five experimental treatments on stuttering. *Journal of Speech and Hearing Research, 22,* 132–46.

Martin, R. R., & Haroldson, S. K. (1981). Stuttering identification: Standard definition and moment of stuttering. *Journal of Speech and Hearing Research, 24,* 59–63.

Martin, R. R., & Haroldson, S. K. (1982). Contingent self-stimulation for stuttering. *Journal of Speech and Hearing Disorders, 47,* 407–13.

Martin, R. R., & Haroldson, S. K. (1988). An experimental increase in stuttering frequency. *Journal of Speech and Hearing Research, 31,* 272–74.

Martin, R. R., & Haroldson, S. K. (1992). Stuttering and speech naturalness: Audio and audiovisual judgments. *Journal of Speech and Hearing Research, 35,* 521–28.

Martin, R. R., Haroldson, S. K., & Kuhl, P. (1972a). Disfluencies in child-child and child-mother speaking situations. *Journal of Speech and Hearing Research, 15,* 753–56.

Martin, R. R., Haroldson, S. K., & Kuhl, P. (1972b). Disfluencies of young children in two speaking situations. *Journal of Speech and Hearing Research, 15,* 831–36.

Martin, R., Haroldson, S. K., & Triden, K. A. (1984). Stuttering and speech naturalness. *Journal of Speech and Hearing Research, 49,* 53–58.

Martin, R. R., Haroldson, S. K., & Woessner, G. L. (1988). Perceptual scaling of stuttering severity. *Journal of Fluency Disorders, 13,* 27–47.

Martin, R. R., Johnson, L. J., Siegel, G. M., & Haroldson, S. K. (1985). Auditory stimulation, rhythm, and stuttering. *Journal of Speech and Hearing Research, 28,* 487–95.

Martin, R. R., Kuhl, P., & Haroldson, S. (1972). An experimental treatment with two preschool stuttering children. *Journal of Speech and Hearing Research, 15,* 743–52.

Martin, R. R., Lawrence, B. A., Haroldson, S. K., & Gunderson, D. (1981). Stuttering and oral stereognosis. *Perceptual and Motor Skills, 53,* 155–62.

Martin, R., Parlour, S. F., & Haroldson, S. (1990). Stuttering and level of linguistic demand: The Stocker Probe. *Journal of Fluency Disorders, 15,* 93–106.

Martin, R., St. Louis, K., Haroldson, S., & Hasbrouck, J. (1975). Punishment and negative reinforcement of stuttering using electric shock. *Journal of Speech and Hearing Research, 18,* 478–90.

Martin, R. R., & Siegel, G. M. (1966a). The effects of response contingent shock on stuttering. *Journal of Speech and Hearing Research, 9,* 340–52.

Martin, R. R., & Siegel, G. M. (1966b). The effects of simultaneously punishing stuttering and rewarding fluency. *Journal of Speech and Hearing Research, 9,* 466–75.

Martin, R. R., & Siegel, G. M. (1969). The effects of a neutral stimulus (buzzer) on motor responses and disfluencies in normal speakers. *Journal of Speech and Hearing Research, 12,* 179–84.

Martin, R. R., Siegel, G. M., Johnson, L. J., & Haroldson, S. K. (1984). Sidetone amplification, noise, and stuttering. *Journal of Speech and Hearing Research, 276,* 518–27.

Martyn, M. M., & Sheehan, J. (1968). Onset of stuttering and recovery. *Behavior Research Therapy, 6,* 295–307.

Martyn, M. M., Sheehan, J., & Slutz, K. (1969). Incidence of stuttering and other speech disorders among the retarded. *American Journal of Mental Deficiency, 74,* 206–11.

Maske-Cash, W. S., & Curlee, R. F. (1995). Effect of utterance length and meaningfulness on the speech initiation times of children who stutter and children who do not stutter. *Journal of Speech and Hearing Research, 38,* 18–25.

Mast, V. R. (1952). Level of aspiration as a method of studying the personality of adult stutterers. [Abstract]. *Speech Monographs, 19,* 196.

Masters, R. S. W. (1992). Knowledge, knerves and know-how: The role of explicit versus implicit knowledge in the breakdown of complex motor skill under pressure. *British Journal of Psychology, 83,* 345–58.

Matoyan, D. S. (2001). Asymmetry of tactile perception and interhemispheric interactions in stutterers. *Human Physiology, 27,* 184–89.

Mattingly, S. C. (1970). The performance of stutterers and nonstutterers on two tasks of dichotic listening. [Abstract]. *ASHA,* 12, 427.

Max, L., & Caruso, A. J. (1998). Adaptation of stuttering frequency during repeated readings: associated changes in acoustic parameters of perceptually fluent speech. *Journal of Speech, Language, and Hearing Research, 41,* 1265–81.

Max, L., Caruso, A. J., & Gracco, V. L. (2003). Kinematic analyses of speech, orofacial nonspeech, and finger movements in stuttering and nonstuttering adults. *Journal of Speech, Language and Hearing Research, 46,* 215–33.

Max, L., Caruso, A. J., & Vandevenne, A. (1997). Decreased stuttering frequency during repeated readings: A motor learning perspective. *Journal of Fluency Disorders, 22,* 17–33.

Max, L., & Gracco, V. L. (2005). Coordination of oral and laryngeal movements in the perceptually fluent speech of adults who stutter. *Journal of Speech, Language and Hearing Research, 48,* 524–42.

Max, L., Guenther, F., Gracco, V., Ghosh, S., & Wallace, M. (2004). Unstable or insufficiently activated internal models and feedback-biased motor control as sources of dysfluency: A theoretical model of stuttering. *Contemporary Issues in Communication Sciences and Disorders, 31,* 105–22.

Max, L., & Yudman, E. M. (2003). Accuracy and variability of isochronous rhythmic timing across motor systems in stuttering versus nonstuttering individuals. *Journal of Speech, Language and Hearing Research, 46,* 146–64.

Maxwell, D. L. (1981). Social and vocational attitudes toward stuttering. *Proceedings of the 18th Congress of the International Association for Logopedics and Phoniatrics.* Washington, DC: American Speech and Language Hearing Association.

Maxwell, D. L. (1982). Cognitive and behavioral self-control strategies: Applications for the clinical management of adult stutterers. *Journal of Fluency Disorders, 7,* 403–32.

Maxwell, R. D. H., & Paterson, J. W. (1958). Meprobamate in the treatment of stuttering. *British Medical Journal,* No. 5075, 873–74.

May, A. E., & Hackwood, A. (1968). Some effects of masking and eliminating low frequency feedback on the speech of stammerers. *Behavior Research Therapy, 6,* 219–23.

Mayberry, R. I., Jaques, J., & DeDe, G. (1998). What stuttering reveals about the development of the gesture-speech relationship. *New Directions for Child Development,* 79, 77–87.

Mazzucchi, A., Moretti, G., Carpeggiani, P., Parma, M., & Paini, P. (1981). Clinical observations on acquired stuttering. *British Journal of Disorders of Communication, 16,* 19–30.

McAllister, A. H. (1937). *Clinical studies in speech therapy.* London: University of London Press.

McAllister, J., & Kingston, M. (2005). Final part-word repetitions in school-age children: Two case studies. *Journal of Fluency Disorders, 30,* 255–67.

McAuliffe, M., & Bernstein Ratner, N. (2007). In-the-canal auditory feedback device results in reduced stuttering 12-months post-fitting in a group of nine participants. *Evidence-Based Communication Assessment and Intervention,* 1, 27–29.

McCall, W. V. (1994). Sertraline-induced stuttering. *The Journal of Clinical Psychiatry, 55,* 316.

McClean, M. D. (1987). Surface recording of the perioral reflexes: Preliminary observations on stutterers and nonstutterers. *Journal of Speech and Hearing Research, 30,* 283–87.

McClean, M., Goldsmith, H., & Cerf, A. (1984). Lower-lip EMG and displacement during bilabial disfluencies in adult stutterers. *Journal of Speech and Hearing Research, 27,* 342–49.

McClean, M. D., Kroll, R. M., & Loftus, N. S. (1990). Kinematic analysis of lip closure in stutterers' fluent speech. *Journal of Speech and Hearing Research, 33,* 755–60.

McClean, M. D., Kroll, R. M., & Loftus, N. S. (1991). Correlation of stuttering severity and kinematics of lip closure. In H. F. M. Peters, W. Hulstijn, & C. W. Starkweather (Eds.), *Speech motor control and stuttering.* Amsterdam: Elsevier.

McClean, M.D., & McLean, A., Jr. (1985). Case report of stuttering acquired in association with phenytoin use for post-head-injury seizures. *Journal of Fluency Disorders, 10,* 241–55.

McClean, M. D., & Runyan, C. M. (2000). Variations in the relative speeds of orofacial structures with stuttering severity. *Journal of Speech, Language and Hearing Research, 43,* 1524–32.

McClean, M., & Tasko, S. (2004). Correlation of orofacial speeds with voice acoustic measures in the fluent speech of persons who stutter. *Experimental Brain Research, 159,* 310–18.

McClean, M. D., Tasko, S. M., & Runyan, C. M. (2004). Orofacial movements associated with fluent speech in persons who stutter. *Journal of Speech, Language and Hearing Research, 47,* 294–303.

McClure, J. A., & Yaruss, S. (2003). Stuttering survey suggests success of attitude-changing treatment. *ASHA Leader, 8,* 3.

McCroskey, R. L. (1957). Effect of speech on metabolism: A comparison between stutterers and nonstutterers. *Journal of Speech and Hearing Disorders, 22,* 46–52.

McDearmon, J. R. (1968). Primary stuttering at the onset of stuttering: A reexamination of data. *Journal of Speech and Hearing Research, 11,* 631–37.

McDevitt, S. C., & Carey, W. (1978). A measure of temperament in 3–7-year-old children. *Journal of Child Psychology and Psychiatry and Allied Disciplines 19,* 245–53.

McDonald, E. T., & Frick, J. V. (1954). Store clerks' reaction to stuttering. *Journal of Speech and Hearing Disorders, 19,* 306–11.

McDonald, J.D., Martin, R.R. (1973). Stuttering and Disfluency as Two Reliable and Unambiguous Response Classes, *Journal of Speech and Hearing Research, 16,* 691–699.

McDonough, A. N., & Quesal, R. W. (1988). Locus of control orientation of stutterers and nonstutterers. *Journal of Fluency Disorders, 13,* 97–106.

McDowell, E. D. (1928). *The educational and emotional adjustments of stuttering children.* New York: Columbia University of Teachers College.

McFarland, D. H., Smith, A., Moore, C. A., & Weber, C. M. (1986). Relationship between amplitude of tremor and reflex responses of the human jaw-closing system. *Brain Research, 366,* 272–78.

McFarlane, S. C., & Lavorato, A. S. (1983). Relationship between voice reaction time and stuttering severity. [Abstract]. *ASHA, 25,* 102.

McFarlane, S. C., & Prins, D. (1978). Neural response time of stutterers and nonstutterers in selected oral motor tasks. *Journal of Speech and Hearing Research, 21,* 768–78.

McFarlane, S. C., & Shipley, K. G. (1981). Latency of vocalization onset for stutterers and nonstutterers under conditions of auditory and visual cuing. *Journal of Speech and Hearing Disorders, 46,* 307–12.

McGee, S. R., Hutchinson, J. M., & Deputy, P. N. (1981). The influence of the onset of phonation on the frequency of disfluency among children who stutter. *Journal of Speech and Hearing Research, 24,* 269–72.

McGuire, R. A., Loren, C., & Rastatter, M. P. (1986). Naming reaction times to tachistoscopically presented pictures: Some evidence for right hemisphere encoding capacity. *Perceptual and Motor Skills, 62,* 303–06.

McHale, A. (1967). An investigation of personality attributes of stammering, enuretic and school-phobic children. *British Journal of Educational Psychology, 37,* 400–03.

McIntyre, M. E., Silverman, F. H., & Trotter, W. D. (1974). Transcendental meditation and stuttering: A preliminary report. *Perceptual and Motor Skills, 39,* 294.

McKay, K. M., Imel, Z. E., & Wampold, B. E. (2006). Psychiatrist effects in the psychopharmacological treatment of depression. *Journal of Affective Disorders, 92,* 287–90.

McKinnon, D., McLeod, S., & Reilly, S. (2007). The prevalence of stuttering, voice, and speech-sound disorders in primary school students in Australia. *Language, Speech, and Hearing Services in Schools, 38,* 5–15.

McKinnon, S. L., Hess, C. W., & Landry, R. G. (1986). Reactions of college students to speech disorders. *Journal of Communication Disorders, 19,* 75–82.

McKnight, R. C., & Cullinan, W. L. (1987). Subgroups of stuttering children: Speech and voice reaction times, segmental durations, and naming latencies. *Journal of Fluency Disorders, 12,* 217–33.

McLaughlin, S. F., & Cullinan, W. L. (1989). Disfluencies, utterance length, and linguistic complexity in non-stuttering children. *Journal of Fluency Disorders, 14,* 17–36.

McLean, A. E., & Cooper, E. B. (1978). Electromyographic indications of laryngeal-area activity during stuttering expectancy. *Journal of Fluency Disorders, 3,* 205–19.

McLean-Muse, A., Larson, C. R., & Gregory, H. H. (1988). Stutterers' and nonstutterers' voice fundamental frequency changes in response to auditory stimuli. *Journal of Speech and Hearing Research, 31,* 549–55.

McLelland, J. K., & Cooper, E. B. (1978). Fluency-related behaviors and attitudes of 178 young stutterers. *Journal of Fluency Disorders, 3,* 253–63.

McMillan, M. O., & Pindzola, R. H. (1986). Temporal disruptions in the "accurate" speech of articulatory defective speakers and stutterers. *Journal of Motor Behavior, 18,* 179–86.

Mehta, M. (1985). Comparison of abbreviated and full relaxation therapy in systematic desensitization of stutterers. *Journal of Personality and Clinical Studies, 1,* 7–10.

Meline, T. (2006). Selecting studies for systematic review: inclusion and exclusion criteria. *Contemporary Issues in Communication Sciences and Disorders, 33,* 21–27.

Mellon, C., Hanson, M., Hasstedt, S., Leppert, M., & White, R. (1991). *Early findings from the study of a large pedigree segregating a stuttering phenotype.* Paper presented at the Proceedings of the 8th International Congress of Human Genetics, Washington, DC

Melnick, K. S., & Conture, E. G. (2000). Relationship of length and grammatical complexity to the systematic and nonsystematic speech errors and stuttering of children who stutter. *Journal of Fluency Disorders, 25,* 21–45.

Melnick, K. S., Conture, E. G., & Ohde, R. N. (2003). Phonological priming in picture naming of young children who stutter. *Journal of Speech, Language and Hearing Research, 46,* 1428–43.

Meltzer, A. (1992). Horn stuttering. *Journal of Fluency Disorders, 17,* 257–64.

Meltzer, H. (1934). Personality differences among stutterers as indicated by the *Rorschach Test. American Journal of Orthopsychiatry, 4,* 262–80.

Meltzer, H. (1935). Talkativeness in stuttering and nonstuttering children. *Journal of Genetic Psychology, 46,* 371–90.

Meltzer, H. (1944). Personality differences between stuttering and nonstuttering children as indicated by the *Rorschach Test. Journal of Psychology, 17,* 39–59.

Menzies, R. G., Onslow, M., & Packman, A. (1999). Anxiety and stuttering: exploring a complex relationship. *American Journal of Speech-Language Pathology, 8,* 3–10.

Merits-Patterson, R., & Reed, C. G. (1981). Disfluencies in the speech of language-delayed children. *Journal of Speech and Hearing Research, 24,* 55–58.

Messenger, M., Onslow, M., Packman, A., & Menzies, R. (2004). Social anxiety in stuttering: measuring negative social expectancies. *Journal of Fluency Disorders, 29,* 201.

Metfessel, M., & Warren, N. D. (1934). Overcompensation by the non-preferred hand in an action-current study of simultaneous movements of the fingers. *Journal of Experimental Psychology, 17,* 246–56.

Métraux, R. W. (1950). Speech profiles of the pre-school child 18 to 54 months. *Journal of Speech and Hearing Disorders, 15,* 37–53.

Metz, D. E., Conture, E. G., & Caruso, A. (1979). Voice onset time, frication, and aspiration during stutterers' fluent speech. *Journal of Speech and Hearing Research, 22,* 649–56.

Metz, D. E., Conture, E. G., & Colton, R. H. (1976). Temporal relations between the respiratory and laryngeal systems prior to stuttered disfluencies [Abstract]. *ASHA, 18,* 664.

Metz, D. E., Onufrak, J. A., & Ogburn, R. S. (1979). An acoustical analysis of stutterers' speech prior to and at the termination of speech therapy. *Journal of Fluency Disorders, 4,* 249–54.

Metz, D. E., Samar, V. J., & Sacco, P. R. (1983). Acoustic analysis of stutterers' fluent speech before and after therapy. *Journal of Speech and Hearing Research, 26,* 531–36.

Metz, D. E., Schiavetti, N., & Sacco, P. R. (1990). Acoustic and psychopohysical dimensions of the perceived speech naturalness of nonstutterers and postreatment stutterers. *Journal of Speech and Hearing Disorders, 55,* 516–25.

Meyer, B. C. (1945). Psychosomatic aspects of stuttering. *Journal of Nervous and Mental Disorders, 101,* 127–57.

Meyer, V., & Mair, J. M. M. (1963). A new technique to control stammering: A preliminary report. *Behavior Research Therapy, 1,* 251–54.

Meyers, S. C. (1986). Qualitative and quantitative differences and patterns of variability in disfluencies emitted by preschool stutterers and nonstutterers during dyadic conversations. *Journal of Fluency Disorders, 11,* 293–306.

Meyers, S. C. (1989). Nonfluencies of preschool stutterers and conversational partners: Observing reciprocal relationships. *Journal of Speech and Hearing Disorders, 54,* 106–12.

Meyers, S. C. (1990). Verbal behaviors of preschool stutterers and conversational partners: Observing reciprocal relationships. *Journal of Speech and Hearing Disorders, 55,* 706–12.

Meyers, S. C., & Freeman, F. J. (1985a). Are mothers of stutterers different? An investigation of social-communicative interaction. *Journal of Fluency Disorders, 10,* 193–209.

Meyers, S. C., & Freeman, F. J. (1985b). Interruptions as a variable in stuttering and disfluency. *Journal of Speech and Hearing Research, 28,* 428–35.

Meyers, S. C., & Freeman, F. J. (1985c). Mother and child speech rates as a variable in stuttering and disfluency. *Journal of Speech and Hearing Research, 28,* 436–44.

Meyers, S. C., Hall, N. E., & Aram, D. M. (1990). Fluency and language recovery in a child with a left-hemisphere lesion. *Journal of Fluency Disorders, 15,* 159–73.

Meyers, S. C., Hughes, L. F., & Schoeny, Z. G. (1989). Temporal-phonemic processing skills in adult stutterers and nonstutterers. *Journal of Speech and Hearing Research, 32,* 274–80.

Miles, S., & Bernstein Ratner, N. (2001). Parental language input to children at stuttering onset.

Journal of Speech, Language and Hearing Research, 44, 1116–30.

Milisen, R. (1937). Expectancy reactions in stutterers. *Abstracts of the Proceedings of the American Speech Correction Association, 7,* 52–55.

Milisen, R. (1938). Frequency of stuttering with anticipation of stuttering controlled. *Journal of Speech Disorders, 3,* 2097–14.

Milisen, R., & Johnson, W. (1936). A comparative study of stutterers, former stutterers and normal speakers whose handedness has been changed. *Archives of Speech, 1,* 61–86.

Millard, S. K. (1998). The value of single subject research. *International Journal of Language and Communication Disorders, 33,* 370–74.

Miller, B., & Guitar, B. (2007, in press). Long-term outcome of the Lidcombe Program for early stuttering intervention. *American Journal of Speech-Language Pathology.*

Miller, J. A., & Miller, T. W. (1977). Adaptation effect in nonfluent speech behavior of controlled stutterers and nonstutterers. *Journal of Fluency Disorders, 2,* 305–10.

Miller, N. E. (1944). Experimental studies of conflict. In J. McV. Hunt (Ed.), *Personality and the behavior disorders.* New York: Ronald Press.

Miller, S., & Watson, B. C. (1992). The relationship between communication attitude, anxiety, and depression in stutterers and nonstutterers. *Journal of Speech and Hearing Research, 35,* 789–98.

Mills, A. W., & Streit, H. (1942). Report of a speech survey. Holyoke, Massachusetts. *Journal of Speech Disorders, 7,* 161–67.

Miltenberger, R. G., Wagaman, J. R., & Arndorfer, R. E. (1996). Simplified treatment and long term follow-up for stuttering in adults: A study of two cases. *Journal of Behavior Therapy and Experimental Psychiatry, 27,* 181–88.

Minifie, F. D., & Cooker, H. S. (1964). A disfluency index. *Journal of Speech and Hearing Disorders, 29,* 189–92.

Moleski, R., & Tosi, D. J. (1976). Comparative psychotherapy: Rational-emotive therapy versus systematic desensitization in the treatment of stuttering. *Journal of Consulting and Clinical Psychology, 44,* 309–11.

Molt, L. F. (1991). Selected acoustic and physiologic measures of speech motor coordination in stuttering and nonstuttering children. In H. F. M. Peters, W. Hulstijn, & C. W. Starkweather (Eds.), *Speech motor control and stuttering.* Amsterdam: Elsevier.

Molt, L. F., & Guilford, A. M. (1979). Auditory processing and anxiety in stutterers. *Journal of Fluency Disorders, 4,* 255–67.

Molt, L. F., & Luper, H. L. (1983). Latency of slow cortical auditory evoked responses in stutterers. [Abstract]. *ASHA, 25,* 164.

Moncur, J. P. (1952). Parental domination in stuttering. *Journal of Speech and Hearing Disorders, 17,* 155–65.

Moncur, J. P. (1955). Symptoms of maladjustment differentiating young stutterers from nonstutterers. *Child Development, 26,* 91–96.

Montgomery, A. A., & Cooke, P. A. (1976). Perceptual and acoustic analysis of repetitions in stuttered speech. *Journal of Communication Disorders, 9,* 317–30.

Montgomery, B. M., & Fitch, J. L. (1988). The prevalence of stuttering in the hearing-impaired school age population. *Journal of Speech and Hearing Disorders, 53,* 131–35.

Montgomery, C. S. (2006). The treatment of stuttering: From the hub to the spoke: Description and evaluation of an integrated therapy program. In N. Bernstein Ratner & J. Tetnowski (Eds.), *Current issues in stuttering research and practice* (pp. 159–204). Mahwah, NJ: Lawrence Erlbaum Associates.

Moore, M. A. S., & Adams, M. R. (1985). The Edinburgh masker: A clinical analog study. *Journal of Fluency Disorders, 10,* 281–90.

Moore, S. E., & Perkins, W. H. (1990). Validity and reliability of judgments of authentic and simulated stuttering. *Journal of Speech and Hearing Disorders, 55,* 383–91.

Moore, W. E. (1938). A conditioned reflex study of stuttering. *Journal of Speech Disorders, 3,* 163–83.

Moore, W. E. (1946). Hypnosis in a system of therapy for stutterers. *Journal of Speech Disorders, 11,* 117–22.

Moore, W. E. (1954). Relations of stuttering in spontaneous speech to speech content and to adaptation. *Journal of Speech and Hearing Disorders, 19,* 208–16.

Moore, W. E. (1959). A study of the blood chemistry of stutterers under two hypnotic conditions. *Speech Monographs, 26,* 64–68.

Moore, W. E., Soderberg, G., & Powell, D. (1952). Relations of stuttering in spontaneous speech to speech content and verbal output. *Journal of Speech and Hearing Disorders, 17,* 371–76.

Moore, W. H., Jr. (1976). Bilateral tachistoscopic word perception of stutterers and normal subjects. *Brain and Language, 3,* 434–42.

Moore, W. H., Jr. (1978). Some effects of progressively lowering electromyographic levels with feedback procedures on the frequency of stuttered verbal behaviors. *Journal of Fluency Disorders, 3,* 127–38.

Moore, W. H., Jr. (1984a). Central nervous system characteristics of stutterers. In R. F. Curlee & W. H. Perkins (Eds.) *Nature and treatment of stuttering: new directions* (pp. 49–72). San Diego: College-Hill.

Moore, W. H., Jr. (1984b). Hemispheric alpha asymmetries during an electromyographic biofeedback procedure for stuttering: A single-subject experimental design. *Journal of Fluency Disorders, 9,* 143–62.

Moore, W. H., Jr. (1986). Hemispheric alpha asymmetries of stutterers and nonstutterers for the recall and recognition of words and connected reading passages: Some relationships to severity of stuttering. *Journal of Fluency Disorders, 11,* 71–89.

Moore, W. H., Jr., & Boberg, E. (1987). Hemispheric processing and stuttering. In L. Rustin, H. Purser, & D. Rowley (Eds.), *Progress in the treatment of fluency disorders* (pp. 19–42). London: Taylor and Francis.

Moore, W. H., Jr., Craven, D. C., & Faber, M. M. (1982). Hemispheric alpha asymmetries of words with positive, negative, and neutral arousal values preceding tasks of recall and recognition: Electrophysiological and behavioral results from stuttering males and nonstuttering males and females. *Brain and Language, 17,* 211–24.

Moore, W. H., Jr., Cunko, C., & Flowers, P. (1979). Cumulative integrated electromyographic activity of selected speech-related muscle groups of nonstutterers during massed oral readings. *Journal of Fluency Disorders, 4,* 149–61.

Moore, W. H., Jr., Flowers, P., & Cunko, C. (1981). Some relationships between adptation and electromyographic activity at laryngeal and masseter sites in stutterers. *Journal of Fluency Disorders, 6,* 81–94.

Moore, W. H., Jr., & Haynes, W. O. (1980). Alpha hemispheric asymmetry and stuttering: Some support for a segmentation dysfunction hypothesis. *Journal of Speech and Hearing Research, 23,* 229–47.

Moore, W. H., Jr., & Lang, M. K. (1977). Alpha asymmetry over the right and left hemispheres of stutterers and control subjects preceding massed oral readings: A preliminary investigation. *Perceptual and Motor Skills, 44,* 223–30.

Moore, W. H., Jr., & Lorendo, L. C. (1980). Hemispheric alpha asymmetries of stuttering males and nonstuttering males and females for words of high and low imagery. *Journal of Fluency Disorders, 5,* 11–26.

Moore, W. H., Jr., & Ritterman, S. I. (1973). The effects of response contingent reinforcement and response contingent punishment upon the frequency of stuttered verbal behavior. *Behavior Research Therapy, 11,* 43–48.

Morávek, M., & Langová, J. (1962). Some electrophysiological findings among stutterers and clutterers. *Folia Phoniatrica, 14,* 305–16.

Morávek, M., & Langová, J. (1967). Problem of the development of the initial tonus in stuttering. *Folia Phoniatrica, 19,* 109–16.

Morgan, M. D., Cranford, J. L., & Burk, K. (1997). P300 event-related potentials in stutterers and nonstutterers. *Journal of Speech, Language, and Hearing Research, 40,* 1334–40.

Morgenstern, J. J. (1953). Psychological and social factors in children's stammering. Ph.D. Dissertation, University of Edinburgh.

Morgenstern, J. J. (1956). Socio-economic factors in stuttering. *Journal of Speech and Hearing Disorders, 21,* 25–33.

Morley, A. (1937). An analysis of associated and predisposing factors in the symptomatology of stuttering. *Psychology Monographs, 49,* 50–107.

Morley, M. E. (1952). A ten-year survey of speech disorders among university students. *Journal of Speech and Hearing Disorders, 17,* 25–31.

Morley, M. E. (1957). *The development and disorders of speech in childhood.* Edinburgh: Livingstone.

Morris, D. W. (1938). Position as a factor of attentional clearness in relation to stuttering. *Journal of Speech Disorders, 3,* 141–58.

Moser, H. M. (1938). A qualitative analysis of eye-movements during stuttering. *Journal of Speech Disorders, 3,* 131–39.

Moss, G. J., & Oakley, D. A. (1997). Stuttering modification using hypnosis: An experimental single-case study. *Contemporary Hypnosis, 14,* 126–31.

Moss, S. E. (1976). The influence of varying degrees of voicing on the adaptation effect in the repeated oral readings of stutterers. *Australian Journal of Human Communication Disorders, 4,* 127–32.

Mouradian, M. S., Paslawski, T., & Shuaib, A. (2000). Return of stuttering after stroke. *Brain and Language, 73,* 120–23.

Movsessian, P. (2005). Neuropharmacology of theophylline induced stuttering: The role of dopamine, adenosine and GABA. *Medical Hypotheses, 64,* 290–97.

Mowrer, D. (1975). An instructional program ot increase fluent speech of stutterers. *Journal of Fluency Disorders, 1,* 25–35.

Mowrer, D. E. (1978). Effect of audience reaction upon fluency rates of six stutterers. *Journal of Fluency Disorders, 3,* 193–203.

Mowrer, D. E. (1998). Alternative research strategies for the investigation of stuttering. *Journal of Fluency Disorders, 23,* 89–97.

Muellerleile, S. (1981). Portable delayed auditory feedback device: A preliminary report. *Journal of Fluency Disorders, 6,* 361–63.

Mulder, L. J. M., & Spierings, E. L. H. (2003). Stuttering relieved by divalproex sodium. *Neurology, 61,* 714.

Mulligan, H. F., Anderson, T. J., Jones, R. D., Williams, M. J., & Donaldson, I. M. (2001). Dysfluency and involuntary movements: a new look at developmental stuttering. *The International Journal of Neuroscience, 109,* 23–46.

Muma, J. R. (1971). Syntax of preschool fluent and disfluent speech: A transformational analysis. *Journal of Speech and Hearing Research, 14,* 428–41.

Murdoch, B. E., Killin, H., & McCaul, A. (1989). A kinematic analysis of respiratory function in a group of stutterers pre- and posttreatment. *Journal of Fluency Disorders, 14,* 323–50.

Muroi, A., Hirayama, K., Tanno, Y., Shimizu, S., Watanabe, T., & Yamamoto, T. (1999). Cessation of stuttering after bilateral thalamic infarction. *Neurology, 53,* 890–91.

Murphy, A. T. (1953). An electroencephalographic study of frustration in stutterers. [Abstract] *Speech Monographs, 20,* 148–49.

Murphy, A. T., & FitzSimons, R. M. (1960). *Stuttering and personality dynamics.* New York: Ronald Press.

Murphy, M. & Baumgartner, J. M. (1981). Voice initiation and termination time in stuttering and nonstuttering children. *Journal of Fluency Disorders, 6,* 257–64.

Murphy, W. (1999). A preliminary look at shame, guilt, and stuttering. In N. Bernstein Ratner & E. C. Healey (Eds.), *Stuttering research and practice: Bridging the gap.* (pp. 131–43). Mahwah, NJ: Lawrence Erlbaum Associates.

Murray, E. (1932). Dysintegration of breathing and eye-movements in stutterers during silent reading and reasoning. *Psychology Monographs, 43,* 218–75.

Murray, F. P. (1969). An investigation of variably induced white noise upon moments of stuttering. *Journal of Communication Disorders, 2,* 109–14.

Murray, H. L., & Reed, C. G. (1977). Language abilities of preschool stuttering children. *Journal of Fluency Disorders, 2,* 171–76.

Murray, K. S., Empson, J. A. C., & Weaver, S. M. (1987). Rehearsal and preparation for speech in stutterers: A psychophysiological study. *British Journal of Disorders of Communication, 22,* 145–50.

Murray, M. G., & Newman, R. M. (1997). Paroxetine for treatment of obsessive-compulsive disorder and comorbid stuttering. *The American Journal of Psychiatry, 154,* 1037.

Murray, T. J., Kelly, P., Campbell, L., & Stefanik, K. (1977). Haloperidol in the treatment of stuttering. *British Journal of Psychiatry, 130,* 370–73.

Myers, F. L. (1978). Relationship between eight physiological variables and severity of stuttering. *Journal of Fluency Disorders, 3,* 181–91.

Mysak, E. D. (1960). Servo theory and stuttering. *Journal of Speech and Hearing Disorders, 25,* 188–95.

Mysak, E. D. (1966). *Speech pathology and feedback theory.* Springfield, IL: Charles C. Thomas.

Nagafuchi, M., & Saso, S. (1986). Stuttering following stroke. [Abstract]. *Folia Phoniatrica, 38,* 333.

Nail-Chiwetalu, B. J., & Bernstein Ratner, N. (2006). Information literacy for speech-language pathologists: A key to evidence-based practice. *Language, Speech, and Hearing Services in Schools, 37,* 157–67.

Nail-Chiwetalu, B. J., & Bernstein Ratner, N. (2007). Assessment of the information-seeking abilities and needs of practicing speech-language pathologists. *Journal of the Medical Library Association, 95,*182–88.

Namasivayam, A., & Lieshout, P. H. H. M. v. (2004). Kinematic changes following static perturbation in people who stutter. In A. Packman, A. Meltzer, & H. F. M. Peters (Eds.), *Theory, research and therapy in fluency disorders* (pp. 331–38). Nijmegen: Nijmegen University Press.

Natke, U. (2000). Reduction of stuttering frequency using frequency-shifted and delayed auditory feedback [German]. *Folia Phoniatrica, 52,* 151–59.

Natke, U., Grosser, K. J., & Kalveram, T. (2001). Fluency, fundamental frequency, and speech rate under frequency-shifted auditory feedback in stuttering and nonstuttering persons. *Journal of Fluency Disorders, 26,* 227–41.

Natke, U., Grosser, K. J., Sandrieser, P., & Kalveram, K. T. (2002). The duration component of the stress effect in stuttering. *Journal of Fluency Disorders, 27,* 305–19.

Natke, U., Sandrieser, P., Pietrowsky, R., & Kalveram, K. T. (2006). Disfluency data of German preschool children who stutter and comparison children. *Journal of Fluency Disorders, 31,* 165–76.

Natke, U., Sandrieser, P., van Ark, M., Pietrowsky, R., & Kalveram, K. T. (2004). Linguistic stress, within-world position, and grammatical class in relation to early childhood stuttering. *Journal of Fluency Disorders, 29,* 109–22.

Naylor, R. V. (1953). A comparative study of methods of estimating the severity of stuttering. *Journal of Speech and Hearing Disorders, 18,* 30–37.

Neaves, A. I. (1970). To establish a basis for prognosis in stammering. *British Journal of Disorders of Communication, 5,* 46–58.

Neelley, J. N. (1961). A study of the speech behavior of stutterers and nonstutterers under normal and delayed auditory feedback. *Journal of Speech and Hearing Disorders, Supplement 7,* 63–82.

Neelley, J. N., & Timmons, R. J. (1967). Adaptation and consistency in the disfluent speech behavior of young stutterers and nonstutterers. *Journal of Speech and Hearing Research, 10,* 250–56.

Neilson, M., & Neilson, P. (1987). Speech motor control and stuttering: a computational model of adaptive sensory-motor processing. *Speech Communication, 6,* 325–33.

Neilson, M. D., & Neilson, P. D. (1979). Systems analysis of tracking performance in stutterers and normals. [Abstract]. *ASHA, 21,* 770.

Neilson, P. D., Andrews, G., Guitar, B. E., & Quinn, P. T. (1979). Tonic Stretch reflexes in lip, tongue, and Jaw muscles. *Brain Research, 178,* 311–27.

Neilson, P. D., & Neilson, M. D. (2005). An overview of adaptive model theory: Solving the problems of redundancy, resources, and nonlinear interactions in human movement control. *Journal of Neural Engineering, 2,* S279–312.

Neilson, P. D., Neilson, M. D., O'Dwyer, N. J., & Summers, J. J. (1992). Adaptive model theory: Application to disorders of motor control. In J. Summers (Ed.), *Approaches to the study of motor control and learning* (pp. 495–548). Amsterdam: North-Holland.

Neilson, P. D., Quinn, P. T., & Neilson, M. D. (1976). Auditory tracking measures of hemispheric asymmetry in normals and stutterers. *Australian Journal of Human Communication Disorders, 4,* 121–26.

Nelson, S. E. (1939). Personal contact as a factor in the transfer of stuttering. *Human Biology, 11,* 393–401.

Nelson, S. E., Hunter, N., & Walter, M. (1945). Stuttering in twin types. *Journal of Speech Disorders, 10,* 335–43.

Nessel, E. (1958). Die verzögerte Sprachrückkopplung (Lee Effekt) bei Stotterern. *Folia Phoniatrica, 10,* 199–204.

Netski, A. L., & Piasecki, M. (2001). Lithium-induced exacerbation of stutter. *The Annals of Pharmacotherapy, 35,* 961.

Neumann, K., Euler, H. A., Gudenberg, A. W. v., Giraud, A.-L., Lanfermann, H., Gall, V., et al. (2003). The nature and treatment of stuttering as revealed by fMRI: A within- and between-group comparison. *Journal of Fluency Disorders, 28,* 381–411.

Neumann, K., Preibisch, C., Euler, H. A., von Gudenberg, A. W., Lanfermann, H., Gall, V., et al. (2005). Cortical plasticity associated with stuttering therapy. *Journal of Fluency Disorders, 30,* 23–39.

Newman, L. L., & Smit, A. B. (1989). Some effects of variations in response time latency on speech rate, interruptions, and fluency in children's speech. *Journal of Speech and Hearing Research, 32,* 635–44.

Newman, P. W. (1954). A study of adaptation and recovery of the stuttering response in self-formulated speech. *Journal of Speech and Hearing Disorders, 19,* 450–58.

Newman, P. W. (1963). Adaptation performances of individual stutterers: Implications for research. *Journal of Speech and Hearing Research, 6,* 293–94.

Newman, P. W., Bunderson, K., & Brey, R. H. (1985). Brain stem electrical responses of stutterers and normals by sex, ears, and recovery. *Journal of Fluency Disorders, 10,* 59–67.

Newman, P. W., Channell, R., & Palmer, M. L. (1986). A comparative study of the independence of unilateral ocular motor control in stutterers and nonstutterers. *Journal of Fluency Disorders, 11,* 105–16.

Newman, P. W., Fawcett, K. D., & Russon, K. V. (1986). Cognitive processing in stuttering as related to translating slurvian. *Journal of Fluency Disorders, 11,* 251–56.

Newman, P. W., Harris, R. W., & Hilton, L. M. (1989). Vocal jitter and shimmer in stuttering. *Journal of Fluency Disorders, 14,* 87–95.

Newman, R., Bernstein Ratner, N., Jusczyk, A. M., Jusczyk, P. W., & Dow, K. A. (2006). Infants' early ability to segment the conversational speech signal predicts later language development: A retrospective analysis. *Developmental Psychology, 42,* 643–55.

Newman, R. S., & Bernstein Ratner, N. (2007). The role of selected lexical factors on confrontation naming accuracy, speed, and fluency in adults who do and do not stutter. *Journal of Speech, Language and Hearing Research, 50,* 196–213.

Newton, K. R., Blood, G. W., & Blood, I. M. (1986). Simultaneous and staggered dichotic word and digit tests with stutterers and nonstutterers. *Journal of Fluency Disorders, 11,* 201–16.

Nippold, M. A. (2001). Phonological disorders and stuttering in children: What is the frequency of co-occurrence? *Clinical Linguistics and Phonetics, 15,* 219–28.

Nippold, M. A. (2002). Stuttering and phonology: Is there an interaction? *American Journal of Speech-Language Pathology, 11,* 99–111.

Nippold, M. A. (2004). Phonological and language disorders in children who stutter: Impact on treatment recommendations. *Clinical Linguistics and Phonetics, 18,* 145–59.

Nippold, M. A., Schwarz, I. E., & Jescheniak, J.-D. (1991). Narrative ability in school-age stuttering boys: A preliminary investigation. *Journal of Fluency Disorders, 16,* 289–308.

Nissani, M., & Sanchez, E. A. (1997). Stuttering caused by gabapentin. *Annals of Internal Medicine, 126,* 410.

Norbut, C. A. (1976). Perception of specific disfluency types by normal-speaking children. [Abstract]. *ASHA, 18,* 631.

Norcross, K., & Andrews, G. (1973). Instruments for measuring stuttering. *Australian Journal of Human Communication Disorders, 1,* 47–49.

Norman, D. A., & Waugh, N. C. (1968). Stimulus and response interference in recognition memory experiments. *Journal of Experimental Psychology, 78,* 551–59.

Novák, A. (1975). Results of the treatment of severe forms of stuttering in adults. *Folia Phoniatrica, 27,* 278–82.

Novák, A. (1978). The influence of delayed auditory feedback in stutterers. *Folia Phoniatrica, 30,* 278–85.

Nowack, W. J., & Stone, R. E. (1987). Acquired stuttering and bilateral cerebral disease. *Journal of Fluency Disorders, 12,* 141–46.

Nuck, M. E., Blood, G. W., & Blood, I. M. (1987). Fluent and disfluent normal speakers' responses on a synthetic sentence identification (SSI) task. *Journal of Communication Disorders, 20,* 161–69.

Nudelman, H. B., Herbrich, K. E., Hess, K. R., & Hoyt, B. D. (1992). A model of the phonatory response time of stutterers and fluent speakers to frequency-modulated tones. *Journal of the Acoustical Society of America, 92,* 1882–88.

Nudelman, H. B., Herbrich, K. E., Hoyt, B. D., & Rosenfield, D. B. (1987). Dynamic characteristics of vocal frequency tracking in stutterers and nonstutterers. In H. F. M. Peters & W. Hulstijn (Eds.), *Speech motor dynamics in stuttering* (pp. 161–69). New York: Springer.

Nudelman, H. B., Herbrich, K. E., Hoyt, B. D., & Rosenfield, D. B. (1989). A neuroscience model of stuttering. *Journal of Fluency Disorders, 14,* 399–427.

Nutall, E. C., & Scheidel, T. M. (1965). Stutterers' estimates of normal apprehensiveness toward speaking. *Speech Monographs, 32,* 455–57.

Nwokah, E. E. (1988). The imbalance of stuttering behavior in bilingual speakers. *Journal of Fluency Disorders, 13,* 357–73.

O'Brian, S., Onslow, M., Cream, A., & Packman, A. (2003). The Camperdown Program: Outcomes of a new prolonged-speech treatment model. *Journal of Speech, Language and Hearing Research, 46,* 933–46.

O'Brian, S., Packman, A., & Onslow, M. (2004). Self-rating of stuttering severity as a clinical tool. *American Journal of Speech-Language Pathology, 13,* 219–26.

O'Brian, S., Packman, A., Onslow, M., Cream, A., O'Brian, N., & Bastock, K. (2003). Is listener comfort a viable construct in stuttering research? *Journal of Speech, Language and Hearing Research, 46,* 503–10.

O'Brian, S., Packman, A., Onslow, M., & O'Brian, N. (2003). Generalizability theory II: Application to perceptual scaling of speech naturalness in adults who stutter. *Journal of Speech, Language and Hearing Research, 46,* 718–23.

O'Brian, S., Packman, A., Onslow, M., & O'Brian, N. (2004). Measurement of stuttering in adults: comparison of stuttering-rate and severity-scaling methods. *Journal of Speech, Language, and Hearing Research, 47,* 1081–87.

Oelschlaeger, M. L., & Brutten, G. J. (1975). Response-contingent positive stimulation of the part-word repetitions displayed by four stutterers. *Journal of Fluency Disorders, 1,* 10–17.

Oelschlaeger, M. L., & Brutten, G. J. (1976). The effect of instructional stimulation on the frequency of repetitions, interjections, and words spoken during the spontaneous speech of four stutterers. *Behavior Therapist, 7,* 37–46.

Okalidou, A., & Kampanaros, M. (2001). Teacher perceptions of communication impairment at screening stage in preschool children living in Patras, Greece. *International Journal of Language and Communication Disorders, 36,* 489–502.

Okasha, A., Bishry, Z., Kamel, M., & Hassan, A. H. (1974). Psychosocial study of stammering in Egyptian children. *British Journal of Psychiatry, 124,* 531–33.

Okasha, A., Moneim, S. A., Bishry, Z., Kamel, M., & Moustafa, M. (1974). Electroencephalographic study of stammering. *British Journal of Psychiatry, 124,* 534–35.

O'Keefe, B. M., & Kroll, R. M. (1980). Clinicians' molar and molecular stuttering analyses of expanded and nonexpanded speech. *Journal of Fluency Disorders, 5,* 43–54.

Olsen, L. T., Steelman, M. L., Buffalo, M. D., & Montague, J. (1999). Preliminary information on stuttering characteristics contrasted between African American and White children. *Journal of Communication Disorders, 32,* 97–108.

Onslow, M. (2004). Ryan's programmed therapy for stuttering in children and adults. *Journal of Fluency Disorders, 29,* 351–60.

Onslow, M., Adams, R., & Ingham, R. (1992). Reliability of speech naturalness ratings of stuttererd speech during treatment. *Journal of Speech and Hearing Research, 35,* 994–1001.

Onslow, M., Andrews, C., & Lincoln, M. (1994). A control/experimental trial of an operant treatment for early stuttering. *Journal of Speech And Hearing Research, 37,* 1244–59.

Onslow, M., Bernstein Ratner, N., & Packman, A. (2001). Changes in linguistic variables during operant, laboratory control of stuttering in children. *Clinical Linguistics and Phonetics, 15,* 651–62.

Onslow, M., & Costa, L. (1996). Speech outcomes of a prolonged-speech treatment for stuttering. *Journal of Speech and Hearing Research, 39,* 734–50.

Onslow, M., Costa, L., Andrews, C., Harrison, E., & Packman, A. (1996). Speech outcomes of a prolonged-speech treatment for stuttering. *Journal of Speech and Hearing Research, 39,* 734–49.

Onslow, M., Costa, L., & Rue, S. (1990). Direct early intervention with stuttering: Some preliminary data. *Journal of Speech and Hearing Disorders, 55,* 405–16.

Onslow, M., Gardner, K., Bryant, K. M., Stuckings, C. L., & Knight, T. (1992). Stuttered and normal speech events in early childhood: The validity of a behavioral data language. *Journal of Speech and Hearing Research, 35,* 79–87.

Onslow, M., Hayes, B., Hutchins, L., & Newman, D. (1992). Speech naturalness and prolonged-speech treatments for stuttering: Further variables and data. *Journal of Speech and Hearing Research, 35,* 274–82.

Onslow, M., & Ingham, R. J. (1987). Speech quality measurement and the management of stuttering. *Journal of Speech and Hearing Disorders, 52,* 2–17.

Onslow, M., Menzies, R. G., & Packman, A. (2001). An operant intervention for early stuttering. *Behavior Modification, 25,* 116–40.

Onslow, M., O'Brian, S., Packman, A., Rousseau, I., & Bothe, A. K. (2004). Long-term follow up of speech outcomes for a prolonged-speech treatment for stuttering: The effects of paradox on stuttering treatment research. In A. Bothe (Ed.), *Evidence-based treatment of stuttering: Empirical bases and clinical applications* (pp. 231–44). Mahwah, NJ: Lawrence Erlbaum Associates.

Onslow, M., & Packman, A. (1997). Control of children's stuttering with response-contingent time-out: behavioral, perceptual, and acoustic data. *Journal of Speech, Language, and Hearing Research, 40,* 121–33.

Onslow, M., & Packman, A. (1999). The Lidcombe Program of early stuttering intervention. In N. Bernstein Ratner & E. C. Healey (Eds.), *Stuttering research and practice: Bridging the gap* (pp. 193–210). Mahwah, NJ: Lawrence Erlbaum Associates.

Onslow, M., & Packman, A. (2002). Stuttering and lexical retrieval: inconsistencies between theory and data. *Clinical Linguistics and Phonetics, 16*(4), 295–98.

Onslow, M., Packman, A., & Beer, T. (2003). The motor learning hypothesis and stuttering adaptation. *Asia Pacific Journal of Speech, Language and Hearing, 8,* 193–99.

Onslow, M., Packman, A., & Harrison, E. (2003). *The Lidcombe program of early stuttering intervention: A clinician's guide.* Austin, TX: Pro-Ed.

Onslow, M., van Doorn, J., & Newman, D. (1992). Variability of acoustic segment durations after prolonged-speech treatment for stuttering. *Journal of Speech and Hearing Research, 35,* 529–36.

Ooki, S. (2005). Genetic and environmental influences on stuttering and tics in Japanese twin children. *Twin Research and Human Genetics, 8,* 69–75.

Oomen, C. C. E., & Postma, A. (2001). Effects of divided attention on the production of filled pauses and repetitions. *Journal of Speech, Language and Hearing Research, 44*(5), 997–1004.

Ornstein, A. F., & Manning, W. H. (1985). Self-efficacy scaling by adult stutterers. *Journal of Communication Disorders, 18,* 313–20.

Orton, S., & Travis, L. E. (1929). Studies in stuttering: IV. Studies of action currents in stutterers. *Archives of Neurology and Psychiatry, 21,* 61–68.

Osawa, A., Maeshima, S., & Yoshimura, T. (2006). Acquired stuttering in a patient with Wernicke's aphasia. *Journal of Clinical Neuroscience, 13,* 1066–69.

Öst, L.-G., Götestam, K. G., & Melin, L. (1976). A controlled study of two behavioral methods in the treatment of stuttering. *Behavior Therapist, 7,* 587–92.

Ota, M., & Nagasawa, T. (2004a). Developmental features of the self-esteem of children who stutter: Comparison with the self-esteem of children who do not stutter. *Japanese Journal of Special Education, 42,* 259–70.

Ota, M., & Nagasawa, T. (2004b). Survey of the adolescent experience of adults who stutter: Implications for enhancing the positive self-evaluation of young children who stutter. *Japanese Journal of Special Education, 41,* 465–74.

Ota, M., & Nagasawa, T. (2005). Developmental features of the self-esteem of dhildren who stutter: Competence in school and discussions of stuttering with their family. *Japanese Journal of Special Education, 43,* 255–65.

Otto, F. M., & Yairi, E. (1975). An analysis of speech disfluencies in Down's syndrome and in normally intelligent subjects. *Journal of Fluency Disorders, 1,* 26–32.

Oxtoby, E. T. (1955). Frequency of stuttering in relation to induced modification following expectancy of stuttering. In W. Johnson & R. R. Leutenegger (Eds.), *Stuttering in children and adults.* Minneapolis: University of Minnesota Press.

Őzge, A., Toros, F., & Çömelekoglu, U. (2004). The role of hemispheral asymmetry and regional activity of quantitative EEG in children with stuttering. *Child Psychiatry and Human Development, 34,* 269–80.

Pachman, J. S., Oelschlaeger, M. L., Hughes, A., & Hughes, H. (1978). Toward identifying effective agents in use of biofeedback to decelerate stuttering behavior. *Perceptual and Motor Skills, 46,* 1006.

Packman, A., Kingston, M., Huber, A., Onslow, M., & Jones, M. (2003). Predicting treatment time with the Lidcombe Program: replication and meta-analysis. *International Journal of Language and Communication Disorders, 38,* 165–78.

Packman, A., & Lincoln, M. (1996). Early stuttering and the Vmodel. *Australian Journal of Human Communication Disorders, 24,* 45–52.

Packman, A., & Onslow, M. (1994). Prolonged speech and modification of stuttering: Perceptual, acoustic, and electroglottographic data. *Journal of Speech and Hearing Research, 37,* 724–38.

Packman, A., Onslow, M., & Menzies, R. (2000). Novel speech patterns and the treatment of stuttering. *Disability & Rehabilitation, 22*(1/2), 65–79.

Packman, A., Onslow, M., Richard, F., & van Doorn, J. (1996). Syllabic stress and variability: A model of stuttering. *Clinical Linguistics and Phonetics, 10,* 235–63.

Paden, E. (2005). Development of phonological ability. In E. Yairi & N. Ambrose (Eds.), *Early childhood stuttering: for clinicians by clinicians* (pp. 197–234). Austin, TX: Pro-Ed.

Paden, E. P., Ambrose, N. G., & Yairi, E. (2002). Phonological progress during the first 2 years of stuttering. *Journal of Speech, Language and Hearing Research, 45,* 256–68.

Paden, E. P., & Yairi, E. (1996). Phonological characteristics of children whose stuttering persisted or recovered. *Journal of Speech and Hearing Research, 39,* 981–91.

Paden, E. P., & Yairi, E. (1999). Early childhood stuttering II: initial status of phonological abilities. *Journal of Speech, Language and Hearing Research, 42,* 1113–25.

Palen, C., & Peterson, J. M. (1982). Word frequency and children's stuttering: The relationship to sentence structure. *Journal of Fluency Disorders, 7,* 55–62.

Palmer, M. F., & Gillette, A. M. (1938). Sex differences in the cardiac rhythms of stutterers. *Journal of Speech Disorders, 3,* 3–12.

Palmer, M. F., & Gillette, A. M. (1939). Respiratory cardiac arrhythmia in stuttering. *Journal of Speech Disorders, 4,* 133–40.

Palmer, M. F., & Osborn, C. D. (1940). A study of tongue pressures of speech defective and normal speaking individuals. *Journal of Speech Disorders, 5,* 133–40.

Panconcelli-Calzia, G. (1955). Die Bedingtheit des Lombardschen Versuches in der Stimm-und-Sprachheilkunde, *Acta Oto-Laryngolical, 45,* 244–51.

Panelli, C. A., McFarlane, S. C., & Shipley, K. G. (1978). Implications of evaluating and intervening with incipient stutterers. *Journal of Fluency Disorders, 3,* 41–50.

Paola Canevini, M., Chifari, R., & Piazzini, A. (2002). Improvement of a patient with stuttering on levetiracetam. *Neurology, 59,* 1288.

Pape-Neumann, J. (2004). [Results of the test-phase of PEVOS, Program for the Evaluation of Stuttering Therapia] [German]. *Forum Logopadie, 18,* 18–22.

Parker, C. S., & Christopherson, F. (1963). Electronic aid in the treatment of stammer. *Medical Electronics and Biological Engineering, 1,* 121–25.

Parker, H. T. (1932). *Defects of speech in school children.* Educational Research Series No. 15. Melbourne, Australia: Melbourne University Press.

Parson, B. S. (1924). *Lefthandedness.* New York: Macmillan.

Patterson, B. R., Neupauer, N. C., Burant, P., Koehn, S., & Reed, A. (1996). A preliminary examination of conversation analytic techniques: Rates of inter-transcriber. *Western Journal of Communication, 60,* 76–91.

Patterson, J., & Pring, T. (1991). Listener attitudes to stuttering speakers: No evidence for a gender difference. *Journal of Fluency Disorders, 16,* 201–05.

Pattie, F. A., & Knight, B. B. (1944). Why does the speech of stutterers improve in chorus reading? *Journal of Abnormal Social Psychology, 39,* 362–67.

Patty, J., & Quarrington, B. (1974). The effects of reward on types of stuttering. *Journal of Communication Disorders, 7,* 65–77.

Pauls, D. L., Leckman, J. F., & Coeh, D. J. (1994). Evidence against a genetic relationship between Gilles de la Tourette's syndrome and anxiety, depression, panic and phobic disorders. *British Journal of Psychiatry, 164,* 215–21.

Peacher, W. G., & Harris, W. E. (1946). Speech disorders in World War II: VIII. Stuttering. *Journal of Speech Disorders, 11,* 303–08.

Pearl, S. Z., & Bernthal, J. E. (1980). The effect of grammatical complexity upon disfluency behavior of nonstuttering preschool children. *Journal of Fluency Disorders, 5,* 55–68.

Peins, M. (1961a). Adaptation effect and spontaneous recovery in stuttering expectancy. *Journal of Speech and Hearing Research, 4,* 91–99.

Peins, M. (1961b). Consistency effect in stuttering expectancy. *Journal of Speech and Hearing Research, 4,* 397–98.

Peins, M., McGough, W. E., & Lee, B. S. (1972). Evaluation of a tape-recorded method of stuttering therapy: improvement in a speaking task. *Journal of Speech and Hearing Research, 15,* 364–71.

Peins, M., McGough, W. E., & Lee, B. S. (1984). Double tape recorder therapy for stutterers. In M. Peins (Ed.), *Contemporary approaches in stuttering therapy* (pp. 73–122). Boston: Little, Brown.

Pellowski, M. W., & Conture, E. G. (2002). Characteristics of speech disfluency and stuttering behaviors in 3- and 4-year-old children. *Journal of Speech, Language and Hearing Research, 45,* 20–35.

Pellowski, M. W., & Conture, E. G. (2005). Lexical priming in picture naming of young children who do and do not stutter. *Journal of Speech, Language and Hearing Research, 48,* 278–94.

Perino, M., Famularo, G., & Tarroni, P. (2000). Acquired transient stuttering during a migraine attack. *Headache, 40,* 170–72.

Perkins, D. (1947). An item by item compilation and comparison of the scores of 75 young adult stutterers on the *California Test of Personality.* [Abstract]. *Speech Monographs, 14,* 211.

Perkins, W., Rudas, J., Johnson, L., & Bell, J. (1976). Stuttering: Discoordination of phonation with articulation and respiration. *Journal of Speech and Hearing Research, 19,* 509–22.

Perkins, W. H. (1953). Stuttering as approach-avoidance behavior: A preliminary investigation. [Abstract]. *Speech Monographs, 20,* 149–50.

Perkins, W. H. (1969). Stuttering and discriminative awareness (SRS Research Grant RD-2275-S, Final Report). Washington, DC: Division of Research and Demonstration Grants, Social and Rehabilitation Services, Department of Health, Education, and Welfare.

Perkins, W. H. (1973a). Replacement of stuttering with normal speech: I. Rationale. *Journal of Speech and Hearing Disorders, 38,* 283–94.

Perkins, W. H. (1973b). Replacement of stuttering with normal speech: II. Clinical procedures. *Journal of Speech and Hearing Disorders, 38,* 295–303.

Perkins, W. H. (1979). From psychoanalysis to discoordination. In H. H. Gregory (Ed.), *Controversies about stuttering therapy.* Baltimore: University of Park Press.

Perkins, W. H. (1992). *Stuttering prevented.* San Diego: Singular Publishing Group.

Perkins, W. H. (undated). An alternative to automatic fluency. In J. F. Gruss (Ed.), *Stuttering therapy: Transfer and maintenance.* Memphis: Speech Foundation of America.

Perkins, W. H., Bell, J., Johnson, L., & Stocks, J. (1979). Phone rate and the effective planning time hypothesis of stuttering. *Journal of Speech and Hearing Research, 22,* 747–55.

Perkins, W. H., & Curlee, R. F. (1969). Clinical impressions of portable masking unit effects in stuttering. *Journal of Speech and Hearing Disorders, 34,* 360–62.

Perkins, W. H., & Hagen, C. (1965). The relation between frequency of stuttering and open expressions of aggression. [Abstract]. *ASHA, 7,* 391.

Perkins, W. H., Kent, R. D., & Curlee, R. F. (1991). A theory of neuropsycholinguistic function in stuttering. *Journal of Speech and Hearing Research, 34,* 734–52.

Perkins, W. H., Rudas, J., Johnson, L., Michael, W. B., & Curlee, R. F. (1974). Replacement of stuttering wtih normal speech: III. Clinical effectiveness. *Journal of Speech and Hearing Disorders, 39,* 416–28.

Perlmann, R., & Berko Gleason, J. (1993). The neglected role of fathers in children's communicative development. *Seminars in Speech and Language, 14,* 314–24.

Perozzi, J. A. (1970). Phonetic skill (sound-mindedness) of stuttering children. *Journal of Communication Disorders, 3,* 207–10.

Perozzi, J. A., & Kunze, L. H. (1969). Language abilities of stuttering children. *Folia Phoniatrica, 21,* 386–92.

Perrin, K. L., & Eisenson, J. (1970). An examination of ear preference for speech and nonspeech stimuli in a stuttering population. [Abstract]. *ASHA, 12,* 427.

Pešák, J. (2004). Preliminary experience with formoterol for the treatment of stuttering. *The Annals of Pharmacotherapy, 38,* 1323.

Pešák, J., & Opavský, J. (2000). Decreased serum copper level in developmental stutterers. *European Journal of Neurology, 7,* 748.

Peters, C. A. (1936). A study of mirror reading in speech defectives and normal speakers. *Archives of Speech, 1,* 48–60.

Peters, H. F. M., & Boves, L. (1987). Aerodynamic functions in fluent speech utterances of stutterers and nonstutterers in different speech conditions. In H. F. M. Peters & W. Hulstijn (Eds.), *Speech motor dynamics in stuttering* (pp. 229–44). New York: Springer.

Peters, H. F. M., & Boves, L. (1988). Coordination of aerodynamic and phonatory processes in fluent speech utterances of stutterers. *Journal of Speech and Hearing Research, 31,* 352–61.

Peters, H. F. M., Boves, L., & van Dielen, I. C. H. (1986). Perceptual judgment of abruptness of voice onset in vowels as a function of the amplitude envelope. *Journal of Speech and Hearing Disorders, 51,* 299–308.

Peters, H. F. M., & Hulstijn, W. (1984). Stuttering and anxiety: The difference between stutterers and nonstutterers in verbal apprehension and physiologic arousal during the anticipation of speech and non-speech tasks. *Journal of Fluency Disorders, 9,* 67–84.

Peters, H. F. M., & Hulstijn, W. (1987a). Programming and initiation of speech utterances in stuttering. In H. F. M. Peters & W. Hulstijn (Eds.), *Speech motor dynamics in stuttering* (pp. 185–96). New York: Springer.

Peters, H. F. M., & Hulstijn, W. (eds.) (1987b). *Speech motor dynamics in stuttering.* New York: Springer.

Peters, H. F. M., Hulstijn, W., & Starkweather, C. W. (1989). Acoustic and physiological reaction times of stutterers and nonstutterers. *Journal of Speech and Hearing Research, 32,* 668–80.

Peters, H. F. M., Hulstijn, W., & Starkweather, C. W. (eds.) (1991). *Speech motor control and stuttering.* Amsterdam: Elsevier.

Peters, H. F., Hulstijn, W., & Van Lieshout, P. H. (2000). Recent developments in speech motor research into stuttering. *Folia Phoniatrica, 52,* 103–19.

Peters, R. W., Love, L., Otto, D., Wood, T., & Benignus, V. (1976). Cerebral processing of speech and nonspeech signals by stutterers. *Proceedings of the XVI Congress of the International Society of Logopedics and Phoniatrics.* Basel: Karger.

Peters, R. W., & Simonson, W. E. (1960). Generalization of stuttering behavior through associative learning. *Journal of Speech and Hearing Research, 3,* 9–14.

Peters, T. J. (1968). Oral language skills of children who stutter. [Abstract]. *Speech Monographs, 35,* 325.

Peters, T. J., & Guitar, B. (1991). *Stuttering: An integrated approach to its nature and treatment.* Baltimore: Williams & Wilkins.

Petersen, S., Fox, P., Posner, M., Mintun, M., & Raichle, M. (1988). Positron emission tomographic studies of the cortical anatomy of single word processing. *Nature, 331,* 585–89.

Peterson, H. A. (1969). Affective meaning of words as rated by stuttering and nonstuttering readers. *Journal of Speech and Hearing Research, 12,* 337–43.

Peterson, H. A., Rieck, M. B., & Hoff, R. K. (1969). A test of satiation as a function of adaptation in stuttering. *Journal of Speech and Hearing Research, 12,* 110–17.

Petkov, D., & Iosifov, I. (1960). [Our experience with the treatment of stuttering in a treatment-logopedic camp]. *Zh. Nevropatol. Psikhiat., 60,* 903–04.

Petrosino, L., Fucci, D., Gorman, P., & Harris, D. (1987). Midline and off-midline tongue and right- and left-hand vibrotactile thresholds of stutterers and normal-speaking individuals. *Perceptual and Motor Skills, 65,* 253–54.

Phillips, P. P., & Myers, C. D. (1978). Peer-group social status of children who stutter. [Abstract]. *ASHA, 20,* 735.

Pienaar, W. D. (1968). Body awareness in certain types of speech defective individuals. *Journal of Projective Techniques and Personality Assessment, 32,* 537–41.

Pierce, C. M., & Lipcon, H. H. (1959). Stuttering: Clinical and electroencephalographic findings. *Military Medicine, 124,* 511–19.

Pindzola, R. H. (1986). Acoustic evidence of aberrant velocities in stutterers' fluent speech. *Perceptual and Motor Skills, 62,* 399–405.

Pindzola, R. H. (1987). Durational characteristics of the fluent speech of stutterers and nonstutterers. *Folia Phoniatrica, 39,* 90–97.

Pinsky, S. D., & McAdam, D. W. (1980). Electroencephalographic and dichotic indices of cerebral laterality in stutterers. *Brain and Language, 11,* 374–97.

Pitluk, N. (1982). Aspects of the expressive language of cluttering and stuttering children. *South African Journal of Communication Disorders, 29,* 77–84.

Pitrelli, F. R. (1948). Psychosomatic and Rorschach aspects of stuttering. *Psychiatric Quarterly, 22,* 175–94.

Pittenger, K. (1940). A study of the duration of temporal intervals between successive moments of stuttering. *Journal of Speech Disorders, 5,* 333–41.

Pizzat, F. J. (1951). A personality study of college stutterers. [Abstract]. *Speech Monographs, 18,* 240–41.

Plankers, T. (1999). Speaking in the claustrium: The psychodynamics of stuttering. *International Journal of Psychoanalysis, 80,* 239–56.

Platt, L. J., & Basili, A. (1973). Jaw tremor during stuttering block: An electromyographic study. *Journal of Communication Disorders, 6,* 102–09.

Platzky, R., & Girson, J. (1993). Indigenous healers and stuttering. *South African Journal of Communication Disorders, 40,* 43–48.

Plexico, L., Manning, W. H., & DiLollo, A. (2005). A phenomenological understanding of successful stuttering management. *Journal of Fluency Disorders, 30,* 1–22.

Podolskaya, O.V., & Shklovsky, V. M. (1973). Ob osobennostyakh nefermentativnoi fibrinolitichkoi aktivnosti i obrazovania kompleksov adrenalin-geparin i noradrenalin-geparin v krovi bolnikh logonervozom. *Zh. Nevropatol. Psikhiat., 73,* 711–15.

Ponsford, R. E., Brown, W. S., Marsh, J. T., & Travis, L. E. (1975). Evoked potential correlates of cerebral dominance for speech perception in stutterers and nonstutterers. [Abstract]. *Electroencephalography and Clinical Neurophysiology, 39,* 434.

Pool, K. D., Devous, M. D., Freeman, F. J., Watson, B. C., & Finitzo, T. (1991). Regional cerebral blood flow in developmental stutterers. *Archives of Neurology, 48,* 509–12.

Porfert, A. R., & Rosenfield, D. B. (1978). Prevalence of stuttering. *Journal of Neurology, Neurosurgery, and Psychiatry, 41,* 954–56.

Porter, H.V. K. (1939). Studies in the psychology of stuttering: XIV. Stuttering phenomena in relation to size and personnel of audience. *Journal of Speech Disorders, 4,* 323–33.

Porterfield, C. L. (1969). Adaptive mechanisms of young disadvantaged stutterers and nonstutterers. *Journal of Projective Techniques and Personality Assessment, 33,* 371–75.

Postma, A., & Kolk, H. (1990). Speech errors, disfluencies, and self-repairs of stutterers in two accuracy conditions. *Journal of Fluency Disorders, 15,* 291–303.

Postma, A., & Kolk, H. (1991). Manual reaction times and error rates in stutterers. *Perceptual and Motor Skills, 72,* 627–30.

Postma, A., & Kolk, H. (1992). Error monitoring in people who stutter: Evidence against auditory feedback theories. *Journal of Speech and Hearing Research, 35,* 1024–32.

Postma, A., & Kolk, H. (1993). The Covert Repair Hypothesis: prearticulatory repair processes in normal and stuttered disfluencies. *Journal of Speech and Hearing Research, 36,* 472–87.

Postma, A., Kolk, H., & Povel, D.J. (1990). Speech planning and execution in stutterers. *Journal of Fluency Disorders, 15,* 49–59.

Poulos, M. G., & Webster, W. G. (1991). Family history as a basis for subgrouping people who stutter. *Journal of Speech and Hearing Research, 34,* 5–10.

Prakash, B., Verghese, S. S., & Dhanaraj, G. E. (2002). Temporal dynamics in sound/syllable repetitions of stutterers and normal non-fluent children: a pilot investigation in Tamil. *Asia Pacific Disability Rehabilitation Journal, 13,* 29–37.

Preibisch, C., Neumann, K., Raab, P., Euler, H. A., von Gudenberg, A. W., Lanfermann, H., et al. (2003a). Evidence for compensation for stuttering by the right frontal operculum. *NeuroImage, 20,* 1356–65.

Preibisch, C., Raab, P., Neumann, K., Euler, H. A., von Gudenberg, A. W., Gall, V., et al. (2003b). Event-related fMRI for the suppression of speech-associated artifacts in stuttering. *NeuroImage, 19,* 1076–85.

Prescott, J. (1988). Event-related potential indices of speech motor programming in stutterers and nonstutterers. *Biological Psychology, 27,* 259–73.

Prescott, J., & Andrews, G. (1984). Early and late components of the contingent negative variation prior to manual and speech responses in stutterers and nonstutterers. *International Journal of Psychophysiology, 2,* 121–30.

Preus, A. (1972). Stuttering in Down's syndrome. *Scandanavian Journal of Educational Research, 16,* 89–104.

Preus, A. (1981). *Identifying Subgroups of Stutterers.* Oslo: Universitetsforlaget.

Preus, A. (1983). Nevrogen og psykogen stamming. *Nord. Tidsskr. Logoped. Foniat., 8,* 49–60.

Preus, A., Gullikstad, L., Grøtterød, H., Erlandsen, O., & Halland, J. (1970). En undersøkelse over forekomst av stamming i en lest tekst. *Norsk Tidsskr. Logoped., 16,* 11–18, 22.

Prins, D. (1968). Pre-therapy adaptation of stuttering and its relation to speech meaures of therapy progress. *Journal of Speech and Hearing Research, 11,* 740–46.

Prins, D. (1970). Improvement and regression in stutterers following short-term intensive therapy. *Journal of Speech and Hearing Disorders, 35,* 123–35.

Prins, D. (1972). Personality, stuttering severity, and age. *Journal of Speech and Hearing Research, 15,* 148–54.

Prins, D. (1976). Stutterers' perceptions of therapy improvement and of posttherapy regression: Effects of certain program modifications. *Journal of Speech and Hearing Disorders, 41,* 452–63.

Prins, D. (1983). Continuity, fragmentation, and tension: Hypotheses applied to evaluation and intervention with preschool disfluent children. In D. Prins & R. J. Ingham (Eds.), *Treatment of stuttering in early childhood* (pp. 21–42). San Diego: College-Hill Press.

Prins, D., & Beaudet, R. (1980). Defense preference and stutterers' speech disfluencies: Implications for the nature of the disorder. *Journal of Speech and Hearing Research, 23,* 757–68.

Prins, D., & Hubbard, C. P. (1988). Response contingent stimuli and stuttering: Issues and implications. *Journal of Speech and Hearing Research, 31,* 696–709.

Prins, D., & Hubbard, C. P. (1990). Acoustical durations of speech segments during stuttering adaptation. *Journal of Speech and Hearing Research, 33,* 494–504.

Prins, D., & Hubbard, C. P. (1992). Constancy of interstress intervals in the fluent speech of people who stutter during adaptation trials. *Journal of Speech and Hearing Research, 35,* 799–804.

Prins, D., Hubbard, C. P., & Krause, M. (1991). Syllabic stress and the occurrence of stuttering. *Journal of Speech and Hearing Research, 34,* 1011–16.

Prins, D., & Lohr, F. (1972). Behavioral dimensions of stuttered speech. *Journal of Speech and Hearing Research, 15,* 61–71.

Prins, D., Main, V., & Wampler, S. (1997). Lexicalization in adults who stutter. *Journal of Speech, Language and Hearing Research, 40,* 373–84.

Prins, D., Mandelkorn, T., & Cerf, F. A. (1980). Principal and differential effects of haloperiodol and placebo treatments upon speech disfluencies in stutterers. *Journal of Speech and Hearing Research, 23,* 614–29.

Prins, D., & McQuiston, B. (1964). Differential analysis of pre-therapy adaptation in stutterers and its relation to selected indicies of therapy progress. [Abstract]. *ASHA, 6,* 401.

Prins, D., & Miller, M. (1973). Personality, improvement, and regression in stuttering therapy. *Journal of Speech and Hearing Research, 16,* 685–90.

Prins, D., & Nichols, A. (1974). Client impressions of the effectiveness of stuttering therapy. A comparison of two programs. *British Journal of Disorders of Communication, 9,* 123–33.

Proceedings of the NIDCD Workshop on Treatment Efficacy Research in Stuttering (1993). September 21–22, 1992. *Journal of Fluency Disorders, 18,* 121–361.

Prosek, R. A., Montgomery, A. A., & Walden, B. E. (1988). Constancy of relative timing for stutterers and nonstutterers. *Journal of Speech and Hearing Research, 31,* 654–58.

Prosek, R. A., Montgomery, A. A., Walden, B. E., & Hawkins, D. B. (1987). Formant frequencies of stuttered and fluent vowels. *Journal of Speech and Hearing Research, 30,* 301–05.

Prosek, R. A., Montgomery, A. A., Walden, B. E., & Schwartz, D. M. (1979). Reaction-time measures of stutterers and nonstutterers. *Journal of Fluency Disorders, 4,* 269–78.

Prosek, R. A., & Runyan, C. M. (1982). Temporal characteristics related to the discrimination of stutterers' and nonstutterers' speech samples. *Journal of Speech and Hearing Research, 25,* 29–33.

Prosek, R. A., & Runyan, C. M. (1983). Effects of segment and pause manipulations on the identification of treated stutterers. *Journal of Speech and Hearing Research, 26,* 510–16.

Prosek, R. A., Walden, B. E., Montgomery, A. A., & Schwartz, D. M. (1979). Some correlates of stuttering severity judgments. *Journal of Fluency Disorders, 4,* 215–22.

Pukačová, M. (1973). Psychological characteristics of stuttering children. *Psychologia a Patopsychologia Dietata, 8,* 233–38.

Pukačová, M. (1974). Psychologické charakteristiky balbutikov. *DSH Abstracts, 14,* 308.

Purser, H., & Rustin, L. (1983). The psychology of treatment evaluation: Cognitive-behavioural treatment of adult dysfluency. [Abstract]. *Folia Phoniatrica, 34,* 165–66.

Putney, W. W. (1955). Characteristics of creative drawings for stutterers. Ph.D. Dissertation, Penn State University.

Quarrington, B. (1953). The performance of stutterers on the *Rosenzweig Picture-Frustration Test. Journal of Clinical Psychology, 9,* 189–92.

Quarrington, B. (1956). Cyclical variation in stuttering frequency and some related forms of variation. *Canadian Journal of Psychology, 10,* 179–84.

Quarrington, B. (1959). Measures of stuttering adaptation. *Journal of Speech and Hearing Research, 2,* 105–12.

Quarrington, B. (1962). Some psychological aspects of the adaptation phenomenon in stuttering. *DSH Abstracts, 2,* 355.

Quarrington, B. (1965). Stuttering as a function of the information value and sentence position of words. *Journal of Abnormal Psychology, 70,* 221–24.

Quarrington, B. (1974). The parents of stuttering children: The literature re-examined. *Canadian Psychiatric Association Journal, 19,* 103–10.

Quarrington, B., Conway, J., & Siegel, N. (1962). An experimental study of some properties of stuttered words. *Journal of Speech and Hearing Research, 5,* 387–94.

Quarrington, B., & Douglass, E. (1960). Audibility avoidance in nonvocalized stutterers. *Journal of Speech and Hearing Disorders, 25,* 358–65.

Quarrington, B., Seligman, J., & Kosower, E. (1969). Goal setting behavior of parents of beginning stutterers and parents of nonstuttering children. *Journal of Speech and Hearing Research, 12,* 435–42.

Quesal, R. W. (1988). Inexact use of "disfluency" and "dysfluency" in stuttering research. *Journal of Speech and Hearing Disorders, 53,* 349–51.

Quesal, R. W., & Shank, K. H. (1978). Stutterers and others: A comparison of communication attitudes. *Journal of Fluency Disorders, 3,* 247–52.

Quinan, C. (1921). Sinistrality in relation to high blood pressure and defects of speech. *Archives of International Medicine, 27,* 255–61.

Quinn, P. T. (1971). Stuttering: Some observations on speaking when alone. *Journal of the Australian College of Speech Therapists, 21,* 92–94.

Quinn, P. T. (1972). Stuttering: Cerebral dominance and the dichotic word test. *Medical Journal of Australia, 2,* 639–43.

Quinn, P. T. (1976). Cortical localization of speech in normals and stutterers. *Australian Journal of Human Communication Disorders, 4,* 118–20.

Quinn, P. T., & Andrews, G. (1976). Speech-related middle ear muscle activity in normal speakers and stutterers. *Australian Journal of Human Communication Disorders, 4,* 117.

Quinn, P. T., & Andrews, G. (1977). Neurological stuttering—A clinical entity? *Journal of Neurology, Neurosurgery, & Psychiatry, 40,* 699–701.

Quinn, P. T., & Peachey, E. C. (1973). Haloperidol in the treatment of stutterers. *British Journal of Psychiatry, 123,* 247–48.

Quist, R. W., & Martin, R. R. (1967). The effect of response contingent verbal punishment on stuttering. *Journal of Speech and Hearing Research, 10,* 795–800.

Raczek, B., & Adamczyk, B. (2004). Concentration of carbon dioxide in exhaled air in fluent and nonfluent speech. *Folia Phoniatrica, 56,* 75–82.

Ragsdale, J. D., & Ashby, J. K. (1982). Speech-language pathologists' connotations of stuttering. *Journal of Speech and Hearing Research, 25,* 75–80.

Ragsdale, J. D., & Sisterhen, D. H. (1984). Hesitation phenomena in the spontaneous speech of normal and articulatory-defective children. *Language and Speech, 27,* 235–44.

Rahman, P. (1956), The self-concept and ideal self-concept of stutterers as compared to nonstutterers. M. A. Thesis, Brooklyn College.

Ralston, L. D. (1981). Stammering: A stress index in Caribbean classrooms. *Journal of Fluency Disorders, 6,* 119–33.

Rami, M. K., & Diederich, E. (2005). Effect of reading with reversed speech on frequency of stuttering in adults. *Perceptual and Motor Skills, 100,* 387–93.

Rami, M. K., Kalinowski, J., Rastatter, M. P., Holbert, D., & Allen, M. (2005). Choral reading with filtered speech: effect on stuttering. *Perceptual and Motor Skills, 100,* 421–31.

Ramig, P. R. (1993). High reported spontaneous stuttering recovery rates: fact or fiction? *Language, Speech, and Hearing Services in Schools, 24,* 156–60.

Ramig, P., & Adams, M. R. (1980). Rate reduction strategies used by stutterers and nonstutterers during high- and low-pitched speech. *Journal of Fluency Disorders, 5,* 27–41.

Ramig, P. R., & Adams, M. R. (1981). Vocal changes in stutterers and nonstutterers during high- and low-pitched speech. *Journal of Fluency Disorders, 6,* 15–33.

Ramig, P., Ellis, J., & Pollard, R. (1997). Application of the SpeechEasy to stuttering treatment: Introduction, background, and preliminary observations. In B. Guitar & R. J. McCauley (Eds.), *Stuttering Treatment: Established and Emerging Approaches.* Baltimore: Lippincott, Williams & Wilkins.

Ramig, P. R., Krieger, S. M., & Adams, M. R. (1982). Vocal changes in stutterers and nonstutterers when speaking to children. *Journal of Fluency Disorders, 7,* 369–84.

Randoll, D. (1988). Erfahrungen und Ergebnisse bei der Anwendung des Systematic Fluency Training for Young Children (SFTYC) von R. E. Shine. *Sprachheilarb., 33,* 227–40.

Rantalaka, S.-L., & Petri-Larmi, M. (1976). Haloperidol (Serenase) in the treatment of stuttering. *Folia Phoniatrica, 28,* 354–61.

Rapaport, D. (1946). *Diagnostic psychological testing.* Chicago: The Yearbook Publishers.

Rappaport, B., & Bloodstein, O. (1971). The role of random blackout cues in the distribution of moments of stuttering. *Journal of Speech and Hearing Research, 14,* 874–79.

Rastatter, M., & Dell, C. W. (1985). Simple motor and phonemic processing reaction times of stutterers. *Perceptual and Motor Skills, 61,* 463–66.

Rastatter, M. P., & Dell, C. W. (1987a). Reaction times of moderate and severe stutterers to monaural verbal stimuli: Some implications for neurolinguistic organization. *Journal of Speech and Hearing Research, 30,* 21–27.

Rastatter, M. P., & Dell, C. W. (1987b). Simple visual versus lexical decision vocal reaction times of stuttering and normal subjects. *Journal of Fluency Disorders, 12,* 63–69.

Rastatter, M. P., & Dell, C. (1987c). Vocal reaction times of stuttering subjects to tachistoscopically presented concrete and abstract words: A closer look at cerebral dominance and language processing. *Journal of Speech and Hearing Research, 30,* 306–10.

Rastatter, M. P., & Dell, C. W. (1988). Reading reaction times of stuttering and nonstuttering subjects to unilaterally presented concrete and abstract words. *Journal of Fluency Disorders, 13,* 319–29.

Rastatter, M. P., & Harr, R. (1988). Measurements of plasma levels of adrenergic neurotransmitters and primary amino acids in five stuttering subjects: A preliminary report (biochemical aspects of stuttering). *Journal of Fluency Disorders, 13,* 127–39.

Rastatter, M. P., & Loren, C. A. (1988). Visual coding dominance in stuttering: Some evidence from central tachistoscopic stimulation (tachistoscopic viewing and stuttering). *Journal of Fluency Disorders, 13,* 89–95.

Rastatter, M. P., Loren, C., & Colcord, R. (1987). Visual coding strategies and hemispheric dominance characteristics of stutterers. *Journal of Fluency Disorders, 12,* 305–15.

Rastatter, M. P., McGuire, R. A., & Loren, C. (1988). Linguistic encoding dominance in stuttering: Some evidence for temporal and qualitative hemispheric processing differences. *Journal of Fluency Disorders, 13,* 215–24.

Rastatter, M. P., Stuart, A., & Kalinowski, J. (1998). Quantitative electroencephalogram of posterior cortical areas of fluent and stuttering participants during reading with normal and altered auditory feedback. *Perceptual and Motor Skills, 87,* 623–33.

Ratcliff-Baird, B. J. (1997). *EEG activation patterns in the frontal lobes of stutterers and nonstutterers during working memory tasks.* ProQuest Information & Learning, US.

Ratcliff-Baird, B. (2001). ADHD and stuttering: Similar EEG profiles suggest neurotherapy as an adjunct to traditional speech therapies. *Journal of Neurotherapy,* 5, 5–22.

Ratusnik, D. L., Kiriluk, E., & Ratusnik, C. M. (1979). Relationship among race, social status, and sex of preschoolers' normal dysfluencies: A cross-cultural investigation. *Language, Speech and Hearing Services in Schools, 10,* 171–77.

Razdolsky, V. A. (1965). O sostoyanii rechi v odinochestve u zaikayushchikhsya. *Zh. Nevropatol. Psikhiat., 65,* 1717–20.

Records, M. A., Heimbuch, R. C., & Kidd, K. K. (1977). Handedness and stuttering: A dead horse? *Journal of Fluency Disorders, 2*, 271–82.

Redwine, G. W. (1959). An experimental study of relationships between self-concepts of fourth and eighth grade stuttering and nonstuttering boys. [Abstract]. *Speech Monographs, 26,* 140–41.

Reed, C. G., & Godden, A. L. (1977). An experimental treatment using verbal punishment with two preschool stutterers. *Journal of Fluency Disorders, 2,* 225–33.

Reed, C. G., & Lingwall, J. B. (1976). Some relationships between punishment, stuttering, and galvanic skin responses. *Journal of Speech and Hearing Research, 19,* 197–205.

Reed, C. G., & Lingwall, J. B. (1980). Conditioned stimulus effects on stuttering and GSRs. *Journal of Speech and Hearing Research, 23,* 336–43.

Reeves, L. (2006). The role of self-help/mutual aid in addressing the needs of individuals who stutter. In N. B. Ratner & J. Tetnowski (Eds.), *Current issues in stuttering research and practice* (pp. 255–78). Mahwah, NJ: Lawrence Erlbaum Associates.

Reich, A., Till, J., & Goldsmith, H. (1981). Laryngeal and manual reaction times of stuttering and nonstuttering adults. *Journal of Speech and Hearing Research, 24,* 192–96.

Reimann, A. (1976). Phonetische Untersuchungen über lautabhängige Vokallängen im Sprechen redgestörter Jugendlicher. *Sprachheilarb., 21,* 1–14.

Reis, R., & Adams, M. R. (1978). Comments on "The Adams and Reis Observations Revisited." *Journal of Fluency Disorders, 3,* 299–302.

Rentschler, G. J., Driver, L. E., & Callaway, E. A. (1984). The onset of stuttering following drug overdose. *Journal of Fluency Disorders, 9,* 265–84.

Rescorla, L., & Achenbach, T. M. (2002). Use of the Language Development Survey (LDS) in a national probability sample of children 18 to 35 months old. *Journal of Speech, Language and Hearing Research, 45,* 733–44.

Rescorla, L., & Bernstein Ratner, N. (1996). Phonetic profiles of toddlers with specific expressive language impairment (SLI-E). *Journal of Speech and Hearing Research, 3* 153.

Resick, P. A., Wendiggensen, P., Ames, S., & Meyer, V. (1978). Systematic slowed speech: A new treatment for stuttering. *Behavior Research Therapy, 16,* 161–67.

Resnick, S., & Tureen, P. (1990). Evaluation of fluent and disfluent speech segments by stutters and nonstutterers. *Journal of Fluency Disorders, 15,* 1–8.

Rheinberger, M. B., Karlin, I. W., & Berman, A. B. (1943). Electroencephalographic and laterality studies of stuttering and nonstuttering children. *Nervous Child, 2,* 117–33.

Rhodes R., Shames, G., & Egolf, D. (1971). "Awareness" in verbal conditoning of language themes during therapy with stutterers. *Journal of Communication Disorders, 4,* 30–39.

Riaz, N., Steinberg, S., Ahmad, J., Pluzhnikov, A., Riazuddin, S., Cox, N., et al. (2005). Genomewide significant linkage to stuttering on chromosome 12. *American Journal of Human Genetics, 76,* 647–51.

Richardson, LaV. H. (1944). A personality study of stutterers and non-stutterers. *Journal of Speech Disorders, 9,* 152–60.

Richter, E. (1982). Ein Beitrag zur Ätiologie des Stotterns. *Sprachheilarb., 27,* 239–45.

Rickard, H. C., & Mundy, M. B. (1965). Direct manipulation of stuttering behavior: An experimental-clinical approach. In L. P. Ullmann & L. Krasner (Eds.), *Case studies in behavior modification.* New York: Holt, Rinehart and Winston.

Rieber, R. W. (1975). A study in psycholinguistics and communication disorders. *Linguistics, 160,* 33–70.

Rieber, R. W., Breskini, S., & Jaffe, J. (1972). Pause time and phonation time in stuttering and cluttering. *Journal of Psycholinguistic Research, 1,* 149–54.

Rieber, R. W., Smith, N., & Harris, B. (1976). Neuropsychological aspects of stuttering and cluttering. In R. W. Rieber (Ed.), *The neuropsychology of language.* (pp. 45–66). New York: Plenum Press.

Rieber, R. W., & Wollock, J. (1977). The historical roots of the theory and therapy of stuttering. *Journal of Communication Disorders, 10,* 3–24.

Riley, G. D. (1972). A stuttering severity instrument for children and adults. *Journal of Speech and Hearing Disorders, 37,* 314–20.

Riley, G. D., & Ingham, J. C. (2000). Acoustic duration changes associated with two types of treatment for children who stutter. *Journal of Speech, Language and Hearing Research, 43,* 965–79.

Riley, G. D., & Riley, J. (1980). Motoric and linguistic variables among children who stutter: A factor analysis. *Journal of Speech and Hearing Disorders, 45,* 504–14.

Riley, G. D., & Riley, J. (1984). A component model for treating stuttering in children. In M. Peins (Ed.), *Contemporary approaches in stuttering therapy* (pp. 123–72). Boston: Little, Brown.

Riley, G., & Riley, J. (1986). Oral motor discoordination among children who stutter. *Journal of Fluency Disorders, 11,* 335–44.

Riley, G., & Riley, J. (1991). Treatment implications of oral motor discoordination. In H. F. M. Peters, W. Hulstijn, & C. W. Starkweather (Eds.), *Speech motor control and stuttering.* Amsterdam: Elsevier.

Riley, J. (1983). High self-expectations: Comparing stuttering to dysarticulating children. [Abstract]. *ASHA, 25,* 160.

Riley, J., & Riley, G. (1999). Speech motor training. In M. Onslow & A. Packman (Eds.), *The handbook of early stuttering intervention* (pp. 139–58). San Diego: Singular.

Riley, J., Riley, G., & Maguire, G. (2004). Subjective Screening of Stuttering Severity, locus of control and avoidance: Research edition. *Journal of Fluency Disorders, 29,* 51–63.

Ringel, R. L., & Minifie, F. D. (1966). Protensity estimates of stutterers and nonstutterers. *Journal of Speech and Hearing Research, 9,* 289–96.

Ritterman, S. I., & Reidenbach, J. W., Jr. (1975). Interdigital variability in the palmer sweat indices of adult stutterers. *Journal of Fluency Disorders, 1,* 33–46.

Ritzman, C. H. (1943). A cardiovascular and metabolic study of stutterers and nonstutterers. *Journal of Speech Disorders, 8,* 161–82.

Robb, M., & Blomgren, M. (1997). Analysis of F2 transitions in the speech of stutterers and nonstutterers. *Journal of Fluency Disorders, 22,* 1–16.

Robb, M. P., Lybolt, J. T., & Price, H. A. (1985). Acoustic measures of stutterers' speech following an intensive therapy program. *Journal of Fluency Disorders, 10,* 269–79.

Robbins, M. G. (1971). The effect of varying conditions of rehearsal on the frequency of stuttering. Ph. D. Dissertation, City University of New York.

Robbins, S. D. (1920). A plethysmographic study of shock and stammering in a trephined stammerer. *American Journal of Physiology, 52,* 168–81.

Robbins, S. D. (1935). The role of rhythm in the correction of stammering. *Quarterly Journal of Speech, 21,* 331–43.

Roberts, P. M. (2002). Disfluency patterns in four bilingual adults who stutter. *Journal of Speech-Language Pathology and Audiology, 26,* 5–19.

Roberts, P., & Shenker, R. (2007). Assessment and treatment of stuttering in bilingual speakers. In E. G. Conture & R. Curlee (Eds.), *Stuttering and related disorders of fluency* (3rd ed.) (pp. 183–210). New York: Thieme.

Robey, R. R. (1976). An investigation of the validity of the *Iowa Scale of Attitude Toward Stuttering* in terms of social desirability and acquiescent response set intrusion. [Abstract]. *ASHA, 18,* 682.

Robey, R. R. (2004). A five-phase model for clinical-outcome reseach. *Journal of Communication Disorders, 37,* 401–11.

Robinson, T. L., Jr., & Crowe, T. A. (1998). Culture-based considerations in programming for stuttering intervention with African American clients and their families. *Language, Speech, and Hearing Services in Schools, 29,* 172–79.

Roland, B. C. (1972). Eye-movements of stutterers and nonstutterers during silent, oral, and choral reading. *Perceptual and Motor Skills, 35,* 297–98.

Roman, K. G. (1960). Handwriting and speech. In D. A. Barbara (Ed.), *Psychological aspects of speech and hearing.* Springfield, IL: Charles C. Thomas.

Rommel, D., Häge, A., Kalehne, P., & Johannsen, H. (2000). Development, maintenance and recovery in childhood stuttering: prospective longitudinal data three years after first contact. In K. Baker, L. Rustin, & F. Cook (Eds.), *Proceedings of the Fifth Oxford Dysfluency Conference* (pp. 168–82). Windsor: Chappell Gardner.

Ronson, I. (1975). Linguistic cues in stuttering: Selected sentence types and the anticipatory struggle hypothesis. *Journal of Speech and Hearing Research, 7,* 38–45.

Ronson, I. (1976). Word frequency and stuttering: The relationship to sentence structure. *Journal of Speech and Hearing Research, 19,* 813–19.

Root, A. R. (1926). A survey of speech defectives in the public elementary schools of South Dakota. *Elementary School Journal, 26,* 531–41.

Rosen, S., & Ludlow, C. L. (1990). Treatment of speech and voice disorders with botulinum toxin. *Journal of the American Medical Association, 264,* 2671–76.

Rosenbek, J. C. (1984). Stuttering secondary to nervous system damage. In R. F. Curlee & W. H. Perkins (Eds.), *Nature and treatment of stuttering: new directions* (pp. 31–48). San Diego: College-Hill Press.

Rosenbek, J., Messert, B., Collins, M., & Wertz, R. T. (1978). Stuttering following brain damage. *Brain and Language, 6,* 82–96.

Rosenberg, S., & Curtiss, J. (1944). The effect of stuttering on the behavior of the listener. *Journal of Abnormal Social Psychology, 49,* 355–61.

Rosenberger, P. B., Wheelden, J. A., & Kalotkin, M. (1976). The effect of Haloperidol on stuttering. *American Journal of Psychiatry, 133,* 331–34.

Rosenfield, D. B. (1972). Stuttering and cerebral ischemia. *New England Journal of Medicine,* 287, 991.

Rosenfield, D. B., & Freeman, F. J. (1983). Stuttering onset after laryngectomy. *Journal of Fluency Disorders, 8,* 265–68.

Rosenfield, D. B., & Goodglass, H. (1980). Dichotic testing of cerebral dominance in stutterers. *Brain and Language, 11,* 170–80.

Rosenfield, D. B., McCarthy, M., McKinney, K., Viswanath, N. S., & Nudelman, H. B. (1994). Stuttering induced by theophylline. *Ear, Nose, and Throat Journal, 73,* 914–18.

Rosenfield, D. B., Miller, S. D., & Feltovich, M. (1980). Brain damage causing stuttering. *Transactions of the American Neurological Association, 105,* 181–83.

Rosenfield, D. B., & Nudelman, H. B. (1987). Neuropsychological models of speech dysfluency. In L. Rustin, H. Purser, & D. Rowley (Eds.), *Progress in the treatment of fluency disorders* (pp. 3–18). London: Taylor and Francis.

Rosenfield, D. B., Viswanath, N. S., Callis-Landrun, L., Di Danato, R., & Nudelman, H. B. (1991). Patients with acquired dysfluencies: What they tell us about developmental stuttering. In H. F. M. Peters, W. Hulstijn, & C. W. Starkweather (Eds.), *Speech motor control and stuttering.* Amsterdam: Elsevier.

Ross, F. L. (1955). A comparative study of stutterers and nonstutterers on a psychomotor discrimination task. In W. Johnson & R. R. Leutenegger (Eds.), *Stuttering in children and adults* (pp. 361–66). Minneapolis: University of Minnesota Press.

Rosso, L. J., & Adams, M. R. (1969). A study of the relationship between the latency and consistency of stuttering. *Journal of Speech and Hearing Research, 12,* 389–93.

Roth, C. R., Aronson, A. E., & Davis, L. J., Jr. (1989). Clinical studies in psychogenic stuttering of adult onset. *Journal of Speech and Hearing Disorders, 54,* 634–46.

Rothenberger, P., Johannsen, H., Schulze, H., Amorosa, H., & Rommel, D. (1994). Use of tiapride on stuttering in children and adolescents. *Perceptual and Motor Skills, 79,* 1163–70.

Rotter, J. B. (1939). Studies in the psychology of stuttering: XI. Stuttering in relation to position in the family. *Journal of Speech Disorders, 4,* 143–48.

Rotter, J. B. (1955). A study of the motor integration of stutterers and nonstutterers. In W. Johnson & R. R. Leutenegger (Eds.), *Stuttering in children and adults* (pp. 367–76). Minneapolis: University of Minnesota Press.

Rouma, G. (1906). Enquête scolaire sur les troubles de la parole chez les écoliers Belges. *Int. Arch. Schulhygiene, 2,* 151–89.

Rousey, C. G., Arjunan, K. N., & Rousey, C. L. (1986). Successful treatment of stuttering following closed head injury. *Journal of Fluency Disorders, 11,* 257–61.

Rousey, C. L. (1958). Stuttering severity during prolonged spontaneous speech. *Journal of Speech and Hearing Research, 1,* 40–47.

Rousey, C. L., Goetzinger, C. P., & Dirks, D. (1959). Sound localization ability of normal, stuttering, neurotic, and hemiplegic subjects. *A.M.A. Archives of General Psychiatry, 1,* 640–45.

Rousseau, I., Packman, A., Onslow, M., Harrison, L., & Jones, M. (2007). Language, phonology, and treatment time in the Lidcombe Program: A prospective study in a Phase II trial. *Journal of Communication Disorders, 40,* 382–97.

Rubin, H., & Culatta, R. (1971). A point of view about fluency. *ASHA, 13,* 380–84.

Runyan, C. M., & Adams, M. R. (1978). Perceptual study of the speech of "successfully therapeutized" stutterers. *Journal of Fluency Disorders, 3,* 25–39.

Runyan, C. M., & Adams, M. R. (1979). Unsophisticated judges' perceptual evaluations of the speech of "successfully treated" stutterers. *Journal of Fluency Disorders, 4,* 29–38.

Runyan, C. M., Bell, J. N., & Prosek, R. A. (1990). Speech naturalness ratings of treated stutterers. *Journal of Speech and Hearing Disorders, 55,* 434–38.

Runyan, C. M., & Bonifant, D. C. (1981). A perceptual comparison: All-voiced versus typical reading passage by children. *Journal of Fluency Disorders, 6,* 247–55.

Runyan, C. M., Hames, P. E., & Prosek, R. A. (1982). A perceptual comparison between paired stimulus and single stimulus methods of presentation of the fluent utterances of stutterers. *Journal of Fluency Disorders, 7,* 71–77.

Runyan, C. M., & Runyan, S. E. (1986). A fluency rules therapy program for young children in the public schools. *Language, Speech and Hearing Services in Schools, 17,* 276–84.

Runyan, C., & Runyan, S. (1999). Therapy for school-aged stutterers: An update of the Fluency Rules Program. In R. Curlee (Ed.), *Stuttering and related disorders of fluency* (2nd ed.) (pp. 110–23). New York: Thieme.

Russell, J. C., Clark, A. W., & van Sommers, P. (1968). Treatment of stammering by reinforcement of fluent speech. *Behavior Research Therapy, 6,* 447–53.

Rustin, L., Kuhr, A., Cook, P. J., & James, I. M. (1981). Controlled trial of speech therapy versus oxprenolol for stammering. *British Medical Journal, 283,* 517–19.

Rustin, L., Purser, H., & Rowley, D. (Eds.). (1987). *Progress in the treatment of fluency disorders.* London: Taylor and Francis.

Rustin, L., Ryan, B. P., & Ryan, B.V. (1987). Use of the Monterey Programmed Stuttering Therapy in Great Britain. *British Journal of Disorders of Communication, 22,* 151–62.

Rutherford, B. R. (1938). Speech reeducation for the birth injured. *Journal of Speech Disorders, 3,* 199–206.

Ryan, B. P. (1971). Operant procedures applied to stuttering therapy for children. *Journal of Speech and Hearing Disorders, 36,* 264–80.

Ryan, B. P. (1974). *Programmed therapy for stuttering in children and adults.* Springfield, IL: Charles C. Thomas.

Ryan, B. (1979). Stuttering therapy in a framework of operant conditioning and programmed learning. In H. H. Gregory (Ed.), *Controversies about stuttering therapy* (pp. 129–74). Baltimore: University Park Press.

Ryan, B. P. (1981). Maintenance programs in progress-II. In E. Boberg (Ed.), *Maintenance of fluency: Proceedings of the Banff conference* (pp. 113–46). New York: Elsevier.

Ryan, B. P. (1992). Articulation, language, rate, and fluency characteristics of stuttering and nonstuttering preschool children. *Journal of Speech and Hearing Research, 35,* 333–42.

Ryan, B. P. (2000). Speaking rate, conversational speech acts, interruption, and linguistic complexity of 20 pre-school stuttering and non-stuttering children and their mothers. *Clinical Linguistics and Phonetics, 14,* 25–51.

Ryan, B. P. (2001a). *Programmed therapy for stuttering in children and adults.* Springfield, IL: Charles C. Thomas.

Ryan, B. P. (2001b). A longitudinal study of articulation, language, rate, and fluency of 22 preschool children who stutter. *Journal of Fluency Disorders, 26,* 107–27.

Ryan, B. P. (2004). The author's (Dr. Bruce Ryan) response to Drs. Walter Manning and Mark Onslow. *Journal of Fluency Disorders, 29,* 361–66.

Ryan, B. P., & Van Kirk, B. (1974). The establishment, transfer, and maintenance of fluent speech in 50 stutterers using delayed auditory feedback and operant procedures. *Journal of Speech and Hearing Disorders, 39,* 3–10.

Ryan, B. P., & Van Kirk, B. (1995). Programmed stuttering treatment for children: Comparison of two establishment programs through transfer, maintenance and follow-up. *Journal of Speech and Hearing Research, 38,* 61–75.

Sacco, P. R., & Metz, D. E. (1989). Comparison of period-by-period fundamental frequency of stutterers and nonstutterers over repeated utterances. *Journal of Speech and Hearing Research, 32,* 439–44.

Sackett, D. L., Rosenberg, W. M., Gray, J. A., Haynes, R. B., & Richardson, W. S. (1996). Evidence based medicine: what it is and what it isn't. *British Medical Journal, 312,* 71–72.

Sahin, H. A., Krespi, Y., Yilmaz, A., & Coban, O. (2005). Stuttering due to ischemic stroke. *Behavioural Neurology, 16,* 37–39.

St. Louis, K. O. (Ed.) (1986). *The atypical stutterer: Principles and practices of rehabilitation.* Orlando, FL: Academic Press.

St. Louis, K. O. (1991). The stuttering/articulation connection. In H. F. M. Peters, Hulstijn & C. W. Starkweather (Eds.), *Speech motor control and stuttering.* Amsterdam: Elsevier.

St. Louis, K. O. (1999). Person-first labeling and stuttering. *Journal of Fluency Disorders, 24,* 1–24.

St. Louis, K. O., & Atkins, C. P. (1988). Nonstutterers' perceptions of stuttering and speech difficulty. *Journal of Fluency Disorders, 13,* 375–84.

St. Louis, K. O., Clausell, P. L., Thompson, J. N., & Rife, C. C. (1982). Preliminary investigation of EMG biofeedback induced relaxation with a preschool aged stutterer. *Perceptual and Motor Skills, 55,* 195–99.

St. Louis, K. O., & Hinzman, A. R. (1988). A descriptive study of speech, language, and hearing characteristics of school-aged stutterers. *Journal of Fluency Disorders, 13,* 331–55.

St. Louis, K. O., Hinzman, A. R., & Hull, F. M. (1985). Studies of cluttering: Disfluency and language measures in young possible clutterers and stutterers. *Journal of Fluency Disorders, 10,* 151–72.

St. Louis, K. O., Murray, C. D., & Ashworth, M. S. (1991). Coexisting communication disorders in a random sample of school-aged stutterers. *Journal of Fluency Disorders, 16,* 13–23.

Sakata, R., & Adams, M. R. (1972). Comparisons among various forms of individual stutterers' disfluency. *Journal of Communication Disorders, 5,* 232–39.

Salmelin, R., Schnitzler, A., Schmitz, F., & Freund, H. J. (2000). Single word reading in developmental stutterers and fluent speakers. *Brain, 123,* 1184–1202.

Salmelin, R., Schnitzler, A., Schmitz, F., Jäncke, L., Witte, O. W., & Freund, H. J. (1998). Functional organization of the auditory cortex is different in stutterers and fluent speakers. *Neuroreport, 9,* 2225–29.

Saltuklaroglu, T., Kalinowski, J., Dayalu, V. N., Guntupalli, V. K., Stuart, A., & Rastatter, M. P. (2003). A temporal window for the central inhibition of stuttering via exogenous speech signals in adults. *Neuroscience Letters, 349,* 120–24.

Saltuklaroglu, T., Kalinowski, J., & Guntupalli, V. K. (2004). Towards a common neural substrate in the immediate and effective inhibition of stuttering. *International Journal of Neuroscience, 114,* 435–50.

Samar, V. J., Metz, D. E., & Sacco, P. R. (1986). Changes in aerodynamic characteristics of stutterers' fluent speech associated with therapy. *Journal of Speech and Hearing Research, 29,* 106–13.

Samson, C. L., & Cooper, E. B. (1980). Motor perseverative behavior in adult stutterers and nonstutterers. *Journal of Fluency Disorders, 5,* 359–72.

Sander, E. K. (1961). Reliability of the *Iowa Speech Disfluency Test. Journal of Speech and Hearing Disorders, Monograph Supplement,* 7, 21–30.

Sander, E. K. (1963). Frequency of syllable repetition and "stutterer" judgments. *Journal of Speech and Hearing Disorders, 28,* 19–30.

Sander, E. K. (1968). Interrelations among the responses of mothers to a child's disfluencies. *Speech Monographs, 35,* 187–95.

Santostefano, S. (1960). Anxiety and hostility in stuttering. *Journal of Speech and Hearing Research, 3,* 337–47.

Sasisekaran, J., & De Nil, L. F. (2006). Phoneme monitoring in silent naming and perception in adults who stutter. *Journal of Fluency Disorders, 31,* 284–302.

Sasisekaran, J., De Nil, L. F., Smyth, R., & Johnson, C. (2006). Phonological encoding in the silent speech of persons who stutter. *Journal of Fluency Disorders, 31,* 1–21.

Sayles, D. G. (1971). Cortical excitability, perseveration, and stuttering. *Journal of Speech and Hearing Research, 14,* 462–75.

Scarbrough, H. E. (1943). A quantitative and qualitative analysis of the electroencephalograms of stutterers and non-stutterers. *Journal of Experimental Psychology, 32,* 156–67.

Schaef, R. A. (1955). The use of questions to elicit stuttering adaptation. *Journal of Speech and Hearing Disorders, 20,* 262–65.

Schaeffer, M., & Shearer, W. (1968). A survey of mentally retarded stutterers. *Mental Retardation, 6,* 44–45.

Schäfersküpper, P. (1982). *Pathophysiologie und therapie des stotterns.* Berlin: Marhold.

Schäfersküpper, P., & Dames, M. (1987). Speech rate and syllable durations in stutterers and nonstutterers. In H. F. M. Peters & W. Hulstijn (Eds.), *Speech motor dynamics in stuttering* (pp. 329–36). New York: Springer.

Schäfersküpper, P., & Simon, T. (1983). The mean fundamental frequency in stutterers and nonstutterers during reading and spontaneous speech. *Journal of Fluency Disorders, 8,* 125–32.

Scheier, M. F., & Carver, C. S. (1985). The self-consciousness scale: a revised version for use with general populations. *Journal of Applied Social Psychology,* 15, 687–99.

Schiavetti, N. (1975). Judgments of stuttering severity as a function of type and locus of disfluency. *Folia Phoniatrica, 27,* 26–37.

Schiavetti, N., Martin, R. R., Haroldson, S. K., & Metz, D. E. (1994). Psychophysical analysis of audiovisual judgments of speech naturalness of nonstutterers and stutterers. *Journal of Speech and Hearing Research, 37,* 46–52.

Schiavetti, N., Sacco, P. R., Metz, D. E., & Sitler, R. W. (1983). Direct magnitude estimation and interval scaling of stuttering severity. *Journal of Speech and Hearing Research, 26,* 568–73.

Schiller, F. (1947). Aphasia studied in patients with missile wounds. *Journal of Neurology, Neurosurgery and Psychiatry, 10,* 183–97.

Schilling, A. (1959). Elektronystagmographische Befunde als Hinweis auf zentrale Koordinationsdefekte bei Stotterern. *Arch. Ohr.-Nas.-Kehlk. Heilk., 175,* 457–61.

Schilling, A. (1960). Röntgen-Zwerchfell-Kymogramme bei Stotterern. *Folia Phoniatrica, 12,* 145–53.

Schilling, A. (1962). Organische Faktoren bei der Entstehung des Stotterns. *HNO, 10,* 149–53.

Schilling, A. (1963). Die medikmamentöse Unterstützung der Therapie des Stotterns. *HNO, 11,* 300–04.

Schilling, A., & Biener, W. (1959). Messung der Vibrationsempfindung mittels Audiometer und Ergebnisse dieser Untersuchung bei Stotterern. *Nervenarzt, 30,* 279–81.

Schilling, A., & Göler, D. (1961). Zur Frage der Monotonie-Untersuchung beim Stottern. *Folia Phoniatrica, 13,* 202–18.

Schilling, A., & Krüger, W. (1960). Untersuchungen über die Motorik sprachgestörter Kinder, *HNO, 8,* 205–09.

Schindler, M. D. (1955). A study of educational adjustments of stuttering and nonstuttering children. In W. Johnson & R. R. Leutenegger (Eds.), *Stuttering in children and adults* (pp. 348–57). Minneapolis: University of Minnesota Press.

Schlanger, B. B. (1953). Speech examination of a group of institutionalized mentally handicapped children. *Journal of Speech and Hearing Disorders, 18,* 339–49.

Schlanger, B. B. (1973). *Mental retardation.* New York: Bobbs-Merrill.

Schlanger, B. B., & Gottsleben, R. H. (1957). Analysis of speech defects among the institutionalized mentally retarded. *Journal of Speech and Hearing Disorders, 22,* 98–103.

Schlesinger, I. M., Forte, M., Fried, B., & Melkman, R. (1965). Stuttering, information load, and response strength. *Journal of Speech and Hearing Disorders, 30,* 32–36.

Schlesinger, I. M., Melkman, R., & Levy, R. (1966). Word length and frequency as determinants of stuttering. *Psychonomic Science, 6,* 255–56.

Schmitt, L. S., & Cooper, E. B. (1978). Fundamental frequencies in the oral reading behavior of stuttering and nonstuttering male children. *Journal of Communication Disorders, 11,* 17–23.

Schmoigl, S., & Ladisch, W. (1967). EEG investigation in stutterers. *Electroencephalography and Clinical Neurophysiology, 23,* 184–85.

Schneier, F. R., Wexler, K. B., & Liebowitz, M. R. (1997). Social phobia and stuttering. *The American Journal of Psychiatry, 154,* 131.

Schönhärl, E. (1964). Altersbedingte Wandlungen im Strukturbild des Stotterns. *HNO, 12,* 152–54.

Schreiber, S., & Pick, C. G. (1997). Paroxetine for secondary stuttering: further interaction of serotonin and dopamine. *The Journal of Nervous and Mental Disease, 185,* 465–67.

Schroeder, P. L., & Ackerson, L. (1931). Relation of personality and behavior difficulties to disorders of speech. In R. West (Ed.), *A symposium on stuttering.* Madison, WI: College Typing Company.

Schuell, H. (1946). Sex differences in relation to stuttering: Part I. *Journal of Speech Disorders, 11,* 277–98.

Schuell, H. (1947). Sex differences in relation to stuttering: Part II. *Journal of Speech Disorders, 12,* 23–28.

Schultz, D. A. (1947). A study of nondirective counseling as applied to adult stutterers. *Journal of Speech Disorders, 12,* 421–27.

Schulz, H. (1977). Vergleichende Untersuchung von Sprachbehinderten und Nichtsprachbehinderten Schülern des 3. Schuljahres mit dem Rechentest DRE 3 von Samstag, Sander und Scyhmidt. *Sprachheilarb., 22,* 86–95.

Schulze, H. (1991). Time pressure variables in the verbal parent-child interaction patterns of fathers and mothers of stuttering, phonologically disordered and normal preschool children. In H. F. M. Peters, W. Hulstijn, & C. W. Starkweather (Eds.), *Speech motor control and stuttering.* Amsterdam: Elsevier.

Schwartz, D., & Webster, L. M. (1977). More on the efficacy of a protracted precision fluency shaping program. *Journal of Fluency Disorders, 2,* 205–15.

Schwartz, H. D., & Conture, E. G. (1988). Subgrouping young stutterers: Preliminary behavioral observations. *Journal of Speech and Hearing Disorders, 31,* 62–71.

Schwartz, H. D., Zebrowski, P. M., & Conture, E. (1990). Behaviors at the onset of stuttering. *Journal of Fluency Disorders, 15,* 77–86.

Schwartz, M. (1976). *Stuttering solved.* New York: Lippencott.

Schwenk, K. A., Conture, E. G., & Walden, T. A. (2007) Reaction to background stimulation of preschool children who do and do not stutter. *Journal of Communication Disorders, 40,* 129–41.

Scripture, E. W. (1931). *Stuttering, lisping, and correction of the speech of the deaf* (2nd ed.). New York: Macmillan.

Scripture, M. K., & Kittredge, W. B. (1923). An attempt to determine another etiological factor of stuttering through objective measurement. *Journal of Educational Psychology, 14,* 162–73.

Seaman, R. S. (1956). A study of the responses of stutterers to the items of the *Rosenzweig Picture-Frustration Study.* M. A. Thesis, Brooklyn College.

Sedláček, C. (1948). Reactions of the autonomic nervous system in attacks of stuttering. *Folia Phoniatrica, 1,* 97–103.

Sedláčková, E. (1963). Exploration de l'équilibre végétatif dans le bégaiement et le bredouillement. *Folia Phoniatrica, 15,* 68–77.

Seebach, M. A., & Caruso, A. J. (1979). Voice onset time during fluent speech: Young stutterers and nonstutterers. [Abstract]. *ASHA, 21,* 764.

Segre, R. (1951). Recherches sur l'influence corticale et palido-striale dans les syndromes spasmodiques. *Review Laryngology, Otology and Rhinology, 72,* 279–81.

Seidel, A., Weinstein, R. B., & Bloodstein, O. (1973). The effect of interposed conditions on the consistency of stuttering. *Journal of Speech and Hearing Research, 16,* 62–66.

Seider, R. A., Gladstien, K. L., & Kidd, K. K. (1982). Language onset and concomitant speech and language problems in subgroups of stutterers and their siblings. *Journal of Speech and Hearing Research, 25,* 482–86.

Seider, R. A., Gladstien, K. L., & Kidd, K. K. (1983). Recovery and persistence of stuttering among relatives of stutterers. *Journal of Speech and Hearing Disorders, 48,* 402–09.

Sermas, C. E., & Cox, M. D. (1982). The stutterer and stuttering: Personality correlates. *Journal of Fluency Disorders, 7,* 141–58.

Seth, G. (1934). An experimental study of the control of the mechanism of speech, and in particular that of respiration in stuttering subjects. *British Journal of Psychology, 24,* 375–88.

Seth, G. (1958). Psychomotor control in stammering and normal subjects: An experimental study. *British Journal of Psychology, 49,* 139–43.

Sewell, W., & Mussen, P. (1952). The effects of feeding, weaning and scheduling procedures on childhood adjustment and the formation of oral symptoms. *Child Development, 23,* 185–91.

Shackson, R. (1936). An action current study of muscle contraction latency with special reference to latent tetany in stutterers. *Archives of Speech, 1,* 87–111.

Shaffer, G. L. (1940). Measures of jaw movement and phonation in nonstuttered and stuttered production of voiced and voiceless plosives. *Speech Monographs, 7,* 85–92.

Shames, G. H. (1951). The relationship between the attitude toward stuttering of secondary stutterers and several of their personality charcteristics. [Abstract]. *Speech Monographs, 18,* 241.

Shames, G. H. (1952). An investigation of prognosis and evaluation in speech therapy. *Journal of Speech and Hearing Disorders, 17,* 386–92.

Shames, G. H., & Beams, H. L. (1956). Incidence of stuttering in older age groups. *Journal of Speech and Hearing Disorders, 21,* 313–16.

Shames, G. H., Egolf, D. B., & Rhodes, R. C. (1969). Experimental programs in stuttering therapy. *Journal of Speech and Hearing Disorders, 34,* 30–47.

Shames, G. H., & Florance, C. L. (1980). *Stutter-free speech: A goal for therapy.* Columbus, OH: Merrill.

Shames, G. H., & Rubin, H. (Eds.) (1986). *Stuttering then and now.* Columbus, OH: Merrill.

Shames, G. H., & Sherrick, C. E., Jr. (1965). A discussion of nonfluency and stuttering as operant behavior, *Journal of Speech and Hearing Disorders, 28,* 3–18. (1963). Reprinted in Barabara, D. A. (Ed.), *New directions in stuttering.* Springfield, IL: Charles C. Thomas.

Shane, M. L. S. (1955). Effect on stuttering of alteration in auditory feedback. In W. Johnson & R. R. Leutenegger (Eds.), *Stuttering in children and adults* (pp. 286–97). Minneapolis: University of Minnesota Press.

Shapiro, A. I. (1980). An electromyographic analysis of the fluent and dysfluent utterances of seveal types of stutterers. *Journal of Fluency Disorders, 5,* 203–31.

Shattuck-Hufnagel, S. (1983). Sublexical units and supra-segmental structures in speech production planning. In P. MacNeilage (Ed.), *The production of speech* (pp. 109–36). New York: Springer.

Shaw, C. K., & Shrum, W. F. (1972). The effects of response-contingent reward on the connected speech of children who stutter. *Journal of Speech and Hearing Disorders, 37,* 75–88.

Shearer, W. M. (1966). Speech: Behavior of middle ear muscle during stuttering. *Science, 152,* 1280.

Shearer, W. M., & Baud, H. E. (1970). Adaptation in mentally retarded stutterers and nonstutterers. *Journal of Communication Disorders, 3,* 118–22.

Shearer, W. M., & Simmons, F. B. (1965). Middle ear activity during speech in normal speakers and stutterers. *Journal of Speech and Hearing Research, 8,* 203–07.

Shearer, W. M., & Williams, J. D. (1965). Self-recovery from stuttering. *Journal of Speech and Hearing Disorders, 30,* 288–90.

Sheehan, J. (1951). The modification of stuttering through non-reinforcement. *Journal of Abnormal Social Psychology, 46,* 51–63.

Sheehan, J. G. (1953). Theory and treatment of stuttering as an approach-avoidance conflict. *Journal of Psychology, 36,* 27–49.

Sheehan, J. G. (1958a). Conflict theory of stuttering. In J. Eisenson (Ed.), *Stuttering: A symposium* (pp. 121–66). New York: Harper & Row.

Sheehan, J. G. (1958b). Projective studies of stuttering. *Journal of Speech and Hearing Disorders, 23,* 18–25.

Sheehan, J. G. (1970). *Stuttering: Research and therapy.* New York: Harper & Row.

Sheehan, J. G. (1974). Stuttering behavior: A phonetic analysis. *Journal of Communication Disorders, 7,* 193–212.

Sheehan, J. G. (1975). Conflict theory and avoidance-reduction therapy. In J. Eisenson (Ed.), *Stuttering: A second symposium* (pp. 97–198). New York: Harper & Row.

Sheehan, J. G. (1979). Level of aspiration in female stutterers: Changing times? *Journal of Speech and Hearing Disorders, 44,* 479–86.

Sheehan, J. G. (1984). Problems in the evaluation of progress and outcome. In W. H. Perkins (Ed.), *Stuttering disorders* (pp. 223–40). New York: Thieme-Stratton.

Sheehan, J. G., Cortese, P. A., & Hadley, R. G. (1962). Guilt, shame, and tension in graphic projections of stuuttering. *Journal of Speech and Hearing Disorders, 27,* 129–39.

Sheehan, J. G., Frederick, C. J., Rosevear, W. H., & Spiegelman, M. A. (1954). A validity study of the *Rorschach* prognostic rating scale. *Journal of Projective Techniques, 18,* 233–39.

Sheehan, J., Hadley, R., & Gould, E. (1967). Impact of authority on stuttering. *Journal of Abnormal Psychology, 72,* 290–93.

Sheehan, J. G., & Lyon, M. A. (1974). Role perception in stuttering. *Journal of Communication Disorders, 7,* 113–25.

Sheehan, J. G., & Martyn, M. M. (1966). Spontaneous recovery form stuttering. *Journal of Speech and Hearing Research, 9,* 121–35.

Sheehan, J. G., & Martyn, M. M. (1970). Stuttering and its disappearance. *Journal of Speech and Hearing Research, 13,* 279–89.

Sheehan, J., Martyn, M. M., & Kilburn, K. L. (1968). Speech disorders in retardation. *American Journal of Mental Deficiency, 73,* 251–56.

Sheehan, J. G., & Sheehan, V. M. (1984). Avoidance-reduction therapy: A response-suppression hypothesis. In W. H. Perkins (Ed.), *Stuttering disorders* (pp. 141–52). New York: Thieme-Stratton.

Sheehan, J. G., & Voas, R. B. (1954). Tension patterns during stuttering in relation to conflict, anxiety-binding, and reinforcement. *Speech Monographs, 21,* 272–79.

Sheehan, J. G., & Zelen, S. (1955). A level; of aspiration in stutterers and nonstutterers. *Journal of Abnormal Social Psychology, 51,* 83–86.

Sheehan, J., & Zussman, C. (1951). Rorschachs of stutterers compared with a clinical control. [Abstract]. *American Psychologist, 6,* 500.

Sheets, B.V. (1941). A study of the visual perseverative tendencies in stutterers and normal speakers. M.A. Thesis, University of Utah.

Shenker, R., & Roberts, P. (2007). Long-term outcome of the Lidcombe Program in bilingual children. In J. Au-Yeung & M. Leahy (Eds.), *Research, treatment and self-help in fluency disorders: New horizons. Proceedings of the Fifth World Congress on Fluency Disorders.* (pp. 431–36): International Fluency Association.

Shenker, R. C.(2004). Bilingualism in early stuttering: empirical issues and clinical implications. In A. Bothe (Ed.), *Evidence-based treatment of stuttering: empirical bases and clinical applications* (pp. 81–96). Mahwah, NJ: Lawrence Erlbaum Associates.

Shenker, R. C., & Finn, P. (1985). An evaluation of the effects of supplemental "fluency" traning during maintenance. *Journal of Fluency Disorders, 10,* 257–67.

Sherman, D. (1952). Clinical and experimental use of the *Iowa Scale of Severity of Stuttering. Journal of Speech and Hearing Disorders, 17,* 316–20.

Sherman, D. (1955). Reliability and utility of individual ratings of severity of audible characteristics of stuttering. *Journal of Speech and Hearing Disorders, 20,* 11–16.

Sherman, D., & McDermott, R. (1958). Individual ratings of severity of moments of stuttering. *Journal of Speech and Hearing Research, 1,* 61–67.

Sherman, D., & Trotter, W. D. (1956). Correlation between two measures of the severity of stuttering. *Journal of Speech and Hearing Disorders, 21,* 426–29.

Sherman, D., Young, M., & Gough, K. (1958). Comparison of three measures of stuttering severity. *Proceedings of the Iowa Academy of Sciences, 65,* 381–84.

Sherrard, C. A. (1975). Stuttering as "false alarm" responding. *British Journal of Disorders of Communication, 10,* 83–91.

Shimamori, S., & Ito, T. (2006). Initial syllable weight and frequency of stuttering in Japanese children. *Japanese Journal of Special Education, 43,* 519–27.

Shine, R. E. (1984). Assessment and fluency training and the young stutterer. In M. Peins (Ed.), *Contemporary approaches in stuttering therapy* (pp. 173–216). Boston: Little, Brown.

Shipp, T., Izdebski, K., & Morrissey, P. (1984). Physiologic stages of vocal reaction time. *Journal of Speech and Hearing Research, 27,* 173–78.

Shopwin, C. D. (1959). An experimental investigation of the passive-dependency component in adult male stutterers. [Abstract]. *Speech Monographs, 26,* 143.

Shriberg, L. D., Tomblin, J. B., & McSweeny, J. L. (1999). Prevalence of speech delay in 6-year-old children and comorbidity with language impairment. *Journal of Speech, Language and Hearing Research, 42,* 1461–81.

Shrum, W. F. (1962). A comparison of the effect of masking noise and increased vocal intensity on the frequency of stuttering. [Abstract]. *ASHA, 4,* 408.

Shtremel, A. Kh. (1963). Zaikanie v syndrome levoi temennoi doli. *Zh. Nevropatol. Psikhiat., 63,* 828–32.

Shugart, Y. Y., Mundorff, J., Kilshaw, J., Doheny, K., Doan, B., Wanyee, J., et al. (2004). Results of a genome-wide linkage scan for stuttering. *American Journal of Medical Genetics, 124A,* 133–35.

Shulman, E. (1955). Factors influencing the variability of stuttering. In W. Johnson & R. R. Leutenegger (Eds.), *Stuttering in children and adults* (pp. 207–17). Minneapolis: University of Minnesota Press.

Shumak, I. C. (1955). A speech situation rating sheet for stutterers. In W. Johnson & R. R. Leutenegger (Eds.), *Stuttering in children and adults* (pp. 341–47). Minneapolis: University of Minnesota Press.

Sichel, R. N. (1973). Initial phoneme in relation to disfluency in the spontaneous speech of nonstuttering preschool children. M. S. Thesis, Brooklyn College.

Siegel, G. M. (1970). Punishment, stuttering, and disfluency. *Journal of Speech and Hearing Research, 13,* 677–714.

Siegel, G. M., & Hanson, B. (1972). The effect of response-contingent neutral stimuli on normal speech disfluency. *Journal of Speech and Hearing Research, 15,* 123–33.

Siegel, G. M., & Haugen, D. (1964). Audience size and variations in stuttering behavior. *Journal of Speech and Hearing Research, 7,* 381–88.

Siegel, G. M., Lenske, J., & Broen, P. (1969). Suppression of normal speech disfluencies through response cost. *Journal of Applied Behavior Analysis, 2,* 265–76.

Siegel, G. M., & Martin, R. R. (1965a). Experimental modification of disfluency in normal speakers. *Journal of Speech and Hearing Research, 8,* 235–44.

Siegel, G. M., & Martin, R. R. (1965b). Verbal punishment of disfluencies in normal speakers. *Journal of Speech and Hearing Research, 8,* 245–51.

Siegel, G. M., & Martin, R. R. (1966). Punishment of disfluencies in normal speakers. *Journal of Speech and Hearing Research, 9,* 208–18.

Siegel, G. M., & Martin, R. R. (1967). Verbal punishment of disfluencies during spontaneous speech. *Language and Speech, 10,* 244–51.

Siegel, G. M., & Martin, R. R. (1968). The effects of verbal stimuli on disfluencies during spontaneous speech. *Journal of Speech and Hearing Research, 11,* 358–64.

Silverman, E.-M. (1971). Situational variability of preschoolers' disfluency: Preliminary study. *Perceptual and Motor Skills, 33,* 1021–22.

Silverman, E.-M. (1972a). Generality of disfluency data collected from preschoolers. *Journal of Speech and Hearing Research, 5,* 84–92.

Silverman, E.-M. (1972b). Preschoolers' speech disfluency: Single syllable word repetition. *Perceptual and Motor Skills, 35,* 1002.

Silverman, E.-M. (1973a). Clustering: A characteristic of preschoolers' speech disfluency. *Journal of Speech and Hearing Research, 16,* 578–83.

Silverman, E.-M. (1973b). The influence of preschoolers' speech usage on their disfluency frequency. *Journal of Speech and Hearing Research, 16,* 474–81.

Silverman, E.-M. (1974). Word position and grammatical function in relation to preschoolers' speech disfluency. *Perceptual and Motor Skills, 39,* 267–72.

Silverman, E.-M. (1975). Effect of selected word attributes on preschoolers' speech disfluency: Initial phoneme and length. *Journal of Speech and Hearing Research, 18,* 430–34.

Silverman, E.-M. (1980). Communication attitudes of women who stutter. *Journal of Speech and Hearing Disorders, 45,* 533–39.

Silverman, E.-M. (1982). Speech-language clinicians' and university students' impressions of women and girls who stutter. *Journal of Fluency Disorders, 7,* 469–78.

Silverman, E.-M., & Vfan Opens, K. (1980). An investigation of sex bias in classroom teachers' speech and language referrals. *Language, Speech and Hearing Services in Schools, 11,* 169–74.

Silverman, E.-M., & Williams, D. E. (1968). A comparison of stuttering and nonstuttering children in terms of five measures of oral language development. *Journal of Communication Disorders, 1,* 305–09.

Silverman, E.-M., & Zimmer, C. H. (1979). Women who stutter: Personality and speech characteristics. *Journal of Speech and Hearing Research, 22,* 553–64.

Silverman, E.-M., & Zimmer, C. H. (1982). Demographic characteristics and treatment experiences of women and men who stutter. *Journal of Fluency Disorders, 7,* 273–85.

Silverman, E.-M., Zimmer, C. H., & Silverman, F. H. (1974). Variability of stutterers' speech disfluencies: The menstrual cycle. *Perceptual and Motor Skills, 38,* 1037–38.

Silverman, F. H. (1970a). Concern of elementary-school stutterers about their stuttering. *Journal of Speech and Hearing Disorders, 35,* 361–63.

Silverman, F. H. (1970b). Course of nonstutterers' disfluency adaptation during 15 consecutive oral readings of the same material. *Journal of Speech and Hearing Research, 13,* 382–86.

Silverman, F. H. (1970c). Distribution of instances of disfluency in consecutive readings of different passages by nonstutterers. *Journal of Speech and Hearing Research, 13,* 874–82.

Silverman, F. H. (1970d). A note on the degree of adaptation by stutterers and nonstutterers during oral reading. *Journal of Speech and Hearing Research, 13,* 173–77.

Silverman, F. H. (1971). The effect of rhythmic auditory stimulation on the disfluency of nonstutterers. *Journal of Speech and Hearing Research, 14,* 350–55.

Silverman, F. H. (1972). Disfluency and word length. *Journal of Speech and Hearing Research, 15,* 788–91.

Silverman, F. H. (1974). Disfluency behavior of elementary-school stutterers and nonstutterers. *Language, Speech and Hearing Services in Schools, 5,* 32–37.

Silverman, F. H. (1975). How "typical" is a stutterer's stuttering in a clinical environment? *Perceptual and Motor Skills, 40,* 458.

Silverman, F. H. (1976a). Do elementary-school stutterers talk less than their peers? *Language, Speech and Hearing Services in Schools, 7,* 90–92.

Silverman, F. H. (1976b). Long-term impact of a miniature metronome on stuttering: An interim report. *Perceptual and Motor Skills, 42,* 1322.

Silverman, F. H. (1980a). Dimensions of improvement in stuttering. *Journal of Speech and Hearing Research, 23,* 137–51.

Silverman, F. H. (1980b). The stuttering problem profile: A task that assists both client and clinician in defining therapy goals. *Journal of Speech and Hearing Disorders, 45,* 119–23.

Silverman, F. H. (1988). The "monster" study. *Journal of Fluency Disorders, 13,* 225–31.

Silverman, F. H. (1990). Are professors likely to report having "beliefs" about the intelligence and competence of students who stutter? *Journal of Fluency Disorders, 15,* 319–21.

Silverman, F. H., & Bohlman, P. (1988). Flute stuttering. *Journal of Fluency Disorders, 13,* 427–28.

Silverman, F. H., & Bloom, C. M. (1973). Spontaneous recovery of nonstutters' disfluency following adaptation. *Journal of Speech and Hearing Research, 16,* 452–55.

Silverman, F. H., & Goodban, M. T. (1972). The effect of auditory masking on the fluency of normal speakers. *Journal of Speech and Hearing Research, 15,* 543–46.

Silverman, F. H., & Paynter, K. K. (1990). Impact of stuttering on perception of occupational competence. *Journal of Fluency Disorders, 15,* 87–91.

Silverman, F. H., & Silverman E.-M. (1971). Stutter-like behavior in the manual communication of the deaf. *Perceptual and Motor Skills, 33,* 45–46.

Silverman, F. H., & Trotter, W. D. (1973). Impact of pacing speech with a miniature electronic metronome upon the manner in which a stutterer is perceived. *Behavior Therapist, 4,* 414–19.

Silverman, F. H., & Umberger, F. G. (1974). Effect of pacing speech with a miniature electronic metronome on the frequency and duration of selected disfluency behaviors in the spontaneous speech of adult stutterers. *Behavior Therapist, 5,* 410–14.

Silverman, F. H., & Williams, D. E. (1967a). Loci of disfluencies in the speech of nonstutterers during oral reading. *Journal of Speech and Hearing Research, 10,* 790–94.

Silverman, F. H., & Williams, D. E. (1967b). Loci of disfluencies in the speech of stutterers. *Perceptual and Motor Skills, 24,* 1085–86.

Silverman, F. H., & Williams, D. E. (1968). A proportional measure of stuttering adaptation. *Journal of Speech and Hearing Research, 11,* 444–46.

Silverman, F. H., & Williams, D. E. (1971). The adaptation effect for six types of speech disfluency. *Journal of Speech and Hearing Research, 14,* 525–30.

Silverman, F. H., & Williams, D. E. (1972a). Performance of stutterers on a single-word adaptation task. *Perceptual and Motor Skills, 34,* 565–66.

Silverman, F. H., & Williams, D. E. (1972b). Prediction of stuttering by school-age stutterers. *Journal of Speech and Hearing Research, 15,* 189–93.

Silverman, F. H., & Williams, D. E. (1972c). Use of revision by elementary-school stutterers and nonstutterers. *Journal of Speech and Hearing Research, 16,* 584–85.

Silverman, L. H., Klinger, H., Lustbader, L., Farrell, J., & Martin, A. D. (1972). The effects of subliminal drive stimulation on the speech of stutterers. *Journal of Nervous and Mental Disorders, 155,* 14–21.

Silverman, S. W., & Bernstein Ratner, N. (1997). Syntactic complexity, fluency, and accuracy of sentence imitation in adolescents. *Journal of Speech, Language, and Hearing Research, 40,* 95–106.

Silverman, S. W., & Bernstein Ratner, N. (2002). Measuring lexical diversity in children who stutter: application of vocd. *Journal of Fluency Disorders, 27,* 289–305.

Simon, C. T. (1945). Complexity and breakdown in speech situations. *Journal of Speech Disorders, 10,* 199–203.

Široký, A., Langová, J., Morávek, M., & Šváb, L. (1978). The occurrence of the saddle-formed nystagmus in stutterers. *Activitas Nervosa Superior, 20,* 146–48.

Skalbeck, O. M. (1957). The relationship of expectancy of stuttering to certain other designated variables associated with stuttering. [Abstract]. *Speech Monographs, 24,* 146.

Slorach, N., & Noehr, B. (1973). Dichotic listening in stuttering and dyslalic children. *Cortex, 9,* 295–300.

Smith, A. (1989). Neural drive to muscles in stuttering. *Journal of Speech and Hearing Research, 32,* 252–64.

Smith, A. (1999). Stuttering: A unified approach to a multifactorial, dynamic disorder. In N. Bernstein Ratner & E. Charles Healey (Eds.), *Stuttering research and practice: Bridging the gap* (pp. 27–44). Mahwah, NJ: Lawrence Erlbaum Associates.

Smith, A., Denny, M., Shaffer, L. A., Kelly, E. M., & Hirano, M. (1996). Activity of intrinsic laryngeal muscles in fluent and disfluent speech. *Journal of Speech and Hearing Research, 39,* 329–48.

Smith, A., Denny, M., & Wood, J. (1991). Instability in speech muscle systems in stuttering. In H. F. M. Peters, W. Hulstijn, & C. W. Starkweather (Eds.), *Speech motor control and stuttering.* Amsterdam: Elsevier.

Smith, A. & Kelly, E. (1997). Stuttering: A dynamic, multifactorial model. In R. Curlee & G. Siegal (Eds.), *Nature and treatment of stuttering: New directions* (2nd ed.) (pp. 204–18). Boston: Allyn & Bacon.

Smith, A., & Kleinow, J. (2000). Kinematic correlates of speaking rate changes in stuttering and normally fluent adults. *Journal of Speech, Language and Hearing Research, 43,* 521–36.

Smith, A., & Luschei, E. S. (1983). Assessment of oral-motor reflexes in stutterers and normal speakers: Preliminary observations. *Journal of Speech and Hearing Research, 26,* 322–28.

Smith, A., Luschei, E., Denny, M., Wood, J., Hirano, M., & Badylak, S. (1993). Spectral analyses of activity of laryngeal and orofacial muscles in stutterers. *Journal of Neurology, Neurosurgery, and Psychiatry, 56,* 1303–11.

Smith, A. M. (1953). Treatment of stutterers with carbon dioxide. *Disorders of the Nervous System, 14,* 243–44.

Smith, K. M., Blood, I. M., & Blood, G. W. (1990). Auditory brainstem responses of stutterers and nonstutterers during speech production. *Journal of Fluency Disorders, 15,* 211–22.

Smits-Bandstra, S., De Nil, L., & Rochon, E. (2006). The transition to increased automaticity during finger sequence learning in adult males who stutter. *Journal of Fluency Disorders, 31,* 22–42.

Smits-Bandstra, S., De Nil, L. F., & Saint-Cyr, J. A. (2006). Speech and nonspeech sequence skill learning in adults who stutter. *Journal of Fluency Disorders, 31,* 116–36.

Snidecor, J. C. (1947). Why the Indian does not stutter. *Quarterly Journal of Speech, 33,* 493–95.

Snidecor, J. C. (1955). Tension and facial appearance in stuttering. In W. Johnson & R. R. Leutenegger (Eds.), *Stuttering in children and adults* (pp. 377–80). Minneapolis: University of Minnesota Press.

Snyder, G. J. (2001). Exploratory research in the measurement and modification of attitudes toward stuttering. *Journal of Fluency Disorders, 26,* 149–60.

Snyder, M. A. (1958). Stuttering and coordination: An investigation of the relationship between the stutterer's coordination and his speech difficulty. *Logos, 1,* 36–44.

Soderberg, G. A. (1960). A study of the effects of delayed side-tone on four aspects of stutterers' speech during oral reading and spontaneous speech. [Abstract]. *Speech Monographs, 27,* 252–53.

Soderberg, G. A. (1962a). Phonetic influences upon stuttering. *Journal of Speech and Hearing Research, 5,* 315–20.

Soderberg, G. A. (1962b). What is "average" stuttering? *Journal of Speech and Hearing Disorders, 27,* 85–86.

Soderberg, G. A. (1966). The relations of stuttering to word length and word frequency. *Journal of Speech and Hearing Research, 9,* 584–89.

Soderberg, G. A. (1967). Linguistic factors in stuttering. *Journal of Speech and Hearing Research, 10,* 801–10.

Soderberg, G. A. (1968). Delayed auditory feedback and stuttering. *Journal of Speech and Hearing Disorders, 33,* 260–67.

Soderberg, G. A. (1969a). A comparison of adaptation trends in the oral reading of stutterers, inferior speakers and superior speakers. *Journal of Communication Disorders, 2,* 99–108.

Soderberg, G. A. (1969b). Delayed auditory feedback and the speech of stutterers: A review of studies. *Journal of Speech and Hearing Disorders, 34,* 20–29.

Soderberg, G. A. (1971). Relations of word information and word length to stuttering disfluencies. *Journal of Communication Disorders, 4,* 9–14.

Soderberg, G. A., & MacKay, D. G. (1972). The function relating stuttering to phoneme frequency and transition probability, *Journal of Verbal Learning and Verbal Behavior, 11,* 83–91.

Solomon, N. D. (1952). A comparison of rigidity of behavior manifested by a group of stutterers compared with "fluent" speakers in oral and other performances as measured by the Einstellung-effect. [Abstract]. *Speech Monographs, 19,* 198.

Sommer, I. E. C., Ramsey, N. F., Mandl, R. C., & Kahn, R. S. (2002). Language lateralization in monozygotic twin pairs concordant and discordant for handedness. *Brain, 125,* 2710–18.

Sommer, M., Koch, M. A., Paulus, W., Weiller, C., & Büchel, C. (2002). Mechanisms of disease. Disconnecting of speech-relevant brain areas in persistent developmental stuttering. *Lancet, 360,* 380–83.

Sommers, R. K., Brady, W. A., & Moore, W. H., Jr. (1975). Dichotic ear preferences of stuttering children and adults. *Perceptual and Motor Skills, 41,* 931–38.

Sovăk, M. (1935). Das vegetative Nervensystem bei Stotterern. Monatsschr. *Ohrenheilk. Laryngo-Rhinol., 69,* 666–80.

Spadino, E. J. (1941). *Writing and laterality characteristics of stuttering children.* New York: Columbia University Teachers College.

Sparks, G., Grant, D. E., Millay, K., Walker-Batson, D., & Hynan, L. S. (2002). The effect of fast speech rate on stuttering frequency during delayed auditory feedback. *Journal of Fluency Disorders, 27,* 187–202.

Spencer, E., Packman, A., Onslow, M., & Ferguson, A. (2005). A preliminary investigation of the impact of stuttering on language use. *Clinical Linguistics and Phonetics, 19,* 191–201.

Spencer, G. (1976). The status of environmental and group cohesiveness in the treatment of stuttering. *Australian Journal of Human Communication Disorders, 4,* 140–45.

Spielberger, C. D. (1956). The effects of stuttering behavior and response set on recognition thresholds. *Journal of Personality, 25,* 33–45.

Spriestersbach, D. C. (1940). An exploratory study of the motility of the peripheral oral structures in relation to defective and superior consonant articulation. M. A. Thesis, University of Iowa.

Spriestersbach, D. C. (1951). An objective approach to the investigation of social adjustment of male stutterers. *Journal of Speech and Hearing Disorders, 16,* 250–57.

Springer, S., & Deutsch, G. (1997). *Left brain, right brain* (5th ed.). New York: Worth.

Stager, S.V. (1990). Heterogeneity in stuttering: Results from auditory brainstem response testing. *Journal of Fluency Disorders, 15,* 9–19.

Stager, S.V., Calis, K., Grothe, D., Bloch, M., Berensen, N. M., Smith, P. J., et al. (2005). Treatment with medications affecting dopaminergic and serotonergic mechanisms: Effects on fluency and anxiety in persons who stutter. *Journal of Fluency Disorders, 30,* 319–35.

Stager, S.V., Denman, D.W., & Ludlow, C. L. (1997). Modifications in aerodynamic variables by persons who stutter under fluency-evoking conditions. *Journal of Speech, Language, and Hearing Research, 40,* 832–47.

Stager, S.V., Jeffries, K. J., & Braun, A. R. (2003). Common features of fluency-evoking conditions studied in stuttering subjects and controls: An H(2)15O PET study. *Journal of Fluency Disorders, 28,* 319–35.

Stager, S.V., & Ludlow, C. L. (1998). The effects of fluency-evoking conditions on voicing onset types in persons who do and do not stutter. *Journal of Communication Disorders, 31,* 33–52.

Stager, S.V., Ludlow, C. L., Gordon, C.T., Cotelingam, M., & Rapoport, J. L. (1995). Fluency changes in persons who stutter following a double blind trial of clomipramine and desipramine. *Journal of Speech and Hearing Research, 38,* 516–25.

Stang, H. (1984). Stationäre mehrdimensionale Verhaltenstherapie bei stotternden Kindern und Jugendlichen—Ein Erfahrungsbericht. *Sprache-Stimme-Gehör, 8,* 16–19.

Stansfield, J. (1990). Prevalence of stuttering and cluttering in adults with mental handicaps. *Journal of Mental Deficiency Research, 34,* 287–307.

Stansfield, J. (1995). Word-final disfluencies in adults with learning difficulties. *Journal of Fluency Disorders, 20,* 1–10.

Starbuck, H. B., & Steer, M. D. (1953). The adaptation effect in stuttering speech behavior and normal speech behavior. *Journal of Speech and Hearing Disorders, 18,* 252–55.

Starbuck, H. B., & Steer, M. D. (1954). The adaptation effect in stuttering and its relation to thoracic and abdominal breathing. *Journal of Speech and Hearing Disorders, 19,* 440–49.

Stark, R. E., & Pierce, B. R. (1970). The effects of delayed auditory feedback on a speech-related task in stutterers. *Journal of Speech and Hearing Research, 13,* 245–53.

Starkweather, C.W. (1971). The case against base rate comparisons in stuttering experimentation. *Journal of Communication Disorders, 4,* 247–58.

Starkweather, C.W. (1984). A multiprocess behavioral approach to stuttering therapy. In W. H. Perkins (Ed.), *Stuttering disorders* (pp. 129–46). New York: Thieme-Stratton.

Starkweather, C.W. (1987). *Fluency and stuttering.* Englewood Cliffs, NJ: Prentice-Hall.

Starkweather, C.W., Armson, J. M., & Amster, B. J. (1987). An approach to the study of motor speech mechanisms in stuttering. In L. Rustin, H. Purser, & D. Rowley (Eds.), *Progress in the treatment of fluency disorders* (pp. 43–58). London: Taylor and Francis.

Starkweather, C.W., Franklin, S., & Smigo, T. M. (1984). Vocal and finger reaction times in stutterers and nonstutterers: Differences and correlations. *Journal of Speech and Hearing Research, 27,* 193–96.

Starkweather, C.W., & Gottwald, S. R. (1990). The demands and capacities model II: Clinical applications. *Journal of Fluency Disorders, 15,* 143–57.

Starkweather, C.W., Gottwald, S., & Halfond, M. (1990). *Stuttering prevention: A clinical method.* Englewood Cliffs, NJ: Prentice-Hall.

Starkweather, C.W., Hirschman, P., & Tannenbaum, R. S. (1976). Latency of vocalization onset: Stutterers versus nonstutterers. *Journal of Speech and Hearing Research, 19,* 481–92.

Starkweather, C.W., & Lucker, J. (1978). Tokens for stuttering. *Journal of Fluency Disorders, 3,* 167–80.

Starkweather, C.W., & Myers, M. (1979). Duration of subsegments within the intervocalic interval in stutterers and nonstutterers. *Journal of Fluency Disorders, 4,* 205–14.

Starr, H. E. (1922). The hydrogen ion concentration of the mixed saliva considered as an index of fatigue and of emotional excitation, and applied to a study of the metabolic etiology of stammering. *American Journal of Psychology, 33,* 394–418.

Starr, H. E. (1928). Psychological concomitants of high alveolar carbon dioxide: A psychobiochemical study of the etiology of stammering. *Psychological Clinic, 17,* 1–12.

Stassi, E. J. (1961). Disfluency of normal speakers and reinforcement. *Journal of Speech and Hearing Research, 4,* 358–61.

Steer, M. D. (1935). A qualitative study of breathing in young stutterers. *Speech Monographs, 2,* 152–56.

Steer, M. D. (1936). The general intelligence of college stutterers. *School and Society, 44,* 862–64.

Steer, M. D. (1937). Symptomatologies of young stutterers. *Journal of Speech Disorders, 2,* 3–13.

Steer, M. D., & Johnson, W. (1936). An objective study of the relationship between psychological factors and the severity of stuttering. *Journal of Abnormal Social Psychology, 31,* 36–46.

Stefankiewicz, S. P., & Bloodstein, O. (1974). The effect of a four-week interval on the consistency of stuttering. *Journal of Speech and Hearing Research, 17,* 141–45.

Stein, M. B., Baird, A., & Walker, J. R. (1996). Social phobia in adults with stuttering. *The American Journal of Psychiatry, 153,* 278–80.

Stephen, S. C. G., & Haggard M. P. (1980). Acoustic properties of masking/delayed feedback in the fluency of stutterers and controls. *Journal of Speech and Hearing Research, 23,* 527–38.

Stephenson-Opsal, D., & Bernstein Ratner, N. (1988). Maternal speech rate modification and childhood stuttering. *Journal of Fluency Disorders, 13,* 49–56.

Stern, E. (1948). A preliminary study of bilingualism and stuttering in four Johannesburg schools. *Journal of Logopaedics, 1,* 15–25.

Sternberg, M. L. (1946). Auditory factors in stuttering. M.A., Thesis, University of Iowa.

Stewart, C., Evans, W. B., & Fitch, J. L. (1985). Oral form perception skills of stuttering and nonstuttering children measured by stereognosis. *Journal of Fluency Disorders, 10,* 311–16.

Stewart, J. L. (1960). The problem of stuttering in certain North American Indian societies. *Journal of Speech and Hearing Disorders, Monograph Supplement 6.*

Stewart, T., & Brosh, H. (1997). The use of drawings in the management of adults who stammer. *Journal of Fluency Disorders, 22,* 35–50.

Stewart, T., & Richardson, G. (2004). A qualitative study of therapeutic effect from a user's perspective. *Journal of Fluency Disorders, 29,* 95–108.

Stidham, K. R., Olson, L., Hillbratt, M., & Sinopoli, T. (2006). A new antistuttering device: treatment of stuttering using bone conduction stimulation with delayed temporal feedback. *The Laryngoscope, 116,* 1951–55.

Still, A. W., & Griggs, S. (1979). Changes in the probability of stuttering following a stutter: A test of some recent models. *Journal of Speech and Hearing Research, 22,* 565–71.

Stock, E. (1966). Untersuchungen zur Intonation bei Stotterern. *Folia Phoniatrica, 18,* 447–61.

Stocker, B., & Gerstman, L. J. (1983). A comparison of the probe technique and conventional therapy for young stutterers. *Journal of Fluency Disorders, 8,* 331–39.

Stocker, B., & Parker, E. (1977). The relationship betwen auditory recall and dysfluency in young stutterers. *Journal of Fluency Disorders, 2,* 177–87.

Stocker, B., & Usprich, C. (1976). Stuttering in young children and level of demand. *Journal of Childhood Communication Disorders, 1,* 116–31.

Stockman, I. J., Woods, D. R., & Tishman, A. (1981). Listener agreement on phonetic segments in early infant vocalizations. *Journal of Psycholinguistic Research, 10,* 593–617.

Story, R. S., Alfonso, P. J., & Harris, K. S. (1996). Pre- and posttreatment comparison of the kinematics of the fluent speech of persons who stutter. *Journal of Speech and Hearing Research, 39,* 991–1005.

Straus, S. E., & Sackett, D. L. (1998). Using research findings in clinical practice. *British Medical Journal, 317,* 339.

Streifler, M., & Gumpertz, F. (1955). Cerebral potentials in stuttering and cluttering. *Confinia Neurological, 15,* 344–59.

Stromsta, C. (1965). A spectrographic study of dysfluencies labeled as stuttering by parents. *De Tehrapia Vocis et Loquelae, Vol. 1, XIII Congress of the International Society of Logopedics and Phoniatrics.*

Stromsta, C. (1972). Interaural phase disparity of stutterers and nonstutterers. *Journal of Speech and Hearing Research, 15,* 771–80.

Stromsta, C. (1986). *Elements of stuttering.* Oshtemo, MI: Atsmonts Publishing.

Stromsta, C. (1987). Acoustic and electrophysiologic correlates of stuttering and early developmental reactions. In H. F. M. Peters & W. Hulstijn (Eds.), *Speech motor dynamics in stuttering* (pp. 267–77). New York: Springer.

Stromsta, C., & Fibiger, S. (1981). Physiological correlates of the core behavior of stuttering. *Proceedings of the 18th Congress of the International Association for Logopedics and Phoniatrics.* Washington, DC: American Speech and Language Hearing Association.

Stromsta, C. P. (1957). A methodology related to the determination of the phase angle of bone-conducted speech sound energy of stutterers and nonstutterers. [Abstract]. *Speech Monographs, 24,* 147–48.

Strother, C. R. (1937). A study of the extent of dyssynergia occurring during stuttering spasm. *Psychology Monographs, 49,* 108–27.

Strother, C. R., & Kriegman, L. S. (1943). Diadochokinesis in stutterers and nonstutterers. *Journal of Speech Disorders, 8,* 323–35.

Strother, C. R., & Kriegman, L. S. (1944). Rhythmokinesis in stutterers and nonstutterers. *Journal of Speech Disorders, 9,* 239–44.

Stuart, A. (1999). The distraction hypothesis and the practice of pseudoscience: A reply to Bloodstein. *Journal of Speech, Language, and Hearing Research, 42,* 913–14.

Stuart, A., & Kalinowski, J. (1996). Fluency effect of frequency alterations of plus/minus one-half and one-quarter octave shifts in feedback of people who stutter. *Journal of Speech and Hearing Research, 39,* 396–402.

Stuart, A., Kalinowski, J., Armson, J., Stenstrom, R., & Jones, K. (1996). Fluency effect of frequency alterations of plus/minus one-half and one-quarter octave shifts in auditory feedback of people who stutter. *Journal of Speech and Hearing Research, 39,* 396–401.

Stuart, A., Kalinowski, J., & Rastatter, M. P. (1997). Effect of monaural and binaural altered auditory feedback on stuttering frequency. *The Journal of the Acoustical Society of America, 101,* 3806–09.

Stuart, A., Kalinowski, J., Rastatter, M. P., & Lynch, K. (2002). Effect of delayed auditory feedback on normal speakers at two speech rates. *The Journal of the Acoustical Society of America, 111,* 2237–41.

Stuart, A., Kalinowski, J., Rastatter, M. P., Saltuklaroglu, T., & Dayalu, V. (2004). Investigations of the impact of altered auditory feedback in-the-ear devices on the speech of people who stutter: initial fitting and 4-month follow-up. *International Journal of Language & Communication Disorders, 39,* 93–113.

Stuart, A., Kalinowski, J., Saltuklaroglu, T., & Guntupalli, V. K. (2006). Investigations of the impact of altered auditory feedback in-the-ear devices on the speech of people who stutter: One-year follow-up. *Disability and Rehabilitation, 28,* 757–65.

Subramanian, A., & Yairi, E. (2006). Identification of traits associated with stuttering. *Journal of Communication Disorders,* 39, 200–16.

Subramanian, A., Yairi, E., & Amir, O. (2003). Second formant transitions in fluent speech of persistent and recovered preschool children who stutter. *Journal of Communication Disorders, 36,* 59–75.

Supprian, T., Retz, W., & Deckert, J. (1999). Clozapine-induced stuttering: epileptic brain activity? *The American Journal of Psychiatry, 156,* 1663–64.

Suresh, R., Ambrose, N., Roe, C., Pluzhnikov, A., Wittke-Thompson, J. K., Ng, M. C.Y., et al. (2006). New complexities in the genetics of stuttering: significant sex-specific linkage signals. *American Journal of Human Genetics, 78,* 554–63.

Susca, M., & Healey, E. C. (2001). Perceptions of simulated stuttering and fluency. *Journal of Speech, Language and Hearing Research, 44,* 61–73.

Sussman, H. M. (1982). Contrastive patterns of inter-hemispheric interference to verbal and spatial concurrent tasks in right-handed, left-handed and stuttering populations. *Neuropsychologia, 20,* 675–84.

Sussman, H. M., & MacNeilage, P. F. (1975). Hemispheric specialization for speech production and perception in stutterers. *Neuropsychologia, 13,* 19–26.

Suter, C. B., Hutchinson, J. M., & Mallard, A. R. (1979). Visible correlates of stuttering severity. [Abstract]. *ASHA, 21,* 733.

Sutton, S., & Chase, R. A. (1961). White noise and stuttering. *Journal of Speech and Hearing Research, 4,* 72.

Šváb, L., Gross, J., & Langová, J. (1972). Stuttering and social isolation: Effect of social isolation with different levels of monitoring on stuttering frequency (a pilot study). *Journal of Nervous and Mental Disorders, 155,* 1–5.

Swift, W. J., Swift, E. W., & Arellano, M. (1975). Haloperidol as a treatment for adult stuttering. *Comprehensive Psychiatry, 16,* 61–67.

Szelag, E., Garwarska-Kolek, D., Herman, A., & Stasiek, J. (1993). Brain lateralization and severity of stuttering in children. *Acta Neurobiologiae Experimentalis, 53,* 263–67.

Szelag, E., Herman-Jeglińska, A., & Garwarska-Kolek, D. (1997). Hemispheric asymmetries in stutterers: Disorder severity and neuroticism? *Acta Psychologica, 95,* 299–315.

Tanaka, Y., Nishida, H., Hayashi, R., Inuzuka, T., & Otsuki, M. (2006). [Callosal disconnection syndrome due to acute disseminated enchephalomyelitis]. *Rinsho Shinkeigaku (Clinical Neurology), 46,* 50–54.

Tanberg, M. C. (1955). A study of the role of inhibition in the moment of stuttering. In W. Johnson & R. R. Leutenegger (Eds.), *Stuttering in children and adults* (pp. 335–40). Minneapolis: University of Minnesota Press.

Tanenbaum, S. (2005). Evidence-based practice as mental health policy: Three controversies and a caveat. *Mental Health, 24,* 163–73.

Tapia, F. (1969). Haldol in the treatment of children with tics and stutterers—and an incidental finding. *Psychiatric Quarterly,* 43, 647–49.

Tasko, S. M., McClean, M. D., & Runyan, C. M. (2007). Speech motor correlates of treatment-related changes in stuttering severity and speech naturalness. *Journal of Communication Disorders, 40,* 42–65.

Tatchell, R. H., Van den Berg, S., & Lerman, J. W. (1983). Fluency and eye contact as factors influencing observers' perceptions of stutterers. *Journal of Fluency Disorders, 8,* 221–31.

Tate, M. W., & Cullinan, W. L. (1962). Measurement of consistency of stuttering. *Journal of Speech and Hearing Research, 5,* 272–83.

Tate, M. W., Cullinan, W. L., & Ahlstrand, A. (1961). Measurement of adaptation in stuttering. *Journal of Speech and Hearing Research,* 4, 321–39.

Tatham, M. A. A. (1973). Implications on stuttering of a model of speech production. In Y. Lebrun & R. Hoops (Eds.), *Neurolinguistic approaches to stuttering.* The Hague: Mouton.

Tawadros, S. M. (1957). An experiment in the group psychotherpay of stutterers. *International Journal of Sociometry, 1,* 181–89.

Taylor, I. K. (1966a). The properties of stuttered words. *Journal of Verbal Learning and Verbal Behavior, 5,* 112–18.

Taylor, I. K. (1966b). What words are stuttered? *Psychological Bulletin,* 65, 233–42.

Taylor, I. K., & Taylor, M. M. (1967). Test of predictions from the conflict hypothesis of stuttering. *Journal of Abnormal Psychology, 72,* 431–33.

Taylor, W. L., Lore, J. I., & Waldman, I. N. (1970). Latencies of semantic aphasics, stutterers and normal controls to cloze items requiring unique and non-unique oral responses. *Proceedings of the Annual Convention of the American Psychological Association, 78,* 75–76.

Telser, E. B. (1971). An assessment of word finding skills in stuttering and nonstuttering children. *Dissertation Abstracts International,* 32 (6-B), 3693–94.

Ten Cate, M. J. (1902). Über die Untersuchung der Atmungsbewegung bei Sprachfehlern. *Monatsschr. Sprachheilk., 12,* 247, 321.

Tetnowski, J. A., & Schagen, A. J. (2001). A comparison of listener and speaker perception of stuttering events. *Journal of Speech-Language Pathology and Audiology, 25,* 8–18.

Thomas, J. D. (1976). A psychophysiologic and personality assessment of stutterers as measured by conditionability, extraversion, and neuroticism. [Abstract]. *ASHA, 18,* 637.

Thompson, A. H. (1985). A test of the distraction explanation of disfluency modification in stuttering. *Journal of Fluency Disorders, 10,* 35–50.

Thorn, K. F. (1949). A study of the personality of stutterers as measured by the *MMPI.* Ph.D. Dissertation, University of Minnesota.

Throneburg, R. N., & Yairi, E. (1994). Temporal dynamics of repetitions during the early stage of childhood stuttering: an acoustic study. *Journal of Speech and Hearing Research, 37,* 1067–75.

Throneburg, R. N., Yairi, E., & Paden, E. P. (1994). Relation between phonologic difficulty and the occurrence of disfluences in the early stage of stuttering. *Journal of Speech and Hearing Research, 37,* 504–09.

Thürmer, U. St., Thumfart, W., & Kittel, G. (1983). Elektromyographische Untersuchungsbefunde bei Stotterern. *Sprache-Stimme-Gehör, 7,* 125–27.

Tiffany, W. R. (1963). Sound mindedness: Studies in the measurement of "phonetic ability." *Western Speech, 27,* 5–15.

Tiffany, W. R., & Hanley, C. N. (1956). Adaptation to delayed sidetone. *Journal of Speech and Hearing Disorders, 21,* 164–72.

Till, J. A., Reich, A., Dickey, S., & Sieber, J. (1983). Phonatory and manual reaction times of stuttering and nonstuttering children. *Journal of Speech and Hearing Research, 26,* 171–80.

Timmons, B. A., & Boudreau, J. P. (1978a). Delayed auditory feedback and the speech of stuttering and nonstuttering children. *Perceptual and Motor Skills, 46,* 551–55.

Timmons, B. A., & Boudreau, J. P. (1978b). Speech disfluencies and delayed auditory feedback reactions of stuttering and nonstuttering children. *Perceptual and Motor Skills, 47,* 859–62.

Timmons, R. J. (1967). A study of adaptation and consistency in a response-contingent punishment situation. [Abstract]. *Speech Monographs, 34,* 311–12.

Tippett, D. C., & Siebens, A. A. (1991). Distinguishing psychogenic from neurogenic dysfluency when neurologic and psychologic factors coexist. *Journal of Fluency Disorders, 16,* 3–12.

Toomey, G. L., & Sidman, M. (1970). An experimental analogue of the anxiety-stuttering relationship. *Journal of Speech and Hearing Research, 13,* 122–29.

Tornick, G. B., & Bloodstein, O. (1976). Stuttering and sentence length. *Journal of Speech and Hearing Research, 19,* 651–54.

Toscher, M. M., & Rupp, R. R. (1978). A study of the central auditory processes in stutterers using the Synthetic Sentence Identification (SSI) test battery. *Journal of Speech and Hearing Research, 21,* 779–92.

Trajkovski, N., Andrews, C., O'Brian, S., Onslow, M., & Packman, A. (2006). Treating stuttering in a preschool child with syllable-timed speech: A case report. *Behaviour Change, 23,* 1–8.

Trautman, L. S., Healey, E. C., Brown, T. A., Brown, P., & Jermano, S. (1999). A further analysis of narrative skills of children who stutter. *Journal of Communication Disorders, 32,* 297–314.

Trautman, L. S., Healey, E. C., & Norris, J. A. (2001). The effects of contextualization on fluency in three groups of children. *Journal of Speech, Language and Hearing Research, 44,* 564–77.

Travis, L. E. (1927a). Dysintegration of the breathing movements during stuttering. *Archives of Neurology and Psychiatry, 18,* 673–90.

Travis, L. E. (1927b). A phono-photographic study of the stutterer's voice and speech. *Psychology* (pp. 916–46). *Monographs, 36,* 109–41.

Travis, L. E. (1928a). A comparative study of the performances of stutterers and normal speakers in mirror tracing. *Psychology Monographs, 39,* 45–50.

Travis, L. E. (1928b). The influence of the group upon the stutterer's speed in free association. *Journal of Abnormal Social Psychology, 23,* 45–51.

Travis, L. E. (1931). *Speech pathology.* New York: D. Appleton-Century.

Travis, L. E. (1934). Dissociation of the homologous muscle function in stuttering. *Archives of Neurology and Psychiatry, 31,* 127–33.

Travis, L. E. (1957). The unspeakable feelings of people, with special reference to stuttering. In L. E. Travis (Ed.), *Handbook of speech pathology* (pp.916–46). New York: Appleton-Century-Crofts.

Travis, L. E., & Fagan, L. B. (1928). Studies in stuttering: III. A study of certain reflexes during stuttering. *Archives of Neurology and Psychiatry, 19,* 1006–13.

Travis, L. E., & Herren, R. Y. (1929). Studies in stuttering: V. A study of simultaneous antitropic movements of the hands of stutterers. *Archives of Neurology and Psychiatry, 22,* 487–94.

Travis, L. E., Johnson, W., & Shover, J. (1937). The relation of bilingualism to stuttering. *Journal of Speech Disorders, 2,* 185–89.

Travis, L. E., & Knott, J. R. (1936). Brain potentials from normal speakers and stutterers. *Journal of Psychology, 2,* 137–50.

Travis, L. E., & Knott, J. R. (1937). Bilaterally recorded brain potentials from normal speakers and stutterers. *Journal of Speech Disorders, 2,* 239–41.

Travis, L. E., & Lindsley, D. B. (1933). An action current study of handedness in relation to stuttering. *Journal of Experimental Psychology, 16,* 258–70.

Travis, L. E, & Malamud, W. (1937). Brain potentials from normal subjects, stutterers, and schizophrenic patients. *American Journal of Psychiatry, 93,* 929–36.

Travis, L. E., Malamud, W., & Thayer, L. R. (1934). The relationship between physical habitus and stuttering. *Journal of Abnormal Social Psychology, 29,* 132–40.

Travis, L. E., Tuttle, W. W., & Cowan, D. W. (1936). A study of the heart rate during stuttering. *Journal of Speech Disorders, 1,* 21–26.

Travis, V. (1936). A study of the horizontal dysintegration of breathing during stuttering. *Archives of Speech, 1,* 157–69.

Treon, M., & Tamayo, F. M.V. (1975). The separate and combined effects of GSR biofeedback and delayed auditory feedback on stuttering: A preliminary study. *Journal of Fluency Disorders, 1,* 3–9.

Trombly, T. (1965). Responses of stutterers and normal speakers to a level of aspiration inventory. *Central States Speech Journal, 16,* 179–81.

Trombly, T. W. (1959). A comparative study of stutterers' levels of aspiration for speech and non-speech performances. [Abstract]. *Speech Monographs, 26,* 143–44.

Trotter, W. D. (1955). The severity of stuttering during successive readings of the same material. *Journal of Speech and Hearing Disorders, 20,* 17–25.

Trotter, W. D. (1956). Relationship between severity of stuttering and word conspicuousness. *Journal of Speech and Hearing Disorders, 21,* 198–201.

Trotter, W. D., & Bergmann, M. F. (1957). Stutterers' and nonstutterers' reactions to speech situations. *Journal of Speech and Hearing Disorders, 22,* 40–45.

Trotter, W. D., & Brown, L. (1958). Speaking time behavior of the stutterer before and after speech therapy. *Journal of Speech and Hearing Research, 1,* 48–51.

Trotter, W. D., & Lesch, M. M. (1967). Personal experiences with a stutter-aid. *Journal of Speech and Hearing Disorders, 32,* 270–72.

Trotter, W. D., & Silverman, F. H. (1973). Experiments with the stutter-aid. *Perceptual and Motor Skills, 36,* 1129–30.

Trotter, W. D., & Silverman, F. H. (1974). Does the effect of pacing speech with a miniature metronome on stuttering wear off? *Perceptual and Motor Skills, 39,* 429–30.

Tsunoda, T., & Moriyama, H. (1972). Specific pattern of cerebral dominance for various sounds in adult stutterers. *Journal of Auditory Research, 12,* 216–27.

Tuck, A. E. (1979). An alaryngeal stutterer: A case history. *Journal of Fluency Disorders, 4,* 239–43.

Turgut, N., Utku, U., & Balci, K. (2002). A case of acquired stuttering resulting from left parietal infarction. *Acta Neurologica Scandinavica, 105,* 408–10.

Turnbaugh, K. R., Guitar, B. E., & Hoffman, P. R. (1979). Speech clinicians' attribution of personality traits as a function of stuttering severity. *Journal of Speech and Hearing Research, 22,* 37–45.

Turnbaugh, K., Guitar, B., & Hoffman, P. (1981). The attribution of personality traits: The stutterer and nonstutterer. *Journal of Speech and Hearing Research, 24,* 288–91.

Tuthill, C. (1940). A quantitative study of extensional meaning with special reference to stuttering. *Journal of Speech Disorders, 5,* 189–91.

Tuthill, C. (1946). A quantitative study of extensional meaning with special reference to stuttering. *Speech Monographs, 13,* 81–98.

Twitmyer, E. B. (1930). Stammering in relation to hemo-respiratory factors. *Quarterly Journal of Speech, 16,* 278–83.

Tyre, T. E., Maisto, S. A., & Companik, P. J. (1973). The use of systematic desensitization in the treatment of chronic stuttering behavior. *Journal of Speech and Hearing Disorders, 38,* 514–19.

Uenishi, S., Mori, T., & Mizumachi, T. (1973). Changes of maximum blood pressure in stutterers. *DSH Abstracts,* 13, 299.

Ulliana, L., & Ingham, R. J. (1984). Behavioral and nonbehavioral variables in the measurement of stutterers' communication attitudes. *Journal of Speech and Hearing Research, 49,* 83–93.

Umeda, K. (1962a). Electroencephalographic study of stutterers. *DSH Abstracts, 2,* 356.

Umeda, K. (1962b). A psychophysiological study of stutterers. *DSH Abstracts, 2,* 266.

Uys, I. C. (1970). 'n Ondersoek na sekere biolinguistiese verskynels by hakkel. *Journal of the South African Logopedic Society, 17,* 67–78.

Vaane, E., & Janssen, P. (1978). Different types of disfluencies and some phonological factors. *Logoped. Foniat., 50,* 14–20.

Valyo, R. A. (1964). PGSR responses of stutterers and nonstutterers during periods of silence and verbalization. [Abstract]. *ASHA, 6,* 422.

Van Borsel, J., Achten, E., Santens, P., Lahorte, P., & Voet, T. (2003). fMRI of developmental stuttering: A pilot study. *Brain and Language, 85,* 369–77.

Van Borsel, J., & de Britto Pereira, M. M. (2005). Assessment of stuttering in a familiar versus an unfamiliar language. *Journal of Fluency Disorders, 30,* 109–24.

Van Borsel, J., Dhooge, I., Verhoye, K., Derde, K., & Curfs, L. (1999). Communication problems in Turner syndrome: A sample survey. *Journal of Communication Disorders, 32,* 435–44.

Van Borsel, J., Geirnaert, E., & Van Coster, R. (2005). Another case of word-final disfluencies. *Folia Phoniatrica 57,* 148–62.

Van Borsel, J., Goethals, L., & Vanryckeghem, M. (2004). Disfluency in Tourette Syndrome: Observational study in three cases. *Folia Phoniatrica, 56,* 358–66.

Van Borsel, J., Jozefien, M., Charlotte, M., Rijke, R., Evy Van, L., & Tineke Van, R. (2006). Prevalence of stuttering in regular and special school populations in Belgium based on teacher perceptions. *Folia Phoniatrica, 58,* 289–302.

Van Borsel, J., Maes, E., & Foulon, S. (2001). Stuttering and bilingualism: A review. *Journal of Fluency Disorders, 26,* 179–205.

Van Borsel, J., Reunes, G., & Van den Bergh, N. (2003). Delayed auditory feedback in the treatment of stuttering: clients as consumers. *International Journal of Language and Communication Disorders, 38,* 119–30.

Van Borsel, J., Van Der Made, S., & Santens, P. (2003). Thalamic stuttering: A distinct clinical entity? *Brain and Language, 85,* 185–90.

Van Borsel, J., Van Lierde, K., Van Cauwenberge, P., Guldemont, I., & Van Orshoven, M. (1998). Severe acquired stuttering following injury of the left supplementary motor region: A case report. *Journal of Fluency Disorders, 23,* 49–58.

Van Dusen, C. R. (1937). A study of the relation of the relative size of the two hands to speech. *Speech Monographs, 4,* 127–34.

Van Dusen, C. R. (1939). A laterality study of nonstutterers and stutterers. *Journal of Speech Disorders, 4,* 261–65.

van Lieshout, P. H., & Hulstijn, W. (1996). From planning to articulation in speech production: What differentiates a person who stutters. *Journal of Speech and Hearing Research, 39,* 546–65.

van Lieshout, P. H., Hulstijn, W., & Peters, H. F. M. (1991). Word size and word complexity: Differences in speech reaction time between stutterers and nonstutterers in a picture and word naming task. In H. F. M. Peters, W. Hulstijn, & C. W. Starkweather (Eds.), *Speech motor control and stuttering.* Amsterdam: Elsevier.

van Lieshout, P. H., Hulstijn, W., & Peters, H. F. (1996). Speech production in people who stutter: Testing the motor plan assembly hypothesis. *Journal of Speech and Hearing Research, 39,* 76–92.

van Lieshout, P. H., Peters, H. F. M., Starkweather, C. W., & Hulstijn, W. (1993). Physiological differences between stutterers and nonstutterers in perceptually fluent speech: EMG amplitude and duration. *Journal of Speech and Hearing Research, 36,* 55–63.

van Lieshout, P. H., Starkweather, C. W., Hulstijn, W., & Peters, H. F. (1995). Effects of linguistic correlates of stuttering on EMG activity in nonstuttering speakers. *Journal of Speech and Hearing Research, 38,* 360–72.

Van Riper, C. (1934). A new test of laterality. *Journal of Experimental Psychology, 17,* 305–13.

Van Riper, C. (1935). The quantitative measurement of laterality. *Journal of Experimental Psychology, 18,* 372–82.

Van Riper, C. (1936). Study of the thoracic breathing of stutterers during expectancy and occurrence of stuttering spasm. *Journal of Speech Disorders, 1,* 61–72.

Van Riper, C. (1937a). The effect of devices for minimizing stuttering on the creation of symptoms. *Journal of Abnormal Social Psychology, 32,* 185–92.

Van Riper, C. (1937b). The effect of penalty upon frequency of stuttering spasms. *Journal of Genetic Psychology, 50,* 193–95.

Van Riper, C. (1937c). The influence of empathic response on the frequency of stuttering. *Psychology Monographs, 49,* 244–46.

Van Riper, C. (1937d). The preparatory set in stuttering. *Journal of Speech Disorders, 2,* 149–54.

Van Riper, C. (1938). A study of the stutterer's ability to interrupt stuttering spasms. *Journal of Speech Disorders, 3,* 117–19.

Van Riper, C. (1939). *Speech correction: principles and methods.* New York: Prentice-Hall.

Van Riper, C. (1954). *Speech correction: Principles and methods* (3rd ed.). Englewood Cliffs, NJ: Prentice-Hall.

Van Riper, C. (1958). Experiments in stuttering therapy. In J. Eisenson (Ed.), *Stuttering: a symposium* (pp. 273–390). New York: Harper & Row.

Van Riper, C. (1963). *Speech correction: Principles and methods, 4th ed.* Englewood Cliffs, NJ: Prentice-Hall.

Van Riper, C. (1970). The use of DAF in stuttering therapy. *British Journal of Disorders of Communication, 5,* 40–45.

Van Riper, C. (1971). *The nature of stuttering.* Englewood Cliffs, NJ: Prentice-Hall.

Van Riper, C. (1972). *Speech correction: Principles and methods* (5th ed.). Englewood Cliffs, NJ: Prentice-Hall.

Van Riper, C. (1973). *The treatment of stuttering.* Englewood Cliffs, NJ: Prentice-Hall.

Van Riper, C. (1982). *The nature of stuttering* (2nd ed.). Englewood Cliffs, NJ: Prentice-Hall.

Van Riper, C., and Hull, C. J. (1955). The quantitative measurement of the effect of certain situations on stuttering. In W. Johnson & R. R. Leutenegger

(Eds.). *Stuttering in children and adults* (pp. 199–206). Minneapolis: University of Minnesota Press.

Van Riper, C., & Milisen, R. L. (1939). A study of the predicted duration of the stutterer's blocks as related to their actual duration. *Journal of Speech Disorders,* 4, 339–46.

Vanryckeghem, M. (1995). The Communication Attitude Test: A concordancy investigation of stuttering and nonstuttering children and their parents. *Journal of Fluency Disorders, 20,* 191–203.

Vanryckeghem, M., & Brutten, G. (1992). *The Communication Attitude Test:* A test-retest reliability investigation. *Journal of Fluency Disorders, 17,* 177–90.

Vanryckeghem, M., & Brutten, G. J. (1996). The relationship between communication attitude and fluency failure of stuttering and nonstuttering children. *Journal of Fluency Disorders, 21,* 109–18.

Vanryckeghem, M., & Brutten, G. J. (2007). *The KiddyCAT: Communication Attitude Test for Preschool and Kindergarten Children Who Stutter.* San Diego: Plural Publishing.

Vanryckeghem, M., Brutten, G. J., & Hernandez, L. M. (2005). A comparative investigation of the speech-associated attitude of preschool and kindergarten children who do and do not stutter. *Journal of Fluency Disorders, 30,* 307–18.

Vanryckeghem, M., Brutten, G. J., Uddin, N., & Van Borsel, J. (2004). A comparative investigation of the speech-associated coping responses reported by adults who do and do not stutter. *Journal of Fluency Disorders, 29,* 237–50.

Vanryckeghem, M., Glessing, J. J., Brutten, G. J., & McAlindon, P. (1999). The main and interactive effect of oral reading rate on the frequency of stuttering. *American Journal of Speech-Language Pathology, 8,* 165–70.

Vanryckeghem, M., Hylebos, C., Brutten, G. J., & Peleman, M. (2001). The relationship between communication attitude and emotion of children who stutter. *Journal of Fluency Disorders, 26*(1), 1.

Van Wyk, M. (1978). 'N oudiovisuele analise van woorddeelherhalings by hakkelaars. *South African Journal of Communication Disorders, 25,* 64–79.

Vartanov, A. V., Glozman, Z. M., Kiselnikov, A. A., & Karpova, N. L. (2005). Cerebral organization of verbal action in stutterers. *Human Physiology, 31,* 132–36.

Vasić, N., & Wijnen, F. (2005). Stuttering as a monitoring deficit. In R. J. Hartsuiker, R. Bastiaanse, A. Postma, & F. Wijnen (Eds.), *Phonological encoding and monitoring in normal and pathological speech* (pp. 226–47). Hove: Psychology Press.

Vaughn, C.-L. D., & Webster, W. G. (1989). Bimanual handedness in adults who stutter. *Perceptual and Motor Skills, 68,* 375–82.

Venkatagiri, H. S. (1980). The relevance of DAF-induced speech disruption to the understanding of stuttering. *Journal of Fluency Disorders, 5,* 87–98.

Venkatagiri, H. S. (1981). Reaction time for voiced and whispered /a/ in stutterers and nonstutterers. *Journal of Fluency Disorders, 6,* 265–71.

Venkatagiri, H. S. (1982a). A comparison of DAF-induced disfluencies with stuttering. *Journal of Communication Disorders, 15,* 385–93.

Venkatagiri, H. S. (1982b). The influence of linguistic stress on stuttering. [Abstract]. *ASHA, 24,* 730.

Venkatagiri, H. S. (1982c). Reaction time for /s/ and /z/ in stutterers and nonstutterers: A test of discoordination hypothesis. *Journal of Communication Disorders, 15,* 55–62.

Venkatagiri, H. S. (2004). Slower and incomplete retrieval of speech motor plans is the proximal source of stuttering: Stutters occur when syllable motor plans stored in memory are concatenated to produce the utterance motor plan. *Medical Hypotheses, 62,* 401–05.

Venkatagiri, H. S. (2005). Recent advances in the treatment of stuttering: A theoretical perspective. *Journal of Communication Disorders, 38,* 375–93.

Victor, C., & Johannsen, H. S. (1984). Untersuchung zur zerebralen Dominanz für Sprache bei Stotterer mittels Tachistoskopie. *Sprache-Stimme-Gehör, 8,* 74–77.

Villarreal, J. J. (1945). The semantic aspects of stuttering in non-stutterers: Additional data. *Quarterly Journal of Speech, 31,* 477–79.

Viswanath, N. S. (1989). Global- and local-temporal effects of a stuttering event in the context of a clausal utterance. *Journal of Fluency Disorders, 14,* 245–69.

Viswanath, N. S. (1991). Temporal structure is reorganized when an utterance contains a stuttering event. In H. F. M. Peters, W. Hulstijn, & C. W. Starkweather (Eds.). *Speech motor control and stuttering.* Amsterdam: Elsevier.

Viswanath, N., Lee, H. S., & Chakraborty, R. (2004). Evidence for a major gene influence on persistent developmental stuttering. *Human Biology, 76,* 401–12.

Viswanath, N. S., Karmonik, C., King, D., Rosenfield, D. B., & Mawad, M. (2003). Functional Magnetic Resonance Imaging (fMRI) of a stutterer's brain during overt speech. *Journal of Neuroimaging, 13,* 280–81.

Voelker, C. H. (1942). On the semantic aspects of stuttering in nonstutterers. *Quarterly Journal of Speech, 28,* 78–80.

von Gudenberg, A. W. (2006). Kassel Stuttering Therapy: evaluation of a computer-aided therapy [German]. *Forum Logopadie, 20,* 6–11.

Wagaman, J. R., & Miltenberger, R. G. (1993). Analysis of a simplified treatment for stuttering in children. *Journal of Applied Behavior Analysis, 26,* 53–62.

Wagaman, J. R., & Miltenberger, R. G. (1995). Long-term follow-up of a behavioral treatment for stuttering children. *Journal of Applied Behavior Analysis, 28,* 233–35.

Walker, S. T., & Walker, J. M. (1973). Differences in heart-rate variability between stutterers and nonstutterers following arousal. *Perceptual and Motor Skills, 36,* 926.

Wall, M. J. (1980). A comparison of syntax in young stutterers and nonstutterers. *Journal of Fluency Disorders, 5,* 345–52.

Wall, M. J. (1982). Language-based therapies for the young child stutterer. *Journal of Childhood Communication Disorders, 6,* 40–49.

Wall, M. J., Starkweather, C. W., & Cairns, H. S. (1981). Syntactic influences on stuttering in young child stutterers. *Journal of Fluency Disorders, 6,* 283–98.

Wall, M. J., Starkweather, C. W., & Harris, K. S. (1981). The influence of voicing adjustments on the location of stuttering in the spontaneous speech of young child stutterers. *Journal of Fluency Disorders, 6,* 299–310.

Walla, P., Mayer, D., Deecke, L., & Thurner, S. (2004). The lack of focused anticipation of verbal information in stutterers: a magnetoencephalographic study. *NeuroImage, 22,* 1321–27.

Walle, E. L. (1971). Intracarotid sodium amytal testing on normal, chronic adult stutterers. *Journal of Speech and Hearing Disorders, 36,* 561.

Wallen, V. (1960). A Q-technique study of the self-concepts of adolescent stutterers and nonstutterers. [Abstract]. *Speech Monographs, 27,* 257–58.

Wallin, J. E. W. (1916). A census of speech defectives among 89,057 public-school pupils—a preliminary report. *School and Society, 3,* 213–16.

Walnut, F. (1954). A personality inventory item analysis of individuals who stutter and individuals who have other handicaps. *Journal of Speech and Hearing Disorders, 19,* 220–27.

Walton, D., & Mather, M. D. (1963). The relevance of generalization techniques to the treatment of stammering and phobic symptoms. *Behavior Research Therapy, 1,* 121–25.

Wampold, B. E. (2001). *The great psychotherapy debate: Models, methods and findings.* Mahwah, NJ: Lawrence Erlbaum Associates.

Wampold, B. E., & Bhati, K. S. (2004). Attending to the omissions: A historical examination of evidence-based practice movements. *Professional Psychology: Research and Practice, 35,* 563–70.

Wampold, B. E., & Brown, G. S. (2005). Estimating variability in outcomes attributable to therapists: A naturalistic study of outcomes in managed care. *Journal of Consulting and Clinical Psychology, 73,* 914–23.

Wampold, B. E., Lichtenberg, J. W., & Waehler, C. A. (2005). A broader perspective: Counseling psychology's emphasis on evidence. *Journal of Contemporary Psychotherapy, 35,* 27–38.

Wampold, B. E., Minami, T., Tierney, S. C., Baskin, T. W., & Bhati, K. S. (2005). The placebo is powerful: Estimating placebo effects in medicine and psychotherapy from randomized clinical trials. *Journal of Clinical Psychology, 61,* 835–54.

Ward, D. (1967). A study of the responses of listeners to dysfluencies of speech. [Abstract]. *Speech Monographs, 34,* 312.

Ward, D. (1997). Intrinsic and extrinsic timing in stutterers' speech: Data and implications. *Language and Speech, 40,* 289–310.

Watkins, R. V. (2005). Language abilities of young children who stutter. In E. Yairi & N. Ambrose (Eds.), *Early childhood stuttering: for clinicians by clinicians* (pp. 235–52). Austin, TX: Pro-Ed.

Watkins, R. V., & Yairi, E. (1997). Language production abilities of children whose stuttering persisted or recovered. *Journal of Speech, Language and Hearing Research, 40*(2), 385–99.

Watkins, R. V., Yairi, E., & Ambrose, N. G. (1999). Early childhood stuttering III: Initial status of expressive language abilities. *Journal of Speech, Language and Hearing Research, 42,* 1125–35.

Watson, B. C., & Alfonso, P. J. (1982). A comparison of LRT and VOT values between stutterers and nonstutterers. *Journal of Fluency Disorders, 7,* 219–41.

Watson, B. C., & Alfonso, P. J. (1983). Foreperiod and stuttering severity effects on acoustic laryngeal reaction time. *Journal of Fluency Disorders, 8,* 183–205.

Watson, B. C., & Alfonso, P. J. (1987). Physiological bases of acoustic LRT in nonstutterers, mild stutterers, and severe stutterers. *Journal of Speech and Hearing Research, 30,* 434–47.

Watson, B. C., Freeman, F. J., Chapman, S. B., Miller, S., Finitzo, T., Pool, K. D., & Devous, M. D., Sr. (1991). Linguistic performance deficits in stutterers: Relation to laryngeal reaction time profiles. *Journal of Fluency Disorders, 16,* 85–100.

Watson, B. C., Freeman, F. J., Devous, M. D., Sr., Chapman, S. B., Finitzo, T., & Pool, K. D. (1994). Linguistic performance and regional cerebral blood flow in persons who stutter. *Journal of Speech and Hearing Research, 37,* 1221–28.

Watson, B. C., Pool, K. D., Devous, M. D., Sr., Freeman, F. J., & Finitzo, T. (1992). Brain blood flow related to acoustic laryngeal reaction time in adult developmental stutterers. *Journal of Speech and Hearing Research, 35,* 555–61.

Watson, J. B., Gregory, H. H., & Kistler, D. J. (1987). Development and evaluation of an inventory to assess adult stutterers' communication attitudes. *Journal of Fluency Disorders, 12,* 429–50.

Watson, J. B. (1987). Profiles of stutterers' and nonstutterers' affective, cognitive, and behavioral communication attitudes. *Journal of Fluency Disorders, 12,* 389–405.

Watson, J. B. (1988). A comparison of stutterers' and nonstutterers' affective, cognitive, and behavioral self-reports. *Journal of Speech and Hearing Research, 31,* 377–85.

Watts, F. (1971). The treatment of stammering by the intensive practice of fluent speech. *British Journal of Disorders of Communication, 6,* 144–47.

Webber, M. J., Packman, A., & Onslow, M. (2004). Effects of self-modelling on stuttering. *International Journal of Language and Communication Disorders, 39,* 509–22.

Weber, C. M., & Smith, A. (1990). Autonomic correlates of stuttering and speech assessed in a range of experimental tasks. *Journal of Speech and Hearing Research, 33,* 690–706.

Weber-Fox, C. (2001). Neural systems for sentence processing in stuttering. *Journal of Speech, Language and Hearing Research, 44,* 814–25.

Weber-Fox, C., Spencer, R. M. C., Spruill III, J. E., & Smith, A. (2004). Phonologic processing in adults who stutter: Electrophysiological and behavioral evidence. *Journal of Speech, Language and Hearing Research, 47,* 1244–58.

Webster, L. M., & Brutten, G. (1972). An audiovisual behavioral analysis of the stuttering moment. *Behavior Therapist, 3,* 555–60.

Webster, L. M., & Gould, W. J. (1975). The effect on stuttering of selectively anesthetizing certain nerve tracts. In L. M. Webster & L. C. Furst (Eds.), *Vocal tract dynamics and dysfluency.* New York: Speech and Hearing Institute.

Webster, R. L. (1970). Stuttering: A way to eliminate it and a way to explain it. In R. Ulrich, T. Stachnik, & J. Mabry (Eds.), *Control of human behavior, Vol. 2.* Glenview, IL: Scott, Foresman.

Webster, R. L. (1974). A behavioral analysis of stuttering: Treatment and theory. In K. S. Calhoun, H. E. Adams, & K. M. Mitchell (Eds.), *Innovative treatment methods in psychopathology.* New York: Wiley.

Webster, R. L. (1975). An operant response shaping program for the establishment of fluency in stutterers. *DSH Abstracts, 15,* 136.

Webster, R. L. (1979a). Empirical considerations regarding stuttering therapy. In H. H. Gregory (Ed.), *Controversies about stuttering therapy* (pp. 209–40). Baltimore: University Park Press.

Webster, R. L. (1979b). Masking influences on speech onset latencies in stutterers and normals. [Abstract]. *ASHA, 21,* 693.

Webster, R. L. (1980). Evolution of a target-based behavioral therapy for stuttering. *Journal of Fluency Disorders, 5,* 303–20.

Webster, R. L. (1991). Manipulation of vocal tone: Implications for stuttering. In H. F. M. Peters,

W. Hulstijn, & C. W. Starkweather (Eds.), *Speech motor control and stuttering.* Amsterdam: Elsevier.

Webster, R. L., & Dorman, M. F. (1970). Decreases in stuttering frequency as a function of continuous and contingent forms of auditory masking. *Journal of Speech and Hearing Research, 13,* 82–86.

Webster, R. L., & Dorman, M. F. (1971). Changes in reliance on auditory feedback cue as a function of oral practice. *Journal of Speech and Hearing Research, 14,* 307–11.

Webster, R. L., & Lubker, B. B. (1968a). Interrelationships among fluency producing variables in stuttered speech. *Journal of Speech and Hearing Research, 11,* 754–66.

Webster, R. L., & Lubker, B. B. (1968b). Masking of auditory feedback in stutterers' speech. *Journal of Speech and Hearing Research, 11,* 221–22.

Webster, R. L., Schumacher, S. J., & Lubker, B. B. (1970). Changes in stuttering frequency as a function of various intervals of delayed auditory feedback. *Journal of Abnormal Psychology, 75,* 45–49.

Webster, W. G. (1985). Neuropsychological models of stuttering: I. Representation of sequential response mechanisms. *Neuropsychologia,* 23, 263–67.

Webster, W. G. (1986a). Neuropsychological models of stuttering: II. Interhemispheric interference. *Neuropsychologia, 24,* 737–41.

Webster, W. G. (1986b). Response sequence organization and reproduction by stutterers. *Neuropsychologia, 24,* 813–21.

Webster, W. G. (1987). Rapid letter transcription performance by stutterers. *Neuropsychologia, 25,* 845–47.

Webster, W. G. (1988). Neural mechanisms underlying stuttering: evidence from bimanual handwriting performance. *Brain and Language, 33,* 226–44.

Webster, W. G. (1989a). Sequence initiation performance by stutterers under conditions of response competition. *Brain and Language, 36,* 286–300.

Webster, W. G. (1989b). Sequence reproduction deficits in stutterers tested under nonspeeded response conditions. *Journal of Fluency Disorders, 14,* 79–86.

Webster, W. G. (1990a). Concurrent cognitive processing and letter sequence transcription deficits in stutterers. *Canadian Journal of Psychology, 44,* 1–13.

Webster, W. G. (1990b). Evidence in bimanual finger-tapping of an attentional component to stuttering. *Behavioral Brain Research, 37,* 93–100.

Webster, W. G. (1993). Hurried hands and tangled tongues: Implications of current research for the management of stuttering. In E. Boberg (Ed.), *Neuropsychology of stuttering* (pp. 73–111). Alberta: University of Alberta Press.

Webster, W. G. (1997). Principles of brain organization related to lateralization of language and speech motor functions in normal speakers and stutterers. In W. Hulstijn, H. F. M. Peters, & P. H. H. M. v. Lieshout (Eds.), *Speech production: Motor control, brain research and fluency disorders* (pp. 119–39). Amsterdam: Elsevier.

Webster, W. G. (1998). Brain models and the clinical management of stuttering. *Journal of Speech-Language Pathology and Audiology, 22,* 220–30.

Webster, W. G., & Poulos, M. (1987). Handedness distributions among adults who stutter. *Cortex, 23,* 705–08.

Webster, W. G., & Ryan, C. R. R. (1991). Task complexity and manual reaction times in people who stutter. *Journal of Speech and Hearing Research, 34,* 708–14.

Weinberg, B. (1964). Stuttering among blind and partially sighted children. *Journal of Speech and Hearing Disorders, 29,* 322–26.

Weiner, A. E. (1984a). Patterns of vocal fold movement during stuttering. *Journal of Fluency Disorders, 9,* 31–49.

Weiner, A. E. (1984b). Stuttering and syllable stress. *Journal of Fluency Disorders, 9,* 301–05.

Weiner, A. E. (1984c). Vocal control therapy for stutterers. In M. Peins (Ed.), *Contemporary approaches in stuttering therapy.* Boston: Little, Brown.

Weisberger, S. E. (1967). An analysis of stuttering as a function of the stutterer's response to an array of standard projective stimuli involving themes of sexuality, aggression, and parental authority. [Abstract]. *Speech Monographs, 34,* 313.

Weisel, A., & Spektor, G. (1998). Attitudes toward own communication and toward stutterers. *Journal of Fluency Disorders, 23,* 157–72.

Weiss, A. L. (2002). Recasts in parents' language to their school-age children who stutter: A preliminary study. *Journal of Fluency Disorders, 27,* 243–67.

Weiss, A. L., & Zebrowski, P. M. (1991). Patterns of assertiveness and responsiveness in parental interactions with stuttering and fluent children. *Journal of Fluency Disorders, 16,* 125–41.

Weiss, A. L., & Zebrowski, P. M. (1992). Disfluencies in the conversations of young children who stutter: Some answers about questions. *Journal of Speech and Hearing Research, 35,* 1230–38.

Weiss, A. L., & Zebrowski, P. M. (1994). The narrative productions of children who stutter: A preliminary view. *Journal of Fluency Disorders, 19,* 39–63.

Weiss, D. A. (1964). *Cluttering.* Englewood Cliffs, NJ: Prentice-Hall.

Welch, I. L. (1961). An investigation of the listening proficiency of stutterers. [Abstract]. *Speech Monographs, 28,* 125–26.

Well, C. D., & Terrell, S. L. (1986). Attitudes and reactions of preschool and school-age children toward a child speaker with stuttering patterns. [Abstract]. *Folia Phoniatrica, 38,* 369.

Wells, B. G., & Moore, W. H., Jr. (1990). EEG alpha asymmetries in stutterers and nonstutterers: effects of linguistic variables on hemispheric processing and fluency. *Neuropsychologia, 28,* 1295–1305.

Wells, G. B. (1979). Effect of sentence structure on stuttering. *Journal of Fluency Disorders, 4,* 123–29.

Wells, G. B. (1983). A feature analysis of stuttered phonemes. *Journal of Fluency Disorders, 8,* 119–24.

Wells, P. G., & Malcolm, M. T. (1971). Controlled trial of the treatment of 36 stutterers. *British Journal of Psychiatry, 119,* 603–04.

Wendahl, R. W., & Cole, J. (1961). Identification of stuttering during relatively fluent speech. *Journal of Speech and Hearing Research, 4,* 281–86.

Wepman, J. M. (1939). Familial incidence in stammering. *Journal of Speech Disorders, 4,* 199–204.

Wertenbroch, W. (1976). Die Behandlung von Stotterern mit Haloperidol. *Sprachheilarb., 21,* 78–82.

West, R. (1931). The phenomenology of stuttering. In R. West (Ed.), *A symposium on stuttering.* Madison, WI: College Typing Company.

West, R. (1958). An agnostic's speculations about stuttering. In J. Eisenson (Ed.), *Stuttering: a symposium* (pp. 167–222). New York: Harper & Row.

West, R., & Ansberry, M. (1968). *The rehabilitation of speech* (4th ed.). New York: Harper & Row.

West, R., Ansberry, M., & Carr, A. (1957). *The rehabilitation of speech* (3rd ed.). New York: Harper & Bros.

West, R., Kennedy, L., & Carr, A. (1947). *The rehabilitation of speech* (rev. ed.). New York: Harper & Bros.

West, R., Nelson, S., & Berry, M. F. (1939). The heredity of stuttering. *Quarterly Journal of Speech, 25,* 23–30.

West, R. & Nusbaum, E. (1929). A motor test for dysphemia. *Quarterly Journal of Speech, 15,* 469–79.

Westby, C. E. (1979). Language performance of stuttering and nonstuttering children. *Journal of Communication Disorders, 12,* 133–45.

Westphal, G. (1933). An experimental study of certain motor abilities of stutterers. *Child Development, 4,* 214–21.

Weuffen, M. (1961). Untersuchung der Wortfindung bei normalsprechenden und stotternden Kindern und Jugendlichen im Alter von 8 bis 16 Jahren. *Folia Phoniatrica, 13,* 255–68.

Wevrick, P., & Mervyn, J. (1999). Natural histories in preschool children who stutter. *Journal of Speech-Language Pathology and Audiology, 23,* 173–83.

Wexler, K. B. (1982). Developmental disfluency in 2-, 4-, and 6-year-old boys in neutral and stress situations. *Journal of Speech and Hearing Research, 25,* 229–34.

Wexler, K. B., & Mysak, E. D. (1982). Disfluency characteristics of 2-, 4-, and 6-year-old males. *Journal of Fluency Disorders, 7,* 37–46.

White, P. A., & Collins, S. R. C. (1984). Stereotype formation by inference: A possible explanation for the "stutterer" stereotype. *Journal of Speech and Hearing Research, 27,* 567–70.

White House Conference Committee Report on Child Health and Protection, Section III. (1931). *Special Education: The Handicapped and the Gifted.* New York: D. Appleton Century.

Wiechmann, J., & Richter, E. (1966). Die Häufigkeit des Stotterns beim Singen. *Folia Phoniatrica, 18,* 435–46.

Wieneke, G., & Janssen, P. (1948). Effect of speaking rate on speech timing variability. In H. F. M. Peters, W. Hulstijn, & C. W. Starkweather (Eds.) (1991). *Speech motor control and stuttering.* Amsterdam: Elsevier.

Wieneke, G., & Janssen, P. (1987). Duration variations in the fluent speech of stutterers and nonstutterers.

In H. F. M. Peters & W. Hulstijn (Eds.), *Speech motor dynamics in stuttering* (pp. 345–52). New York: Springer.

Wieneke, G., & Janssen, P. (1991). Effect of speaking rate on speech timing variability. In H. F. M. Peters, W. Hulstijn, & W. Starkweather (Eds.), *Speech motor control and stuttering* (pp. 325–31). Amsterdam: Exerpta Medica.

Wiener, N. (1948). *Cybernetics.* New York: Wiley.

Wijnen, F. (1990). The development of sentence planning. *Journal of Child Language, 17,* 651–75.

Wijnen, F., & Boers, I. (1994). Phonological priming effects in stutterers. *Journal of Fluency Disorders, 19,* 1–20.

Wilkenfeld, J. R., & Curlee, R. F. (1997). The relative effects of questions and comments on children's stuttering. *American Journal of Speech-Language Pathology, 6,* 79–89.

Wilkie, T., & Beilby, J. (1996). Post-treatment stuttering severity under different assessment conditions. *Australian Journal of Human Communication Disorders, 24,* 19–27.

Wilkins, C., Webster, R. L., & Morgan, B. T. (1984). Cerebral lateralization of visual stimulus recognition in stutterers and fluent speakers. *Journal of Fluency Disorders, 9,* 131–41.

Williams, A. M., & Marks, C. J. (1972). A comparative analysis of the *ITPA* and *PPVT* performance of young stutterers. *Journal of Speech and Hearing Research, 15,* 323–29.

Williams, D. E. (1955). Masseter muscle action potentials in stuttered and nonstuttered speech. *Journal of Speech and Hearing Disorders, 20,* 242–61.

Williams, D. E. (1957). A point of view about "stuttering." *Journal of Speech and Hearing Disorders, 22,* 390–97.

Williams, D. E. (1962). Modification of stuttering behavior by the use of electric shock. *Asha, 4,* 408–09.

Williams, D. E., & Kent, L. R. (1958). Listener evaluations of speech interruptions. *Journal of Speech and Hearing Research, 1,* 124–31.

Williams, D. E., Melrose, B. M., & Woods, C. L. (1969). The relationship between stuttering and academic achievement in children. *Journal of Communication Disorders, 2,* 87–98.

Williams, D. E., & Silverman, F. H. (1968). Note concerning articulation of school-age stutterers. *Perceptual and Motor Skills, 27,* 713–14.

Williams, D. E., Silverman, F. H., & Kools, J. A. (1968). Disfluency behavior of elementary-school stutterers and nonstutterers: The adaptation effect. *Journal of Speech and Hearing Research, 11,* 622–30.

Williams, D. E., Silverman, F. H., & Kools, J. A. (1969a). Disfluency behavior of elementary-school stutterers and nonstutterers: The consistency effect. *Journal of Speech and Hearing Research, 12,* 301–07.

Williams. D. E., Silverman, F. H., & Kools, J. A. (1969b). Disfluency behavior of elementary-school stutterers and nonstutterers: Loci of instances of disfluency. *Journal of Speech and Hearing Research, 12,* 308–18.

Williams, D. E., Wark, M., & Minifie, F. D. (1963). Ratings of stuttering by audio, visual, and audiovisual cues. *Journal of Speech and Hearing Research, 6,* 91–100.

Williams, D. F., & Brutten, G. J. (1994). Physiologic and aerodynamic events prior to the speech of stutterers and nonstutterers. *Journal of Fluency Disorders, 19,* 83–111.

Williams, H. G., & Bishop, J. H. (1992). Speed and consistency of manual movements of stutterers, articulation-disordered children, and children with normal speech. *Journal of Fluency Disorders, 17,* 191–203.

Williams, J. D., & Martin, R. B. (1974). Immediate versus delayed consequences of stuttering responses. *Journal of Speech and Hearing Research, 17,* 569–75.

Wilson, D. M. (1950). A study of the personalities of stuttering children and their parents as revealed through projection tests. Ph.D. Dissertation, University of Southern California.

Wilson, L., Onslow, M., & Lincoln, M. (2004). Telehealth adaptation of the lidcombe program of early stuttering intervention: Five Case Studies. *American Journal of Speech-Language Pathology, 1,* 81–93.

Wilson, R. G. (1950). A study of expressive movements in three groups of adolescent boys, stutterers, non-stutterers, maladjusted and normals, by means of three measures of personality, *Mira's Myokinetic Psychodiagnosis,* the *Bender-Gestalt,* and figure drawing. Ph.D. Dissertation, Western Reserve University.

Wingate, M. E. (1959). Calling attention to stuttering. *Journal of Speech and Hearing Research, 2,* 326–35.

Wingate, M. E. (1962a). Evaluation and stuttering. Part I: Speech characteristics of young children. *Journal of Speech and Hearing Disorders, 27,* 106–15.

Wingate, M. E. (1962b). Personality needs of stutterers. *Logos, 5,* 35–37.

Wingate, M. E. (1964). Recovery from stuttering. *Journal of Speech and Hearing Disorders, 29,* 312–21.

Wingate, M. E. (1966a). Behavioral rigidity in stutterers. *Journal of Speech and Hearing Research, 9,* 626–29.

Wingate, M. E. (1966b). Prosody in stuttering adaptation. *Journal of Speech and Hearing Research, 9,* 550–56.

Wingate, M. E. (1967a). Slurvian skill of stutterers. *Journal of Speech and Hearing Research, 10,* 844–48.

Wingate, M. E. (1967b). Stuttering and word length. *Journal of Speech and Hearing Research, 10,* 146–52.

Wingate, M. E. (1969). Sound and pattern in "artificial" fluency. *Journal of Speech and Hearing Research, 12,* 677–86.

Wingate, M. E. (1970). Effect on stuttering of changes in audition. *Journal of Speech and Hearing Research, 13,* 861–73.

Wingate, M. E. (1971). Phonetic ability in stuttering. *Journal of Speech and Hearing Research, 14,* 189–94.

Wingate, M. E. (1972). Deferring the adaptation effect. *Journal of Speech and Hearing Research, 15,* 547–50.

Wingate, M. E. (1975). Expectancy as basically a short-term process. *Journal of Speech and Hearing Research, 18,* 31–42.

Wingate, M. E. (1976). *Stuttering: Theory and treatment.* New York: Irvington.

Wingate, M. E. (1977). Criteria for stuttering. *Journal of Speech and Hearing Research, 20,* 596–600.

Wingate, M. E. (1979a). The first three words. *Journal of Speech and Hearing Research, 22,* 604–12.

Wingate, M. E. (1979b). The loci of stuttering: grammar or prosody? *Journal of Communication Disorders, 12,* 283–90.

Wingate, M. E. (1981a). Questionnaire study of laryngectomee stutterers. *Journal of Fluency Disorders, 6,* 273–81.

Wingate, M. E. (1981b). Sound pattern in artificial fluency: Spectrographic evidence. *Journal of Fluency Disorders, 6,* 95–118.

Wingate, M. E. (1982). Early position and stuttering occurrence. *Journal of Fluency Disorders, 7,* 243–58.

Wingate, M. E. (1984a). The recurrence ratio. *Journal of Fluency Disorders, 9,* 21–29.

Wingate, M. E. (1984b). Stutter events and linguistic stress. *Journal of Fluency Disorders, 9,* 295–300.

Wingate, M. E. (1986). Adaptation, consistency and beyond: I. Limitations and contradictions. *Journal of Fluency Disorders, 11,* 1–36.

Wingate, M. E. (1988). *The structure of stuttering: A psycholinguistic analysis.* New York: Springer-Verlag.

Wingate, M. E. (2001). SLD is not stuttering. *Journal of Speech, Language and Hearing Research, 44,* 381–84.

Wingate, M. E., & Hamre, C. E. (1967). Stutterers' projection of listener reaction. *Journal of Speech and Hearing Research, 10,* 339–43.

Winitz, H. (1961). Repetitions in the vocalizations of children in the first two years of life. *Journal of Speech and Hearing Disorders, Monograph Supplement 7,* 55–62.

Winkelman, N. W., Jr. (1954). Chlorpromazine in the treatment of neuropsychiatric disorders. *Journal of the American Medical Association, 155,* 18–21.

Winkler, L. E., & Ramig, P. (1986). Temporal characteristics in the fluent speech of child stutterers and nonstutterers. *Journal of Fluency Disorders, 11,* 217–29.

Winslow, M., & Guitar, B. (1994). The effects of structured turn-taking on disfluencies: A case study. *Language, Speech, and Hearing Services in Schools, 25,* 251–57.

Wischner, G. J. (1947). Stuttering behavior and learning: A program of research. Ph.D. Dissertation, University of Iowa.

Wischner, G. J. (1950). Stuttering behavior and learning: A preliminary theoretical formulation. *Journal of Speech and Hearing Disorders, 15,* 324–35.

Wischner, G. J. (1952a). Anxiety-reduction as reinforcement in maladaptive behavior: Evidence in stutterers' representations of the moment of difficulty. *Journal of Abnormal Social Psychology, 47,* 566–71.

Wischner, G. J. (1952b). An experimental approach to expectancy and anxiety in stuttering behavior. *Journal of Speech and Hearing Disorders, 17,* 139–54.

Witt, M. H. (1925). Statistische Erhebungen über den Einfluss des Singens und Flüsterns auf das Stottern, *Vox, 11,* 41–43.

Wohl, M.T. (1951). The incidence of speech defect in the population. *Speech, 15,* 13–14.

Wohl, M.T. (1968). The electronic metronome—an evaluative study. *British Journal of Disorders of Communication, 3,* 89–98.

Wohl, M.T. (1970). The treatment of non-fluent utterance—a behavioural approach. *British Journal of Disorders of Communication, 5,* 66–76.

Wolk, L. (1981). Vocal tract dynamics in an adult stutterer. *South African Journal of Communication Disorders, 28,* 38–52.

Wolk, L., Blomgren, M., & Smith, A. B. (2000). The frequency of simultaneous disfluency and phonological errors in children: a preliminary investigation. *Journal of Fluency Disorders, 25,* 269–81.

Wolk, L., Edwards, M. L., & Conture, E. G. (1993). Coexistence of stuttering and disordered phonology in young children. *Journal of Speech and Hearing Research, 36,* 906–17.

Wolpe, J. (1958). *Psychotherapy by reciprocal inhibition.* Stanford, CA: Stanford University Press.

Wong, A., Gottesman, I., & Petronis, A. (2005). Phenotypic differences in genetically identical organisms: the epigenetic perspective. *Human Molecular Genetics, 14,* R11-R18.

Wong, C.Y. Y., & Bloodstein, O. (1977). Effect of adjacency on the distribution of new stutterings in two successive readings. *Journal of Speech and Hearing Research, 20,* 35–39.

Wood, F., Stump, D., McKeehan, A., Sheldon, S., & Proctor, J. (1980). Patterns of regional cerebral blood flow during attempted reading aloud by stutterers both on and off haloperidol medication: Evidence for inadequate left frontal activation during stuttering. *Brain and Language, 9,* 141–44.

Woods, C. L. (1974). Social position and speaking competence of stuttering and normally fluent boys. *Journal of Speech and Hearing Research, 17,* 740–47.

Woods, C. L. (1978). Does the stigma shape the stutterer? *Journal of Communication Disorders, 11,* 483–87.

Woods, C. L., & Williams, D. E. (1971). Speech clinicians' conceptions of boys and men who stutter. *Journal of Speech and Hearing Disorders, 36,* 225–34.

Woods, C. L., & Williams, D. E. (1976). Traits attributed to stuttering and normally fluent males. *Journal of Speech and Hearing Research, 19,* 267–78.

Woods, S., Shearsby, J., Onslow, M., & Burnham, D. (2002). Psychological impact of the Lidcombe Program of early stuttering intervention. *International Journal of Language and Communication Disorders, 37,* 31–40.

Woolf, G. (1967). The assessment of stuttering as struggle, avoidance, and expectancy. *British Journal of Disorders of Communication, 2,* 158–71.

Wright, L., Ayre, A., & Grogan, S. (1998). Outcome measurement in adult stuttering therapy: A self-rating profile. *International Journal of Language and Communication Disorders, 33,* 378.

Wu, J. C., Maguire, G., Riley, G., Fallon, J., LaCasse, L., Chin, S., et al. (1995). A positron emission tomography [18F] deoxyglucose study of developmental stuttering. *Neuroreport, 6,* 501–05.

Wu, J. C., Maguire, G., Riley, G., Lee, A., Keator, D., Tang, C., et al. (1997). Increased dopamine activity associated with stuttering. *Neuroreport, 8,* 767–70.

Wulff, J. (1935). Lippen- Kiefer- Zungen- und Handreaktionen auf Reizdarbietungen nach unterschiedlichen Zeitintervallen bei normalsprechenden und bei stotternden Kindern im Alter von etwa 14 Jahren. *Vox, 21,* 40–45.

Wyatt, G. L. (1958). A developmental crisis theory of stuttering. *Language and Speech, 1,* 250–64.

Wyatt, G. L. (1969). *Language learning and communication disorders in children.* New York: Free Press.

Wyatt, G. L., & Herzan, H. M. (1962). Therapy with stuttering children and their mothers. *American Journal of Orthopsychiatry, 23,* 645–59.

Wynia, B. L. (1964). The consistency effect in the speech repetitions of normal speaking young children. M. S., Thesis, Pennsylvania State University.

Wynne, M. K., & Boehmler, R. M. (1982). Central auditory function in fluent and disfluent normal speakers. *Journal of Speech and Hearing Research, 25,* 54–57.

Yairi, E. (1972). Disfluency rates and patterns of stutterers and nonstutterers. *Journal of Communication Disorders, 5,* 225–31.

Yairi, E. (1976). Effects of binaural and monaural noise on stuttering. *Journal of Auditory Research, 16,* 114–19.

Yairi, E. (1981). Disfluencies of normally speaking two-year-old children. *Journal of Speech and Hearing Research, 24,* 490–95.

Yairi, E. (1982). Longitudinal studies of disfluencies in two-year-old children. *Journal of Speech and Hearing Research, 25,* 155–60.

Yairi, E. (1983). The onset of stuttering in two- and three-year-old children: A preliminary report. *Journal of Speech and Hearing Disorders, 48,* 171–77.

Yairi, E., & Ambrose, N. (1992a). A longitudinal study of stuttering in children: A preliminary report. *Journal of Speech and Hearing Research, 35,* 755–60.

Yairi, E., & Ambrose, N. (1992b). Onset of stuttering in preschool children: Selected factors. *Journal of Speech and Hearing Research, 35,* 782–88.

Yairi, E., & Ambrose, N. (1996). Genetics of stuttering: A critical review. *Journal of Speech & Hearing Research, 39,* 771–85.

Yairi, E., & Ambrose, N. G. (1999). Early childhood stuttering I: persistency and recovery rates. *Journal of Speech, Language and Hearing Research, 42,* 1097–113.

Yairi, E., & Ambrose, N. (2005). *Early childhood stuttering: For clinicians by clinicians.* Austin, TX: Pro-Ed.

Yairi, E., Ambrose, N., & Cox, N. (1996). Genetics of stuttering: a critical review. *Journal of Speech and Hearing Research, 39,* 771–84.

Yairi, E., Ambrose, N., & Niermann, R. (1993). The early months of stuttering: A developmental study. *Journal of Speech and Hearing Research, 36,* 521–28.

Yairi, E., Ambrose, N., Paden, E. P., & Throneburg, R. N. (1996). Predictive factors of persistence and recovery: Pathways of childhood stuttering. *Journal of Communication Disorders, 29,* 51–77.

Yairi, E., & Clifton, N. F., Jr. (1972). Disfluent speech behavior of preschool children, high school seniors, and geriatric persons. *Journal of Speech and Hearing Research, 15,* 714–19.

Yairi, E., & Hall, K. D. (1993). Temporal relations within repetitions of preschool children near the onset of stuttering: a preliminary report. *Journal of Communication Disorders, 26,* 231–44.

Yairi, E., & Jennings, S. M. (1974). Relationship between the disfluent speech behavior of normal speaking preschool boys and their parents. *Journal of Speech and Hearing Research, 17,* 94–98.

Yairi, E., & Lewis, B. (1984). Disfluencies at the onset of stuttering. *Journal of Speech and Hearing Research, 27,* 155–59.

Yairi, E., & Williams, D. E. (1970). Speech clinicians' stereotypes of elementary school boys who stutter. *Journal of Communication Disorders, 3,* 161–70.

Yairi, E., & Williams, D. E. (1971). Reports of parental attitudes by stuttering and by nonstuttering children. *Journal of Speech and Hearing Research, 14,* 596–604.

Yannatos, G. (1960). L'hydroxyzine dans la thérapeutique des bégaiements. J. Franc. *ORL, 9,* 293–96.

Yaruss, J. S. (1997). Utterance timing and childhood stuttering. *Journal of Fluency Disorders, 22,* 263–86.

Yaruss, J. S. (1999). Utterance length, syntactic complexity, and childhood stuttering. *Journal of Speech, Language and Hearing Research, 42,* 329–44.

Yaruss, J. S. (2000). Converting between word and syllable counts in children's conversational speech samples. *Journal of Fluency Disorders, 25,* 305–16.

Yaruss, J. S. (2001). Evaluating treatment outcomes for adults who stutter. *Journal of Communication Disorders, 34,* 163–82.

Yaruss, J. S., Coleman, C., & Hammer, D. (2006). Treating preschool children who stutter: description and preliminary evaluation of a family-focused treatment approach. *Language, Speech and Hearing Services in Schools, 37,* 118–36.

Yaruss, J. S., & Conture, E. G. (1993). F2 transitions during sound/syllable repetitions of children who stutter and predictions of stuttering chronicity. *Journal of Speech and Hearing Research, 36,* 883–96.

Yaruss, J. S., & Conture, E. G. (1995). Mother and child speaking rates and utterance lengths in adjacent fluent utterances: Preliminary observations. *Journal of Fluency Disorders, 20,* 257–78.

Yaruss, J. S., & Conture, E. G. (1996). Stuttering and phonological disorders in children: Examination of the Covert Repair Hypothesis. *Journal of Speech and Hearing Research, 39,* 349–64.

Yaruss, J. S., LaSalle, L. R., & Conture, E. G. (1998). Evaluating stuttering in children: Diagnostic data. *American Journal of Speech-Language Pathology, 7,* 62–76.

Yaruss, J. S., & Logan, K. J. (2002). Evaluating rate, accuracy, and fluency of young children's diadochokinetic productions: A preliminary investigation. *Journal of Fluency Disorders, 27,* 65–87.

Yaruss, J. S., Max, M. S., Newman, R., & Campbell, J. H. (1998). Comparing real-time and transcript-based techniques for measuring stuttering. *Journal of Fluency Disorders, 23,* 137–51.

Yaruss, J. S., Newman, R. M., & Flora, T. (1999). Language and disfluency in nonstuttering children's conversational speech. *Journal of Fluency Disorders, 24,* 185–207.

Yaruss, J. S., & Quesal, R. W. (2006). *Overall Assessment of the Speaker's Experience of Stuttering (OASES):* Documenting multiple outcomes in stuttering treatment. *Journal of Fluency Disorders, 31,* 90–115.

Yaruss, J. S., Quesal, R. W., & Murphy, B. (2002). National Stuttering Association members' opinions about stuttering treatment. *Journal of Fluency Disorders, 27,* 227–43.

Yaruss, J. S., Quesal, R. W., Reeves, L., Molt, L. F., Kluetz, B., Caruso, A. J., et al. (2002). Speech treatment and support group experiences of people who participate in the National Stuttering Association. *Journal of Fluency Disorders, 27,* 115–33.

Yates, A. J. (1963). Delayed auditory feedback. *Psychology Bulletin, 60,* 213–32.

Yeakle, M. K., & Cooper, E. B. (1986). Teacher perceptions of stuttering. *Journal of Fluency Disorders, 11,* 345–59.

Yeoh, H. K., Lind, C. R. P., & Law, A. J. J. (2006). Acute transient cerebellar dysfunction and stuttering following mild closed head injury. *Child's Nervous System, 22,* 310–13.

Yeudall, L. T. (1985). A neuropsychological theory of stuttering. *Seminars in Speech and Language, 6,* 197–223.

Yonovitz, A., & Shepherd, W. T. (1977). Electrophysiological measurement during a time-out procedure in stuttering and normal speakers. *Journal of Fluency Disorders, 2,* 129–39.

Yoshiyuki, H. (1984). Phonatory initiation, termination, and vocal frequency change reaction times of stutterers. *Journal of Fluency Disorders, 9,* 115–24.

Yoss, K. A., & Darley, F. L. (1974). Developmental apraxia of speech in children with defective articulation. *Journal of Speech and Hearing Research, 17,* 399–416.

Young, M. A. (1961). Predicting ratings of severity of stuttering. *Journal of Speech and Hearing Disorders, Monograph Supplement 7,* 31–54.

Young, M. A. (1964). Identification of stutterers from recorded samples of their fluent speech. *Journal of Speech and Hearing Research, 7,* 302–03.

Young, M. A. (1965). Audience size, perceived situational difficulty, and stuttering frequency. *Journal of Speech and Hearing Research, 8,* 401–07.

Young, M. A. (1969a). Observer agreement: Cumulative effects of rating many samples. *Journal of Speech and Hearing Research, 12,* 135–43.

Young, M. A. (1969b). Observer agreement: Cumulative effects of repeated ratings of the same samples and of knowledge of group results. *Journal of Speech and Hearing Research, 12,* 144–55.

Young, M. A. (1970). Anchoring and sequence effects for the category scaling of stuttering severity. *Journal of Speech and Hearing Research, 13,* 360–68.

Young, M. A. (1974). Stuttering severity and instructions to increase speaking rate. *Illinois Speech and Hearing Journal, 8,* 3–6.

Young, M. A. (1975a). Comment on "stuttering frequency and the onset of phonation." *Journal of Speech and Hearing Research, 18,* 600–02.

Young, M. A. (1975b). Observer agreement for marking moments of stuttering. *Journal of Speech and Hearing Research, 18,* 530–40.

Young, M. A. (1975c). Onset, prevalence, and recovery from stuttering. *Journal of Speech and Hearing Disorders, 40,* 49–58.

Young, M. A. (1980). Comparison of stuttering frequencies during reading and speaking. *Journal of Speech and Hearing Research, 23,* 216–17.

Young, M. A. (1981). A reanalysis of "stuttering therapy: the relation between attitude change and long-term outcome." *Journal of Speech and Hearing Disorders, 46,* 221–22.

Young, M. A. (1984). Identification of stuttering and stutterers. In R. F. Curlee & W. H. Perkins (Eds.), *Nature and treatment of stuttering: New directions* (pp. 12–30). San Diego: College-Hill Press.

Young, M. A. (1994). Evaluating differences between stuttering and nonstuttering speakers: The group difference design. *Journal of Speech and Hearing Research,* 37, 522–34.

Young, M. A., & Downs, T. D. (1968). Testing the significance of the agreement among observers. *Journal of Speech and Hearing Research, 11,* 5–17.

Young, M. A. & Prather, E. M. (1962). Measuring severity of stuttering using short segments of speech. *Journal of Speech and Hearing Research, 5,* 256–62.

Yovetich, W. S. (1984). Message therapy: Language approach to stuttering therapy with children. *Journal of Fluency Disorders, 9,* 11–20.

Yovetich, W. S., Booth, J. C., & Tyler, R. S. (1977). The effect of dysfluencies on attention in stutterers and nonstutterers. *Human Communication, 1,* 29–39.

Yovetich, W. S., & Dolgoy, S. (2001). The impact of listeners' facial expressions on the perceptions of speakers who stutter. *Journal of Speech-Language Pathology and Audiology, 25,* 145–51.

Yovetich, W. S., Leschied, A. W., & Flicht, J. (2000). Self-esteem of school-age children who stutter. *Journal of Fluency Disorders, 25,* 143–53.

Zackheim, C. T., & Conture, E. G. (2003). Childhood stuttering and speech disfluencies in relation to children's mean length of utterance: A preliminary study. *Journal of Fluency Disorders, 28,* 115–43.

Zaleski, T. (1965). Rhythmic skills in stuttering children. *De Therapia Vocis et Loquelae, Vol. I. of the XIII Congress of the International Society of Logopedics and Phoniatrics.*

Zaliouk, D., & Zaliouk, A. (1965). Stuttering, a differential approach in diagnosis and therapy. *De Therapia Vocis et Loquelae, Vol. I. of the XIII Congress of the International Society of Logopedics and Phoniatrics.*

Zaner, A. R. (1950). Speech defects noted among amputees. M. A. Thesis, University of Wisconsin.

Zebrowski, P. M. (1991). Duration of the speech disfluencies of beginning stutterers. *Journal of Speech and Hearing Research, 34,* 483–91.

Zebrowski, P. M. (1994). Duration of sound prolongation and sound/syllable repetition in children who stutter. *Journal of Speech and Hearing Research, 37,* 254–64.

Zebrowski, P. M. (2007). Treatment factors that influence therapy outcomes of children who stutter In R. Curlee & E. G. Conture (Eds.) *Stuttering and related disorders of fluency* (3rd ed.) (pp. 23–38). New York: Thieme.

Zebrowski, P. M., & Conture, E. G. (1989). Judgments of disfluency by mothers of stuttering and normally disfluent children. *Journal of Speech and Hearing Research, 32,* 625–34.

Zebrowski, P. M., Conture, E. G., & Cudahy, E. A. (1985). Acoustic analysis of young stutterers' fluency: Preliminary observations. *Journal of Fluency Disorders, 10,* 173–92.

Zebrowski, P. M., Weiss, A. L., Savelkoul, E. M., & Hammer, C. S. (1996). The effect of maternal rate reduction on the stuttering, speech rates and linguistic productions of children who stutter: Evidence from individual dyads. *Clinical Linguistics and Phonetics, 10,* 189–206.

Zeffiro, T., & Frymiare, J. (2006). Functional neuroimaging of speech production. In M. Trazxler & M. Gernsbacher (Eds.), *Handbook of psycholinguistics* (2nd ed.) (pp. 125–50). Amsterdam: Elsevier.

Zeharia, A., Mukamel, M., Carel, C., Weitz, R., Danziger, Y., & Mimouni, M. (1999). Conversion reaction: Management by the paediatrician. *European Journal of Pediatrics, 158,* 160–65.

Zelaznik, H. N., Smith, A., & Franz, E. A. (1994). Motor performance of stutterers and nonstutterers on timing and force control tasks. *Journal of Motor Behavior, 26,* 340–47.

Zelaznik, H. N., Smith, A., Franz, E. A., & Ho, M. (1997). Differences in bimanual coordination associated with stuttering. *Acta Psychologica, 96,* 229–43.

Zelen, S. L., Sheehan, J. G., & Bugental, J. F. T. (1954). Self-perceptions in stuttering. *Journal of Clinical Psychology, 10,* 70–72.

Zenner, A. A., Ritterman, S. I., Bowen, S. K., & Gronhovd, K. D. (1978). Measurement and comparison of anxiety levels of parents of stuttering, articulatory defective, and normal-speaking children. *Journal of Fluency Disorders, 3,* 273–83.

Zenner, A. A., Webster, L. M., & Fitzgerald, R. G. (1974). The consistency of behaviors in stutterers and nonstutterers during massed oral readings of the same material: A difference measure. [Abstract]. *ASHA, 16,* 567.

Zerneri, L. (1966). Tentatives d'application de la voix retardée ("delayed speech feedback") dans la thérapie du bégaiement. J. Franc. *ORL, 15,* 415–18.

Zibelman, R. (1982). Avoidance-reduction therapy for stuttering. *American Journal of Psychotherapy, 36,* 489–96.

Zimmermann, G. (1980a). Articulatory behaviors associated with stuttering: Cinefluoro-graphic analysis. *Journal of Speech and Hearing Research, 23,* 108–21.

Zimmermann, G. (1980b). Articulatory dynamics of fluent utterances of stutterers and nonstutterers. *Journal of Speech and Hearing Research, 23,* 95–107.

Zimmermann, G. (1980c). Stuttering: A disorder of movement. *Journal of Speech and Hearing Research, 23,* 122–36.

Zimmermann, G., Liljeblad, S., Frank, A., & Cleeland, C. (1983). The Indians have many terms for it: Stuttering among the Bannock-Shoshoni. *Journal of Speech and Hearing Research, 26,* 315–18.

Zimmermann, G. N. (1985). The Bannock-Shoshoni still have terms for it: Whither Stewart. *Journal of Speech and Hearing Research, 28,* 315–16.

Zimmermann, G. N., & Hanley, J. M. (1983). A cinefluorographic investigation of repeated fluent productions of stutterers in an adaptation procedure. *Journal of Speech and Hearing Research, 26,* 35–42.

Zimmermann, G. N., & Knott, J. R. (1974). Slow potentials of the brain related to speech processing in normal speakers and stutters. *Electroencephalography and Clinical Neurophysiology, 37,* 599–607.

Zimmermann, G. N., Smith, A., & Hanley, J. M. (1981). Stuttering: In need of a unifying conceptual framework. *Journal of Speech and Hearing Research, 24,* 25–31.

Zimmerman, S., & Kalinowski, J. (1997). Effect of altered auditory feedback on people who stutter during scripted telephone conversations. *Journal of Speech, Language and Hearing Research, 40,* 1130–35.

Zsilavecz, U. (1981). Cybernetic functioning in stuttering. *South African Journal of Communication Disorders, 28,* 60–66.

Author Index

Subject Index

d

e

f

t